# Veterinary Diseases: Diagnosis, Treatment and Prevention

# Veterinary Diseases: Diagnosis, Treatment and Prevention

Edited by Lauren Boyle

AMERICAN
MEDICAL PUBLISHERS
www.americanmedicalpublishers.com

American Medical Publishers,
41 Flatbush Avenue,
1st Floor, New York,
NY 11217, USA

Visit us on the World Wide Web at:
www.americanmedicalpublishers.com



ISBN: 978-1-63927-525-0



**Cataloging-in-Publication Data**

Veterinary diseases : diagnosis, treatment and prevention / edited by Lauren Boyle.
p. cm.
Includes bibliographical references and index.
ISBN 978-1-63927-525-0
1. Veterinary medicine. 2. Veterinary medicine--Diagnosis. 3. Animals--Diseases--Treatment.
4. Animals--Diseases--Prevention. I. Boyle, Lauren.

SF745 .V48 2022
636.089--dc23

# Table of Contents

# Preface

Animal diseases can be caused by a variety of pathogens, such as bacteria, fungi, viruses, etc. Some bacterial diseases are anthrax, diphtheria, Lyme disease, salmonellosis and rickettsioses, while fungal diseases include aspergillosis, blastomycosis, candidiasis and dermatophytosis. Animals are susceptible to genetic diseases, such as complex vertebral malformation, hyperinsulinism hyperammonemia syndrome, foal immunodeficiency syndrome and hyperkalemic periodic paralysis, among others. The field of veterinary medicine is concerned with the diagnosis, treatment and prevention of all veterinary diseases. The diagnosis of disease is possible through an examination of body fluids and animal tissue. This is under the scope of veterinary pathology. It may be further divided into anatomical and clinical pathology. Anatomical pathology deals with the diagnosis of disease based on a microscopic, molecular and gross examination of organs, tissues and whole bodies. The diagnosis of disease through a laboratory analysis of bodily fluids, such as urine, blood or cavitary effusions is under the scope of clinical pathology. Some common interventions to achieve good animal health include vaccination against animal diseases, such as rabies, dental prophylaxis, etc. Specialties in veterinary medicine include areas like anesthesiology, cardiology, dermatology, dentistry, etc. This book outlines the diagnosis, treatment and prevention of veterinary diseases in detail. It will help the readers in keeping pace with the rapid changes in veterinary science and medicine.

Various studies have approached the subject by analyzing it with a single perspective, but the present book provides diverse methodologies and techniques to address this field. This book contains theories and applications needed for understanding the subject from different perspectives. The aim is to keep the readers informed about the progresses in the field; therefore, the contributions were carefully examined to compile novel researches by specialists from across the globe.

Indeed, the job of the editor is the most crucial and challenging in compiling all chapters into a single book. In the end, I would extend my sincere thanks to the chapter authors for their profound work. I am also thankful for the support provided by my family and colleagues during the compilation of this book.

**Editor**

# 1

# Progression of experimental chronic Aleutian mink disease virus infection

Trine Hammer Jensen[1,2,3*], Mariann Chriél[1] and Mette Sif Hansen[1]

**Abstract**

**Background:** Aleutian mink disease virus (AMDV) is found world-wide and has a major impact on mink health and welfare by decreasing reproduction and fur quality. In the majority of mink, the infection is subclinical and the diagnosis must be confirmed by serology or polymerase chain reaction (PCR). Increased knowledge based on a systematically description of clinical signs, pathology and histopathology might be a tool to reduce the risk of infection from subclinically infected mink to AMDV free herds. The aim of this study was to give a histopathological description of the progression of a chronic experimental infection with a currently circulating Danish strain of AMDV, Saeby/DEN/799.1/05. These results were compared with the pathogenesis of previously published AMDV stains.

**Results:** This experimental AMDV infection resulted in only decreased appetite and soft or discolored feces, primarily within the first 8 weeks after AMDV inoculation. Gross pathology revealed few and inconsistent findings mainly associated with the liver, spleen and kidneys. The majority of the AMDV inoculated wild type mink ($n = 41$) developed various histopathological changes consistent with AMDV infection in one or more organs: infiltrations of mononuclear cells in liver, kidney and brain, reduced density of lymphocytes and increased numbers of plasma cells in lymph nodes and spleen. Natural infection, as occurred in the sentinel sapphire mink (four of six mink), progressed similar to the experimentally inoculated mink.

**Conclusions:** Experimental AMDV inoculation mainly resulted in subclinical infection with unspecific clinical signs and gross pathology, and more consistent histopathology appearing at any time after AMDV inoculation during the 24 weeks of observation. Thus, the observed histopathology substantiates AMDV infection and no correlation to time of inoculation was found. This confirms that diagnosing AMDV infection requires serology and/or PCR and the Saeby/DEN/799.1/05 AMDV strain results in histopathology consistent with other AMDV strains.

**Keywords:** Aleutian mink disease virus, AMDV, Mink, Chronic experimental infection, Histopathology

## Background

Aleutian mink disease virus (AMDV) is a parvovirus infecting mink (*Neovison vison*) world-wide [1–4]. AMDV infection is characterized by plasmacytosis, hypergammaglobulinaemia and immune complex formation [5]. The outcome of AMDV infection depends on host factors such as genotype and the age of the mink, viral load and the virus strain [6–8]. In juvenile mink, AMDV infection may cause acute pneumonia with high mortality [9–11]. In adult mink, one or more of the following conditions can occur as acute though mainly chronic lesions: glomerulonephritis [5, 12], arteritis [13], hepatitis [14] and meningoencephalitis [15, 16]. In naïve mink, acute pneumonia [9–11] and facial swelling (unpublished observations, the authors) can be the predominant clinical sign of all age groups. Classical chronic symptoms of AMDV infection is single white hairs in the fur ("sprinklers") [17], reduced reproductive performance including reduced litter size and abortions [10]. Histologically, evidence of AMDV infection is interstitial pneumonia with alveolar hyaline membranes in mink kits [10] or plasma cell infiltrations in various organs in adult mink [5, 11]. However, polymerase chain reaction (PCR) or serology must be applied to confirm the diagnosis [1, 18–20].

*Correspondence: trine@bio.aau.dk
[2] Present Address: Department of Chemistry and Bioscience, Aalborg University/Aalborg Zoo, Frederik Bajers Vej 7H, 9100 Aalborg, Denmark
Full list of author information is available at the end of the article

Most AMDV infected farmed mink develop subclinical infections, but this is not well documented in recent literature [21]. Subclinically infected mink poses the main risk of transmitting AMDV to uninfected mink farms. Previous experimental studies on AMDV histopathology involve older strains of AMDV and focus on specific organs [22, 23] and not on the disease progression in the whole organism. The aim of the present study was to describe lesions and disease progression induced by a currently circulating Danish AMDV strain, Saeby/DEN/799.1/05. These results would be of practical diagnostic value and would in comparison with previously described AMDV strains reveal if potential consistent clinical signs or lesions could indicate the time of infection. During this chronic experimental AMDV infection of Danish farmed mink, the mink were monitored daily for clinical signs and evaluated for gross pathology and histopathology 2, 4, 8, 16 and 24 weeks after inoculation.

## Methods

### Mink

Mink (*Neovison vison*) were purchased from two farms on Zealand (Denmark), an island that at the time of purchase and during this study had been free of AMDV for more than a decade. The mink (42 wild type mink and 6 sapphire mink) were tested negative for antibodies against AMDV by counter-current immunoelectrophoresis (CIEP) before they were moved to the experimental facility at the National Veterinary Institute (NVI), Technical University of Denmark. The mink were all females because they were easier to handle in terms of size and temper. Twelve one-year-old wild type mink were used for a short term infection experiment. Half of the mink ($n = 15$ wild type mink, $n = 3$ sapphire mink) used in the chronic infection experiment were five-months-old and the other half of the mink ($n = 15$ wild type mink, $n = 3$ sapphire mink) were 15-months-old. The farms had no records of previous AMDV, mink enteritis virus or other serious infectious diseases and no records of any vaccinations. The care and use of the animals was in accordance with the guidelines and approved by The Animal Experiments Inspectorate (approval number 2009/561-1755).

The 48 mink were housed indoor in four isolation rooms designed for animal experiments with 12 mink cages in one row in each room. Each mink was housed individually in standard mink wire mesh cages with a wooden nest box with straw. A standard commercial mink diet from the local mink feed producer were given to the mink daily. Upon arrival at the animal experimental facility, all mink were clinically assessed and the mink had 2 days for acclimatization before AMDV inoculation at day 0. Mink exhibiting clinical signs according to clinical endpoints (weight loss, anorexia, compromised welfare, or severe gastrointestinal, respiratory or urinary symptoms) at any time during the experiment were euthanized. One wild type mink was euthanized before the AMDV inoculation for health reasons and thus not included in the data analysis. Two sapphire mink were included in each group as sentinels. Sapphire mink carry the Aleutian gene making them more susceptible to Aleutian disease (AD) [7, 8].

### Experimental infections with AMDV

A short term experiment of 1 month with 12 one-year-old wild type female mink was performed to determine the lowest dilution of the AMDV organ homogenate for induction of chronic infection. The mink were divided into four groups of three mink that were anesthetized by intramuscular injection with ketamine (10–15 mg/kg) and xylazine (0.5–1 mg/kg), followed by intraperitoneal injection of 1 ml of the AMDV organ homogenate undiluted, diluted in PBS with 4 % penicillin/streptomycin 1:100, 1:1000 or 1:10,000. The homogenate consisted of spleens from farmed mink naturally infected in 2009 with the currently most prevalent Danish AMDV strain Saeby/DEN/799.1/05 [4] as described by Jensen et al. [24]. The mink were observed daily and clinically scored as described below. Blood samples, fecal samples and oro-nasal swabs were collected weekly.

Two weeks after AMDV inoculation one mink from each of the four groups were euthanized by cardiac injection of pentobarbital preceded by ketamine/xylazine anesthesia. The remaining eight mink were euthanized 4 weeks after AMDV inoculation (Fig. 1). All mink were necropsied and organs were examined macroscopically, sampled and stored at −80 °C. One mink delivered two mink kits 12 days after AMDV inoculation from which oro-nasal swabs and organs were sampled.

A long term chronic infection experiment of 6 months was initiated by intraperitoneal inoculation of 29 wild type female mink, and six sapphire female mink were used as sentinels as described by Jensen et al. [24]. The 35 mink were divided in three groups with 11, 12 and 12 mink in each and euthanized after 8, 16 and 24 weeks respectively (Fig. 2). Details of this experiment are described by Jensen et al. [24]. In short, during the experiment blood samples were taken weekly to test for AMDV antibodies by CIEP and AMDV DNA by PCR for the first 8 weeks and then every second week till the end of the experiment at 24 weeks after AMDV inoculation. Oro-nasal swabs and feces were collected at the same days and tested for AMDV DNA. At the end of the experiment the mink were euthanised, necropsied and all organs were examined for AMDV DNA by PCR.

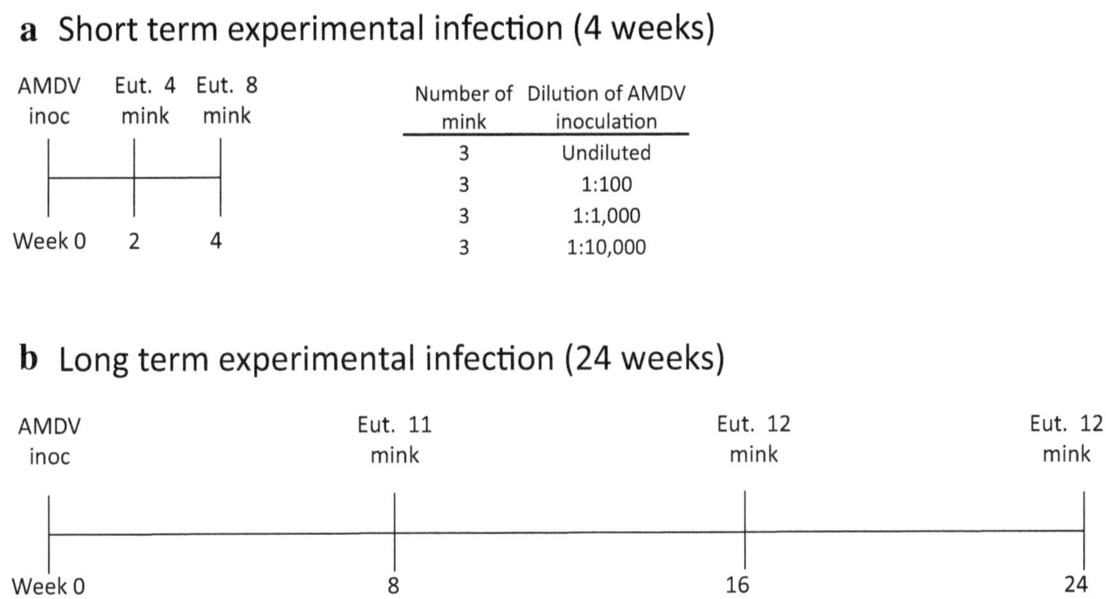


**Fig. 1** Mink inoculated with Aleutian mink disease virus (AMDV) and euthanized 2 and 4 weeks later (**a**) and 8, 16 and 24 weeks later (**b**). The mink in experiment A were given different dilutions of AMDV as shown in the table. One mink from each dilution group was euthanized after 2 weeks and the rest after 4 weeks. The mink in experiment B were inoculated with a 1:10,000 dilution of the AMDV homogenate. *Inoc* inoculated, *Eut* euthanized

### Scoring of clinical signs

Every day each mink were clinically assessed and scored according to: (a) general condition, (b) respiration, (c) appetite, (d) feces. A score of 0–3 was given for each category depending on the clinical status with 0 describing the normal general condition with: (a) curiosity and free movements, (b) normal respiration with a moist nose, (c) eating all feed at once, and (d) formed dark normal feces. The score 1 was given for slight symptoms such as: (a) slightly depressed, slow and reduced movements, (b) labored respiration, (c) not eating all feed at once, (d) scarce dry or soft feces. The score 2 was given for moderate symptoms such as: (a) depression, only moves when forced, (b) decreased appetite, (c) labored respiration with sneezing and/or nasal discharge, and (d) either very scarce, dry feces or mild to moderate diarrhea. The score 3 was given for severe clinical signs involving (a) apathy/lethargy, (b) heavy respiratory sounds with nasal discharge and coughing, (c) anorexia, and (d) no feces or severe diarrhea. Finally, the content of blood in the urine was scored visually with 0 if unapparent or 3 if hematuria.

### Histopathology, detection of AMDV DNA and antibodies

At necropsy samples of lung, liver, spleen, duodenum, jejunum, mesenteric lymph node, kidney and brain (cerebrum and cerebellum) were fixed by immersion in 10 % neutral buffered formalin, processed by routine histology methods, embedded in paraffin wax and cut in 3–5 μm sections. Not all organs were collected from every mink (Table 4). The sections were mounted on conventional glass slides and stained with hematoxylin and eosin for histopathological examination. The tissue sections were evaluated blinded and systematically for the following AMDV associated lesions [23]: perivascular infiltration of mononuclear cells (lymphocytes, plasma cells and macrophages) in the lungs; bile duct proliferation and/or infiltration of mononuclear cells in the portal areas of the liver; infiltration of mononuclear cells in lamina propria and/or around blood vessels in the intestines; infiltration of mononuclear cells in the kidney; infiltration of mononuclear cells in plexus choroideus and/or perivascular cuffing of mononuclear cells in the meninges or brain parenchyma.

Lesions in lung, liver, intestine, kidney and brain were scored as: suspected (one small, focal infiltration of mononuclear cells); mild (few and small infiltrations); moderate (several small or few disseminated infiltrations); or massive (multifocal disseminated infiltrations). The spleen was evaluated for the following AMDV associated lesions: activation of lymphoid follicles with necrotic cells and macrophages; and reduced density (depletion) of lymphoid cells in lymphoid follicles and/or diffusely in the spleen. In the mesenteric lymph node, the following lesions were described: reduced density of lymphoid cells in lymphoid follicles; reduced density of lymphocytes in medulla and increased numbers of plasma cells in

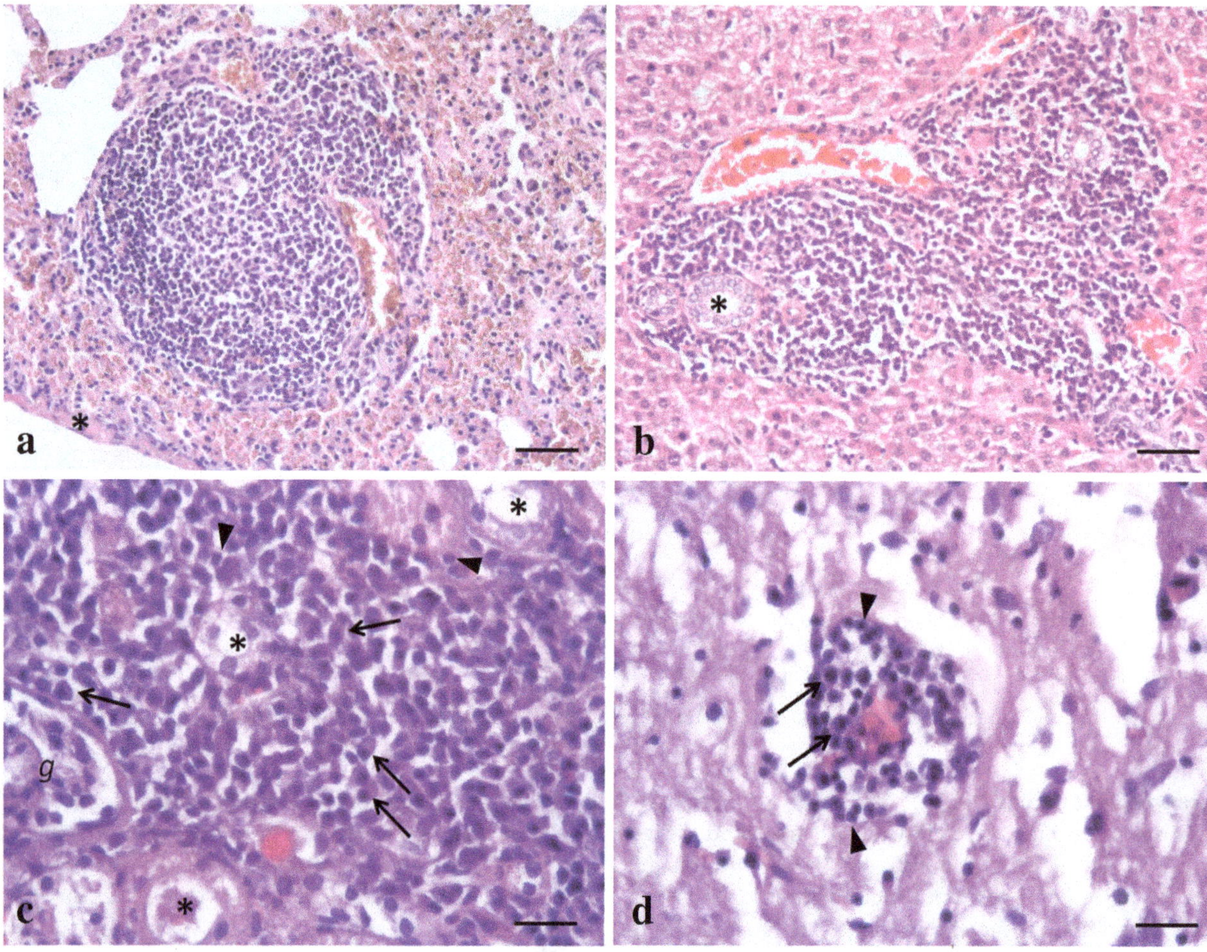


**Fig. 2** Histopathological findings in wild type mink experimentally inoculated with AMDV. **a** Massive perivascular infiltration of mononuclear cells in the lung 8 weeks after AMDV inoculation. Pleura (*asterisk*). *HE* Hematoxylin and eosin. *Scale bar* 50 µm. **b** Massive infiltration of mononuclear cells in a portal triad of the liver 4 weeks after AMDV inoculation. Bile duct (*asterisk*). HE, *scale bar* 50 µm. **c** Massive interstitial infiltration of mononuclear cells in the cortex of the kidney 16 weeks after AMDV inoculation. Plasma cells (*arrow*), lymphocytes (*arrowhead*), kidney tubule (*asterisk*), glomerulus (*g*). HE, *scale bar* 20 µm. **d** Moderate non-suppurative perivascular cuffing in white matter of cerebrum 16 weeks after AMDV inoculation. Plasma cells (*arrow*), lymphocytes (*arrowhead*). HE, *scale bar* 20 µm

medulla and sinuses; increased numbers of macrophages, mainly in the medulla of the lymph node.

Due to the limited number of mink in each dilution group in the short term study, the histopathology of the mink euthanized at 2 weeks after AMDV inoculation (n = 4) is described collectively and likewise for the mink euthanized at 4 weeks (n = 8). In addition, the histopathological changes are described collectively for the infected sentinel sapphire mink (n = 4) without regard for the differences in duration of the infection since the exact time of infection is not known.

QIAamp Blood Mini kit (Qiagen, Hilden, Germany) was used to isolate total DNA from mink organs, blood samples stabilized with EDTA and swab samples in PBS. Total DNA from fecal samples was isolated with QIAamp DNA Stool Mini Kit (Qiagen, Hilden, Germany). All samples were tested by PCR as described by Jensen et al. [18]. Sera were tested by CIEP at Kopenhagen Diagnostic (Kopenhagen Fur, Copenhagen, Denmark, [24]).

## Results

### Short term experimental infection with AMDV

The 12 mink inoculated with four different dilutions (undiluted, 1:100, 1:1000 and 1:10,000) of the AMDV organ homogenate developed antibodies as detected by CIEP after 2–3 weeks. These antibodies persisted until the animals were euthanized (Table 1). Too few mink were inoculated with each of the four dilutions (n = 3) to draw any solid conclusions between the groups. However, the mink given the undiluted AMDV organ homogenate all (n = 3) had seroconverted 2 weeks after AMDV inoculation whereas only one had seroconverted after

**Table 1 Short term experimental infection with different dilutions of Aleutian mink disease virus (AMDV) organ homogenate**

| Dilution of AMDV organ | Antibody detected by CIEP | | Virus excretion oro-nasal | | Virus excretion fecal | | |
|---|---|---|---|---|---|---|---|
| Homogenate | W2 | W3 + 4[a] | W3 | W4 | W2 | W3 | W4 |
| 1:10,000 | 1/3 | 2/2 | 0/2 | 0/2 | 1/3 | 2/2 | 2/2 |
| 1:1000 | 2/3 | 2/2 | 1/2 | 2/2 | 2/3 | 2/2 | 2/2 |
| 1:100 | 2/3 | 2/2 | 1/2 | 1/2 | 1/3 | 2/2 | 2/2 |
| Undiluted | 3/3 | 2/2 | 0/2 | 0/2 | 2/3 | 0/2 | 1/2[b] |
| In total | 8/12 | 8/8 | 2/8 | 3/8 | 6/12 | 6/8 | 7/8 |
| Kits 3w old (n = 2) | na | na | na | 2 | na | na | na |

Number of AMDV positive mink after AMDV inoculation out of total number of mink

*CIEP* counter current immunoelectrophoresis, *w* week, *na* not assessed

[a] Week (W) 3 and 4 were merged because the results were the same

[b] Rectal swab was positive

AMDV inoculation with a 1:10,000 dilution (Table 1). AMDV DNA was found in fecal samples in all mink from 2 to 4 weeks after inoculation (Table 1). AMDV DNA was found in oro-nasal swabs 3 weeks after AMDV inoculation of mink with 1:100 and 1:1000 AMDV organ homogenate dilutions, and in the two kits 4 weeks after inoculation of the mothers. No AMDV DNA was found in oro-nasal swabs from mink inoculated with the undiluted and 1:10,000 dilution of the AMDV organ homogenate (Table 1). Viremia results are not shown because different blood preparations from different experimental days were used for PCR (plasma, serum, buffy coat and full blood) which made the results incomparable. No significant clinical signs related to AMDV infection were observed (data not shown). At necropsy 2 weeks after AMDV inoculation all mink (n = 4) had pale or enlarged livers, this was only seen in two of eight mink 4 weeks after AMDV inoculation (Table 2). In addition, splenomegaly was seen in six of eight mink 4 weeks after AMDV inoculation (Table 2).

**Table 2 Necropsy findings of Aleutian mink disease virus (AMDV) inoculated mink (n = 47, including sentinels)**

| Weeks after AMDV | Mink with gross pathological changes | | | |
|---|---|---|---|---|
| Inoculation | Fur[a] | Liver[b] | Spleen[c] | Kidney[d] |
| 2 weeks | 0 | 4/4 | 0/4 | 0/4 |
| 4 weeks | 0 | 2/8 | 6/8 | 0/8 |
| 8 weeks | 0 | 9/11 | 7/11 | 4/11 |
| 16 weeks | 0 | 10/12 | 6/12 | 1/12 |
| 24 weeks | 2/12 | 3/12 | 2/12 | 0/12 |

[a] Abnormal fur colour with sprinklers

[b] Abnormal livers were pale and some mink also had congestive hepatopathy

[c] Enlarged spleen

[d] Either pale cortex, enlarged or both

AMDV was found by PCR in all types of examined organs after euthanasia, though not with the same frequency (Table 3). Most consistently, AMDV was found in the spleen, mesenteric lymph node, kidney, liver and bone marrow, all mink euthanized after 4 weeks had virus in these organs (Table 3).

A summary of the histopathology results of the short term study are presented in Table 4. Solid conclusions were difficult to obtain due to the small number of mink in these first weeks. Briefly, the majority of the mink had depletion of lymphoid cells in the spleen and mesenteric lymph nodes within the first 4 weeks after inoculation with AMDV. Activation of the lymphoid follicles in the spleen was another frequent finding at 4 weeks after AMDV inoculation (five of eight mink). Increased numbers of plasma cells and/or macrophages in the mesenteric lymph nodes were observed in about half of the AMDV inoculated mink. All mink (n = 12) had periportal infiltration of mononuclear cells in the liver, with a tendency of more pronounced lesions at 4 weeks, whereas lung- and kidney lesions were only seen at 4 weeks after inoculation. In the brain only mild lesions of non-suppurative perivascular cuffing and leptomeningitis was seen in five of eight mink at 4 weeks and one of four mink at 2 weeks. The cellular infiltration in lung, kidney, liver and brain was a mixture of plasma cells, lymphocytes and macrophages. Both mink kits had non-suppurative interstitial pneumonia without hyaline membranes, and one of them had massive periportal infiltration of mononuclear cells in the liver, whereas the other had bile duct proliferation.

### Chronic experimental infection with AMDV

In total, 3894 mink days were scored, meaning every day each mink was observed in total of all mink in the experiment. Overall, at 92.7 % of the mink days the mink were

**Table 3 Aleutian mink disease virus (AMDV) DNA detected with PCR in organs of mink**

| Organs | Number of mink with AMDV positive organs | | |
|---|---|---|---|
| | 2 weeks | 4 weeks | 4 weeks, kits 3w old[a] |
| Spleen | 4/4 | 8/8 | 2/2 |
| Mesenteric lymph node | 3/4 | 8/8 | 2/2 |
| Liver | 4/4 | 8/8 | 2/2 |
| Lung | 2/4 | 6/8 | 2/2 |
| Kidney | 3/4 | 8/8 | 2/2 |
| Intestine | 3/4 | 7/8 | 2/2 |
| Brain | 2/4 | 6/8 | na |
| Bone marrow | 3/4 | 8/8 | na |

The groups of mink inoculated with different AMDV dilutions were merged in the table because the results of the small groups were similar

*na* not assessed

[a] Two mink kits were born the first week of the experiment. The organs of these two kits were tested with PCR for AMDV DNA 3 weeks later

clinically normal. During 7.3 % of the mink days, abnormal clinical scores were recorded, primarily within the first 8 weeks (September and October) of the experiment (data not shown because of unspecific findings). At the majority of mink days with abnormal scoring, the mink were generally in good condition (n = 233 mink days, 82 %), but either having soft or discolored feces (n = 142, 50.2 %) or decreased appetite (n = 46, 16.3 %). The majority of the mink with compromised general condition was in addition observed to have slightly decreased appetite (30 of 50 mink days, data not shown). No hematuria was observed.

Three mink (one wild type and two sapphire mink) were euthanized during the experiment due to reaching the clinical endpoints. About five weeks after AMDV inoculation one wild type female (from the group of mink 8 weeks in the experiment) had decreased appetite, was reluctant to move and had soft feces. Three days later, it had labored respiration and was euthanized. The necropsy findings were pale liver and enlarged pale congested kidneys. The results from this mink were included in the 8 weeks group. One sapphire female, developed an ulcer on the nose appearing around 8 weeks after the experiment started and was treated with antibiotics. Later it developed conjunctivitis and 1 week later was slow and had slightly decreased appetite, it deteriorated with anorexia and diarrhea and was euthanized. At necropsy, the liver was pale and hemolytic *Staphylococci* sp. was cultured. Another sapphire mink had slightly decreased appetite 16 weeks after the experiment started and developed nasal and ocular discharged and was euthanized few days later. At gross necropsy, the findings were gingivitis, enlarged congested spleen and the kidneys had pale cortex.

In general, few pathological findings were observed at necropsy (Table 2). The majority of the findings were pale liver and splenomegaly 8–16 weeks after AMDV inoculation, less frequently pale or enlarged kidneys were seen (Table 2). Two of the mink euthanized 24 weeks after AMDV inoculation had single "sprinklers". Details of serology and virology results of the chronic experimental infection are described by Jensen et al. [24]. In short, the mink seroconverted 2–3 weeks after AMDV inoculation and remained seropositive throughout the 24 weeks of experiment. The majority of the mink had a transient viremia developing 1–3 weeks after AMDV inoculation and two mink had persistent viremia for 24 weeks. AMDV excretion was detected in feces and oro-nasal swabs at various and intermittent time intervals [24].

### Histopathology observed 8, 16 and 24 weeks after AMDV inoculation

Histopathological changes typical for AMDV infection was seen in all organs from mink in the long term study, a summary of these results are presented in Table 4 and Fig. 2. The majority of the mink had histopathological changes in the liver and kidney, and less consistently in the lung and intestine (Table 4). The involvement of the different organs and the extent of the lesions varied within and between the groups of animals. There was no statistical significant difference throughout the study period (early compared to late) in the number of histopathological findings in the lung, liver, kidney or brain (data not shown).

Two of the sentinel sapphire mink did not become viremic or developed antibodies and these two mink had no AMDV associated histopathological changes. Nevertheless, one of them developed slight depletion of lymphocytes and had increased numbers of plasma cells and macrophages in the mesenteric lymph node. Infiltration of mononuclear cells was seen in liver and kidney of the four viremic sentinel mink, and two of these had perivascular infiltrations in the lung. Other findings were perivascular cuffings (one mink) and mononuclear infiltrations in plexus choroideus (one mink) in the brain, and intestinal perivascular infiltrations of mononuclear cells (one mink).

The two wild type mink with persistent viremia throughout the 24 weeks of the study had histopathological changes similar to the other mink. They both had few and small infiltrations with monocular cells in the lungs and moderate in the liver. One of the mink had moderate multifocal infiltrations in the kidneys and some dilated tubuli and mild non-suppurative leptomeningitis.

**Table 4 Scoring of histopathological changes in Aleutian mink disease virus (AMDV) inoculated mink**

| Tissue | Score/lesion | Sentinel | Post inoculation week | | | | |
|---|---|---|---|---|---|---|---|
| | | | 2 | 4 | 8 | 16 | 24 |
| Lung | Suspect | – | – | – | – | – | – |
| | Mild | – | – | 2 | 2/9 | 2/10 | – |
| | Moderate | 1 | – | – | – | 2/10 | – |
| | Massive | 1 | – | 2 | 2/9 | – | – |
| | Total | 2/4 (50 %) | 0/4 | 4/8 (50 %) | 4/9 (44 %) | 4/10 (40 %) | 0/10 |
| Liver | Suspect | – | – | – | 1/9 | 3/9 | 1/9 |
| | Mild | – | 2 | 2 | 2/9 | 4/9 | 3/9 |
| | Moderate | 3 | 2 | 2 | 5/9 | 1/9 | 3/9 |
| | Massive | 1 | – | 4 | 1/9 | – | – |
| | Total | 4/4 (100 %) | 4/4 (100 %) | 8/8 (100 %) | 9/9 (100 %) | 8/9 (89 %) | 7/9 (78 %) |
| Intestine | Suspect | – | – | – | – | – | – |
| | Mild | – | – | – | – | – | 1/10 |
| | Moderate | 1 | – | – | 3/7 | – | – |
| | Massive | – | – | – | – | – | – |
| | Total | 1/4 (25 %) | 0/4 | 0/7 | 3/7 (43 %) | 0/10 | 1/10 (10 %) |
| Kidney | Suspect | – | – | – | 1/9 | 3/10 | 2/10 |
| | Mild | 1 | – | 2 | 2/9 | 1/10 | 2/10 |
| | Moderate | – | – | 2 | 2/9 | 1/10 | 2/10 |
| | Massive | 3 | – | 2 | 1/9 | 3/10 | – |
| | Total | 4/4 (100 %) | 0/4 | 6/8 (75 %) | 6/9 (67 %) | 8/10 (80 %) | 6/10 (60 %) |
| Brain | Suspect | – | – | – | 1/9 | – | – |
| | Mild | 2 | 1 | 5 | 6/9 | 3/10 | 6/10 |
| | Moderate | – | – | – | – | 2/10 | – |
| | Massive | – | – | – | – | – | – |
| | Total | 2/4 (50 %) | 1/4 (25 %) | 5/8 (63 %) | 7/9 (78 %) | 5/10 (50 %) | 6/10 (60 %) |
| Spleen | LF act[a] | – | – | 5/8 | 2/9 | 4/10 | – |
| | LF dep[b] | 3/4 | 3/4 | 1/8 | – | 2/10 | 2/10 |
| | Dif. dep[c] | 2/4 | – | 1/8 | 1/9 | 2/10 | 3/10 |
| | Stasis | 1/4 | 2/4 | 2/8 | 2/9 | 2/10 | 1/10 |
| | Total[d] | 4/4 (100 %) | 4/4 (100 %) | 8/8 (100 %) | 3/9 (33 %) | 8/10 (80 %) | 4/10 (40 %) |
| Mesenteric lymph node | LF dep | 3/4 | 3/4 | 4/7 | 4/9 | 1/9 | 1/9 |
| | Plasma cells[e] | 2/4 | 3/4 | 3/7 | 3/9 | 3/9 | 7/9 |
| | Macrop[f] | 2/4 | 1/4 | 3/7 | – | 3/9 | 3/9 |
| | Total[g] | 4/4 (100 %) | 3/4 (75 %) | 7/7 (100 %) | 6/9 (67 %) | 5/10 (50 %) | 7/9 (78 %) |

No. of animals with lesion/no. of tissues examined

In lung, liver, intestine, kidney and brain the grade of the lesions/infiltrations of mononuclear cells were scored semi quantitatively as follows; Suspect: single small lesion. Mild, moderate and massive, respectively: small, moderate, massive lesion/infiltration of mononuclear cells

[a] Activation of lymphoid follicles (LF act) with presence of necrotic cells and macrophages

[b] Depletion of lymphoid cells in LF (LF dep)

[c] Diffuse depletion of lymphoid cells (Dif dep)

[d] Total number of mink with histological changes in the spleen

[e] Reduced density of lymphocytes and increased numbers of plasma cells in the sinuses (plasma cells)

[f] Increased numbers of macrophages, mainly in the medulla (macrop)

[g] Total number of mink with histopathological changes in the mesenteric lymph node

The other mink had mineral deposits in the renal tubuli and mild infiltrations with mononuclear cells in the intestines.

Two mink were euthanized during the infection experiment due to clinical disease, one wild type mink after 5 weeks and a sapphire mink after 18 weeks. These two mink had histopathological changes similar to the others: Moderate non-suppurative perivascular infiltrations of mononuclear cells in the lungs, and liver. Mild infiltrations in the intestines and massive infiltrations in the kidneys. In addition, the sapphire mink also had mild mononuclear cell infiltrations in the brain. No correlation between histopathology and AMDV DNA in the organs compared to the other mink could be established.

## Discussion

The AMDV infection induced in this study provide a model for chronic AMDV infection in mink with a 1:10,000 dilution of an organ homogenate with the currently circulating Danish AMDV strain, Saeby/DEN/799.1/05. Surprisingly, even with undiluted AMDV organ homogenate the mink did not become clinically affected within four weeks, indicating that the Saeby/DEN/799.1/05 is not dose dependent. In the short time study, irrespective of the inoculation dosage, the mink developed antibodies 2–4 weeks after AMDV inoculation, like in the long term study [24]. Similar, all mink in the short term study excreted AMDV viral DNA in feces as shown for the long term study [24]. AMDV DNA excretion in oro-nasal secretions was detected in the mink inoculated with AMDV diluted 1:1000 and 1:100, but not undiluted and diluted 1:10,000 supporting the previously observed inconsistency in excretion [24, 25]. AMDV DNA was found in all examined organs 2 and 4 weeks after AMDV inoculation, which is consistent with another study where AMDV DNA also was found in spleen, lymph nodes, bone marrow, liver, kidney, lung and intestines 10 days after inoculation with a Canadian AMDV field strain [19]. However, the number of mink in the short term experiment was low but the apparent lack of doses dependent response in infection confirms earlier studies [7, 20] and contradicts an older study of dose dependency in AMDV infection [25]. The lowest dilution of AMDV organ homogenate was chosen for the long term experiment because the lowest dilution was enough to induce chronic infection which was the aim of the study. Using a higher dilution of the AMDV organ homogenate potentially could induce an acute infection although the short term study did not indicate it. Given the ethical considerations of an animal experiment and economic expenses no such risk were taken and the lowest AMDV organ homogenate dilution was used. Unexpectedly, one mink delivered two kits which were kept for 3 weeks and both of these kits were subclinically infected with AMDV, i.e. the organs were PCR positive and they excreted AMDV DNA. The kits did not present symptoms in contrast to previous findings [10, 11] maybe because of their short life.

The clinical signs observed in this study were scarce with 93 % of all observations representing unaffected mink in good condition, probably due to the chronic subclinical course of the experimental infection. This was also observed in another experimental infection study [12] and under commercial farm conditions (unpublished observation, authors). Secondly, mink were euthanized within short time after showing the first symptoms for animal welfare reasons, so clinical AD was not observed in progression. The initial diffuse symptoms of decreased appetite corresponded to what Eklund et al. [25] observed. The three mink euthanized for welfare reasons were most likely suffering from AD, although hemolytic Staphylococcus was cultured in the liver from one of the mink. This relatively low disease rate is comparable to what has been observed in other chronic experimental AMDV infection of non-Aleutian genotype mink [5, 8, 12, 20]. Also in farms with chronic AMDV infection clinical signs and mortality in general is relatively limited [26] and the reason why commercial mink farms can produce despite AMDV infection. Interestingly, the majority of the clinical signs in the present study were observed in the first 2 months of the experiment, September and October. The relatively high prevalence of symptoms in these months can be related to stress after being moved to the experimental facility and change to winter fur (October). In commercial farms the antibiotic usage is commonly prescribed in these months which indicate this is a stressful period for the mink under production conditions, too [27].

Notably, no central nervous system (CNS) symptoms were observed despite the infiltrations of mononuclear cells in cerebrum, cerebellum, meninges and plexus choroideus. This is consistent with a study of Irish mink farms without neurologic disease, but non-suppurative meningoencephalitis [16], but contrary to an American field study of farmed mink with neurologic symptoms caused by non-suppurative meningoencephalitis [15]. The absence of CNS symptoms might be explained by the apparently less severe CNS lesions in the present study compared to the lesions described by Dyer et al. [15] which could be a time related issue.

The sentinel sapphire mink were included in the comparison of clinical signs and gross pathology after natural transmission of the virus knowing that they were not infected at the same time as the other mink. However, they showed the same symptoms and pathology as the experimentally inoculated mink. Clinical disease led to euthanasia of two of six sapphire mink and only one of 29 wild type mink presumably due to the sapphire genotype [7, 8]. Overall, the sapphire mink were too few for firm conclusions in itself, but they represented important results as sentinels in the experimental infection. Compared to previous studies it was expected that the sapphire mink would be more affected by AMDV than the wild type mink [7, 8, 28]. Not only the mink genotype but also virus strain of AMDV has been associated with different virulence [6–8]. The AMDV-Utah and AMDV-TR caused progressive disease in sapphire and pastel mink whereas AMDV-Pullman caused only progressive disease in 2/3 of the sapphire mink and not at all in the pastel mink [8]. Hadlow et al. found no consistent difference in clinical signs between the AMDV strains [7]. However, it is believed that many of the field strains of AMDV has a lower virulence [19, 20, 26] compared to the AMDV strains used in older studies [6].

The gross pathology observed in this study was similar regardless of how long time after AMDV inoculation the mink were euthanized with exception of: (1) the white sprinkle hairs that was observed only 24 weeks after AMDV inoculation, and (2) the kidney lesions were not observed until 2 months after AMDV inoculation. In general, few pathological changes are observed in chronic AMDV infected mink [14], which might represents the unspecific symptoms observed.

The AMDV associated histopathology seen in the present study corresponds to that seen by others [14–16, 28, 29]. No pathognomonic lesions exist for AD, but infiltration of mononuclear cells in several organs raises a strong suspicion of AD. The earliest histopathological sign of AMDV infection was seen in the liver at 2 weeks after inoculation, which has also been shown by others [28]. This might be related to the intraperitoneal route of inoculation, causing the virus to reach the liver as the first organ compared to for example the lung or the kidneys. This is further supported by the fact that no AMDV related lesions were seen in the lung or kidney of the mink 2 weeks in experiment, whereas these tissues developed AMDV related lesions later in the experimental infection. Furthermore, the liver was the organ that most often had lesions in all groups of mink, followed by the kidneys, brain, lung and intestines, respectively. This is in contrast to the prevalence of AMDV DNA in the organs, where the intestines were much more frequently positive compared to liver tissue at all time points [24] and indicates that the lesions are not caused by the viral infection itself, but the increased antibody production.

In the short term study the lesions were seen more frequent and pronounced in the mink euthanized 4 weeks after AMDV inoculation compared to the mink euthanized after 2 weeks, which reflects the time it takes to develop the lesions. The histopathological changes seemed to decrease from weeks 8 to 24 in the long term study with the exception of fur/skin affection, the same tendency was seen in regard to gross lesions. However, these differences were not statistically significant and the small sample size excludes firm conclusions. Histology is an important and sensitive tool in regard of suspicion and diagnostics of AD; however, final diagnosis must always be confirmed by PCR and/or antibody detection. Due to the variations in the progression of the lesions, histology cannot be used to conclude the time of infection.

## Conclusions

The currently circulating AMDV strain Saeby/DEN/799.1/05 cause few clinical signs with low mortality after experimental infection. The clinical signs observed were primarily decreased appetite and soft and/or discolored feces. The gross pathology was mainly associated with liver, spleen and kidney. Histopathological changes were seen in all organs but most frequently in liver, kidney and brain. No specific time of onset or pathognomonic lesions was observed. These findings are consistent with previous studies of AMDV and highlight the unpredictable disease pattern of AMDV and the necessity of supplementary and more sensitive tests like PCR and/or serology to confirm the diagnosis.

### Authors' contributions

THJ conceived the study, carried out the practical work and drafted the manuscript. MSH did all the histopathological work and wrote part of the manuscript. MC participated in the design of the study, did the analysis of the clinical signs and contributed significantly to the manuscript. All authors read and approved the final manuscript.

### Author details

[1] National Veterinary Institute, Technical University of Denmark, Bülowsvej 27, 1870 Frederiksberg C, Denmark. [2] Present Address: Department of Chemistry and Bioscience, Aalborg University/Aalborg Zoo, Frederik Bajers Vej 7H, 9100 Aalborg, Denmark. [3] Aalborg Zoo, Mølleparkvej 63, 9000 Aalborg, Denmark.

### Acknowledgements

The animal care staff at the National Veterinary Institute (NVI), Lindholm is acknowledged for taking good care of the animals and skillful assistance. The laboratory technicians at NVI, Aarhus and Annie Ravn Pedersen at NVI, Copenhagen are acknowledged for excellent help with processing the samples. Jens Nielsen and Åse Uttenthal are acknowledged for good advice and helpful discussions about the animal experiments. The Danish Fur Breeders Research Foundation is acknowledged for the financial support of these experiments.

### Competing interests

The authors declare that they have no competing interests.

### References

1. Knuuttila A, Uzcategui N, Kankkonen J, Vapalahti O, Kinnunen P. Molecular epidemiology of Aleutian mink disease virus in Finland. Vet Microbiol. 2009;133:229–38.
2. Sang Y, Ma J, Hou Z, Zhang Y. Phylogenetic analysis of the VP2 gene of Aleutian mink disease parvoviruses isolated from 2009 to 2011 in China. Virus Genes. 2012;45:31–7.
3. Farid AH, Zillig ML, Finley GG, Smith GC. Prevalence of the Aleutian mink disease virus infection in Nova Scotia, Canada. Prev Vet Med. 2012;106:332–8.

4. Christensen LS, Gram-Hansen L, Chriél M, Jensen TH. Diversity and stability of Aleutian mink disease virus during bottleneck transitions resulting from eradication in domestic mink in Denmark. Vet Microbiol. 2011;149:64–71.
5. Porter DD, Larsen AE, Porter HG. Aleutian disease of mink. Adv Immunol. 1980;29:261–86.
6. Alexandersen S. Pathogenesis of disease caused by Aleutian mink disease parvovirus. APMIS Suppl. 1990;14:1–32.
7. Hadlow WJ, Race RE, Kennedy RC. Comparative pathogenicity of four strains of Aleutian disease virus for pastel and sapphire mink. Infect Immun. 1983;41:1016–23.
8. Oie KL, Durrant G, Wolfinbarger JB, Martin D, Costello F, Perryman S, et al. The relationship between capsid protein (VP2) sequence and pathogenicity of Aleutian mink disease parvovirus (ADV): a possible role for raccoons in the transmission of ADV infections. J Virol. 1996;70:852–61.
9. Larsen S, Alexandersen S, Lund E, Have P, Hansen M. Acute interstitial pneumonitis caused by Aleutian disease virus in mink kits. Acta Pathol Microbiol Immunol Scand [A]. 1984;92:391–3.
10. Alexandersen S. Acute interstitial pneumonia in mink kits: experimental reproduction of the disease. Vet Pathol. 1986;23:579–88.
11. Alexandersen S, Larsen S, Aasted B, Uttenthal A, Bloom ME, Hansen M. Acute interstitial pneumonia in mink kits inoculated with defined isolates of Aleutian mink disease parvovirus. Vet Pathol. 1994;31:216–28.
12. Alexandersen S, Bloom ME, Wolfinbarger J. Evidence of restricted viral replication in adult mink infected with Aleutian disease of mink parvovirus. J Virol. 1988;62:1495–507.
13. Porter DD, Larsen AE, Porter HG. The pathogenesis of Aleutian disease of mink. 3. Immune complex arteritis. Am J Pathol. 1973;71:331–44.
14. Valdovska A, Pilmane M. Histopathologic and immunohistochemical lesions in liver of mink infected with Aleutian disease virus. Pol J Vet Sci. 2011;14:69–76.
15. Dyer NW, Ching B, Bloom ME. Nonsuppurative meningoencephalitis associated with Aleutian mink disease parvovirus infection in ranch mink. J Vet Diagn Invest. 2000;12:159–62.
16. Jahns H, Daly P, McElroy MC, Sammin DJ, Bassett HF, Callanan JJ. Neuropathologic features of Aleutian disease in farmed mink in Ireland and molecular characterization of Aleutian mink disease virus detected in brain tissues. J Vet Diagn Invest. 2010;22:101–5.
17. Farid AH, Ferns LE. Aleutian mink disease virus infection may cause hair depigmentation. Scientifur. 2011;35:55–9.
18. Jensen TH, Christensen LS, Chriel M, Uttenthal A, Hammer AS. Implementation and validation of a sensitive PCR detection method in the eradication campaign against Aleutian mink disease virus. J Virol Methods. 2011;171:81–5.
19. Farid AH, Hussain I, Arju I. Detection of Aleutian mink disease virus DNA and antiviral antibodies in American mink (*Neovison vison*) 10 days post-inoculation. J Vet Diagn Invest. 2015;27:287–97.
20. Jackson MK, Ellis LC, Morrey JD, Li ZZ, Barnard DL. Progression of Aleutian disease in natural and experimentally induced infections of mink. Am J Vet Res. 1996;57:1753–8.
21. An SH, Ingram DG. Transmission of Aleutian disease from mink with inapparent infections. Am J Vet Res. 1978;39:309–13.
22. Johnson MI, Henson JB, Gorham JR. The influence of genotype on the development of glomerular lesions in mink with Aleutian disease virus. Am J Pathol. 1975;81:321–36.
23. Mori S, Nose M, Miyazawa M, Kyogoku M, Wolfinbarger JB, Bloom ME. Interstitial nephritis in Aleutian mink disease. Possible role of cell-mediated immunity against virus-infected tubular epithelial cells. Am J Pathol. 1994;144:1326–33.
24. Jensen TH, Hammer AS, Chriél M. Monitoring chronic infection with a field strain of Aleutian mink disease virus. Vet Microbiol. 2014;168:420–7.
25. Eklund CM, Hadlow WJ, Kennedy RC, Boyle CC, Jackson TA. Aleutian disease of mink: properties of the etiologic agent and the host responses. J Infect Dis. 1968;118:510–26.
26. Jackson MK, Winslow SG, Dockery LD, Jones JK, Sisson DV. Investigation of an outbreak of Aleutian disease on a commercial mink ranch. Am J Vet Res. 1996;57:1706–10.
27. Chriél M, Harslund J, Jensen TH, Jakobsen E, Hammer AS, Lassen-Nielsen AM. Antimicrobials in mink-consumption and resistance patterns. Proceedings of the 10th International Scientific Congress in fur animal production. Scientifur. 2012;32:165–71.
28. Henson JB, Gorham JR, McGuire TC, Crawford TB. Pathology and pathogenesis of Aleutian disease. Front Biol. 1976;44:175–205.
29. Bloom ME, Kanno H, Mori S, Wolfinbarger JB. Aleutian mink disease: puzzles and paradigms. Infect Agents Dis. 1994;3:279–301.

# 2

# Bovine trypanosomosis: changes in parasitemia and packed cell volume in dry and wet seasons

Efrem Degneh[1], Workineh Shibeshi[2], Getachew Terefe[1*], Kaleab Asres[3] and Hagos Ashenafi[1]

**Abstract**

**Background:** Animal trypanosomosis is one of the major disease problems affecting agricultural productivity in Ethiopia. The impact of the disease is believed to vary with season and agro-ecologies in line with fly vector distribution. A cross-sectional study on bovine trypanosomosis was conducted from November 2015 to June 2016, in seven selected villages of Gidami district, Oromia Regional State, western Ethiopia. A total of 930 blood samples were collected and subjected to parasitological and hematological analysis.

**Result:** The overall prevalence of bovine trypanosomosis was 14.1%. The seasonal prevalence shows 9.06% in early dry and 18.4% in early rainy seasons. Three trypanosome species, *Trypanosoma congolense, Trypanosoma vivax* and *Trypanosoma brucei* were identified in the examined animals. *T. congolense* followed by *T. vivax* were the predominant species (respectively 59.0 and 35.9% in early dry season and 62.0 and 22.8% in early rainy season). The prevalence of *T. vivax* remained similar in both early dry and early rainy seasons in both lowland and midland agroecologies whereas *T. congolense* was more dominant in the lowland area in both seasons compared to mid land study sites. The disease was more prevalent in lowland (23.9%) compared to midland (11.1%) during early rainy season ($P < 0.001$) whereas no significant difference was observed between the two agroecologies during early dry season ($P = 0.165$). Packed cell volume (PCV) was much lower in parasitemic animals than in aparasitemic cattle whereas the mean PCV value for parasitemic animals (20.36%; 95% CI 19.56 to 21.16) in early dry season was similar to values in early rainy season (20.46%, 95% CI 18.84 to 21.08%). A similar situation was noticed for animals in both low land and mid land study sites.

**Conclusion:** Overall, the detection of trypanosomes in blood was significantly affected by agro-ecology, season and body condition of the animals. Special emphasis should be given to integrated trypanosomosis management in early rainy months where fly population is believed to start increasing.

**Keywords:** Agro-ecology, Gidami, PCV, Prevalence, Season, Bovine trypanosomosis, Western Ethiopia

## Background

African animal trypanosomosis (AAT) is the most important constraint to livestock production in tropical Africa [1–3], and considered as a threat to poverty alleviation programs in the continent [4]. The disease is widely distributed with about 50 million heads of cattle and other livestock species being at risk [5]. It is cyclically transmitted by tsetse flies [6] and mechanically by a number of biting flies [7]. Animal trypanosomosis is most important in cattle, but can also cause serious losses in camels, equines, goats and sheep. In Africa the annual direct and indirect losses due to this disease for livestock are estimated at 4.5 billion USD [8].

Ethiopia is believed to have the largest livestock population in Africa, which is currently estimated to be 54

*Correspondence: getachew_terefe@yahoo.com
[1] Department of Pathology and Parasitology, College of Veterinary Medicine and Agriculture, Addis Ababa University, P.O.Box 34, Debre Zeit, Ethiopia

million cattle, 25.5 million sheep and 24.1 million goats [9]. However, the livestock industry of the country is suffering from debilitating diseases such as trypanosomosis with approximately 15% of all arable land or 220,000 km$^2$ area infested with tsetse flies [10]. Morbidity and mortality losses from ruminant livestock alone are estimated to be USD 200 million [11].

Although a number of studies have reported the prevalence of the disease in many places of the country [12–14], data on the seasonal dynamics of the problem and associated risk factors is scanty for the Gidami district of the Oromia Regional State, western Ethiopia. The Gidami district is one of the districts richly endowed with livestock resources but is ravaged by animal trypanosomosis (District office of Livestock and Fisheries: personal communication). Therefore, the present study was aimed at assessing the prevalences of bovine trypanosomosis and associated risk factors in early dry and early rainy seasons, in order to provide baseline data that can be used in planning and implementation of disease control program in this area.

## Methods

### Study area

This study was conducted from November 2015 to June 2016 in the Gidami District of West/Kellem Wollega Zone of the Oromia Regional State (western Ethiopia). The Gidami district is located 670 km to the west of the capital, Addis Ababa (Fig. 1). The area has two distinct seasons: a dry season extending from November to May; and a wet season which extends from June to September. It has a total area of 219,641 hectares. The altitude of the area ranges from 1200 to 2200 m above sea level. Based on the altitude the area is subdivided into three climatic zones: highland (8%), midland (75%) and lowland (17%). The mean annual rainfall and temperature ranges of the area are 1200 to 2000 mm and 15 to 25 °C respectively. Mixed crop-livestock farming is the main source of livelihoods. The vegetation cover is dominated by savanna grassland, forest, riverine and bush lands. Wild games like buffalos, bush pig, warthog, lions, antelopes, leopard, hyena and monkeys are commonly found in the area. The livestock population of the district has been estimated

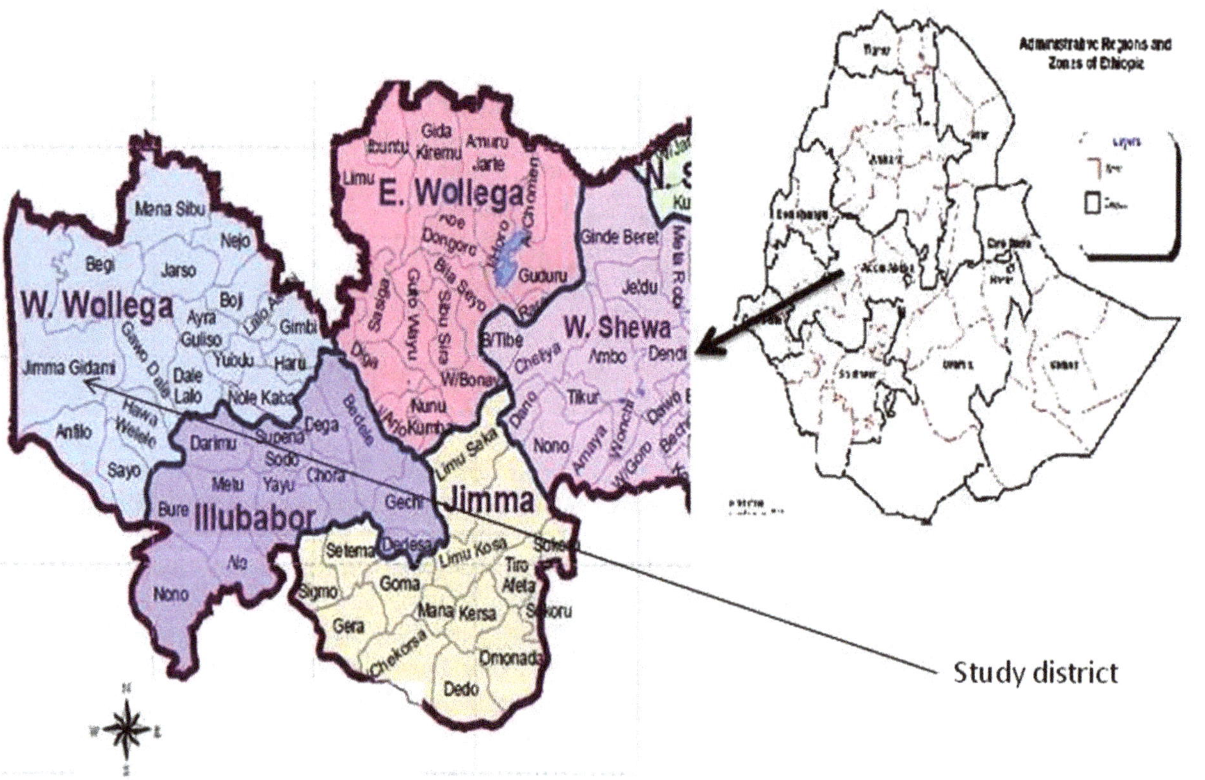


**Fig. 1** Map showing the location of the study area in western Ethiopia

to be around 73,000 cattle, 47,000 sheep, 24,000 goats, 12,000 equines and 140,000 chickens [9]. Communal grazing without any supplementary feeding is the major livestock husbandry system throughout the year.

### Study design and sampling methods

A cross-sectional study was conducted to estimate the prevalence of bovine trypanosomosis in the study area. Seven peasant associations were selected purposively based on livestock population and accessibility from two agro-climatic zones: four from lowland (<1600 m above sea level) and the rest three from midland (>1600 m above sea level). Animals were bled during early dry (November and December) and early rainy (May and June) seasons of the year. A systematic random sampling technique was employed to sample every other individual animal caught at communal grazing points of each village. The sample size was determined based on the expected prevalence of 16.9% as previously reported by Kebede [15] for the nearby district, Sayo Nole in West Wollega, and absolute desired precision of 5% at 95% confidence level as described by Thrusfield [16]. Accordingly, 215 animals were required to be sampled in each study season (total = 430). However, because of adequate availability of animals, this number was increased to 930 to improve the precision. Accordingly, a total of 514 animals from the lowland area (230 and 284 in dry and wet season respectively) and 416 animals from the midland areas (200 and 216 in dry and wet season respectively) were sampled.

### Study population

The study population consisted of all zebu cattle above 1 year of age, which were usually kept under an extensive husbandry system. A total of 930 animals (500 males and 430 females) were systematically selected in early dry and early rainy seasons. The age of animals was determined by dentition [17] and conventionally categorized as young (1 to 3 years) and adult (>3 years). The body condition score of animals was recorded by classifying animals into three groups as good, medium, and poor based on the appearance of ribs and vertebral spinous processes [18].

### Blood sampling and examination

Blood samples were collected by puncturing the superficial ear vein of each animal into heparinized capillary tubes and centrifuged immediately in a hematocrit centrifuge. Packed cell volume (PCV) was measured for each sample. Animals with PCV less than 24% were considered to be anemic [19, 20]. The contents of the capillary tubes (including about 1 mm above and below the buffy coat) were examined using buffy coat technique to reveal trypanosomes under 40× magnifications under the light microscope [21–23]. From trypanosome positive samples thin blood smears were made and stained with Giemsa for species identification by light microscopy. The trypanosome species were distinguished using their size, position of the kinetoplast, presence of undulating membranes and length of the free flagella according to [20, 24].

### Data analysis

Data collected from each study animal and laboratory analyses were entered into a Microsoft excel spreadsheet and un-coded. SPSS version 20 was used for the analysis and interpretation of the data. The prevalence of trypanosomosis was calculated as the number of infected individuals divided by the number of individuals examined and multiplied by 100. The difference in prevalence between altitude, season, sex, age and body condition score was compared by Chi square test. Student's t-test was used to compare the mean PCVs between parasitemic and aparasitemic animals, among seasons and agroecologies. Generally, $P < 0.05$ was considered to be statistically significant.

## Results

### Parasitological findings

Out of 930 examined cattle, 131 were positive for trypanosomosis using the buffy coat technique with an overall prevalence of 14.08% (95% CI 11.9 to 16.5%). The prevalence was significantly higher in low land than in mid land, during early rainy season than in early dry season and in animals with poor and moderate body condition compared to those with good body condition ($P < 0.001$). Similarly, the prevalence of the infection in poor body conditioned animals was significantly higher than in animals with medium body condition (Table 1). There was a notable increase in the prevalence of bovine trypanosomes in low land areas during early rainy season as compared to the mid land ($P < 0.001$) whereas no significant difference was detected between low land and mid land areas during early dry season ($P = 0.165$) (Table 2). Three trypanosome species, *T. congolense, T. vivax* and *T. brucei* were identified in the study animals. *T. congolense* was the predominant species (59 and 62%) followed by *T. vivax* (35.9 and 22.8%) in early dry and early rainy seasons respectively (Fig. 2).

### Packed cell volume

Statistical analysis of the PCV values indicated that the overall mean PCV was significantly lower for trypanosomosis positive animals (20.48%, 95% CI 19.97 to 20.99%) compared with that of negative animals (25.77%, 95% CI 25.48 to 26.07%) irrespective of season of sampling and agro-ecology ($P < 0.001$). On the other hand, there was no notable difference between mean PCVs of

**Table 1 Prevalence of bovine trypanosomosis with different potential risk factors in Gidami district, Oromia Regional State, western Ethiopia**

| Potential risk factors | No of animals | Prevalence (%) | 95% CI | $\chi^2$ value | P-value |
|---|---|---|---|---|---|
| Altitude | | | | | |
| Low land | 514 | 18.09 | 14.76 to 21.42 | 15.24 | 0.0001 |
| Middle land | 416 | 9.13 | 6.36 to 11.9 | | |
| Season | | | | | |
| Early dry | 430 | 9.07 | 6.36 to 11.78 | 16.61 | <0.0001 |
| Early rainy | 500 | 18.4 | 15 to 21.80 | | |
| Body condition | | | | | |
| Poor | 294 | 27.9 | 22.77 to 33.03 | 39.16<br>14.95 | <0.0001<br>0.0001 |
| Medium | 458 | 10.3 | 7.52 to 13.08 | | |
| Good | 177 | 1.1 | −0.44 to 2.64 | | |
| Sex | | | | | |
| Male | 500 | 14.4 | 11.32 to 17.48 | 0.09 | 0.766 |
| Female | 430 | 13.72 | 10.47 to 16.97 | | |
| Age | | | | | |
| 1–3 years | 291 | 11.34 | 7.7 to 14.98 | 2.64 | 0.104 |
| >3 years | 639 | 15.34 | 11.55 to 16.73 | | |

**Table 2 Prevalence of bovine trypanosomosis during early rainy and early dry seasons in low land and midland areas of Gidami district, western Ethiopia**

| Season | No. of animals | Prevalence (%) | 95% CI | $\chi^2$ value | P-value |
|---|---|---|---|---|---|
| Early rainy season | | | | | 0.0003 |
| Low land | 284 | 23.9 | 18.94 to 28.86 | 13.36 | |
| Mid land | 216 | 11.11 | 6.92 to 15.30 | | |
| Early dry season | | | | | 0.1649 |
| Low land | 230 | 10.86 | 6.84 to 14.88 | 1.93 | |
| Mid land | 200 | 7 | 3.46 to 10.54 | | |

trypanosomosis positive animals when lowland and midland agroecologies ($P = 0.331$) as well as early rainy and early dry seasons ($P = 0.379$) were compared (Table 3). Strong association between prevalence of trypanosomosis and anemia (expressed in terms of reduction in PCV below 25%) was observed ($P < 0.001$) in both sampling seasons and agroecologies (Table 4). Among the trypanosomosis positive animals, 92.3 and 91.3% fall in anemic category in early dry and early rainy seasons respectively while 90.3 and 94.7% of them were anemic respectively in lowland and midland sampling sites.

## Discussion

The present study revealed that trypanosomosis is widespread in Gidami District with an overall prevalence of 14.08% (95% CI 11.9 to 16.5%). This result was slightly lower than the findings of Kebede [15] who reported an overall prevalence of 16.9% in the nearby Sayo Nole District. The fact that there were no vector control intervention practices in the study area during the study period suggest that any reduction could be attributed to difference in season of sampling and/or changes in ecological/climatic conditions that affect vector fly density/distribution overtime [25]. Higher prevalence values were also reported by Cherenet et al. [26] and Mulaw et al. [27] respectively with 25.7 and 28.1% proportions from different parts of Ethiopia. On the other hand, the prevalence reported here is in close agreement with the report of Feyissa et al. [28] in selected Villages of Humbo District, southern Ethiopia (14.2%) and higher than the 2.86% reported by Biyazen et al. [29]. Such variations may exist because of differences in agro-ecology, sampling season, vector infection rate, animal susceptibility and practice of trypanocidal drug use and fly control operations which may obviously impact on epidemiological situations of the disease [30–32].

The findings in the present study is in agreement with the fact that the most pathogenic trypanosome species for cattle, i.e., *T. congolense* and *T. vivax*, are abundant in most parts of western Ethiopia ([10, 27], in Ethiopia in general as well as in other parts of Africa [33–35]. The high proportion of *T. congolense* is similar with the previous report of Duguma et al. [36] in south-western Ethiopia (76%), Ameen et al. [37] in Ogbomoso Area of Oyo State, Nigeria who reported only *T. congolense* infection and Dawud and Molalegne [38] at Mao-Komo district of Benshangul Gumuz regional state (63.2%). The high ratio of *T. congolense* may be ascribed to the

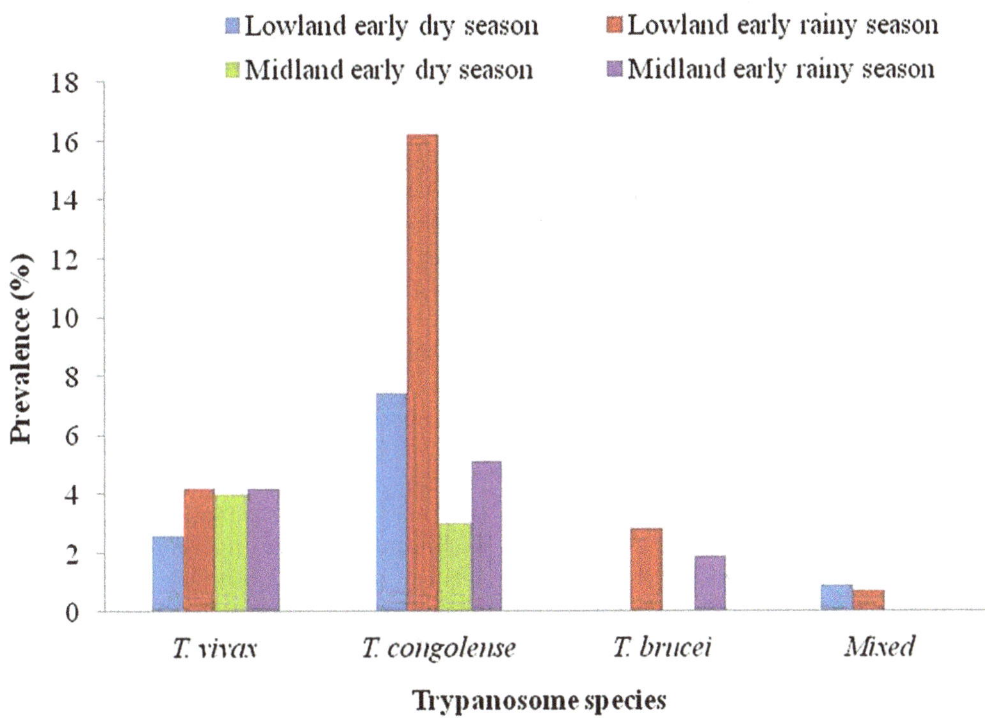


**Fig. 2** *Trypanosome* species identified during the study period in Gidami District, western Ethiopia

**Table 3 Comparison of PCV of parasitologically positive animals according to sampling season and agro-ecology**

| Risk factors | Category | No. of parasitemic animals | % PCV | 95% CI | *t*. value | P-value |
|---|---|---|---|---|---|---|
| Season | Early dry | 39 | 20.36 | 19.53 to 21.19 | −0.308 | 0.379 |
| | Early rainy | 92 | 20.53 | 19.89 to 21.17 | | |
| Agro-ecology | Low land | 93 | 20.41 | 19.81 to 21.00 | −0.439 | 0.331 |
| | Mid land | 38 | 20.66 | 19.64 to 21.68 | | |

**Table 4 Comparison of trypanosome prevalence between anemic and non-anemic cattle during early dry and early rainy seasons from lowland and midland study areas**

| Category | Anemia status[a] | No. of animals examined | % positive animals | 95% CI | $\chi^2$ value | *P*-value |
|---|---|---|---|---|---|---|
| Early dry | Anemic | 179 | 20.10 | 14.20 to 26.0 | 36.51 | <0.0001 |
| | Non-anemic | 251 | 1.20 | 0.0 to 2.5 | | |
| Early rainy | Anemic | 274 | 30.66 | 25.2 to 36.1 | 60.03 | <0.0001 |
| | Non-anemic | 226 | 3.54 | 1.1 to 5.9 | | |
| Low land | Anemic | 271 | 31.00 | 25.5 to 36.5 | 67.87 | <0.0001 |
| | Non-anemic | 243 | 3.70 | 1.20 to 5.50 | | |
| Mid land | Anemic | 182 | 19.78 | 14.00 to 25.60 | 44.178 | <0.0001 |
| | Non-anemic | 234 | 0.85 | 0.00 to 2.00 | | |

[a] Anemic: PCV ≤24%, non-anemic: PCV >24%

more efficient transmission of this species by major cyclical vectors (tsetse flies) than *T. vivax* in tsetse infested areas [33].

Although the rate of infection with trypanosomes was high in both study periods, it was significantly higher at the beginning of the rainy season, particularly with *T.*

*congolense*. This agrees with the reports of Majekodunmi et al. [31]. Although fly burden was not assessed in this study, the high incidence of trypanosome infections at the beginning of the rainy season may be explained by the increasing density of tsetse and other biting flies during this time of the year [39]. It is also possible that the cumulative effect of feed shortage during the dry season preceding the sampling may have reduced immunity of the animals while favoring higher infection prevalence. Holmes et al. [40] and Katunguka-Rwakishaya et al. [41] reported that high protein intake reduces the pathologic effect of trypanosomosis and enhances recovery following treatment with trypanocidal drugs. On the other hand, our finding does not agree with the report of Ameen et al. [37] which indicated higher rate of *T. congolense* infection in dry season than in wet season which probably is explained by the reason given by the authors. They suggested that presence of few ponds in the dry season might have forced the animals to come close together and also created a favorable ground for the tsetse flies.

The prevalence of bovine trypanosomosis is also known to be affected by agro-ecological conditions such as altitude [42]. In this study, the prevalence of trypanosomosis was significantly higher in lowland areas compared to those in mid-land study sites during the early rainy season. This suggests the possible development of optimum vegetation, temperature and humidity favorable for tsetse fly breeding and survival [35]. This finding agrees with other studies done elsewhere [43]. The absence of difference in prevalence of the disease during early dry season may suggest that the two agro-ecologies did have adequate vegetation for the animals to graze and exposure to fly infestation have started declining.

Body condition of the cattle was another factor that has shown strong association with trypanosomosis prevalence. Animals with poor body condition were found more affected by trypanosomes than other cattle with good body condition. This finding is in line with previous reports [44–47]. This might be attributed to reduced resistance of those animals having poor body condition or related to the progressive weight loss arising from debilitating nature of the disease itself [48].

In line with other previous studies on bovine trypanosomosis [42, 44, 49, 50], anemia was significantly more severe in trypanosome infected cattle (as evidenced by lower mean PCV) compared to trypanosomosis negative animals. This is further supported by the fact that majority of trypanosomosis positive animals had PCV values lower than 25% and the non-anemic category had very low proportion of trypanosome positive cases. On the other hand, the majority of the animals classified as anemic had no detectable trypanosomes suggesting that other anemia causing factors such as poor nutrition, helminthiasis etc. could be responsible for the reduction in PCV. In this regards, our findings agree with the reports in other previous studies [51–53]. It may also be partly due to the low sensitivity of parasitological diagnostic method used in this study [49, 54, 55] which has resulted in some trypanosome positive animals with lower PCV to be wrongly categorized as negative for trypanosomes. Trypanosomes become very difficult to detect when the parasitemia is lower than 60 trypanosomes/mL blood [56, 57].

## Conclusions

The current study indicated that the prevalence of trypanosomosis is significant to the level that it can limit livestock production in the Gidami District of Ethiopia. Two pathogenic species, *T. congolense* and *T. vivax* were mainly responsible for the disease in the study area. Significant variation in prevalence was also observed between seasons, agro-ecology and animal body condition scores. Anemia was characteristic of the infection in both lowland and mid land agroecologies irrespective of the sampling season. The situation warrants the initiation and intensification of tsetse fly control activities especially in the early wet season where *T. congolense* is most dominant.

**Authors' contributions**

ED drafted the proposal and the manuscript, collected, analyzed and interpreted the data. WS supervised the project and edited the manuscript. GT supported the analyses and interpretation of the results and edited the manuscript. KA drafted the proposal and edited the manuscript. HA supervised the project and edited the manuscript. All authors read and approved the final manuscript.

**Author details**

[1] Department of Pathology and Parasitology, College of Veterinary Medicine and Agriculture, Addis Ababa University, P.O.Box 34, Debre Zeit, Ethiopia. [2] Department of Pharmacology and Clinical Pharmacy, School of Pharmacy, College of Health Sciences, Addis Ababa University, P.O.Box 9086, Addis Ababa, Ethiopia. [3] Department of Pharmaceutical Chemistry and Pharmacognosy, School of Pharmacy, College of Health Sciences, Addis Ababa University, P.O.Box 9086, Addis Ababa, Ethiopia.

**Acknowledgements**

The authors would like to thank Wollega University and Addis Ababa University (College of Health Sciences, School of Pharmacy: Trypanosomosis thematic research project) for the finical support to conduct this investigation. We also thank management and technical staff of Bedele Regional Veterinary Laboratory for allowing access to laboratory facility and cooperation during sample collection from the field. Gidami district Livestock Development and Health Office is also acknowledged for its invaluable support and collaboration during the study period.

**Competing interests**

The authors declare that they have no competing interests.

**Funding**

This research was part of a PhD research project and was partially supported by the Office of the Director for Graduate programs (Addis Ababa University) and the thematic research project, Trypanosomosis, located at the College of Health Sciences (Addis Ababa University).

**References**

1. Courtin F, Jamonneau V, Duvallet G, Garcia A, Coulibaly B, Doumenge JP, et al. Sleeping sickness in West Africa (1906–2006): changes in spatial repartition and lessons from the past. Trop Med Int Health. 2008;13:334–44.
2. Holt HR, Selby R, Mumba C, Napier GB. Guitian assessment of animal African trypanosomiasis (AAT) vulnerability in cattle-owning communities of sub-Saharan Africa. Parasit Vectors. 2016;9:53. doi:10.1186/s13071-016-1336-5.
3. Shaw AP. Assessing the economics of animal trypanosomosis in Africa-history and current perspectives. Onderstepoort J Vet Res. 2009;76:27–32.
4. Oluwafemi RA. Tsetse/trypanosomosis challenges and rural poverty in Africa: implications for food security and MDG1, Review. RJAEM. 2014;3:158–61.
5. Mattioli RC, Feldmann G, Hendrickx W, Wint J, Jannin J, Slingenbergh J. Tsetse and trypanosomiasis intervention policies supporting sustainable animal agricultural development. Food Agric Environ. 2004;2:310–4.
6. Steverding D. The history of African trypanosomiasis. Parasit Vectors. 2008;1:3. doi:10.1186/1756-3305-1-3.
7. Desquesnes M, Dia ML. *Trypanosoma vivax*: mechanical transmission in cattle by one of the most common African tabanids, Atylotus agrestis. Exp Parasitol. 2003;103:35–43.
8. Affognon HD. Economic analysis of trypanocide use in villages under risk of drug resistance in West Africa, PhD Thesis, University of Hannover, Germany. 2007.
9. CSA (Central Statistical Agency). Agricultural sample survey, volume II: report on livestock and livestock characteristics (Private peasant holdings). statistical bulletin 570. Addis Ababa: Federal Democratic Republic of Ethiopia; 2013.
10. Abebe G. Trypanosomosis in Ethiopia. Ethiop J Biol Sci. 2005;4:75–121.
11. Abebe G, Jobre Y. Trypanosomosis: a threat to cattle production in Ethiopia. Rev Med Vet. 1996;147:897–902.
12. Birhanu H, Fikru R, Said M, Kidane W, Gebrehiwot T, Hagos A, et al. Epidemiology of *Trypanosoma evansi* and *Trypanosoma vivax* in domestic animals from selected districts of Tigray and Afar regions, Northern Ethiopia. Parasit Vectors. 2015;8:212. doi:10.1186/s13071-015-0818-1.
13. Lelisa K, Shimelis S, Bekele J, Shiferaw D. Bovine trypanosomosis and its fly vectors in three selected settlement areas of Hawa-Gelan district, western Ethiopia. Onderstepoort J Vet Res. 2014;81:715. doi:10.4102/ojvr.v81i1.715.
14. Leta S, Alemayehu G, Seyoum Z, Bezie M. Prevalence of bovine trypanosomosis in Ethiopia: a meta-analysis. Parasit Vectors. 2016;9:139. doi:10.1186/s13071-016-1404-x.
15. Kebede B. Prevalence of bovine trypanosomosis and apparent density of tsetse flies in Sayo nole District Western Oromia. Ethiop Vet Sci Tech. 2015;6:254. doi:10.4172/2157-7579.1000254.
16. Thrusfield M. Veterinary Epidemiology. 3rd ed. Blackwell science Ltd: London; 2005. p. 228–46.
17. DeLahunta A, Hable RE. Teeth. In: DeLahunt A, Hable RE, editors. Applied veterinary anatomy. Philadelphia: W.B. Saunders Company; 1986.
18. Nicholson MJ, Butterworth MH. A guide to condition scoring of zebu cattle. ILCA: Addis Ababa Ethiopia; 1986. p. 212–35.
19. Van den Bossche P, Shumba W, Makhambera P. The distribution and epidemiology of bovine trypanosomosis in Malawi. Vet Parasitol. 2000;88:163–76.
20. OIE. Standardized techniques for the diagnosis of tsetse transmitted trypanosomiasis. In: OIE Terrestrial ManualRome, Italy. 2008: 49.
21. Eisler MC, Brandt J, Bauer B, Clausen PH, Delespaux V, Holmes PH, et al. Standardized tests in mice and cattle for the detection of drug resistance in tsetse-transmitted trypanosomes of African domestic cattle. Vet Parasitol. 2001;97:171–82.
22. Chappuis F, Loutan L, Simarro P, Lejon V, Buscher P. Options for the field diagnosis of human African trypanosomiasis. Clinic Microbiol Rev. 2005;10:133–46.
23. Murray M, Murray PK, McIntyre WIM. An improved technique for the diagnosis of African trypanosomosis. Trans R Soc Trop Med Hyg. 1977;71:325–6.
24. Picozzi K, Tilly A, Fevre EM, Coleman P, Magona JW, Odiit M, et al. The diagnosis of trypanosome infections: applications of novel technology for reducing disease risk. Afr J Biotechnol. 2002;1:39–45.
25. Patz JA, Graczyk TK, Geller N, Vittor AY. Effects of environmental change on emerging parasitic diseases. Int J Parasitol. 2000;30:1395–405.
26. Cherenet T, Sani RA, Speybroeck N, Panandam JM, Nadzr S, Van den Bossche P. A comparative longitudinal study of bovine trypanosomiasis in tsetse-free and tsetse-infested zones of the Amhara region, northwest Ethiopia. Vet Parasitol. 2006;140:251–8.
27. Mulaw S, Addis M, Fromisa A. Study on the prevalence of major trypanosome affecting bovine in tsetse infested Asosa District of Benshagul-Gumuz Regional State, western Ethiopia. Global Vet. 2011;7:330–6.
28. Feyissa B, Samson A, Mihreteab B. Bovine trypanosomosis in selected villages of Humbo District. South Ethiop Global Vet. 2011;7:192–8.
29. Biyazen H, Duguma R, Asaye M. Trypanosomosis, its risk factors, and anemia in cattle population of Dale Wabera District of Kellem Wollega Zone, Western Ethiopia. J Vet Med. 2014;. doi:10.1155/2014/374191.
30. Geiger A, Ponton F, Simo G. Adult blood-feeding tsetse flies, trypanosomes, microbiota and the fluctuating environment in Sub-Saharan Africa. ISMEJ. 2015;9:1496–507.
31. Majekodunmi AO, Fajinmi A, Dongkum C, Picozzi K, Thrusfield MV, Welburn SC. A longitudinal survey of African animal trypanosomiasis in domestic cattle on the Jos Plateau, Nigeria: prevalence, distribution and risk factors. Parasit Vectors. 2013;6:239. doi:10.1186/1756-3305-6-239.
32. Reifenberg JM, Cuisance D, Frezil JL, Cuny G, Uvallet GD. Comparison of the susceptibility of different *Glossina* species to simple and mixed infections with *Trypanosoma* (Nannomonas) *congolense* savannah and riverine forest types. Med Vet Entomol. 1997;11:246–52.
33. Leak SGA. Tsetse Biology and Ecology: their role in the epidemiology and control of trypanosomosis. Wallingford: CABI publishing in association with the ILRI; 1999. p. 152–210.
34. McDermott JJ, Woitag T, Sidibe I, Bauer B, Boucader D, Ouedrago D, et al. Field studies on drug- resistant animal trypanosomes in Kenedogou province, Burkina Faso. Acta Trop. 2003;86:93–103.
35. Cherenet T, Sani RA, Panandam JM, Nadzr S, Speybroeck N, Van Den Bossche P. Seasonal prevalence of bovine trypanosomiasis in a tsetse-infested zone and a tsetse-free zone of the Amhara region, north-west Ethiopia. Onderstepoort J Vet Res. 2004;71:307–12.
36. Duguma R, Tasew S, Olani A, Damena D, Alemu D, Mulatu T, et al. Spatial distribution of *Glossina* sp. and *Trypanosoma* sp. in south-western Ethiopia. Parasit Vectors. 2015;8:430. doi:10.1186/s13071-015-1041-9.
37. Ameen SA, Joshua RA, Adedeji OS, Raheem AK, Akingbade AA, Leigh OO. Preliminary studies on prevalence of ruminant trypanosomosis in Ogbomoso Area of Oyo State, Nigeria. Middle East J Sci Res. 2008;3:214–8.
38. Dawud A, Molalegne B. Epidemiological study of bovine trypanosomosis in Mao-Komo. Special District, Benishangul Gumuz Regional State, Western Ethiopia. Global Vet. 2011;6:402–8.
39. Van den Bossche P, De Deken R. Seasonal variations in the distribution and abundance of the tsetse fly, *Glossina morsitans morsitans* in eastern Zambia. Med Vet Entomol. 2002;16:170–6.
40. Holmes PH, Katunguka-Rwakishaya E, Bennison JJ, Wassink GJ, Parkins JJ. Impact of nutrition on the pathophysiology of bovine trypanosomiasis. Parasitology. 2000;120(Suppl):S73–85.
41. Katunguka-Rwakishaya E, Parkins JJ, Fishwick G, Murray M, Holmes PH. The pathophysiology of *Trypanosoma congolense* infection in Scottish Blackface sheep. Influence of dietary protein. Vet Parasitol. 1993;47:189–204.
42. Sinshaw A, Abebe G, Desquesnes M, Yoin W. Biting flies and *Trypanosoma vivax* infection in three highland district bordering Lake Tana, Ethiopia. Vet. Parasitol. 2006;142:35–46.
43. Mamoudou A, Zoli A, Mbahin N, Tanenbe C, Clausen BP, Marcotty H, et al. Prevalence and incidence of bovine trypanosomosis on the Adamaoua plateau in Cameroon 10 years after the tsetse eradication campaign. Vet Parasitol. 2006;142:16–22.
44. Molalegne B, Yeshitila A, Asmamaw A. Prevalence of bovine trypanosomosis in selected areas of Jabi Tehnan District, West Gojjam

of Amhara Regional State, North-western Ethiopia. Global Vet. 2010;5:243–7.
45. Teka W, Terefa D, Wondimu A. Prevalence study of bovine trypanosomiasis and tsetse density in selected villages of Arbaminch, Ethiopia. J Vet Med Anim Health. 2012;4:36–41.
46. Dinka H, Abebe G. Small ruminants trypanosomosis in southwest of Ethiopia. Small Rumin Res. 2005;57:239–43.
47. Tafese W, Melaku A, Fentahun T. Prevalence of bovine trypanosomosis and its vectors in two districts of East Wollega Zone, Ethiopia. Onderstepoort J Vet Res. 2012;79:385. doi:10.4102/ojvr.v79i1.385.
48. Radostits OM, Gay CC, Hinchcliff KW, Constable PD. Veterinary medicine: a text book of diseases of cattle, horses, sheep, pigs and goats. 10th ed. New York: Saunders-Elsevier; 2007. p. 1536–96.
49. Marcotty T, Simukoko H, Berkvens D, Vercruysse J, Praet N, Van Den Bossche P. Evaluating the use of packed cell volume as an indicator of trypanosomal infections in cattle in eastern Zambia. Prev Vet Med. 2008;87:288–300.
50. Degu F, Ayalew B, Tewodros F, Mersha C. Occurrence of bovine trypanosomosis, in the Blue Nile river basin, Northwest Ethiopia. Europ J Appl Sci. 2012;4:129–35.
51. Magona JW, Walubengo J, Olaho-Mukani W, Revie CW, Jonsson NN, Eisler MC. A Delphi survey on expert opinion on key signs for clinical diagnosis of bovine trypanosomosis, tick-borne diseases and helminthoses. Bull Anim Health Prod Afr. 2004;52:130–40.
52. Zinsstag J, Ankers P, Ndao M, Bonfoh B, Pfister K. Multiparasitism, production and economics in domestic animals in sub-Saharan West Africa. Parasitol Today. 1998;14:46–9.
53. Mbewe NJ, Namangala B, Sitali L, Vorster I, Michelo C. Prevalence of pathogenic trypanosomes in anemic cattle from trypanosomosis challenged areas of Itezhi-Tezhi district in central Zambia. Parasit Vectors. 2015;8:638. doi:10.1186/s13071-015-1260-0.
54. Simukoko H, Marcotty T, Vercruysse J, Van den Bossche P. Bovine trypanosomiasis risk in an endemic area on the eastern plateau of Zambia. Res Vet Sci. 2011;90:51–4.
55. Naessens J. Bovine trypanotolerance. A natural ability to prevent severe anaemia and haemophagocytic syndrome. Int J Parasitol. 2006;36:521–8.
56. Desquesnes M. Evaluation of a simple PCR technique for the diagnosis of *Trypanosoma vivax* infection in the serum of cattle in comparison to parasitological techniques and antigen-enzyme-linked-immunosorbent assay. Acta Trop. 1997;65:139–48.
57. Luckins AG. Methods for diagnosis of trypanosomiasis in livestock. FAO corporate document repository. 2010. http://www.fao.org/DOCRDP.

# 3

# A novel model for studying ileitis-induced visceral hypersensitivity in goats

Adnan Hassan Tahir, Juan Wan, Manoj Kumar Shah, Habibullah Janyaro, Xiao-Jing Li and Ming-Xing Ding*

**Abstract**

**Background:** Visceral hypersensitivity (VH) is a common condition in many gastrointestinal disorders such as inflammatory bowel diseases (IBDs) in human and animals. Most studies often induce Crohn's disease/colitis to investigate VH in small experimental animals. Although farm animals commonly suffer from IBDs, their VH has not been investigated so far. Because goats can suffer from Johne's disease, a naturally occurring Crohn's-like disease, they may be suitable to be used for studying the mechanism underlying VH in common intestinal disorders of large animals. In the present study, 60 healthy goats of either sex were equally divided into a 2, 4, 6-trinitrobenzenesulfonic acid (TNBS) group and saline group. A volume of 1.2 ml of TNBS-ethanol solution (30 mg TNBS in 40 % ethanol) or an equal volume of isotonic saline was injected into the wall of the terminal ileum through laparotomy. The severity of the developing ileitis was determined according to macro- and microscopic pathologic scores and the levels of myeloperoxidase, interleukin-1β, interleukin-6 and tumor necrosis factor-α, and VH was evaluated with visceromotor responses (VMR) to colorectal distension on days 3, 7, 14, 21 and 28. VMRs were assessed with a continuous ramp distention mode with 6 s for each pressure (20, 40, 60, 80 and 100 mmHg).

**Results:** Compared to the saline group, the TNBS-treated goats showed apparent transmural pathological changes and a significant increase ($P < 0.05$) in macroscopic and microscopic change scores, and levels of myeloperoxidase, interleukin-1β, interleukin-6 and tumor necrosis factor-α in the ileum, and VMR to colorectal distension. The goats exhibited apparent ileitis at days 3 to 21, and VH at days 7 to 28 following TNBS treatment.

**Conclusion:** This experiment successfully established a reproducible ileitis and VH with administration of TNBS-ethanol solution in the ileal wall of goats. This model is useful for studying the pathogenesis of the IBD and the mechanism underlying VH, and for evaluating the efficacy of new therapeutic regimens.

**Keywords:** Inflammatory bowel disease, Johne's disease, Ileitis, TNBS, Visceral hypersensitivity, Visceromotor response

## Background

Inflammatory bowel diseases (IBDs) are a collection of chronic inflammatory disorders of the gastrointestinal tract in human and animals. The major symptoms are visceral hypersensitivity (VH) (visceral pain, altered bowel movement, increased mucosal secretion) with weight loss, malnutrition, fever and lack of appetite [1, 2]. VH is one of the important symptoms in about 50–70 % of patients experiencing the initial onset of IBD.

Johne's disease (JD), a kind of IBDs, is seen in cattle, sheep and goats and is caused by *Mycobacterium avium* subsp. *paratubersulosis*. Gross lesions of JD include intense reddening, mucosal granulomatous inflammation and wall thickening, especially in ileum [3]. This chronic intestinal disease occurs worldwide and causes mortality and productivity loss of ruminants [4, 5]. JD shares many similarities with human Crohn's disease (CD) in terms of symptoms, location and pathological changes. The small intestine, especially the terminal ileum, is the primary location of both diseases [6, 7]. VH is an important characteristic of IBD in humans, but VH in ruminants is rarely reported. Studies have indicated that VH may result from a dysregulated mucosal immunologic

*Correspondence: dmx@mail.hzau.edu.cn
College of Veterinary Medicine, Huazhong Agricultural University, No. 1, Shizishan Street, Hongshan District, Wuhan, Hubei 430070, People's Republic of China

response to one or more antigens present in the enteric flora as well as a genetic predisposition to the development of this response [8–11]. However, its underlying mechanisms are still unknown. Most studies have investigated VH utilizing colitis models; however, such models are not appropriate for studying the exact mechanism by which ileitis induces VH because its location, duration, microbiota and central regulating mechanism are different.

Different chemicals such as acetic acid, formalin, indomethacin, 2, 4, 6-trinitrobenzenesulfonic acid (TNBS), carrageenan and dextran sodium sulfate have been used to study IBD. Among these chemicals, TNBS is the most commonly used. Nowadays, TNBS in combination with ethanol has been used to induce ileitis or colitis in mice [12], rats [13], guinea pigs [14, 15] and pigs [16]. Several studies reported that intracolonic administration of TNBS-ethanol solution can provoke VH in rats [17–19]. So far no VH model of farm animals has been reported.

In the present study, a TNBS-ethanol solution was injected into goat's terminal ileum wall to induce ileitis and VH. The macroscopic and microscopic damage scores, and levels of myeloperoxidase (MPO) and cytokines were detected for evaluating the severity of the induced inflammation. Visceromotor response (VMR) to colorectal distension (CRD) was used to assess VH.

## Methods

### Experimental animals

Goats were thoroughly examined to ascertain their health status. The animals were kept under the same nutritional and managemental conditions. They were dewormed and acclimatized to the environment for 1 week before the initiation of the study. The experiment was approved by the Institutional Animal Care and Use Committee of Huazhong Agricultural University, Wuhan, China (HZAUSH-2015-007), and performed with the guidelines of the Committee for Research and Ethical Issues of the International Association for the Study of Pain.

### Determination of TNBS dosage for model experiment

Eighteen male goats (about 1-year-old) were randomly divided into 6 groups i.e. saline, 40 % ethanol, 30 mg TNBS (Sigma Aldrich company, USA) and TNBS-ethanol solutions (20, 30 or 40 mg in 40 % ethanol), with 3 goats each group. The goats were kept off feed for 12 h prior to the experiment to avoid anaesthesia-induced regurgitation and other respiratory complications. Baseline cardinal parameters like respiratory rate, pulse rate and body temperature were recorded. The animals were premedicated with atropine (0.03 mg/kg, IM), etamsylate (0.02 g/kg, IM) and xylazole (0.10 mg/kg, IM, North China Pharmaceutical Co., Ltd, Hubei, China). Goats were placed on the left lateral recumbency. After the trachea was intubated to avoid aspiration of ruminal contents, anaesthesia was induced via intravenous administration of ketamine HCl (0.5 mg/kg/min, Yao Pharma Co., Ltd, China). The anaesthetic depth was judged according to eyelid and corneal reflexes and painful response to the prickle of the abdominal skin and coronary hooves. A 6-cm incision was performed on the right flank abdomen following aseptic surgical principle, and the distal part of the ileum was identified and exteriorized. Total 1.2 ml of saline, 40 % ethanol, 30 mg TNBS or TNBS-ethanol solutions (20, 30 and 40 mg in 40 % ethanol) was injected into the ileal wall through five points, approximately 15 cm proximal to the ileocecal junction, with a 30-gauge needle. The intestine was then returned to the abdominal cavity. The abdominal wall and peritoneum were closed using standard procedure. The goats were monitored till recovered from anaesthesia. Tramadol hydrochloride (5 mg/kg, IM) was injected to relieve postoperative pain for 2 days. The wound was treated with 1 % povidone iodine solution daily until completely healed. The animals were resubjected to a similar laparotomy on day 7. The ileal mesentery arteries and veins supplying the injected region were ligated with 3-0 chromic catgut. Four intestinal clamps were applied on both sides of the injected part to prevent content leakage. The 6 cm terminal ileum of each goat was excised 15 cm proximal to the ileocecal junction. The ileum segment was flushed with phosphate buffered saline, cut longitudinally and placed flatly on a clean drape sheet. After detection of the macroscopic changes, a 2 × 2 cm tissue block was taken from the approximate part of the ileum segment opposite to the mesentery, and stored in 10 % formalin for histopathological examination. An expert surgical team performed enteric end-to-end anastomosis immediately after the removal of the partial ileal segment and closed the abdomen using standard methods. The goats received tramadol hydrochloride (5 mg/kg, IM) for 3 days and ampicillin (20 mg/kg, IM) for 5 days. After 2 week recovery, the animals were sent to goat farms. The ileitis severity was determined according to gross and microscopical lesions, and the dose of TNBS inducing moderate ileitis was chosen for the model experiment.

### Experimental setup

The experimental setup is illustrated in Fig. 1. Sixty goats (30 males and 30 females, about 1-year-old) were included. The animals were randomly divided into two equal groups receiving TNBS and isotonic saline, respectively. The goats were anesthetized and laporatomized with the methods described above. The distal part of the ileum was exteriorized. For the TNBS group, 1.2 ml of TNBS-ethanol solution (30 mg TNBS in 40 % ethanol)

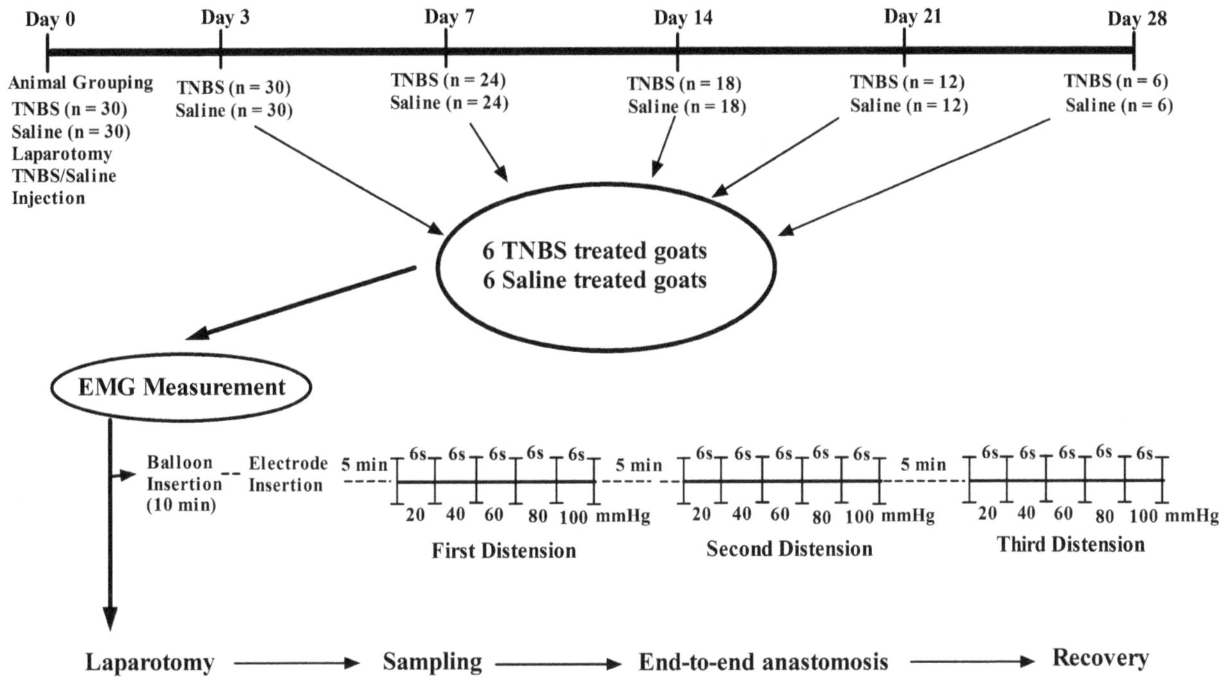


**Fig. 1** Illustration of the experimental design and electromyography protocol

was injected into the ileal wall. In the saline group, the same volume of isotonic saline was injected in the same manner. Animals were weighed at days 0, 3, 7, 14, 21 and 28 following surgery. Six animals were selected from each group at days 3, 7, 14, 21 and 28, respectively, for electromyography (EMG). After EMG, the goats immediately underwent the same laparotomy. The ileum segment was handled as described above. After macroscopic changes were detected, a 2 × 2 cm tissue block was taken from the approximate part of the segment opposite to the mesentery, and preserved in 10 % formalin for histopathological examination. Another 2 × 2 cm tissue block was taken from the distal part opposite to the mesentery, weighed, frozen in liquid nitrogen and finally transferred to store in −80 °C for the measurements of tumor necrosis factor-alpha (TNF-α), interleukin-1 beta (IL-1β), interleukin-6 (IL-6) and MPO. Enteric end-to-end anastomosis and postoperative care were conducted as before.

### Colorectal distension testing

VH was reflected by EMG. EMG was used to record VMR to CRD of goats at days 3, 7, 14, 21 and 28 after surgery as described previously [20]. Briefly, the goats were restrained to keep standing. A manual distension device was made using a T-connector connecting a balloon, a vacuum pump and a sphygmomanometer. The polyethylene balloon (12 cm) was lubricated with paraffin and inserted into the distal colon 10 cm from the anus of goats 10 min before each VMR measurement. Two nickel-steel needles (0.45 mm in diameter and 5 cm in length) were inserted 2 cm apart directly into the external oblique muscle at the center of the left abdomen as electrodes 5 min before each VMR. The electrodes were clamped with adjacent skin, respectively, and connected to an EMG recorder (Nanjing Medease Science and Technology Co., Ltd, China). EMG was amplified and filtered with a processing system MedLab-U/4C501H (Nanjing Medease Science and Technology Co., Ltd, China). The balloon was inflated with the pump. The pressure in the balloon was measured with the sphygmomanometer. In our pretest, goats showed VMR changes when distention pressure increased from 20 to 100 mmHg, and exhibited stronger painful response when pressure reached to 120 mmHg. Therefore, graded pressures (20, 40, 60, 80 and 100 mmHg) were chosen for the model experiment. The balloon was inflated in a continuous ramp distension mode (20, 40, 60, 80 and 100 mmHg). EMG at each stage was recorded for 6 s. The procedure of balloon distension and EMG recordings was repeated every 5 min for 3 times (Fig. 1). Average EMG values for 3 times were analyzed with MedLabV6.3 software (Nanjing Medease Science and Technology Co., Ltd, China) and expressed as millivolt per second (mV/s).

### Macroscopic and microscopic observations

The macroscopic lesions were scored by two independent observers who were unaware of the treatments according to a scale of 0–10 (Table 1). The macroscopic scores were assessed according to adhesion of ileal serosum to the intestinal loops, and mucosal pseudomembrane, hyperemia, ulceration, and wall thickening with a modification of the criteria described by Vadilla et al. [21]. Samples were processed for the histological studies by routine techniques. Six series of 5 μm tissue sections were obtained. Three sections were stained with hematoxylin-eosin (HE). Another 3 were stained with 0.5 % toluidine blue working solution for 3–5 min. Two pathologists were blindly assigned to examine and scored all sections according to crypt depth, inflammatory cells infiltration, submucosal thickness and blood vessel congestion with a modification of the method described previously [21].

### Measurement of cytokines and MPO

The ileal tissue was grinded in liquid nitrogen, and homogenized in 1 ml phosphate buffered solution, pH 7.2 at 4 °C containing PMSF protein inhibitor. Homogenates were shaken at 60 Hz for 90 s, and the solution was centrifuged at 5000×*g* at 4 °C for 15 min. The supernatant was harvested. The protein concentrations were determined using a Nano Drop Spectrophotometer (Thermo Fisher Scientific, Inc., USA). Concentrations of TNF-α, IL-1β, IL-6 and MPO were measured using ELISA kits (Neo Bioscience Inc. Shenzhen, China for cytokines; eBioscience, Inc. USA for MPO) following the manufacturer's instructions. Each sample was analyzed in triplicate and the values are presented as pg/mg.

### Statistical analysis

Experimental data are presented as the mean ± SD. Statistical analyses were performed using SPSS version 18.0 (SPSS Inc., Chicago, IL, USA). The statistical significant difference in macro- and micro-scopic scores between the groups was analyzed with the Mann–Whitney test. The statistical comparisons of other data were performed using independent *t* test. A difference was considered significant if P value was less than 0.05.

## Results

### TNBS dose determination for ileitis

Gross or microscopic lesions were not observed in the ileum of goats of the saline group. The TNBS-alone treated ileums showed minute neutrophil infiltration and increased wall thickness. The severity of ileal inflammation increased with the increase of TNBS dose (0–40 mg) in 40 % ethanol. The gross or microscopic scores in 30 mg TNBS in 40 % ethanol were 5.67 ± 0.57 and 6.33 ± 0.58, respectively and significantly higher ($P < 0.05$) than that in the 20 mg TNBS in 40 % ethanol group (3.33 ± 0.57 and 3.67 ± 0.58, respectively), but lower than that in 40 mg TNBS in 40 % ethanol (8.00 ± 1.00 and 8.67 ± 1.15, respectively). Therefore, 30 mg TNBS in 40 % ethanol induced a moderate ileitis and was chosen for further model experiments.

### Effect of TNBS treatment on body weight

The saline-treated goats showed a decrease in body weight at day 3. The body weight of the TNBS-treated goats decreased at days 3 and 7. But both groups increased body weight at days 14 to 28. Compared with the saline group, body weight in the TNBS group was

**Table 1 Morphological criteria for the assessment of ileal damage**

| Macroscopic changes | | Scores | Microscopic changes | | Scores |
|---|---|---|---|---|---|
| Adhesions | None | 0 | Crypt depth | Normal | 0 |
| | Minimum | 1 | | <50 % reduction | 1 |
| | Involving several bowel loops | 2 | | >50 % reduction | 2 |
| Mucosal hyperemia | Normal | 0 | Inflammatory cells | No infiltration | 0 |
| | Mild | 1 | | Few scattered cells | 1 |
| | Moderate | 2 | | Distributed but not dense | 2 |
| | Severe | 3 | | Dense | 3 |
| Ulcers | None | 0 | Blood vessel congestion | Normal | 0 |
| | Ulceration <2 cm length | 1 | | Mild | 1 |
| | Two ulcers <2 cm | 2 | | Moderate | 2 |
| | More sites of ulceration or one >2 cm | 3 | | Severe | 3 |
| Wall thickness | Normal | 0 | Ulceration | Normal | 0 |
| | 50 % increase | 1 | | Moderate | 1 |
| | 100 % increase | 2 | | Severe | 2 |
| Maximum scores | | 10 | Maximum scores | | 10 |

lower ($P = 0.028$ and 0.021) at days 7 and 14. There was no difference ($P = 0.12$ and 0.622) in body weight between two groups at days 21 and 28 (Fig. 2c).

## Macroscopic and microscopic changes of the TNBS-treated ileum

Gross lesions were not observed at days 3 to 21 after ileal saline injection. In the TNBS group, the ileal mucosa showed apparent congestion, hemorrhage, necrosis and wall thickness with widespread pseudo-membrane adhered to the mucosa at day 3, and light red color, sporadic adhered pseudo-membrane, localized necrosis and apparent wall thickening at day 7, and mild congestion and wall thickening at day 14 (Fig. 2a). No apparent lesions were observed in the adjacent visceral organs and tissues such as large intestines, jejunum and mesentery. Macroscopic lesion scores in the TNBS-treated ileum at days 3, 7 and 14 were 8.43 ± 1.29, 5.54 ± 1.11 and 2.90 ± 1.50, respectively and significantly more severe ($P < 0.05$) than those in the saline group (2.45 ± 0.99, 1.33 ± 0.98 and 0.95 ± 0.79, respectively). However, there was no difference ($P > 0.05$) in macroscopic lesion scores between the saline and TNBS treatments at days 21 and 28 (Fig. 2b).

In the saline-treated goats, there were minute infiltrated inflammatory cells at day 3, but no inflammatory changes at days 7 to 28. In the TNBS group, the ileal wall showed apparent inflammatory cells infiltration and ulceration at day 3, extensive inflammatory cells infiltration, and apparent submucosal and muscular layer ulceration and blood vessel congestion at day 7, extensive inflammatory cells infiltration and granuloma at day 14, and moderate inflammatory cells infiltration and granuloma in the submucosa and muscular layer at day 21. Microscopic lesions were not observed in ileum at day 28 after TNBS treatment. Microscopic lesion scores in the TNBS group at days 3, 7, 14, and 21 were 8.78 ± 0.78, 7.11 ± 0.86, 5.41 ± 1.77 and 3.25 ± 0.52 and therefore significantly more severe ($P < 0.05$) than those of the saline group (2.17 ± 0.75, 1.16 ± 0.75, 0.88 ± 0.61 and 0.5 ± 0.54, respectively). However, there was no difference ($P > 0.05$) in microscopic lesion scores between the two groups at day 28 (Fig. 3). The number of mast cells in the ileum of the TNBS-group at days 3 and 7 were

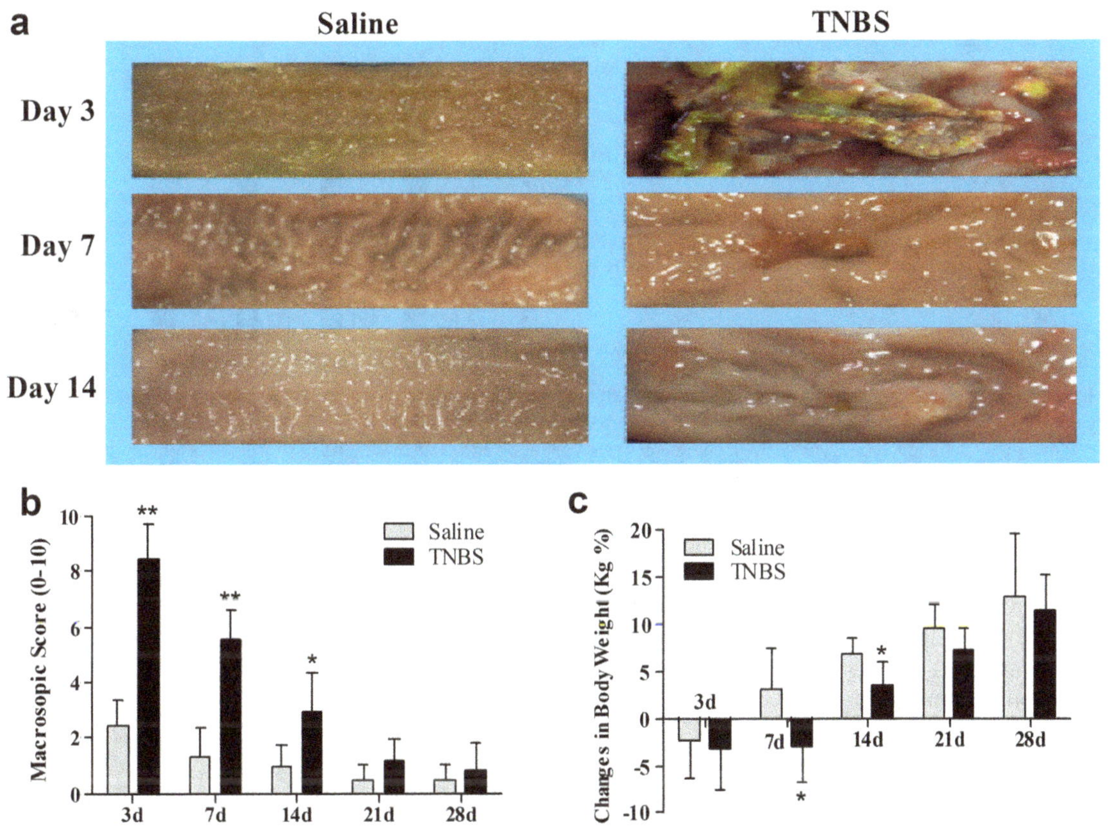


**Fig. 2** Morphologic changes (**a**), macroscopic scores (**b**) and body weight changes (**c**) of the TNBS-treated ileum in goats. TNBS group showed severe inflammation, ulceration and wall thickening at day 3, considerable damage in ileum at day 7, severity of these damages were decreased at day 14. The values are mean ± SD, n = 6. $^*P < 0.05$ and $^{**}P < 0.01$ show significant difference compared with the control

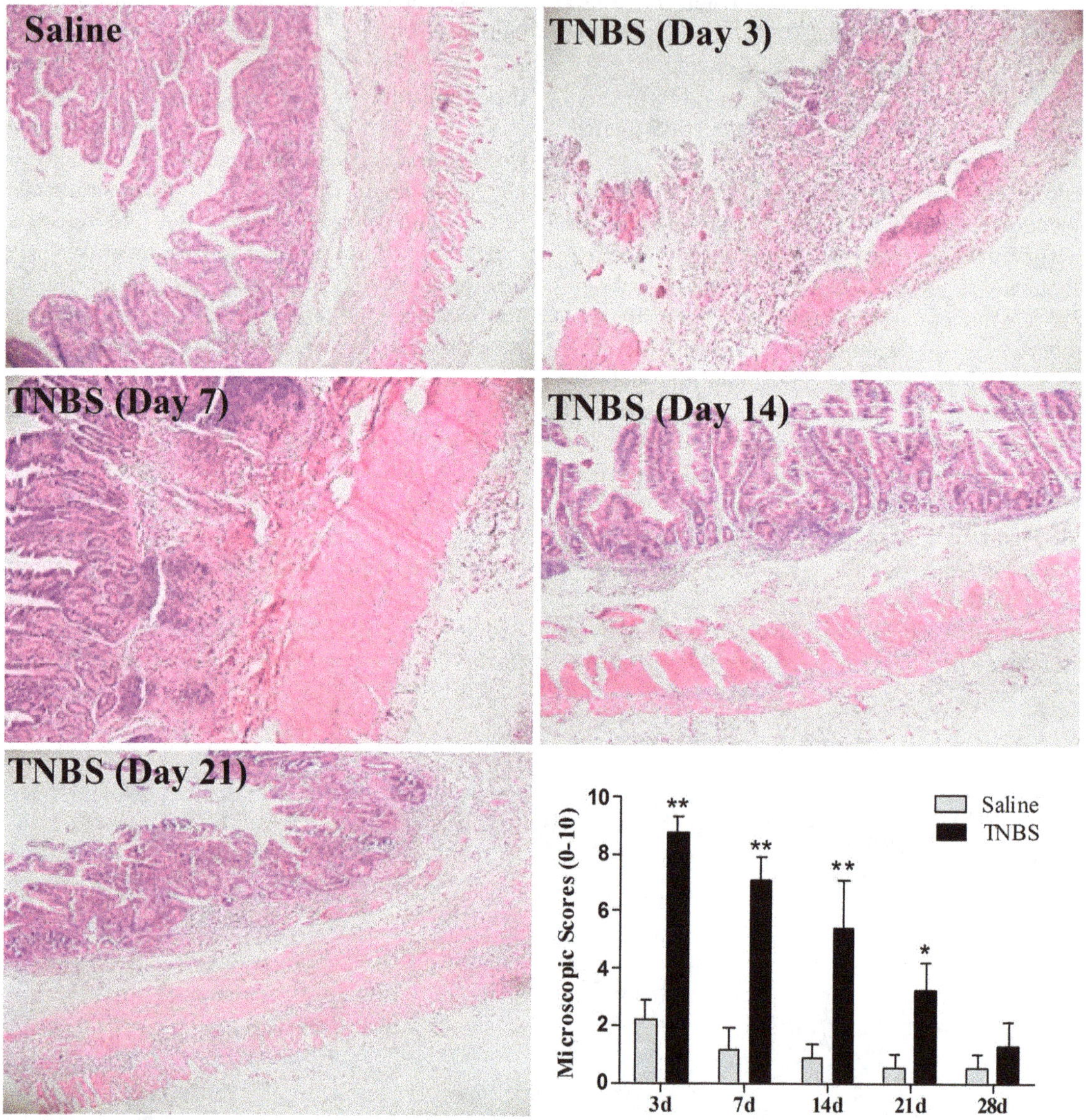


**Fig. 3** Microscopic lesions and microscopic lesion scores of the TNBS-treated ileum in goats. No significant inflammation in saline group, an extensive disruption of mucosal and submucosal layers, and inflammatory cell infiltration at day 3, ulceration of submucosal and muscular layers and inflammatory cell infiltration at day 7, Extensive inflammatory cells infiltration and granulomas at day 14, moderate infiltration of inflammatory cells and granulomas at 21 day after TNBS administration. The values are mean ± SD, n = 6. *$P < 0.05$ and **$P < 0.01$ show significant difference compared with the control

58.63 ± 9.30 and 50.62 ± 11.48 per mm$^2$, compared to 24.33 ± 8.27 and 24.51 ± 5.51 in the saline group ($P < 0.01$). However, there was no difference ($P > 0.05$) in mast cell counts between the saline and TNBS treatments at days 14 to 28 (Fig. 4).

### Concentrations of MPO and cytokines in the ileal tissue

In the saline group, changes were not observed in levels of MPO, TNF-α, IL-1β or IL-6 throughout the experiment. The concentrations of MPO in the TNBS-treated ileum were 2089.03 ± 435.30 pg/mg at day 3 and 1406.27 ± 264.53 pg/mg at day 7, i.e. significantly higher than in the saline group ($P < 0.01$) (977.65 ± 168.47 and 913.47 ± 214.57 pg/mg, respectively). The MPO concentrations between two groups at days 14 to 28 did not differ ($P > 0.05$) (Fig. 5a). Compared with the saline group, concentrations of TNF-α, IL-1β and IL-6 in the TNBS group increased ($P < 0.05$) by 208.67, 364.72 and 330.15 % at day 3, and by 126.69, 168.71 and 209.60 % at day 7. The concentrations of IL-1β and IL-6 in the TNBS

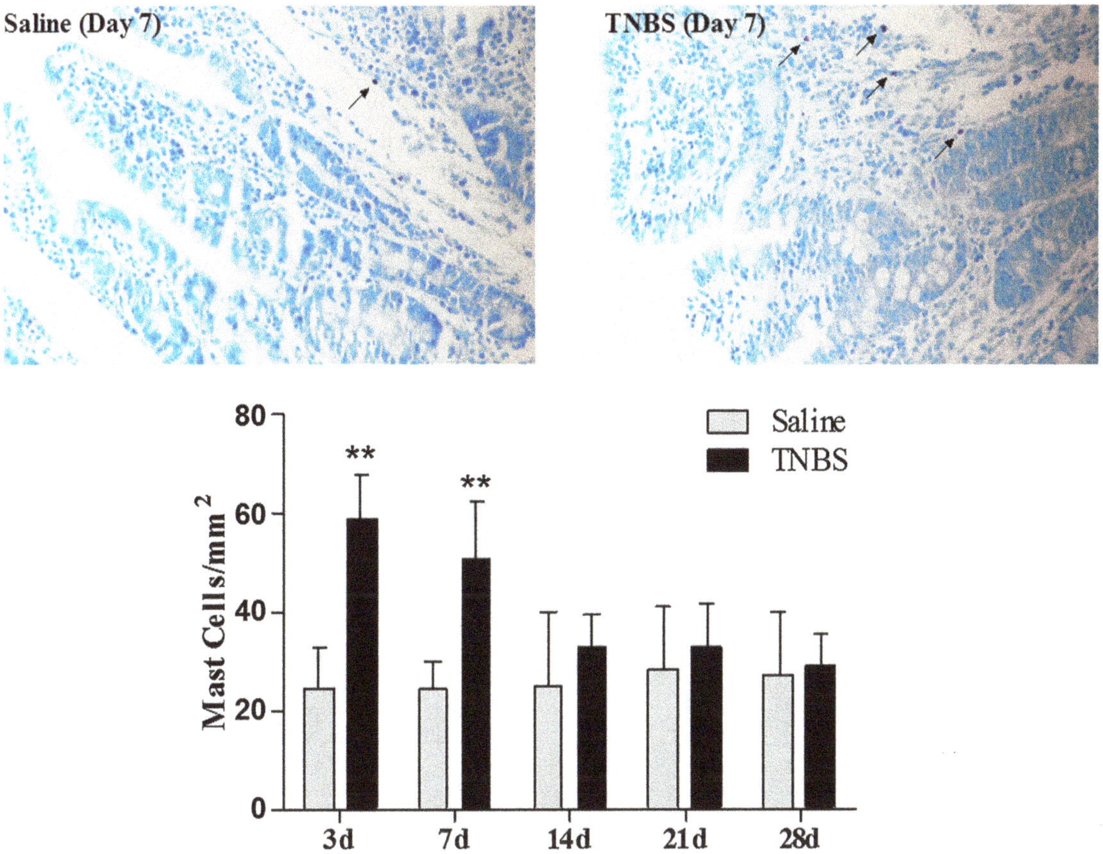


**Fig. 4** Mast cells in the ileal mucosa and mast cells count of the TNBS-treated ileum in goats. Mast cells were stained with 0.5 % toluidine blue (×200). Mast cells in saline group and in TNBS group at day 7 after treatments. The values are mean ± SD, n = 6 **$P < 0.01$ shows significant difference compared with the control

group increased ($P < 0.05$) by 140.22 and 143.93 % at day 14, respectively.

There were no differences ($P > 0.05$) in the concentrations of TNF-α at days 14 to 28 and IL-1β and IL-6 at days 21 to 28 between two groups (Fig. 5b–d).

### Visceromotor response

Graded balloon distension (20, 40, 60, 80 and 100 mmHg) in colorectum resulted in VMR at days 7, 14, 21 and 28. The goats showed signs such as restlessness, rapid breathing, guarding, tail wagging, lips curling, head back to the abdomen and posture change when balloon distension was applied. There was no difference ($P > 0.05$) in VMR between the saline group and TNBS group at day 3. VMRs in the TNBS-treated goats were higher ($P < 0.05$) than those in the saline control in a pressure-dependent manner at days 7 to 28 except for that with 40 mmHg at day 28. Compared with the saline group, VMR in the TNBS group increased ($P < 0.05$) with 40, 60, 80 and 100 mmHg at day 7. VMR in the TNBS-treated goats increased ($P < 0.05$) with 40 mmHg, and reached greatest ($P < 0.01$) with 60, 80 and 100 mmHg at days 14 and 21. At day 28, VMR in the TNBS group increased ($P < 0.05$) with 60 and 80 mmHg, and further increased ($P < 0.01$) with 100 mmHg (Fig. 6).

## Discussion

Rectal instillation of TNBS-ethanol solution is an established model that is used to examine the pathogenesis of acute and chronic colitis, and to determine the mechanisms and efficacy of therapies. Some researchers have administered TNBS to induce ileitis. It seems that the inflammatory response of small intestine to TNBS is different from the well-characterized response of the colon. Most studies have shown that TNBS-induced ileitis lasts several days whereas the colitis persists for several weeks after TNBS administration. The administration and doses of TNBS differ between studies; the methodology is inconsistent, and no standardized protocol exists. Moreels et al. [22] injected 85 mg/kg body weight of TNBS in 40 % ethanol into rat's ileum and found a marked inflammatory reaction occurred at 36 h and lasted up to

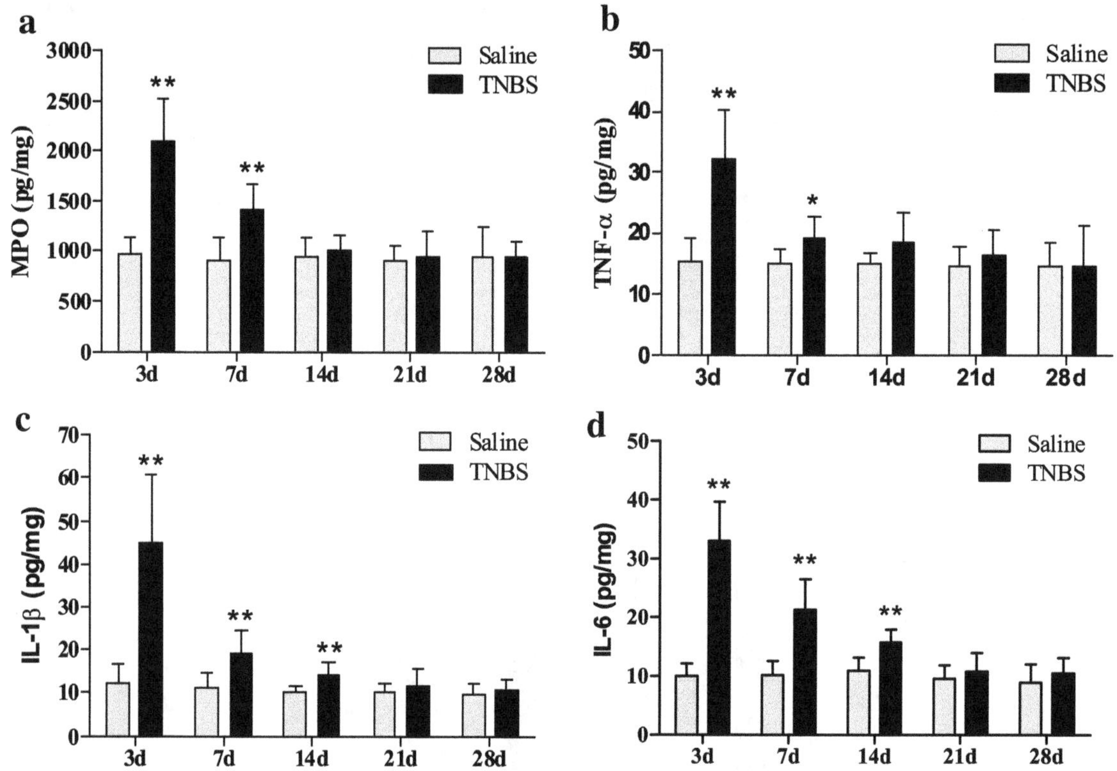


**Fig. 5** Measurement of MPO (**a**) and cytokines level like TNF-α (**b**), IL-1β (**c**) and IL-6 (**d**), and in ileum after TNBS administration (mean ± SD, n = 6). *$P < 0.05$ and **$P < 0.01$ show significant difference compared with the control

7 days according to MPO concentration and macroscopic and microscopic pathologic changes. O'Hara et al. [23] injected 60 mg/kg body weight of TNBS in 30 % ethanol into the ileum of guinea pigs and observed a severe inflammation at day 3. Nurgali et al. [24] translumenally administered 30 mg/kg body weight TNBS in 30 % ethanol in guinea pigs and observed the clinically as well as histologically inflammatory evidences up to 7 days. Merritt et al. [16] injected TNBS-ethanol solutions (0.5–1 g TNBS in 33–75 % ethanol) into the ileal lumen of pigs, and induced ileitis up to 7 days. These studies showed a transient ileitis induced by TNBS in these animals.

Most researchers have administered TNBS-ethanol solution (30 to 150 mg/kg body weight or 10 to 40 mg/rat of TNBS in 30 to 50 % ethanol) into the intestinal lumen to induce colitis or ileitis in rats. Studied showed that 50 % ethanol or 30 mg TNBS alone induced mild colitis for <7 days while 10 to 30 mg TNBS in combination with ethanol (30 or 50 %) caused mild to severe colitis for over 21 days in rats [25, 26]. We injected different TNBS-ethanol solutions (20, 30 and 40 mg TNBS in 40 % ethanol) into the ileal wall of goats, provoked mild to severe ileitis. It is believed that TNBS and ethanol act in concert on the intestinal tissue. TNBS as a hapten can bind intestinal tissue proteins, induce inflammatory and immune responses, and result in VH [17, 27]. Ethanol induces acute inflammation and may contribute to TNBS diffusion. The action of TNBS-ethanol solution in the lumen of the intestines was influenced by many factors. Intestine emptying, mucus secretion and peristalsis may reduce the contact time of TNBS with the ileal mucosa, influence severity and duration of inflammation [16]. To avoid these influences, Czaja et al. [28] injected 4 % paraformaldehyde into the multiple sites of the ileal wall of pigs and found that apparent transient ileitis occurred at day 3. So far ileitis induced by TNBS injection into the ileal wall has not been reported. Our study showed that administration of TNBS-ethanol solution (30 mg TNBS in 40 % ethanol) in the ileal wall caused moderate ileitis of each goat, characterized by weight loss, diarrhea, and histopathologically apparent changes including extensive congestion, hemorrhage, mucosal necrosis, granulomas, diffuse infiltrated neutrophils and lymphocytes in lamina propia, and thickened wall. These symptoms and pathological changes are similar to JD. According to macroscopic and microscopic changes, the TNBS-induced ileitis in our experiment occurred at day 3, persisted till day 21 and disappeared at day 28.

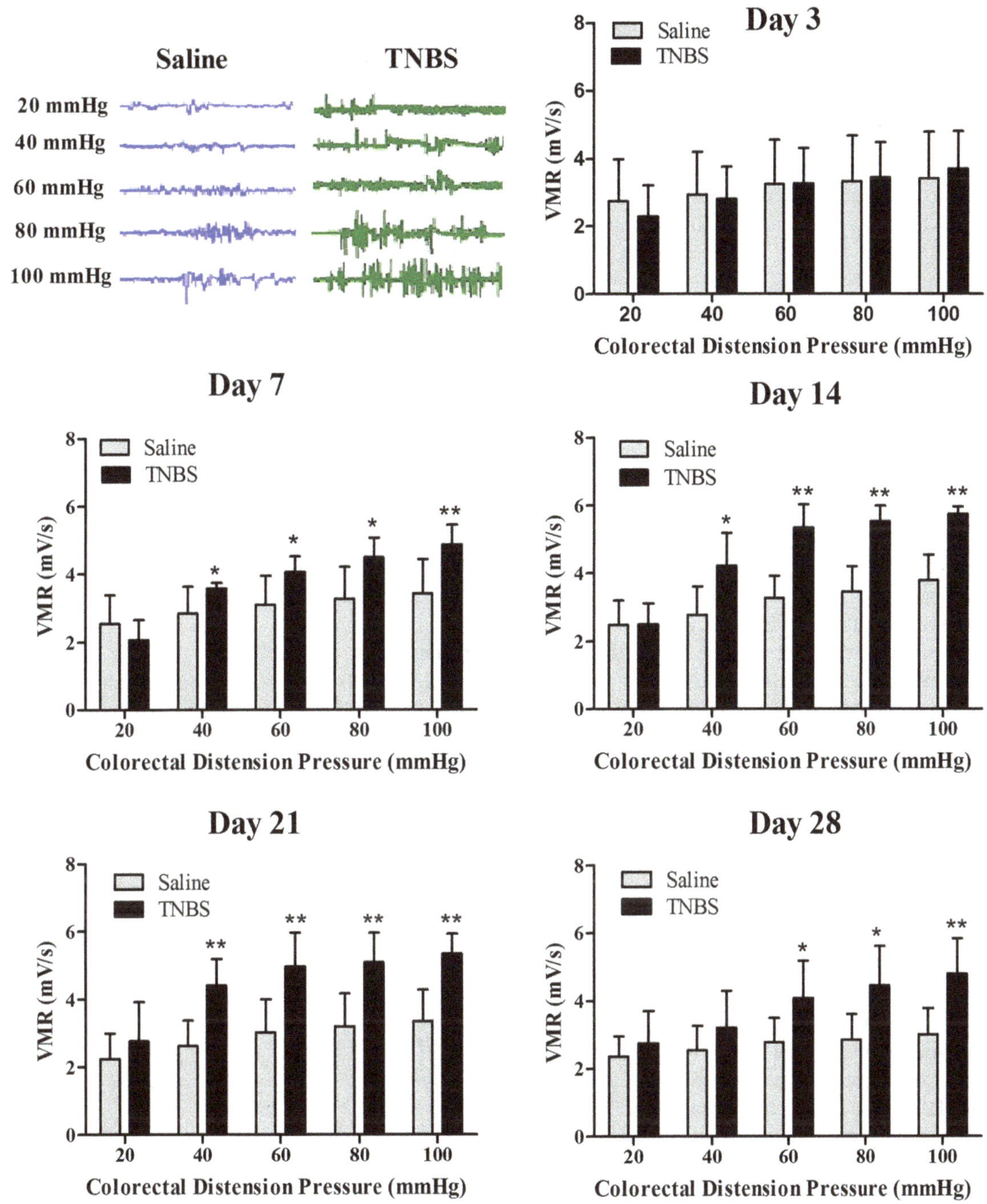


**Fig. 6** Representative electromyography (EMG) traces at day 14 and visceromotor responses (VMR) to colorectal distension (mean ± SD, n = 6) at days 3, 7, 14, 21 and 28 after treatments. $^{*}P < 0.05$ and $^{**}P < 0.01$ show significant difference compared with the control

JD usually occurs in ruminants, and its transmural lesions include thickened wall and granulomas in the small intestine, which is similar to human CD [3]. According to the CD study, microbial invasion and activation of immune response may have an important role in the development of these lesions [29]. Epidemiology suggests some relationship between gut flora and inflammatory granulomas. Ruminants have more bacteria in the cecum than other omnivorous and carnivorous animals. The granuloma development in the present study showed that enteric immune system was activated by a number of microorganisms existing in the ileum and proliferating under the pathological condition or their retrograding from the cecum.

Abdominal pain and discomfort are amongst the most frustrating symptoms for patients suffering from IBD. They not only occur during acute flares of inflammation but also do during remission [30, 31]. Adam et al. [17] intracolonally administered TNBS in Lewis rats, and found VH occurred at day 3, disappeared at day 14, and reappeared at day 28 to 42 after TNBS administration. Zhou et al. [18] used 20 mg TNBS in 50 % ethanol in the colon of Sprague-Dawley rats, observed VH at days 2 to 28. Feng et al. [32] injected TNBS into the colon lumen of mice, and observed VH at days 7 to 14. Shah et al. [20] injected TNBS into the ileal lumen of Sprague-Dawley rats, observed ileitis at day 3, followed by VH at days 7 to 21. The discrepancies in onset time and duration of VH above may be due to different inflammation locations and species. We injected TNBS into the ileal wall of goats, observed a significant VH at days 7 to 28, which is similar to the results of Shah et al. [20]. Because our experiment stopped at day 28, how long the VH lasted needs to be further confirmed.

A single visceral afferent fiber can span over ten spinal cord segments, send terminal branches throughout the superficial and deep dorsal horn, as well as project to the contralateral dorsal horn [33, 34]. Studies showed that VH from the colorectum is mediated via both thoracolumbar and lumbosacral spinal afferent pathways whereas VH from terminal ileum is mainly mediated via thoracolumbar spinal afferent pathways [35–37]. Because there is a viscero-visceral convergence of nociceptive impulses from small and large intestines on the spinal neurons, CRD can be used as a nociceptive stimulator for ileum hypersensitivity. EMG is the most commonly used technique to quantify the abdominal muscle contractions in response to graded CRD.

Studies showed that in biopsies obtained from patients with IBDs, the number of mast cells was increased [38]. Shah et al. [20] found increased mast cells at day 3, followed by VH at day 7 after administration of TNBS into the ileal lumen of rats. Our study showed that administration of TNBS in the ileal wall induced increased mast cells at days 3 to 7, and VH at days 7 to 28 in goats, which is in consistency with the results of Shah et al. [20]. Ohashi et al. [39] injected TNBS into the proximal colon of wild rats and mast cell knockout rats, and found that TNBS induced VH in the wild rats, but not in the mast cell deficient rats. Studies have showed that TNBS-induced VH can be suppressed by an oral treatment with a mast cell stabilizer, doxantrazole, in a dose-dependent manner [40]. The activated mast cells are demonstrated to release inflammatory mediators (cytokines, protease etc.), thereby activate protease-activated receptor-2 (PAR-2). The activation of PAR-2 leads to sensitizing transient receptor potential vanilloid subtype-1 receptors and to trigger the release of substance-P (SP) and calcitonin gene-related peptide (CGRP), which ultimately elicits neurogenic inflammation and hypersensitivity [17, 41, 42]. These studies suggest an important role of mast cells in the initiation and development of VH.

Although the causes of VH is unknown, microbial activation of immune system and induction of pro-inflammatory cytokines such as IL-6, TNF-α and IL-1β seem to be critical in genetically predisposed individuals. Adam et al. [11] reported that VH occurred in Lewis rats with increased IL-6 level, but not in Fisher rats without increased IL-6 level. Deletion of the regulatory sequence consisting of adenosine-uracil multimers in the 3'untranslated region of cytokine-encoding transcripts in mice results in increased transcription and expression of TNF-α upon cell activation. These mice spontaneously develop a granulomatous CD-like disorder and an arthritis-like inflammation [43]. It is demonstrated that TNF-α triggers the subsequent release of IL-1β, which can produce hypersensitivity.

## Conclusions

Injection of 30 mg TNBS in 40 % ethanol into the terminal ileal wall of goats induced apparent inflammation and transmural lesions, which are morphologically very similar to JD and human CD. VMR results showed that VH occurred at day 7 after TNBS injection and lasted up to day 28. This experiment successfully constructed a more economic (compared with TNBS injection into the intestinal lumen) and reproducible ileitis and VH, which is useful for studying the pathogenesis of ruminant's and human IBDs, and the mechanism underlying VH, and for evaluating the efficacy of new therapeutic regimens.

#### Abbreviations

CD: Crohn's disease; CRD: colorectal distension; ELISA: enzyme-linked immunosorbent assay; EMG: electromyography; IBDs: inflammatory bowel diseases; IL-1β: interleukin-1 beta; IL-6: interleukin-6; JD: Johne's disease; MPO: myeloperoxidase; TNBS: 2,4,6-trinitrobenzenesulfonic acid; TNF-α: tumor necrosis factor-alpha; VH: visceral hypersensitivity; VMR: visceromotor response.

#### Authors' contributions

AHT performed the experiments, analyzed the data (including statistical analysis) and drafted the manuscript. JW, MKS, HJ and XL performed the experiments and analysis of data. MXD participated in study design and coordination, and helped to draft the manuscript. All authors read and approved the final manuscript.

#### Acknowledgements

This work supported by the fund from the National Natural Science Foundation of China (Grant No. 31472246).

#### Competing interests

The authors declare that they have no competing interests.

## References


1. Brandhorst G, Weigand S, Eberle C, Raddatz D, Karaus M, Oellerich M, et al. CD4(+) immune response as a potential biomarker of patient reported inflammatory bowel disease (IBD) activity. Clin Chim Acta. 2013;421:31–3.
2. Castaneda AE, Tuulio-Henriksson A, Aronen ET, Marttunen M, Kolho KL. Cognitive functioning and depressive symptoms in adolescents with inflammatory bowel disease. World J Gastroenterol. 2013;19:1611–7.
3. Clarke CJ, Little D. The pathology of ovine paratuberculosis: gross and histological changes in the intestine and other tissues. J Comp Pathol. 1996;114:419–37.
4. Gonda MG, Chang YM, Shook GE, Collins MT, Kirkpatrick BW. Effect of *Mycobacterium paratuberculosis* infection on production, reproduction, and health traits in US Holsteins. Prev Vet Med. 2007;80:103–19.
5. Wadhwa A, Kumar N, Velasco-Villa A, Eda S. Overview of Johne's disease immunology. Vet World. 2013;6:901–4.
6. Crohn BB, Ginzburg L, Oppenheimer GD. Landmark article Oct 15, 1932. Regional ileitis: a pathological and clinical entity. JAMA. 1984;251:73–9.
7. Momotani E, Whipple DL, Thiermann AB, Cheville NF. Role of M cells and macrophages in the entrance of *Mycobacterium paratuberculosis* into domes of ileal Peyer's patches in calves. Vet Pathol. 1988;25:131–7.
8. Garcia-Lafuente A, Antolin M, Guarner F, Crespo E, Salas A, Forcada P, et al. Incrimination of anaerobic bacteria in the induction of experimental colitis. Am J Physiol. 1997;272:G10–5.
9. Blumberg RS, Saubermann LJ, Strober W. Animal models of mucosal inflammation and their relation to human inflammatory bowel disease. Curr Opin Immunol. 1999;11:648–56.
10. Matricon J, Barnich N, Ardid D. Immunopathogenesis of inflammatory bowel disease. Self Nonself. 2010;1:299–309.
11. Adam B, Tsopelas C, Liebregts T, Bartholomeusz FD, Holtmann G. Host immune response determines visceral hyperalgesia in a rat model of post-inflammatory irritable bowel syndrome. J Gastroenterol. 2013;48:1119–27.
12. Cheon GJ, Cui Y, Yeon D-S, Kwon S-C, Park B-G. Mechanisms of motility change on trinitrobenzenesulfonic acid-induced colonic inflammation in mice. Korean J Physiol Pharmacol. 2012;16:437–46.
13. Qin H-Y, Xiao H-T, Wu JCY, Berman BM, Sung JJY, Bian Z-X. Key factors in developing the trinitrobenzene sulfonic acid-induced post-inflammatory irritable bowel syndrome model in rats. World J Gastroenterol. 2012;18:2481–92.
14. Pontell L, Castelucci P. Structural changes in the epithelium of the small intestine and immune cell infiltration of enteric ganglia following acute mucosal damage and local inflammation. Virchows Arch. 2009;455:55–65.
15. Nurgali K, Qu Z, Hunne B, Thacker M, Pontell L, Furness JB. Morphological and functional changes in guinea-pig neurons projecting to the ileal mucosa at early stages after inflammatory damage. J Physiol. 2011;589:325–39.
16. Merritt AM, Buergelt CD, Sanchez LC. Porcine ileitis model induced by TNBS-ethanol instillation. Dig Dis Sci [Internet]. 2002;47:879–85.
17. Adam B, Liebregts T, Gschossmann JM, Krippner C, Scholl F, Ruwe M, et al. Severity of mucosal inflammation as a predictor for alterations of visceral sensory function in a rat model. Pain. 2006;123:179–86.
18. Zhou Q, Price DD, Caudle RM, Verne GN. Visceral and somatic hypersensitivity in TNBS-induced colitis in rats. Dig Dis Sci. 2008;53:429–35.
19. Qian A, Song D, Li Y, Liu X, Tang D, Yao W, et al. Role of voltage gated $Ca^{2+}$ channels in rat visceral hypersensitivity change induced by 2, 4, 6-trinitrobenzene sulfonic acid. Mol Pain. 2013;9:15.
20. Shah MK, Wan J, Janyaro H, Tahir AH, Cui L, Ding M-X. Visceral hypersensitivity is provoked by 2,4,6 trinitrobenzene sulfonic acid-induced ileitis in rats. Front Pharmacol. 2016;7:214. doi:10.3389/fphar.2016.00214.
21. Videla S, Vilaseca J, Medina C, Mourelle M, Guarner F, Salas A, et al. Selective inhibition of phosphodiesterase-4 ameliorates chronic colitis and prevents intestinal fibrosis. J Pharmacol Exp Ther. 2006;316:940–5.
22. Moreels TG, De Man JG, De Winter BY, Lefebvre RA, Herman AG, Pelckmans PA. Effect of TNBS-induced morphological changes on pharmacological contractility of the rat ileum. Eur J Pharma. 2001;423:211–22.
23. O'Hara JR, Lomax AE, Mawe GM, Sharkey KA. Ileitis alters neuronal and enteroendocrine signalling in guinea pig distal colon. Gut. 2007;56:186–94.
24. Nurgali K, Nguyen TV, Matsuyama H, Thacker M, Robbins HL, Furness JB. Phenotypic changes of morphologically identified guinea-pig myenteric neurons following intestinal inflammation. J Physiol. 2007;583:593–609.
25. Morris GP, Beck PL, Herridge MS, Depew WT, Szewczuk MR, Wallace JL. Hapten-induced model of chronic inflammation and ulceration in the rat colon. Gastroenterology. 1989;96:795–803.
26. Boughton-Smith NK, Wallace JL, Morris GP, Whittle BJ. The effect of anti-inflammatory drugs on eicosanoid formation in a chronic model of inflammatory bowel disease in the rat. Br J Pharmacol. 1988;94:65–72.
27. Kim HS, Berstad A. Experimental colitis in animal models. Scand J Gastroenterol. 1992;27:529–37.
28. Czaja K, Kaleczyc J, Sienkiewicz W, Lakomy M. The influence of experimental ileitis on the neuropeptide coding of enteric neurons in the pig. Pol J Vet Sci. 2005;8:155–63.
29. Kamada N, Seo S-U, Chen GY, Núñez G. Role of the gut microbiota in immunity and inflammatory disease. Nat Rev Immunol. 2013;13:321–35.
30. Vermeulen W, De Man JG, Pelckmans PA, De Winter BY. Neuroanatomy of lower gastrointestinal pain disorders. World J Gastroenterol. 2014;20:1005–20.
31. De Schepper HU, De Man JG, Moreels TG, Pelckmans PA, De Winter BY. Review article: gastrointestinal sensory and motor disturbances in inflammatory bowel disease—clinical relevance and pathophysiological mechanisms. Aliment Pharmacol Ther. 2008;27:621–37.
32. Feng B, La J, Tanaka T, Schwartz ES, Mcmurray TP, Gebhart GF, et al. Altered colorectal afferent function associated with TNBS-induced visceral hypersensitivity in mice altered colorectal afferent function associated with TNBS-induced visceral hypersensitivity in mice. Am J Physiol Gastrointest Liver Physiol. 2012;303:G817–24.
33. Foreman RD. Mechanisms of visceral pain: from nociception to targets. Drug Discov Today Dis Mech. 2004;1:457–63.
34. Traub RJ. Sensitization in visceral pain and hyperalgesia. Semin Pain Med. 2003;1:150–8. doi:10.1016/S1537-5897(03)00040-5.
35. Tan LL, Bornstein JC, Anderson CR. Distinct chemical classes of medium-sized transient receptor potential channel vanilloid 1-immunoreactive dorsal root ganglion neurons innervate the adult mouse jejunum and colon. Neuroscience. 2008;156:334–43.
36. Traub RJ. Evidence for thoracolumbar spinal cord processing of inflammatory, but not acute colonic pain. Neuroreport. 2000;11:2113–6.
37. Moore BA, Stewart TMR, Hill C, Vanner SJ. TNBS ileitis evokes hyperexcitability and changes in ionic membrane properties of nociceptive DRG neurons. Am J Physiol Gastrointest Liver Physiol. 2002;282:G1045–51.
38. Gelbmann CM, Mestermann S, Gross V, Köllinger M, Schölmerich J, Falk W. Strictures in Crohn's disease are characterised by an accumulation of mast cells colocalised with laminin but not with fibronectin or vitronectin. Gut. 1999;45:210–7.
39. Ohashi K, Sato Y, Kawai M, Kurebayashi Y. Abolishment of TNBS-induced visceral hypersensitivity in mast cell deficient rats. Life Sci. 2008;82:419–23.
40. Ohashi K, Sato Y, Iwata H, Kawai M, Kurebayashi Y. Colonic mast cell infiltration in rats with TNBS-induced visceral hypersensitivity. J Vet Med Sci. 2007;69:1223–8.
41. Gschossmann JM, Coutinho SV, Miller JC, Huebel K, Naliboff B, Wong HC, et al. Involvement of spinal calcitonin gene-related peptide in the development of acute visceral hyperalgesia in the rat. Neurogastroenterol Motil. 2001;13:229–36.
42. Sun RQ, Tu YJ, Lawand NB, Yan JY, Lin Q, Willis WD. Calcitonin gene-related peptide receptor activation produces PKA- and PKC-dependent mechanical hyperalgesia and central sensitization. J Neurophysiol. 2004;92:2859–66.
43. Kontoyiannis D, Pasparakis M, Pizarro TT, Cominelli F, Kollias G. Impaired on/off regulation of TNF biosynthesis in mice lacking TNF AU-rich elements: implications for joint and gut-associated immunopathologies. Immunity. 1999;10:387–98.

# 4

# Effect of concrete slats, three mat types and out-wintering pads on performance and welfare of finishing beef steers

Bernadette Earley[1*], John D. McNamara[2], Stephen J. Jerrams[2] and Edward G. O'Riordan[3]

**Abstract**

**Background:** The objective was to investigate the effect of placing mats on concrete slatted floors on performance, behaviour, hoof condition, dirt scores, physiological and immunological variables of beef steers, and to compare responses with animals on out-wintering pads. Continental crossbred beef steers [n = 360; mean (±SD) initial live weight 539 kg (42.2)] were blocked by breed and live weight and randomly assigned to one of five treatments; (1) Concrete slats alone, (2) Mat 1 (Natural Rubber structure) (Durapak Rubber Products), (3) Mat 2 (Natural rubber structure) (EasyFix), (4) Mat 3 (modified ethylene vinyl acetate (EVA) foam structure) and (5) Out-wintering pads (OWP's).

**Results:** Animals on the OWPs had a greater ($P < 0.05$) live weight gain ($P < 0.05$) compared with the slat and Mat 2 treatments: results for Mat 1 and Mat 3 were the same ($P > 0.05$) as the other treatments. Animals on the OWPs had reduced lying percentage time compared with all the other treatments. Dry matter (DM) intake was greater for animals on the OWPs compared with all the other treatments. Carcass weight, kill out proportion, carcass fat score, carcass composition score, FCR and physiological responses were similar ($P > 0.05$) among treatments. No incidence of laminitis was observed among treatments. The number of hoof lesions was greater on all mat types ($P < 0.05$) compared with concrete slats and OWP treatments. Dirt scores were greater ($P < 0.05$) for animals on OWPs when measured on days 42, 84, 105, 126 and 150 compared with animals on slats.

**Conclusions:** Under the conditions adopted for the present study, there was no evidence to suggest that animals housed on bare concrete slats were disadvantaged in respect of animal welfare compared with animals housed on other floor types. It is concluded that the welfare of steers was not adversely affected by slats compared with different mat types or OWPs.

**Keywords:** Housing, Animal welfare, Concrete slat, Rubber mat

## Background

There is a shortage of published research on the effect of placing mats on concrete slats in facilities for winter finishing beef cattle. Most previous housing studies reported significant behavioural alterations concerning the welfare of cattle accommodated on fully slatted concrete floors [1–9]. Elmore et al. [1] reported that the addition of slatted rubber mats to concrete pens improved locomotion, leg and joint health, and alterations in behaviour that are indicative of increased traction and reduced discomfort in finishing beef steers. Other studies have measured the growth of finishing cattle in response to a range of space allowances [10–13]. Biological performance is an indicator of animal well-being and previous studies have demonstrated that stress due to reduced space allowance can negatively affect animal performance [13–16]. Schlichting et al. and Schlichting and Smidt [15, 16] reported that the abrasive effect of the concrete slatted floor led to reduced slipping of hooves on contact. A study by Murphy et al. [17] measured the in vitro abrasion on a wear-testing instrument of hoof horn samples of cattle

*Correspondence: bernadette.earley@teagasc.ie
[1] Animal and Bioscience Research Department, Animal & Grassland Research and Innovation Centre, Teagasc, Grange, Dunsany, Co. Meath C15 PW93, Ireland

in relation to breed and housing. The hoof horn of Friesian cattle was softer if they had been housed on concrete slats rather than on straw, but there was no such effect in Hereford cattle. Interest in out-wintering pads (OWPs) as a low cost alternative to indoor housing is another system that has been studied [18]. The OWP's consist of a woodchip lying area constructed over a drainage system, which may or may not be sheltered. Animals have access to feed from a self-feeder at the feed-face of the OWP. The OWP system has been shown, under experimental conditions, to meet environmental guidelines as well as being capable of supporting satisfactory animal performance, health and welfare [18].

The hypothesis of the study was that the provision of a Mat flooring or an out-wintering pad (OWP) would offer protection to the animals' feet, particularly over a 150-day winter period, which would in turn improve hoof health. Furthermore, it was hypothesised that finishing cattle on the mats or OWPs would have enhanced performance compared with concrete slats owing to more comfortable underfoot conditions that would in turn lead to improvements in animal welfare. The objective was to investigate the effect of placing mats on concrete slatted floors on performance, hoof condition and body cleanliness of finishing beef steers, and to compare responses with animals on out-wintering pads. Accordingly, this study examined the behavioural, physiological and immunological responses of the steers by assessing the consequences of the floor type on the welfare of finishing beef cattle that were offered a total mixed ration (TMR) diet.

## Methods

### Environmental conditions

This study was conducted at Teagasc Grange, located in Co. Meath, Ireland (latitude 53.52187, longitude-6.65247). The mean daily air temperature in the housing facility (from November to May) and the ambient environment was continuously recorded using Testo 175 data loggers (Radionics, Dublin, Ireland).

### Animals, experimental design and diet

Continental crossbred beef steers [n = 360; mean (±SD) initial live-weight 539 kg (42.2)] were blocked by breed and live-weight and randomly assigned to one of five treatments; (1) Concrete slats alone, (2) Mat 1 (Natural Rubber structure) (Durapak Rubber Products, Cork, Ireland), (3) Mat 2 (Natural rubber structure) (EasyFix, Galway, Ireland), (4) Mat 3 [modified ethylene vinyl acetate (EVA) foam structure (Mayo, Ireland)] and (5) Out-wintering pads (OWPs) (constructed in 2006). Animals assigned to treatments 1–4 were accommodated in a roofed building with concrete slatted floors. The concrete slats (5 gang/pen) in the pens were supplied by Banagher Concrete Ltd., Offaly, Ireland. Each gang slat had the following dimensions; void length 945 mm × 3 mm; void space 35 mm; slat length 3.5 m; slat rib width 170 mm; slat width 1.18 m. The mats were supplied and fitted to the concrete slats in the cattle pens by the respective suppliers. There were eight pens per treatment, with nine steers per pen at a mean space allowance of 2.73 $m^2$/head, whereas animals accommodated outdoors on the OWPs had a space allowance of 12 $m^2$/head. The shed was dimly lit using infra-red lighting to allow visualisation during the behavioural studies.

### Animal diet

All animals were fed a total mixed ration (TMR) of silage and rolled barley on a 50:50 dry matter (DM) basis. Typically 2000 kg of silage and 500 kg rolled barley was mixed in a 12 cubic meter Abbey Vertical Mixer (VF 12) fitted with a Digistar weighing system. Feed was weighed into each group every day at 9:00 throughout the study and refusals were measured twice weekly. The steers had free access to water drinkers in their pens. Each pen was fitted with a single 2 l nose fill water bowl which was positioned 55 cm above the floor of the pen. The TMR samples offered were submitted to Grange Labs at Teagasc for chemical analysis [dry matter digestibility (DMD), crude protein (CP), ash, neutral detergent fibre (NDF)] and pH analyses [19]. Animals were vaccinated with a Covexin 8 (Merck, Animal Health, MSD Animal Health, Dublin, Ireland) and a Bovilis-Bovipast RSP (Merck, Animal Health, MSD Animal Health, Dublin, Ireland) injections 3 weeks prior to commencement of the study.

### Health

The general health status of the steers was recorded by a trained staff member. A complete record of any clinical symptoms by infection or injury and their veterinary treatment was maintained.

### Hoof condition

The general condition of the four hooves of each animal was recorded prior to (day 0) and at the end of the study (i.e., on retrieval of the hooves post-slaughter of the animals). A single observer, who was experienced in hoof examination assessed the four hooves of each animal on both occasions and preliminary scoring was carried out to verify repeatability of results. The hooves were trimmed on day 0 and again on the retrieval of the hooves post-slaughter, to allow visualization. Both claws per each of the four hooves were examined by the same trained observer for the presence of lesions using the method of Greenough and Vermunt [20]. The dorsal area was examined for equal and unequal size and the plantar area for heel erosion, under run sole, digital dermatitis, inter-digital dermatitis and white line damage. The total number of lesions was averaged over all four hooves and the number each animal had obtained during the study was determined. Animals were observed for any signs of lameness every 3 weeks to coincide with animal live weight recordings. All animals were assessed by the same trained person for abnormal gait and back posture while walking and standing using the method of Sprecher et al. [21] on a scale of 1 (normal) to 5 (abnormally lame).

#### *Animal cleanliness scoring*

All animals were dirt scored on day 0 before assignment to treatment and at 21 day intervals (day 0, 21, 42, 63, 84, 105, 126 and 150) throughout the study. Dirt scoring was carried out by the same person on each occasion and was carried out blind to treatment. The body dirt scoring system used by Earley et al. [22], which was adapted from Scott and Kelly [23] was applied. Using this system, the entire left side of each animal was diagrammatically divided into 16 body segments and each segment was assigned a score between 1 (very clean) and 5 (very dirty) levels of intensity. Each animal was then given an overall dirt score between 16 and 80, which was equal to the sum of the scores for each of the 16 body segments [22].

### Behaviour

An individual Eneo CCTV camera was placed over each pen and the behavioural data were recorded. Behavioural observations were conducted over six 3-week intervals, continuously for 72 h duration. Animals were identified by their natural body markings. During the period of darkness, the shed housing the animals was dimly lit using infra-red lights to allow observation of the animals on the CCTV cameras. The cameras were connected to a video tape recorder (Panasonic AG6040) via a multivision system (Panasonic WJ-FS109, monochrome duplex multiplexer, Lynx, Dunsany, Co. Meath, Ireland) which allowed pictures from all cameras to be viewed on one screen at a time. The pictures from all the cameras were marked with individual pen number, time and date settings. The behavioural analysis was performed by a trained staff member. Steers were observed by instantaneous scan sampling of the CCTV recordings. The interval between scans was 10 min. This interval was chosen based on previous recording of animal behaviours [22, 24]. Each steer was observed for behavioural activity and body contact. Counts of lying, standing, eating and drinking, mounting, head-butting, licking and grooming were recorded. In the behavioural activity category, steers were observed for the following: lying down: head supported by the neck, head not supported by the neck (chin on the floor, on the body or on another steer); standing: with or without moving; eating (head in the trough); drinking; head to head contact except while eating; head contact with the body of another steer; and mounting. In the contact category the criteria were: no body contact with other steers and contact with one, two or three steers; grooming refers to self-grooming and allogrooming constitutes licking another animal.

### Average daily live weight and carcass characteristics

Live weights were measured on day-1 and again on day 0 before assignment to treatment, at 21-day intervals (day 0, 21, 42, 63, 84, 105, 126 and 150) throughout the study and average daily gain (ADG) determined. Animals were slaughtered from day 150 of the experiment onwards. Cold carcass weights were recorded, with carcass conformation and fat scores graded using a video imaging analysis carcass classification system (VBS 2000, E + P, Oranienberg, Germany) based on the EU Beef Carcass Classification Scheme according to the EU beef carcass classification scheme (EC, 2006) [25]. Feed conversion ratio (FCR) was expressed as kilograms of DMI/pen/day divided by kilograms of live weight gain/pen/day.

### Physiological, haematological and immunological variables

Animals were blood sampled via jugular venipuncture on days 0 and 150. For the blood sampling procedure, the animals were moved to a holding pen with a squeeze chute facility and were blood sampled with minimal restraint. Blood sampling was carried out by the same experienced operator on each occasion and the time taken to collect the blood samples was less than 60 s/animal.

#### *Haematological measurements*

Blood samples were collected into (1 × 6 ml) $K_3$ ethylenediaminetetraacetic acid ($K_3$EDTA) tube (Vacuette, Cruinn Diagnostics, Ireland) for haematological cell distributions and haemoglobin content determined using an automated analyser (Celltac MEK-6108 K; Nihon-Kohdon, Tokyo, Japan) and reagents supplied by Celltac (Alpha Technologies, Dublin, Ireland).

#### *Blood metabolites, acute phase proteins and immune measurements*

Heparinized blood samples were collected by jugular venipuncture and the plasma was separated by centrifugation at 1600×*g* at 8 °C for 15 min (except for interferon (IFN)-γ at 300×*g*; at 8 °C for 15 min) and subsequently stored at −20 °C until assayed for subsequent analysis of metabolic variables associated with mobilization of body energy reserves, dehydration and muscle injury [albumin, total protein, creatine kinase (CK), glucose, non-esterified fatty acid (NEFA), βeta-hydroxy butyrate (βHB)], inflammatory biomarkers (the acute phase proteins (fibrinogen, haptoglobin) and a measure of cell mediated immunity interferon-(IFN)γ production [26]).

***Albumin***

The concentration of albumin was determined on an automatic clinical analyser (Olympus AU400 Clinical Analyser, Tokyo, Japan) using the reagents supplied by Olympus (catalogue number OSR6102). The composition of the reagents (at final concentration) required for this test were: succinate buffer (pH 4.2) (100 mmol/l) and bromocresol green (0.2 mmol/l) and following gentle inversion the reagents were ready to use directly from the kit.

***Total protein***

The concentration of total protein in plasma was determined on an automatic clinical analyser (Olympus AU400 Clinical Analyser, Tokyo, Japan) using the reagents supplied by Olympus (catalogue number OSR6132) (Olympus UK Ltd., Voice House, Watford, Hertfordshire, WD24 4JL, UK). The composition of the reagents (at final concentration) required for this test were; sodium hydroxide (200 mmol/l), potassium sodium tartrate (32 mmol/l), copper sulphate (18.8 mmol/l) and potassium iodide (30 mmol/l) and following gentle inversion the reagents were ready to use directly from the kit.

***Creatine kinase (CK)***

The activity of CK was determined on an automatic clinical analyser (Olympus AU400 Clinical Analyser, Tokyo, Japan) using the reagents supplied by Olympus (catalogue number OSR6179). The composition of the reagents (at final concentrations of reactive ingredients) required for this test were: imidazole (pH 6.5) (100 mmol/l), NADP (2 mmol/l), ADP (2 mmol/l), AMP (5 mmol/l), EDTA (2 mmol/l), glucose (20 mmol/l), creatine phosphate (30 mmol/l), n-acetlycysteine (0.2 mmol/l), activator (26 mmol/l), $Mg^{2+}$ (10 mmol/l), diadenosine pentaphosphate (0.01 mmol/l), hexokinase (>4 kU/l) and glucose-6-phosphate dehydrogenase (>2.8 kU/l). Prior to the placement of the reagents on board the instrument, the entire kit contents of R1-2 (4 ml) were transferred to the entire kit contents of R1-1 (22 ml) and mixed by gentle inversion. The second reagent bottle (R2) (6 ml) was ready to use from the kit and was placed directly on the instrument.

***Glucose***

The concentration of glucose was determined on an automatic clinical analyser (Olympus AU400 Clinical Analyser, Tokyo, Japan) using the reagents supplied by Olympus (catalogue number OSR6121). The composition of the reagents (at final concentration of reactive ingredients) required for this test were: piperazine-*N,N'*-bis (ethanesulfonic acid (PIPES) buffer (pH 7.6) (24 mmol/l)), ATP ($\geq$2 mmol/l), $NAD^+$ ($\geq$1.32 mmol/l), $Mg^{2+}$ (2.37 mmol/l), hexokinase ($\geq$0.59 mmol/l), G6P-DH ($\geq$0.59 mmol/l) and required no preparation prior to placement on the instrument.

***Non-esterified fatty acids***

The concentration of non-esterified fatty acids (NEFA) was determined on an automatic clinical analyser (Olympus AU400 Clinical Analyser, Tokyo, Japan) using the reagents supplied by Randox Laboratories (catalogue number FA115) (Randox Labs ltd., Ardmore, Diamond Rd., Crumlin BT29 4QY, Co. Antrim, Ireland). The kit comprised of five reagents. The buffer (R1a) and enzyme diluent (R2a) were ready to use from the kit. The enzyme/coenzymes (R1b) were reconstituted with 10 ml of buffer (R1a) and mixed by gently swirling. Maleimide (R2b) was reconstituted with enzyme diluent (R2a) and was inverted several times to ensure that maleimide was completely dissolved. This was then used immediately to reconstitute enzyme reagent (R2c) which was protected from light and placed on board the instrument for analysis. All reagents were kept at 4 °C prior to and after preparation.

***β-Hydroxy butyrate (βHB)***

The concentration of βHB was determined on an automatic clinical analyser (Olympus AU400 Clinical Analyser, Tokyo, Japan) using the reagents supplied by Randox Laboratories (catalogue number RB 1007). The kit comprised of five reagents: R1a [Buffer (Tris buffer (pH 8.5) 100 mmol/l), EDTA (2 mmol/l), Oxalic acid (20 mmol/l)] and R1b (Enzyme/Coenzyme NAD + 2.5 U/ml; 3-hydroxybutyrate dehydrogenase 0.12 U/ml)). The reagents were stored at 4 °C prior to and after preparation.

***Acute phase protein response (fibrinogen and haptoglobin)***

Blood collected into vacutainer tubes containing lithium heparin and sodium citrate was used to determine the plasma concentration of haptoglobin and fibrinogen, respectively. Plasma was harvested following centrifugation at 1600×*g* at 4 °C for 15 min and stored at −80 °C until assayed. Plasma concentration of haptoglobin was measured using an automatic analyser (spACE, Alfa Wassermann, Inc., West Caldwell, NJ, USA) and commercial assay kit (Tridelta Development Ltd., Wicklow, Ireland) according to the manufacturer's procedure as described by Eckersall et al. [27]. Plasma concentration of fibrinogen was measured using an automatic analyser (spACE, Alfa Wassermann, Inc., West Caldwell, NJ, USA) using a method described by Becker et al. [28].

#### *Immune variable; interferon-γ (IFN-γ)*

Blood samples for IFN-γ determination were collected by jugular venipuncture into aseptic vacutainer tubes containing lithium heparin and the stimulated lymphocyte production of IFN-γ was determined following whole blood culture. Duplicate 1.48 ml aliquots of heparinized blood were cultured in sterile 24-well flat culture plates (Sarstedt Ltd., Drinagh, Wexford, Ireland) with 20 μl of PBS (GibcoBRL, Life Technologies Ltd., Paisley, Scotland) containing either 1 mg/ml of PHA (Sigma-Aldrich, Inc., St. Louis, MO, product No. L-9132) or 1 mg/ml of Concanavalin A (Con A; Sigma-Aldrich; product No. C 5275) or no additive for 24 h at 37 °C in an atmosphere of 5% $CO_2$. Aseptic techniques were practised during this procedure under laminar flow conditions. The culture plates were then centrifuged at 1600×*g*, at 4 °C for 20 min; the supernatant was harvested and frozen at −20 °C until it was assayed for IFN-γ production, using an ELISA procedure [27] (Bovigam, CSL Biosciences, Victoria, Australia; catalogue No. 03000201). The in vitro phytohemagglutinin (PHA)- and Con A-stimulated IFN-γ production was calculated by subtracting the absorbance at 450 nm of wells that received PBS alone from the absorbance of wells that received either PHA or Con A [29].

#### *Physical characteristics of the mats*

The mats were tested to give an assessment of physical parameters: hardness, simulated hoof—mat contact properties and time dependent deformation characteristics at the German Institute for Rubber Technology, (Hannover [DIK]). The proprietary mats, hereafter referred to as Mats 1, 2, and 3, were compared. Testing conformed to current ISO international standards. Each mat had its own distinct pattern on the mat upper surface which would inevitably have had some minor influence on physical test results. Mats 1 and 2 were predominantly made of natural rubber (NR) and Mat 3 comprised a modified ethylene vinyl acetate (EVA) foam structure.

#### *Shore A hardness*

The Shore hardness test for rubber samples is basically a method of indirectly characterising the elastic modulus of a rubber by measuring the elastic indentation caused by a rigid indentor pressed into the surface under specified loading conditions. Theoretically, hardness values range from zero degrees when the modulus is zero, (very soft rubber) up to 100° where the modulus is infinitely high. The Shore A hardness of each sample was measured at room temperature and on a stand mounted digital Shore meter with a timer allowing the values of hardness to be determined consistently throughout testing. In each test a reading of hardness was taken after a 3 s constant force application of a standard indentor to a 6 mm thick specimen prepared in each instance from an actual mat. The values shown in Table 1 were an average of five tests, taken on different parts of the specimen prepared from the mat, but at least 12 mm from the edge of the specimen in all tests. This procedure complies with test standard ISO 7619:1997 (Rubber—determination of indentation hardness by means of pocket hardness meters).

#### *Friction measurements*

The characterisation of friction coefficients was carried out using a Zwick universal testing machine (Type 1445.17, fitted with a 5 kN load cell) which was modified to encompass friction measurements. The tests were conducted over a range of sliding velocities from 0.1 to 30 mm/min and under an applied stress of 18.4 kPa. Under the range of sliding velocities any local interfacial thermal effects due to contact between the mat and the testing surface was negligible. Also, the amount of abrasion of the specimens was minimised by the selection of a low load.

The test specimens used were cut from actual mats and measured 40 × 40 $mm^2$ with a thickness equal to the mat under test. The specimens were bonded to an aluminium alloy plate which was loaded with a 3 kg mass. The plate was then drawn by a stranded steel wire which traversed two pulleys, one of which was connected to the 5 kN load cell allowing the friction force to be measured directly. All tests were carried out at room temperature. For wet friction testing, a consistent level of wetness was ensured

**Table 1 Results from the various tests that were used to characterise the physical properties of the mats**

| | Mat 1 | Mat 2 | Mat 3 |
|---|---|---|---|
| Mean Shore A hardness (±SE) | 64 (0.16) | 70 (0.22) | 61 (0.16) |
| Mean wet friction (μ)* | 0.59 | 0.63 | 0.38 |
| (Maximum) | (0.67) | (0.70) | (0.40) |
| (Minimum) | (0.53) | (0.57) | (0.37) |
| (±SE) | (0.04) | (0.04) | (0.01) |
| Mean dry friction (μ)* | 0.71 | 0.74 | 0.40 |
| (Maximum) | (0.74) | (0.76) | (0.43) |
| (Minimum) | (0.67) | (0.72) | (0.38) |
| (±SE) | (0.02) | (0.01) | (0.02) |
| Compression (mm) | | | |
| As result of applied stress equivalent to application of one hoof | 0.839 | 1.090 | 0.933 |
| Creep (mm) | | | |
| As result of an applied stress equivalent to the application of one hoof for 300 s | 0.095 | 0.138 | 0.292 |

* The mean values of μ displayed are calculated from the three lowest sliding velocities as illustrated in Figs. 1 and 2. This was conducted to eliminate the effect of the phenomenon known as "stick slip" which was a characteristic of the test apparatus rather than of the test materials

by the sample being immersed in a water/detergent (95:5) mixture for each test. Friction tests conformed to an adaptation of ISO 15113:1999, Rubber—determination of frictional properties.

#### *Dry and wet friction*

Samples of Mat 1, Mat 2 and Mat 3 were drawn over the test track surface. Initially the friction force peaked at a point where the adhesion force between the sample and surface began to break down and subsequently a slightly lower approximately constant frictional force was measured as the specimen travelled along the test track. This constant force is termed $F_{const}$ and the friction coefficient was calculated from.

$$\mu = F_{const}/ F_N$$

where μ is the coefficient of friction and $F_N$ is the normal force.

The test was repeated four times at each sliding velocity in planes normal to and in line with the mat surface patterns. An average friction coefficient was calculated for each material and sliding velocity (i.e. eight tests per quoted coefficient of friction).

#### *Compression creep tests*

The mats were subjected to a compression creep test on an MTS 831.50 elastomer testing system (2.5 kN load cell). This test was devised specifically to render useful data in respect of time dependent properties for each product. A force was applied through two flat plates, approximately equivalent to that which a finishing steer would typically exert on a mat due to the downward load transmitted through one hoof. This force was maintained for a period of 300 s to examine how the reaction force in the region of contact on the mat relaxed with time. The applied stress was calculated from an average animal mass (625 kg) divided by four and the surface area of a typical hoof (5300 $mm^2$) as specified by Kirchner and Boxberger [30].

### Statistical analysis

All statistical analyses were performed using SAS software Version 9.3 (SAS Institute Inc. Cary, NC, USA). The pen was the experimental unit for all variables. Data were checked for normality and homogeneity of variance by histograms, q–q plots, and formal statistical tests as part of the UNIVARIATE procedure of SAS (version 9.3; SAS Institute, 2006). Data that were not normally distributed were transformed by raising the variable to the power of lambda. The appropriate lambda value was obtained by conducting a Box-Cox transformation analysis using the TRANSREG procedure of SAS. Data subjected to transformation were used to calculate P-values. Data from the three concrete slat treatments were analysed using a mixed model ANOVA with the MIXED procedure of SAS to examine the effect of treatment on intake, performance traits, hoof lesion scores, physiological and behavioural data. The PDIFF option was applied to evaluate the pair-wise comparisons between the OWP treatment and the concrete slat treatment. The statistical model included the fixed effect of treatment and batch. Data with multiple observations, such as dirt scores, haematological variables and metabolites, were analysed using a repeated measures ANOVA (MIXED procedure of SAS 9.3). Terms for treatment, day and their interaction were included in the model. If the interaction term was not significant ($P > 0.05$) it was subsequently excluded from the final model. The PDIFF option and the Tukey test were applied as appropriate to evaluate pair-wise comparisons between the group means on concrete slats and the associated P values were derived. Data were considered statistically significant when $P < 0.05$. Least square means (Lsmeans) are reported with standard error of the mean.

## Results

### Characteristics of mats

#### *Shore A hardness*

The mean (±SE) Shore A hardness for the three mat types were: Mat 1, 64 (0.16); Mat 2, 70 (0.22); Mat 3, 61 (0.16), respectively (Table 1).

#### *Wet and dry friction results*

A high friction coefficient for both wet and dry conditions is desirable between the hoof of the animal and the rubber mat. The higher the friction coefficient the less likely the animal is to slip when moving about in the pen, which will obviously provide a more comfortable environment for the animal. When the animal has firm and secure footing it will be more likely to move about its environment in a more natural manner to feed as desired without risk of slippage and sustaining injury.

The wet friction results are the most relevant for the normal environment encountered by the mats (Table 1). Figure 1 shows the results of the wet friction tests where, as stated previously, the test track was immersed in water with a 5% detergent mix. There is a clear difference in the friction coefficients for each material with some stick–slip behaviour having a pronounced influence, notably where friction coefficients for Mat 2 declined at greater sliding velocities.

Dry friction test results are shown in Table 1 and Fig. 2 and it was observed that Mats 1 and 2 experienced some stick–slip behaviour at greater velocities. Consistently in both the wet and dry friction tests, the ranking order was Mat 2, Mat 1 and Mat 3 (i.e. Mat 2 was shown to have the highest and Mat 3 the lowest coefficient of sliding friction in contact with a constant rigid surface). Thus Mat 2 exhibited superior friction properties to the other mats tested.

### *Compression creep tests*

The results from the compression creep tests are summarised in Fig. 3. Creep behaviour from a zero datum after the 2 s load application are presented in Fig. 4.

### *Environmental conditions*

The mean (±SE) daily air temperature (°C) recorded in the shed facility (from November to May) was 9.9 (0.03) (min 1.7 max 22.4) and 6.6 (0.04) (min −5.2; max 22.6) for the ambient (outside) temperature.

### *Animal diet*

The mean (±SE) chemical composition and nutritive value of the TMR offered to animals was: crude ash 81.4 g/kg DM (2.09), crude protein 149.8 g/kg DM (1.52), in vitro DM digestibility (DMD) 798.1 g/kg (4.03), neutral detergent fibre (NDF) 450.4 g/kg DM (5.0), pH 4.2 (0.03).

### *Animal cleanliness*

There was a significant treatment, day and treatment × day interaction ($P < 0.05$) for dirt score (Table 2). Dirt scores did not differ ($P > 0.05$) between mat or slat treatments but were lower ($P < 0.05$) than for the OWP treatment with an overall significant treatment × day interaction ($P < 0.001$). Dirt scores were greater ($P < 0.05$) on OWPs on days 42, 84, 105, 126 and 150 compared with slats.

### *Animal health, performance, and hoof lesions*

No animal presented with clinical signs of bovine respiratory disease or required veterinary treatment for any ailment throughout the study period. The daily live weight gain of animals on the OWPs was greater for animals on the OWP compared with animals housed on slats and on Mat 2; Mat 1 and Mat 3 were not different from the other treatments (Table 3). However, carcass weight, kill out proportion, carcass fat score, carcass composition score and FCR were similar among treatments (Table 3). Animals on the OWPs had a greater ($P < 0.05$) dry matter (DM) feed intake compared with animals on the slat and the three mat types (Table 3). DMI was similar ($P > 0.05$) between the slat and mat treatments. The number of hoof lesions was greater on all mat types ($P < 0.05$) compared with concrete slats and OWP treatments (Table 3).

### *Animal behaviour*

Overall (period 1–6 combined), the percentage of animals lying at any one time, was greater ($P < 0.05$) in the animals housed on concrete slats, mats 1, 2 and 3 compared with the animals housed on the OWPs (Table 3). The percentage of animals eating at any one time was lower ($P < 0.05$) on concrete slats and Mat 2 compared with OWPs. The percentage of animals drinking at any one time was lower on OWPs compared with concrete slats and Mat 2 and was not different from Mat 1 and Mat 3.

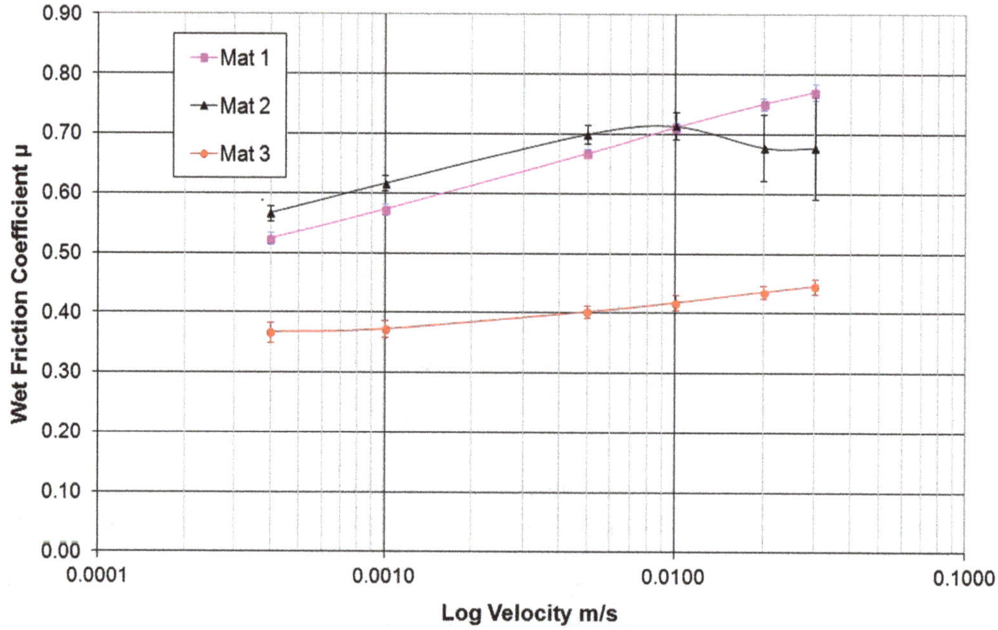


**Fig. 1** Wet friction values measured for a range of sliding velocities

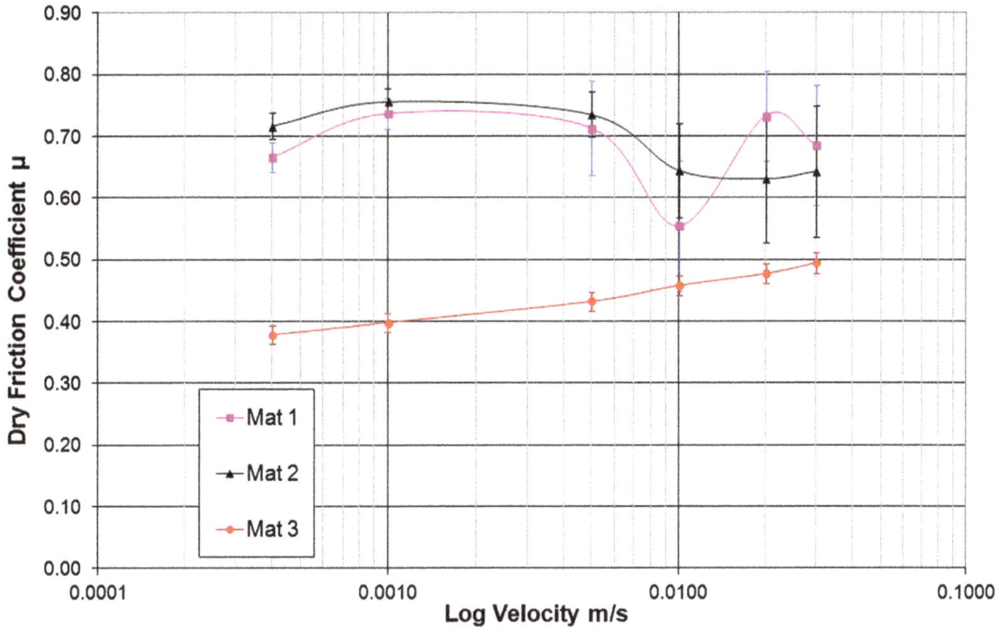


**Fig. 2** Dry friction values measured for a range of sliding velocities

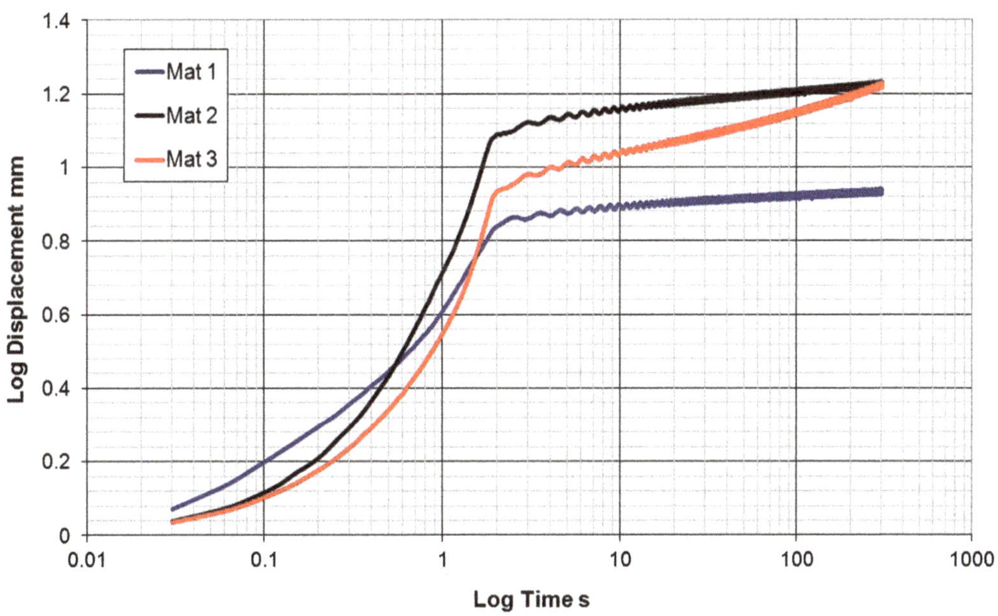


**Fig. 3** Graph showing results of compression tests where a stress equivalent to that exerted by a single hoof exerted upon the Mat

***Physiological variables***

There was no effect of treatment or treatment × day interaction ($P > 0.05$) for plasma concentrations of albumin, total protein, βHB, NEFA, glucose, fibrinogen, haptoglobin, Con-A, PHA-induced IFN-γ and CK activity (Table 4). Day of sampling was significant ($P < 0.05$) for plasma concentrations of albumin, βHB, NEFA, glucose, fibrinogen, haptoglobin, PHA-induced-IFN-γ production and CK activity.

***Haematological variables***

There was no effect of treatment or treatment × day interactions ($P > 0.05$) whereas day ($P < 0.05$) was significant for basophil, eosinophil, leukocyte, lymphocyte,

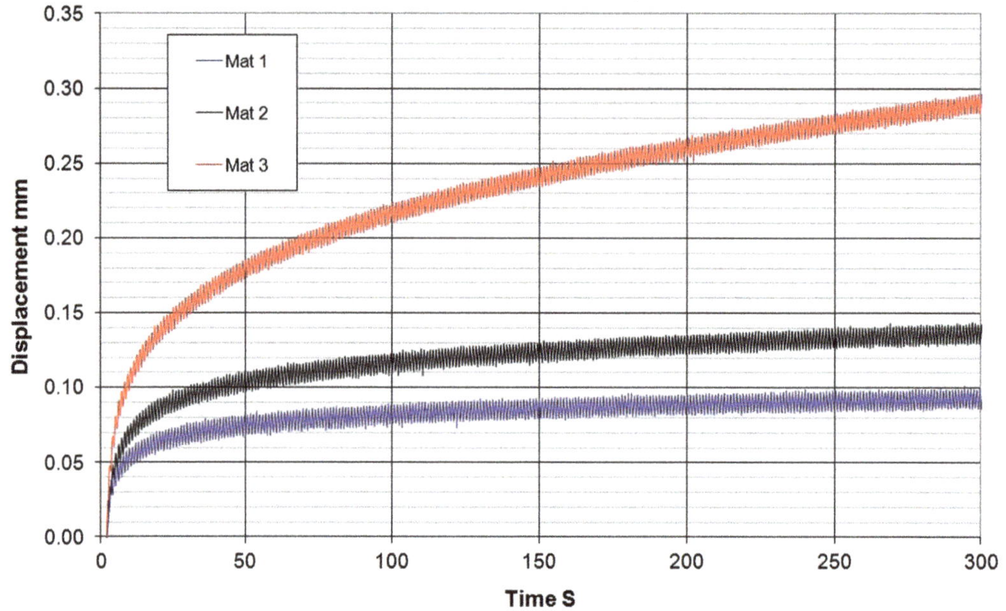


**Fig. 4** Graph showing the results of creep tests where a stress equivalent to that exerted by one hoof was maintained on the Mat for 300 s

**Table 2 Cleanliness scores of finishing beef steers on concrete slats, Mat 1, Mat 2, Mat 3 and OWP's from day 0 to day 150. Values are expressed as Lsmeans (±SE)**

| | d 0 | d 21 | d 42 | d 63 | d 84 | d 105 | d 126 | d 150 | SE |
|---|---|---|---|---|---|---|---|---|---|
| Concrete slats | $37^{a}$ | 45 | $48^{x}$ | 43 | $39^{x}$ | $34^{x}$ | $27^{b,x}$ | $23^{b,x}$ | 0.112 |
| Mat 1 | $37^{a}$ | $45^{b}$ | 48 | 46 | 41 | 33 | $24^{b}$ | $21^{b}$ | 0.112 |
| Mat 2 | $36^{a}$ | $47^{b}$ | $50^{b}$ | $46^{b}$ | 43 | 35 | $27^{b}$ | $22^{b}$ | 0.112 |
| Mat 3 | $37^{a}$ | 48 | $51^{b}$ | $49^{b}$ | 44 | 34 | $26^{b}$ | $22^{b}$ | 0.112 |
| OWP's | $35^{a}$ | 43 | $55^{b,y}$ | 42 | $57^{b,y}$ | $48^{b,y}$ | $40^{y}$ | $32^{y}$ | 0.112 |

Sum of 16 body parts each on a cleanliness scale of 1 (clean) to 5 (dirty)

Interactions; Treatment P = 0.006; Day P < 0.001; Treatment × day P < 0.001

$^{a,b}$ Lsmeans (in rows) that do not have a common superscript differ by P < 0.05

$^{x,y}$ Lsmeans (in columns) that do not have a common superscript differ by P < 0.05

monocyte, neutrophil, red blood cell number, haemoglobin concentration and haematocrit percentage (Table 5). There was no effect of treatment, sampling day or treatment × day interaction (P > 0.05) for white blood cell number.

## Discussion

In the present study, measuring the responses of animals to the different floor types, in terms of performance, hoof score, dirt scores, behaviour, immunological and physiological variables provided an insight into how the animals were coping. The objective of this study was to explore, in systematic fashion, factors affecting the overall performance, and welfare of animals housed on different floor types. The rationale for using TMR feeding was to achieve a relatively stable rumen pH and fermentation pattern throughout the day. This has been reported to promote better cellulose digestion and a greater lipogenic to non-lipogenic volatile fatty acid (VFA) ratio [31, 32]. Animals on the OWPs had a greater live weight gain compared with the slat and Mat 2 treatments: Mat 1 and Mat 3 were the same as the other treatments. Interestingly, carcass weight, kill out proportion, carcass fat score, carcass composition score and FCR were similar among treatments. The similar carcass weight for animals on the slat treatment in the present study is consistent with other studies in Ireland examining the performance and carcass characteristics of finishing animals housed on concrete slats and fed similar diets [32–38].

**Table 3 Intake, performance, slaughter traits, hoof scores, behaviour of finishing beef steers housed on concrete slats, Mat 1, Mat 2, Mat 3 and OWP's**

| | Concrete slats | Mat 1 | Mat 2 | Mat 3 | OWP's | SE | Significance |
|---|---|---|---|---|---|---|---|
| Initial weight (kg) | 538.4 | 538.4 | 538.4 | 538.4 | 539.1 | 9.40 | NS |
| Final weight (kg) | 677.2 | 693.4 | 676.1 | 682.6 | 699.5 | 7.37 | NS |
| Carcass (kg) | 371.9 | 385.8 | 374.7 | 381.1 | 384.7 | 5.00 | NS |
| Live weight gain/day | 0.93[a] | 1.04 | 0.92[a] | 0.97 | 1.08[b] | 0.03 | $P = 0.011$ |
| Kill out proportion (KO) (%) | 55.0 | 55.7 | 55.4 | 55.8 | 55.1 | 0.40 | NS |
| Kidney and channel fat (kg) | 11.2 | 10.7 | 11.4 | 10.9 | 11.2 | 0.37 | NS |
| Carcass composition score[1] | 9.0 | 9.5 | 8.8 | 9.1 | 9.4 | 0.23 | NS |
| Carcass fat score[2] | 10.7 | 10.7 | 10.9 | 10.8 | 10.7 | 0.22 | NS |
| Dry matter intake (DMI) kg/animal/day | 9.1[a] | 9.3[a] | 9.2[a] | 9.2[a] | 10.1[b] | 0.09 | $P < 0.001$ |
| DMI/LWG | 9.9 | 9.0 | 10.0 | 9.5 | 9.5 | 0.34 | NS |
| FCR (kg DMI/kg of LWG gained)[3] | 9.9 | 9.0 | 10.0 | 9.5 | 9.5 | 0.35 | NS |
| Hoof lesions[4] | 20[a] | 33[b] | 32[b] | 30[b] | 24[a,b] | 3.38 | $P = 0.050$ |
| Percent lying time (%) | 49.4[a] | 47.2[a] | 48.7[a] | 45.2[a] | 38.0[b] | 1.11 | $P < 0.001$ |
| Percent eating (%) | 18.1[a] | 20.6 | 18.0[a] | 20.9 | 22.1[b] | 0.94 | $P = 0.003$ |
| Percent drinking time (%) | 0.60[a] | 0.48 | 0.54[a] | 0.51 | 0.38[b] | 0.04 | $P = 0.010$ |

Values are expressed as Lsmeans (SE)

*NS* not statistically significant

[a,b] Lsmeans (in rows) that do not have a common superscript differ by $P < 0.05$

[1] EU Beef Carcass Classification Scheme, scale 1 (poorest) to 15 (best)

[2] EU Beef Carcass Classification Scheme, scale 1 (leanest) to 15 (fattest)

[3] FCR was expressed as kilogram carcass gain per 1000 kg DMI

[4] The total number of hoof lesions/animal at the end of the study

Dry matter intake was greater in the OWPs compared with all other treatments, whereas feed conversion ratio (FCR) was similar across treatments. Studies comparing concrete slats with straw as underfoot conditions in pens for finishing bulls are often confounded by space allowance, as housing systems utilising straw, have a larger total floor area per animal than fully slatted pens [39]. Gygax et al. [40] examined the effects of four space allowances (2.5, 3.0, 3.5 and 4.0 $m^2$) on the behaviour and cleanliness of finishing bulls on fully slatted rubber coated floors and concluded that that increasing space allowance had several beneficial and no negative effects on welfare indicators. In the present study, dirt scores were greater on the OWPs compared with all other treatments. Additionally, animals on the OWPs spent less time lying compared with all treatments. It is reported in the literature that cattle housed on concrete floors tended to lie down or stand up less frequently and displayed more abnormal movements than animals housed on straw [2–4, 13, 18, 41, 42]. Bulls housed on slatted floors were reported to be more hesitant about lying down and were more likely to lie down via the "dog-sitting" position [43]. In addition, Graf [2] recorded a greater incidence of abnormal lying down movements among bulls on slatted concrete floors, but only at low space allowances.

A series of experiments examining the flooring preferences of cattle were conducted by Irps [44, 45]. In one study [44] 15-mo-old cattle spent more time lying on a straw-covered area than on rubber-coated concrete slats and spent the least time lying on uncovered concrete slats when they had access to all three areas. However, when lying times for fattening bulls were measured across three pens, one with rubber-coated concrete slats, one with 50% rubber-coated and 50% plain concrete slats and one with 100% plain concrete slats, there were no differences in lying times across the three systems [46]. Rubber coated slatted floors have been tested as an alternative floor quality in housing systems for finishing bulls [5, 39, 40] and the results indicate that finishing bulls lie down more frequently, slip less and have fewer hock lesions compared with fully slatted concrete floors. Interestingly, Elmore et al. [1] reported that flooring substrate had a large impact on health, hygiene, and postural changes of finishing beef steers, though there was no effect of flooring treatment on time budget behaviour or performance data. In the present study, the number of hoof lesions was greater on all mat types compared with concrete slats and OWP treatments. Although significant differences in numbers of lesions were found, the lesions were not severe enough to be biologically meaningful in terms

**Table 4 Plasma metabolic variables (albumin, globulin, total protein, βHB, NEFA, Glucose, creatine kinase), acute phase proteins (fibrinogen, haptoglobin) and immune variables Concanavalin-A (Con-A) induced and Phytohaemagglutinin (PHA) induced interferon-γ (IFN-γ) of finishing beef steers on day 0 and day 150**

| | Bleed | Concrete slats | Mat 1 | Mat 2 | Mat 3 | OWP | SE | Treatment (T) | Day (D) | T x D |
|---|---|---|---|---|---|---|---|---|---|---|
| Albumin | d 0 | 32.64$^a$ | 32.44$^a$ | 32.90$^a$ | 32.56$^a$ | 32.81$^a$ | 0.143 | NS | P < 0.05 | NS |
| (g/l) | d 150 | 34.16$^b$ | 34.63$^b$ | 34.23$^b$ | 34.54$^b$ | 34.01$^b$ | 0.192 | | | |
| Globulin | d 0 | 41.43 | 41.58 | 41.83 | 41.68 | 42.19 | 0.515 | NS | NS | NS |
| (g/l) | d 150 | 41.02 | 39.92 | 40.59 | 40.39 | 38.88 | 0.505 | | | |
| Total protein | d 0 | 74.06 | 74.02 | 74.72 | 74.24 | 74.99 | 0.552 | NS | NS | NS |
| (g/l) | d 150 | 75.18 | 74.55 | 74.82 | 74.93 | 72.88 | 0.456 | | | |
| βHB | d 0 | 0.27$^a$ | 0.27$^a$ | 0.29$^a$ | 0.27$^a$ | 0.29 | 0.01 | NS | P < 0.05 | NS |
| (mmol/l) | d 150 | 0.23$^b$ | 0.23$^b$ | 0.23$^b$ | 0.22$^b$ | 0.28 | 0.01 | | | |
| NEFA | d 0 | 0.15 | 0.17 | 0.17 | 0.19 | 0.22$^a$ | 0.01 | NS | P < 0.05 | NS |
| (mmol/l) | d 150 | 0.16 | 0.18 | 0.15 | 0.16 | 0.13$^b$ | 0.01 | | | |
| Glucose | d 0 | 3.98$^a$ | 3.93$^a$ | 4.05$^a$ | 4.01$^a$ | 3.99 | 0.03 | NS | P < 0.05 | NS |
| (mmol/l) | d 150 | 4.29$^b$ | 4.21$^b$ | 4.30$^b$ | 4.34$^b$ | 4.12 | 0.03 | | | |
| Creatine kinase | d 0 | 273.5$^a$ | 255.8$^a$ | 266.0$^a$ | 244.0$^a$ | 321.8$^a$ | 11.86 | NS | P < 0.05 | NS |
| (U/l) | d 150 | 165.9$^b$ | 183.3$^b$ | 159.3$^b$ | 166.3$^b$ | 173.8$^b$ | 7.18 | | | |
| Fibrinogen | d 0 | 489.0$^a$ | 483.2$^a$ | 502.3$^a$ | 498.6$^a$ | 511.0$^a$ | 11.04 | NS | P < 0.05 | NS |
| (mg/dl) | d 150 | 382.3$^b$ | 366.0$^b$ | 364.2$^b$ | 348.1$^b$ | 351.2$^b$ | 8.46 | | | |
| Haptoglobin | d 0 | 0.75$^a$ | 0.75$^a$ | 0.76$^a$ | 0.77$^a$ | 0.78$^a$ | 0.02 | NS | P < 0.05 | NS |
| (g of Hb binding capacity/l) | d 150 | 0.64$^b$ | 0.58$^b$ | 0.62$^b$ | 0.58$^b$ | 0.55$^b$ | 0.01 | | | |
| Concanavalin-A (CON-A) induced IFN-γ | d 0 | 1.04 | 1.03 | 0.83 | 0.98 | 0.93 | 0.10 | NS | NS | NS |
| Absorbance @450 nm | d 150 | 0.95 | 1.05 | 0.84 | 1.07 | 0.93 | 0.11 | | | |
| Phytohaemagglutinin (PHA) induced IFN-γ | d 0 | 0.90$^a$ | 0.83$^a$ | 1.06$^a$ | 0.91$^a$ | 0.81$^a$ | 0.09 | NS | P < 0.05 | NS |
| Absorbance @450 nm | d 150 | 0.48$^b$ | 0.52$^b$ | 0.59$^b$ | 0.59$^b$ | 0.58$^b$ | 0.06 | | | |

Values are expressed as Lsmeans (SE)

*NS* not statistically significant, *T* Treatment, *D* Day, *T* × *D* Treatment × day interaction

[a,b] Lsmeans (in rows) that do not have a common superscript differ by P < 0.05

of lameness. No information is available on the effects of high friction floors on cattle locomotion. Phillips and Morris [47–49] and Phillips et al. [50] measured these variables in cows walking on floors with different levels of friction. Phillips and Morris [49] and Phillips et al. [50] reported that floor friction had a considerable impact on the walking pattern of cows. Cows walked quickly with frequent, short steps on low friction floors ($\mu < 0.4$). As $\mu$ increased to 0.5 (mean of static and sliding friction) with aggregates of 0.5 and 1.2 mm, step length increased and the number of steps decreased in order to maintain speed. Increased $\mu$ also may increase the hanging limb phase at the expense of the supporting limb phase, to reduce friction, while maintaining a long stride. Their findings suggest that the optimum coefficient of friction for cattle floors is between 0.4 and 0.5 and significantly Web and Nilsson [51] reported that the incidence of slip increases rapidly as coefficients of static friction for floors decrease below 0.4.

In the present study, the hardness values (Shore A scale measurements to ISO 7619) ranked the mats from hardest to softest (Mat 2, Mat 1, and Mat 3). The coefficients of friction were determined for each material in both wet and dry conditions on a roughened metal test track (an adaptation of ISO 15113). For both wet and dry tests, the ranking was Mat 2, Mat 1, and Mat 3 where the friction coefficients went from highest to lowest. In creep tests under constant compressive loading which replicated a typical stress resulting from the load transmitted under one hoof, the ranking order after load application was 3, 2, 1 (largest to smallest change in deformation). Mat 2 produced the highest coefficient of friction under both wet and dry conditions when subject to sliding motion in contact with a rigid surface. This is considered to be a positive characteristic in respect of comfort and safety and more likely to promote behaviour similar to that in the cow's outdoor environment. If a high coefficient of friction, high static and dynamic deformation and low

**Table 5 Haematological variables of finishing beef steers on day (0) and d 150**

| | Bleed | Concrete slats | Mat 1 | Mat 2 | Mat 3 | OWP | SE | Treatment (T) | Day (D) | T × D |
|---|---|---|---|---|---|---|---|---|---|---|
| WBCP | d 0 | 9.11 | 9.46 | $9.19^{a}$ | $9.61^{a}$ | 9.60 | 0.163 | NS | P < 0.05 | NS |
| ($1 \times 10^3$ μl) | d 150 | 8.85 | 9.03 | $8.66^{b}$ | $8.82^{b}$ | 9.82 | 0.166 | | | |
| Basophil number | d 0 | $0.07^{a}$ | $0.08^{a}$ | $0.07^{a}$ | $0.08^{a}$ | $0.08^{a}$ | $0.002^{a}$ | NS | P < 0.05 | NS |
| ($1 \times 10^3$ μl) | d 150 | $0.06^{b}$ | $0.06^{b}$ | $0.06^{b}$ | $0.06^{b}$ | $0.06^{b}$ | $0.002^{b}$ | | | |
| Eosinophil number | d 0 | $0.07^{a}$ | $0.08^{a}$ | $0.07^{a}$ | $0.08^{a}$ | $0.08^{a}$ | 0.002 | NS | P < 0.05 | NS |
| ($1 \times 10^3$ μl) | d 150 | $0.06^{b}$ | $0.06^{b}$ | $0.06^{b}$ | $0.06^{b}$ | $0.06^{b}$ | 0.002 | | | |
| Leukocyte number | d 0 | 0.07 | 0.05 | 0.06 | 0.05 | $0.09^{a}$ | 0.005 | NS | P < 0.05 | NS |
| ($1 \times 10^3$ μl) | d 150 | 0.05 | 0.05 | 0.06 | 0.05 | $0.05^{b}$ | 0.003 | | | |
| Lymphocyte number | d 0 | 5.29 | 5.24 | 5.11 | 5.58 | 5.47 | 0.098 | NS | P < 0.05 | P < 0.064 |
| ($1 \times 10^3$ μl) | d 150 | 5.67 | $5.73^{b}$ | 5.34 | 5.76 | $6.00^{b}$ | 0.100 | | | |
| Monocyte number | d 0 | $0.55^{a}$ | $0.57^{a}$ | $0.49^{a}$ | $0.54^{a}$ | $0.52^{a}$ | 0.014 | NS | P < 0.05 | P = 0.036 |
| ($1 \times 10^3$ μl) | d 150 | $0.34^{b}$ | $0.38^{b}$ | $0.39^{b}$ | $0.37^{b}$ | $0.41^{b}$ | 0.009 | | | |
| Neutrophil number | d 0 | 2.42 | $2.47^{a}$ | 2.37 | 2.68 | 2.33 | 0.054 | NS | P < 0.05 | NS |
| ($1 \times 10^3$ μl) | d 150 | 2.22 | $2.12^{b}$ | 2.29 | 2.35 | 2.14 | 0.046 | | | |
| Haematocrit | d 0 | $33.39^{a}$ | $33.10^{a}$ | $33.22^{a}$ | $32.27^{a}$ | $33.72^{a}$ | 0.36 | NS | P < 0.05 | NS |
| % | d 150 | $37.60^{b}$ | $37.45^{b}$ | $36.62^{b}$ | $37.00^{b}$ | $36.44^{b}$ | 0.24 | | | |
| Platelet number | d 0 | $447.9^{a}$ | $464.1^{a}$ | $484.2^{a}$ | $485.8^{a}$ | $457.3^{a}$ | $8.65^{a}$ | NS | P < 0.05 | NS |
| ($1 \times 10^3$ μl) | d 150 | $203.4^{b}$ | $185.2^{b}$ | $192.2^{b}$ | $205.9^{b}$ | $195.4^{b}$ | $30.39^{b}$ | | | |
| Red blood cell number | d 0 | $8.19^{a}$ | $8.14^{a}$ | 7.98 | $7.87^{a}$ | 8.29 | 0.101 | NS | P < 0.05 | NS |
| ($1 \times 10^3$ μl) | d 150 | $8.62^{b}$ | $8.62^{b}$ | 8.32 | $8.46^{b}$ | 8.50 | 0.068 | | | |
| Haemoglobin | d 0 | 12.95 | 12.84 | 12.86 | 12.61 | 13.21 | 0.149 | NS | NS | NS |
| (g/dl) | d 150 | 13.36 | 13.27 | 12.98 | 13.15 | 13.08 | 0.139 | | | |

Values are expressed as Lsmeans (SE)

*NS* not statistically significant, *T* Treatment, *D* Day, *T* × *D* Treatment × day interaction

[a,b] Lsmeans (in rows) that do not have a common superscript differ by P < 0.05

hardness were seen as desirable attributes for the mat materials and equal weighting is given to each property, there is little to choose between the performance of each mat.

Without devising specific tests, it is problematic to study the influence of dynamic and static friction when indentation of rubber takes place, as in the situation where a load is transmitted by a hoof. It is essential to minimise the influence of the dynamic properties of apparati if friction data is to be believed. Tests also need to quantify the contributions of bulk friction and adhesive friction [52]. Further research could shed light on these factors.

Alterations in the levels of blood cell constituents are indicative of an attempt to restore homeostasis when adverse physical conditions are encountered by an animal and thus, blood cells are very sensitive indicators of the patho-physiological responses of animals to a stressor [53].

In the present study, lymphocyte functional assays in terms of PHA-induced and Con A-induced IFN-γ production were used to assess cell-mediated immune function. The results showed no change in immune response among treatments in response to stimulation in vitro with the two mitogens, CON-A and PHA, indicating that there was no impairment of immune responsiveness of animals on the slat compared with the other treatments. Induction of a proliferative response induced by antigen in vitro has been shown to be representative of cellular immunocompetence [24]. The secretion of IFN-γ by lymphocytes is critically important in orchestrating an effective immune response, especially cellular immunity [29], and the induction of IFN-γ by Con A and PHA lectins corresponds to the degree of blastogenesis in cattle [54]. In the present study, maintenance of homeostasis was not affected by floor type. There was no effect of floor type on blood metabolite concentrations; thus metabolic homeostasis was maintained across treatments and the metabolite concentrations in the present study were within the normal physiological ranges for cattle [55–57].

## Conclusions

Steers on the OWPs had reduced lying percentage time compared with all the other treatments. Carcass weight, kill out proportion, carcass fat score, carcass composition score, and FCR, and physiological responses were similar among treatments. No incidence of laminitis was observed among treatments. There were a greater number of lesions on the hooves of animals housed on mats compared with bare concrete slats and OWP treatments. Therefore, under appropriate environmental conditions, out-wintering steers on OWP's is a good alternative to wintering indoors on bare concrete slats. However, dirt scores were greater for animals on OWPs on days 42, 84, 105, 126 and 150 compared with slats. Under the conditions of the present study, there is no evidence to suggest that animals housed on bare concrete slats are at an animal welfare disadvantage compared with other floor treatments.

#### Abbreviations

ADF: acid detergent fibre; bHB: beta hydroxy butyrate; CCTV: close circuit television. CK: creatine kinase; Con-A: concanavalin-A; DM: dry matter; DMD: dry matter digestibility; DMI: dry matter intake; IFN-γ: interferon-γ; Lsmeans: least square means; PHA: phytohaemagglutinin A; FCR: feed conversion ratio; NEFA: non-esterified fatty acids; NS: not statistically significant; RBC: red blood cell; SD: standard deviation; SE: standard error; TMR: total mixed ration; WBC: white blood cell.

#### Authors' contributions

BE and EOR designed and planned the study and all authors drafted the manuscript. BE performed the statistical analysis. BE, EOR, JDMcN, SJ participated in interpretation of data. All authors read and approved the final manuscript.

#### Author details

[1] Animal and Bioscience Research Department, Animal & Grassland Research and Innovation Centre, Teagasc, Grange, Dunsany, Co. Meath C15 PW93, Ireland. [2] Centre for Elastomer Research (CER), School of Manufacturing and Design Engineering, Dublin Institute of Technology (DIT), Dublin, Ireland. [3] Livestock Systems Research, Department Animal & Grassland Research and Innovation Centre, Teagasc, Grange, Dunsany, Co. Meath C15 PW93, Ireland.

#### Acknowledgements

The authors thank: Francis Collier, Joe Larkin, Eddie Mulligan, Margaret Murray and Dan Prendiville for excellent technical help and assistance during the study; the farm staff (Seamus Fagan, Liam Kirk, Hugh Mulligan) at Teagasc, Grange, for care and management of the animals; the advice and use of physical test facilities provided by Dr. Thomas Alshuth and Peter Erren of the Deutsches Institut für Kautschuktechnologie e.V. (DIK, Hannover, Germany).

#### Competing interests

The authors declare that they have no competing interests.

#### References

1. Elmore MR, Elischer MF, Claeys MC, Pajor EA. The effects of different flooring types on the behavior, health, and welfare of finishing beef steers. J Anim Sci. 2015;93(3):1258–66.
2. Graf B. Spaltenbodenhaltung bei mastochsen. Landbauforschung Volkenrode Sonderheft. 1979;48:73–88.
3. Graf B. Inwieweit genu¨ gen Laufstallsysteme den artspezifischen Anspru¨ chen von Mastrindern? U¨ berpru¨ fung anhand von Merkmalen des Ausruhverhaltens. In: Aktuelle Arbeiten zur artgema¨ßen Tierhaltung 299, KTBL-Schrift. 1984. p. 9–13.
4. Der Graf B. Einfluss unterschiedlicher Laufstallsysteme auf Verhaltens-merkmale von Matschen. Eidgenossichen Technishen Hochschule: Zurich; 1984. p. 282.
5. Ruis-Heutinck LFM, Smits MCJ, Smits AC, Heeres JJ. Effects of floor type and floor area on behaviour and carpal joint lesions in beef bulls. Improving health and welfare in animal production. In: Proceedings of sessions of the EAAP Commission on Animal Management & Health. The Hague. 21–24 August 2000.
6. Schrader L, Roth H-R, Winterling C, Brodmann N, Langhans W, Geyer H, Graf B. The occurrence of tail tip alterations in fattening bulls kept under different husbandry conditions. Anim Wel. 2001;10:119–30.
7. Schulze Westerath H, Gygax L, Mayer C, Wechsler B. Leg lesions and cleanliness of finishing bulls kept in housing systems with different lying area surfaces. The Vet J. 2007;174:77–85.
8. Mayer C, Thio T, Westerath HS, Ossent P, Gygax L, Wechsler B, Friedli K. Vergleich von Betonspaltenbo¨ den, gummimodifizierten Spaltenbo¨den und Buchten mit Einstreu in der Bullenmast unter dem Gesichtspunkt der Tiergerechtheit. Landbauforschung Vo¨lkenrode-FAL Agricultural Research, Sonderheft. 2007. p 303.
9. Absmanner E, Rouha-Mülleder C, Scharl T, Leisch F, Troxler J. Effects of different housing systems on the behaviour of beef bulls–an on-farm assessment on Austrian farms. Appl Anim Behav Sci. 2009;118:12–9.
10. Ingvartsen KL, Andersen HR. Space allowance and type of housing for growing cattle. Acta Agr Scand A Anim. 1993;43:65–80.
11. Fisher AD, Crowe MA, Prendiville DJ, Enright WJ. Indoor space allowance: effects on growth, behaviour, adrenal and immune responses of finishing beef heifers. Anim Sci. 1997;64:53–62.
12. Fisher AD, Crowe MA, O'Kiely P, Enright WJ. Growth, behaviour, adrenal and immune responses of finishing beef heifers housed on slatted floors at 1.5, 2.0, 2.5 or 3.0 $m^2$ space allowance. Livest Prod Sci. 1997;51:245–54.
13. Hickey MC, Earley B, Fisher AD. The effect of floor type and space allowance on welfare indicators of finishing steers. Irish J of Agri Food Res. 2003;42:89–100.
14. Lowe DE, Steen RWJ, Beattie VE, Moss BW. The effects of floor type systems on the performance, cleanliness, carcass composition and meat quality of housed finishing beef cattle. Livest Prod Sci. 2001;69:33–42.
15. Schlichting MC. Adaption of cattle to different floor types. In: Wierenga HK, Peterse DJ, editors. Cattle housing systems, lameness and behaviour. The Netherlands: Martinus Nijhoff; 1987. p. 87.
16. Schlichting MC, Smidt D. Welfare aspects of housing systems for veal calves and fattening bulls. CEC: Luxembourg; 1987.
17. Murphy PA, Hannan J, Monaghan M. A survey of lameness in beef cattle housed on slats and on straw. In: Wierenga HK, Peterse DJ, editors. Cattle housing systems, lameness and behaviour. The Netherlands: Martinus Nijhoff; 1987. p. 67.
18. Hickey MC, French P, Grant J. Out-wintering pads for finishing beef cattle: animal production and welfare. Anim Sci. 2002;75:447–58.
19. Owens D, McGee M, Boland T, O'Kiely P. Intake, rumen fermentation and nutrient flow to the omasum in beef cattle fed grass silage fortified with sucrose and/or supplemented with concentrate. Anim Feed Sci Technol. 2008;144:23–43.
20. Greenough PR, Vermunt JJ. Evaluation of subclinical lameness in a dairy herd and observations on associated nutritional and management factors. Vet Record. 1991;128:11–7.
21. Sprecher DJ, Hostetler DE, Kaneene JB. A lameness scoring system that uses posture and gait to predict dairy cattle reproductive performance. Theriogenol. 1997;47:1179–87.
22. Earley B, McDonnell B, O'Riordan E. Effect of floor type on the performance, physiological and behavioural responses of finishing beef steers. Acta Vet Scand. 2015;57:1–11.
23. Scott GB, Kelly M. Cattle cleanliness in different housing systems. Farm Build Prog. 1989;1989(95):21–4.
24. Gupta S, Earley B, Nolan M, Formentin E, Crowe MA. Effect of repeated regrouping and relocation on behaviour of steers. Appl Anim Behav Sci. 2008;110(3):229–43.
25. EC. Council Regulation (EC) No 1183/2006 of 24 July 2006 concerning the community scale for the classification of carcasses of adult bovine animals. Off J Eur Union. 2006;L214:1–6.
26. Earley B, Crowe MA. Effects of ketoprofen alone or in combination with local anesthesia during the castration of bull calves on plasma cortisol, immunological, and inflammatory responses. J Anim Sci. 2002;80:1044–52.

27. Eckersall PD, Duthie S, Safi S, Moffatt D, Horadagoda NU, Doyle S, Parton R, Bennett D, Fitzpatrick JL. An automated biochemical assay for haptoglobin: prevention of interference from albumin. Comp Haem Int. 1999;9:117–24.
28. Becker U, Bartl K, Wahlefed AW. A functional photometric assay for plasma fibrinogen. Thromb Res. 1984;1984(35):475–84.
29. Rothel JS, Jones SL, Corner LA, Cox JC, Wood PR. A sandwich enzyme immunoassay for bovine interferon gamma and its use for the detection of tuberculosis in cattle. Aust Vet J. 1990;67:134–7.
30. Kirchner M, Boxberger J. Loading of the claws and the consequences for the design of slatted floor. In: Wierenga HK, Peterse DJ, editors. Cattle housing systems, lameness and behaviour. The Netherlands: Martinus Nijhoff; 1987. p. 37.
31. Kaufmann W. Influence of the composition of the ration and the feeding frequency on pH regulation in the rumen and on feed intake in ruminants. Livest Prod Sci. 1976;3:103–14.
32. Keane MG, Drennan MJ, Moloney AP. Comparison of supplementary concentrate levels with grass silage, separate or total mixed ration feeding, and duration of finishing in beef steers. Livest Prod Sci. 2006;103:169–80.
33. Keane MG, Allen P. Effects of production system intensity on performance, carcass composition and meat quality of beef cattle. Livest Prod Sci. 1998;56:203–14.
34. Keane MG, Allen P. Effects of pasture fertiliser N level on herbage composition, animal performance and on carcass and meat quality traits. Livest Prod Sci. 1999;61:233–44.
35. Keane MG, Allen P. A comparison of Friesian-Holstein, Piemontese × Friesian-Holstein and Romagnola × Friesian-Holstein steers for beef production and carcass traits. Livest Prod Sci. 2002;78:143–58.
36. Caplis J, Keane MG, Moloney AP, O'Mara FP. Effects of supplementary concentrate level with grass silage, and separate or total mixed ration feeding, on performance and carcass traits of finishing steers. Irish J of Agric and Food Res. 2005;44:27–43.
37. Keane MG, Drennan MJ. A comparison of Friesian, Aberdeen Angus × Friesian and Belgian Blue × Friesian steers finished at pasture or indoors. Livest Sci. 2008;115:268–78.
38. Keane MG, Drennan M. Effects of supplementary concentrate level in winter, and subsequent finishing on pasture or indoors, on performance and carcass traits of Holstein-Friesian, Aberdeen Angus × Holstein-Friesian and Belgian Blue × Holstein-Friesian steers. Livest Sci. 2009;121:250–8.
39. Gygax L, Mayer C, Schulze Westerath H, Friedli K, Wechsler B. On-farm assessment of the lying behaviour of finishing bulls kept in housing systems with different floor qualities. Anim Wel. 2007;16:205–8.
40. Gygax L, Siegwart R, Wechsler B. Effects of space allowance on the behaviour and cleanliness of finishing bulls kept in pens with fully slatted rubber coated flooring. Appl Anim Behav Sci. 2007;107:1–12.
41. Andreae U, Smidt D. Behavioural alteration in young cattle on slatted floors. Hohenheimer Arbeiten. 1982;121:51–60.
42. Ruis-Heutinck LFM, Smits MCJ, Smits AC, Heeres JJ. Effects of floor type and floor area on behaviour and carpal joint lesions in beef bulls. In: Blokhuis HJ, Ekkel ED, Wechsler B, editors. Improving health and welfare in animal production, vol. 102. Wageningen: EAAP Publication; 2000. p. 29–36.
43. Andreae U. Zur Aktivita¨tsfrequenz von Mastbullen bei Spaltenbodenhaltung. Landbauforschung Vo¨lkenrode Sonderheft. 1979;48:89–94.
44. Irps H. Results of research projects into flooring preferences of cattle. In: Baxter SH, Baxter MR, MacCormack JAC, editors. Farm animal housing and welfare. The Netherlands: Martinus Nijhoff; 1983. p. 200.
45. Irps H. The influence of the floor on the behaviour and lameness of beef bulls. In: Wierenga HK, Peterse DJ, editors. Cattle housing systems, lameness and behaviour. The Netherlands: Martinus Nijhoff; 1987. p. 73.
46. O'Connell J, Giller PS, Meaney WJ. Weanling training and cubicle usage as heifers. Appl Anim Behav Sci. 1993;37:185–95.
47. Phillips CJC, Morris ID. The locomotion of dairy cows on concrete floors that are dry, wet or covered with a slurry of excreta. J Dairy Sci. 2000;83:1767–72.
48. Phillips CJC, Morris ID. The locomotion of dairy cows on floor surfaces with different frictional properties. J Dairy Sci. 2001;2001(84):623–8.
49. Phillips CJC, Morris ID. The ability of cattle to distinguish between, and their preference for, floors with different levels of friction, and their avoidance of floors contaminated with excreta. Anim Welf. 2002;11:21–9.
50. Phillips CJC, Morris ID, Lomas CA. A novel operant conditioning test to determine whether dairy cows dislike passageways that are dark or covered with slurry. Anim Welf. 2001;2001(10):65–72.
51. Webb NG, Nilsson C. Flooring and injury—an overview. In: Baxter SH, Baxter MR, MacCormack JAD, editors. Farm animal housing and welfare. The Hague: Martinus Nijhoff; 1983. p. 226–59.
52. Jerrams S. Friction and adhesion in rigid surface indentation of nitrile rubber. J Mat Des. 2005;2005:251–8.
53. Jones ML, Allison RW. Evaluation of the ruminant complete blood cell count. Vet Clin N Am Food Anim Pract. 2007;2007(23):377–402.
54. Ishikawa H, Shirahata T, Hasegawa K. Interferon-g production of mitogen stimulated peripheral lymphocytes in perinatal cows. J Vet Med Sci. 1994;56:735–8.
55. Schalm OW. Balliere tindall and cox. Covent Garden: London; 1961. p. 130–1.
56. Schalm OW. Manual of bovine haematology: Anemia's/leukocytes/testing. Santa Barbara: Veterinary Practice Publishing; 1984.
57. Radostits OM, Gay CC, Blood DC, Hinchcliff KW. Veterinary medicine: a textbook of the diseases of cattle, sheep, pigs, goats and horses. 9th ed. London: W.B. Saunders; 2000.

# 5

# Current knowledge on feline injection-site sarcoma treatment

Katarzyna Zabielska-Koczywąs*, Anna Wojtalewicz and Roman Lechowski

**Abstract**

Feline injection-site sarcomas (FISS) are malignant skin tumours of mesenchymal origin, the treatment of which is a challenge for veterinary surgeons. The role of surgery, radiotherapy and chemotherapy in FISS treatment has been studied, and a correlation between "clean" surgical margins and disease-free survival has been shown. In addition, clean surgical margins are one of the most important factors for achieving a low recurrence rate. The most effective method of FISS treatment includes combining radical surgery with pre- or postoperative radiotherapy. Chemotherapy may be used as a palliative method of treatment or may be considered an adjunctive therapy for surgery and radiotherapy. In cats with FISS without metastasis, the use of immunostimulant treatment with Oncept IL-2, intended as a complementary immunotherapy in association with surgery and brachytherapy, may also be considered to reduce the risk of relapse and increase the time to relapse. Additionally, this review focuses on recent advances in FISS treatment, including the use of novel compounds, such as doxorubicin conjugated to glutathione-stabilized gold nanoparticles, liposomal doxorubicin or tyrosine kinase inhibitors.

**Keywords:** Chemotherapy, Clean margin, Immunotherapy, Radical surgery, Radiotherapy

## Background

Feline injection-site sarcomas (FISS) are malignant skin tumours of mesenchymal origin that develop in 1–10 of every 10,000 vaccinated cats. The pathogenesis of this disease is unknown. However, the most accepted hypothesis is that a local post-vaccination (or injection) inflammatory process leads to neoplastic transformation [1]. This hypothesis is supported by histological findings of a central area of necrosis and the presence of inflammatory cells (Fig. 1a), including multinucleated giant cells (Fig. 1b), which have phagocytized a greyish-blue material consistent with the aluminium-based vaccine adjuvant in some cases [2–6].

FISS appear most frequently at the site of vaccinations, especially when vaccines against feline leukaemia virus (FeLV) or rabies have been used [4, 7–10], but the tumour may also develop after injection of various pharmaceutical substances, such as steroidal and non-steroidal anti-inflammatory drugs [8, 11, 12], lufenuron [13] and antibiotics. FISS may also develop after microchip implantation [14, 15] or as a reaction to non-absorbable surgical stitches [16]. FISS treatment is challenging because the local tumour recurrence rate ranges from 14 to 69% [17–20].

## Search strategy

This review was based on a search of the PubMed database (http://www.ncbi.nlm.nih.gov/pubmed) using the terms "feline injection-site sarcoma" OR "feline postvaccinal sarcoma" OR "feline vaccine-associated sarcoma" AND "treatment" OR "therapy". Only papers written in English were included. The abstracts of the obtained hits were evaluated, and the most relevant articles were selected based on our experience in FISS. This systematic review is a synthesis of current knowledge in the field and highlights possible novel methods of FISS treatment that warrant further investigation.

### Clinical staging for treatment decision

The first-line therapy for FISS is aggressive radical surgery. Implementing adjunctive therapies, such as radiation, chemotherapy or immunotherapy, depends on

*Correspondence: katarzyna_zabielska@sggw.pl
Department of Small Animal Diseases with Clinic, Faculty of Veterinary Medicine, Warsaw University of Life Sciences, Nowoursynowska 159c, 02-776 Warsaw, Poland

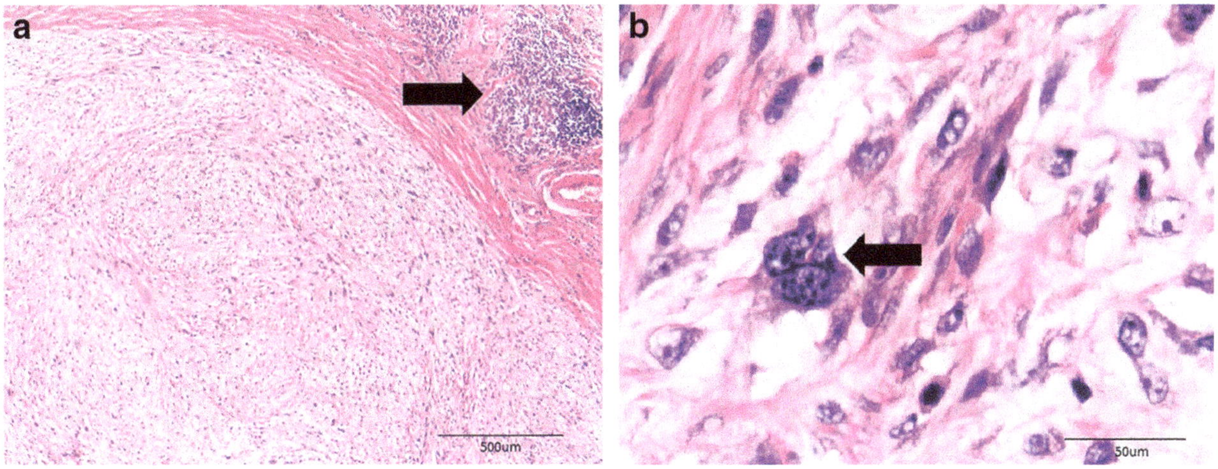


**Fig. 1** Photomicrographs of feline injection-site sarcoma. **a** An inflammatory response (*arrow*) in the peripheral part of the tumour. Haematoxylin and eosin, *bar* 500 µm. **b** A multinucleated giant cell (*arrow*). Haematoxylin and eosin, bar 50 µm

the clinical status of the patient. Initially, computed tomography (CT) or magnetic resonance imaging (MRI) should be performed to determine the actual tumour size because some studies have shown that the tumour may be much larger than estimated by physical examination [21, 22]. The staging of the tumour requires a complete blood count, a serum biochemical panel, urinalysis, 3-view thoracic radiography, lymph node examination by palpation, and ultrasonography of the abdominal cavity and cytology when applicable [23]. Thoracic radiography is performed to exclude metastases to the lungs, which occur in 10–24% of FISS cases. CT has proven useful not only in planning peripheral excision margins [16, 21, 24] but also for the patient following surgical excision because it can provide information about the area that needs to be re-excised or included in the radiation treatment field [25].

## Surgery alone

Aggressive, radical surgery or wide excision is recommended. In practice, this means surgery with at least 3 cm (preferably 5 cm) margins peripherally and one fascial plane deep into the tumour. If the tumour involves adjacent bone structures, such as the scapula, a spinous process or the pelvis, bone structures must be removed during surgery [23]. Marginal excision is rarely curative and often leads to local recurrence and is therefore not recommended. It has been shown that cats subjected to aggressive excision in the first surgery have longer tumour-free intervals than cats with marginal excision (325 days versus 79 days) [26]. It was also shown by Kaplan–Meier's product limit method that there is a significant difference in time to the first recurrence between cats treated with wide excision surgery compared to marginal excision surgery (419 days versus 66 days) [27]. After tumour excision, histopathology of the surgical margins is mandatory to ensure complete excision of the tumour.

Completeness of surgical margins is considered the most important predictive factor for FISS treatment. In a study by Cronin et al. [22], five cats with tumour cells in the margins of the resected tissue showed a median disease-free interval (DFI) of 170 days, while 26 cats with negative tumour margins showed a median DFI of 700 days ($P < 0.0001$). Using post-surgery 3D histological margin status evaluation, Giudice et al. [19] demonstrated that tumours with infiltrated margins recurred approximately 10 times more frequently than those with non-infiltrated margins ($P = 0.001$). The tumour should be resected with at least a 5 cm margin surrounding the palpable tumour edge because it prolongs the disease-free survival time from 499 to 1461 days [20]. It has also been shown that disease-free survival can be prolonged if the surgery is performed by an experienced surgeon from a referral veterinary clinic. The median time to first recurrence was found to be 274 days, compared to 64 days when the surgery was performed at a non-referral institution [27].

The owner should also be informed about the post-surgical complications that may appear. Minor complications, such as chronic constipation and pneumonia, are managed successfully by medical treatment in most cases. Major complications, such as dehiscence of the surgical incisions, e.g., when the tumour is localized in the interscapular region or laryngeal paralysis, requires a second surgical intervention and intensive care treatment.

It must be emphasized that not all tumours can be completely removed surgically, possibly due to significant tumour size or localization in the intra-scapular region with infiltration into the thoracic part of the spine or due to the poor general condition of the animal, such as phase 3 or 4 chronic renal failure.

### Adjuvant radiation

Even radical surgery may be insufficient (the recurrence rate is up to 70%, and the disease-free survival time is approximately only 6 months [4]); therefore, radiotherapy is often used pre- or postoperatively. When radiotherapy is administered prior to surgery, metastatic seeding during surgery is less likely. Kobayashi et al. [28] suggest using pre-operative radiation (using cobalt photons, 3.0 Gy in 16 daily fractions) for cats with FISS for long-term tumour control, especially in cases where tumour cells at the margin of the resected specimen are not identified. Unfortunately, these authors did not assess the influence of pre-operative irradiation on the overall survival of the cats.

On the other hand, Mayer et al. [29] have claimed, based on analysis of the medical history of 76 cats with FISS, that curative radiation therapy in combination with surgery results in long-term survival. These researchers examined the overall survival of cats after pre-operative radiation and postoperative radiation, and they showed that significantly longer overall survival was obtained for cats with postoperative radiation (705 days versus 310 days). However, they maintained that the method of selection for cats for pre-operative radiation may have biased their results.

Eckstein, in his retrospective analysis of radiation therapy in 76 cats with FISS [30], claimed that both post-surgical curative radiation (12 × 4.0 Gy delivered on a Monday–Tuesday–Thursday–Friday schedule or 12 × 5.0 Gy delivered on a Monday–Wednesday–Friday schedule) and coarse fractionated radiotherapy (4 fractions of 8.0 Gy each administered once a week) were effective.

Cronin et al. [22] performed a study on 33 cats with histopathologically confirmed FISS treated with radiation therapy followed by surgery. They showed that obtaining only a negative tumour margin significantly ($P < 0.001$) prolonged DFI (median DFI of 700 days versus 112 days in cats with tumour cells at the margin). All other factors, such as tumour volumes, number of prior tumour excisions and various descriptors of the radiation therapy techniques, played no role in prolonging DFI.

Cohen et al. [31] analysed the medical records of 50 cats with FISS that underwent surgery and electron beam radiation (13 fractions of 400 Gy, given each Monday, Wednesday and Friday); in contrast to the results obtained by Cronin et al. [22], they identified an association between tumour size, the number of prior tumour excisions, median survival time or DFI. Moreover, Cohen et al. [31] showed that the size of tumours before the first surgery was correlated with the median survival time (smaller tumours had longer survival times). In addition, DFI and survival time decreased as the time between surgery and the start of radiotherapy increased. Moreover, the time between the onset of the disease and the initiation of the radiotherapy influenced the survival time, as cats that started radiotherapy earlier showed a longer survival time. On the other hand, while the number of surgical procedures did not influence the median survival time, this factor was crucial for DFI; cats that underwent only one surgery had a longer DFI than cats with more than one surgery (median DFI 469 days and 345 days, respectively). The 1-year and 2-year survival rates were 86 and 44%, respectively.

Nolan et al. [32] analysed the medical records of cats with FISS (each cat had complete local and systemic staging, including CT-based planning) that underwent surgery together with stereotactic body radiation therapy (SBRT) (ranging from 24 to 35 Gy delivered in 3 to 5 fractions either on consecutive or alternative days). These authors concluded that SBRT may be used as a palliative treatment or may be considered for use prior to surgery to downstage the disease. However, their study had some limitations, such as a small population of heterogeneous patients (11 cats), various radiation doses and protocols as well as the lack of a control group of additional anti-cancer treatments after SBRT.

Despite the fact that radiotherapy combined with radical surgery seems to be the most efficient therapy for FISS, the short- and long-term side effects of radiotherapy should be considered prior to the decision to administer treatment. The short-term effects of radiation that appear within a few weeks after the completion of a course of fractionated radiotherapy include dermatological changes (e.g., skin erythema, mucositis) and gastrointestinal tract disorders (e.g., vomiting, diarrhoea) [33]. Some of the early side effects may also be iatrogenic due to inappropriately performed radiation, e.g., skin necrosis due to prolonged exposure or excessive radiation dose. Radiotherapy should therefore be performed only by qualified veterinary surgeons. Although rarely described in veterinary medicine, long-term radiation toxicity effects, such as fibrosis, atrophy, vascular damage, neural damage and a range of endocrine and growth-related effects, are well documented in human medicine [33]. Because these long-term side effects appear mostly within months to years after radiation, the lack of information about them in cats with FISS is likely due to a lack of studies on the long-term monitoring of the health status of cats or their survival times being too short. Thus, studies monitoring the long-term health conditions of cats with FISS that received radiotherapy are needed. Minimal side effects were observed after brachytherapy and SBRT, which indicates that these represent the safest methods of radiotherapy.

### Role of chemotherapy in combined treatment

Chemotherapy should not be used as monotherapy, although it may be considered a palliative treatment or in an adjuvant or neoadjuvant setting in a multimodal approach. Cytostatic drugs that have been used in FISS treatment include doxorubicin, ifosfamide, carboplatin, cyclophosphamide, mitoxantrone and vincristine. However, the effectiveness of chemotherapy in the treatment of FISS remains debatable. One of the most significant issues concerning the interpretation of results from clinical trials assessing the effectiveness of chemotherapy for FISS treatment is that these studies were performed on a very small number of cats. The results of a phase II clinical trial of FISS treatment with ifosfamide (900 mg/m$^2$ body surface area IV, administered twice with a 3-week interval), showing that 11 of 27 cats showed a complete or partial response, suggest that this drug may serve as an efficient adjuvant treatment [34].

### Doxorubicin in multimodal FISS treatment

The results of studies performed in the USA on 71 cats after partial excision of FISS and radiotherapy show a markedly longer remission time in patients that were additionally treated with doxorubicin administered between three to five times at 3-week intervals than in patients with no doxorubicin therapy. Furthermore, the study indicated a definite prolonged remission time in patients treated with doxorubicin, which provided a better quality of life for those patients [35]. Administration of doxorubicin did not, however, prolong the disease-free survival time.

Moreover, when comparing the results of a randomized, multicentre study on 108 cats with FISS treated with either doxorubicin or liposomal doxorubicin (Caelyx) to a historical control group of cats with FISS treated with surgery alone, the cats receiving chemotherapy showed prolonged DFI (388 versus 93 days) [36]. In a pilot study including 10 cats with advanced FISS, it was shown that liposomal doxorubicin used with palliative daily fraction radiotherapy could also be used as a depot radiosensitizer [37]. Additionally, in a study performed on 12 cats with non-resectable FISS, combining doxorubicin with cyclophosphamide resulted in a partial response in 50% of cats and significant improvement in the survival time of responders [38]. Moreover, it has been demonstrated that doxorubicin used in neoadjuvant chemotherapy combined with anatomical resection of the tumour and muscle compartment prolongs both DFI and the tumour-free survival time [39].

A few studies have shown that adding doxorubicin treatment to surgery and radiotherapy or postoperative electron beam therapy has no influence on disease-free survival time, lifetime and tumour remission [17, 31, 40]. However, those studies included small numbers of animals and have low power. As a result, doxorubicin is considered to be the drug of choice for FISS treatment if a patient is classified for adjuvant chemotherapy.

The main impediments to doxorubicin administration, however, are the side effects related to its poor biodistribution and high toxicity. Doxorubicin has a short drug half-life and it is taken up by the mononuclear phagocyte system as quickly as 5 min after intra-venous administration, which leads to a lower drug concentration in the tumour. Moreover, doxorubicin administration in cats causes anaemia, myelosuppression and nephrotoxicity [36]. As a result, cats with diseases such as chronic renal failure, haemolytic anaemia, autoimmune-mediated anaemia or various bone marrow disorders are excluded from doxorubicin administration. New substances, which will overcome these limitations, are under investigation.

### Preclinical trials

In vitro studies have shown good cytotoxic effects of doxorubicin, vincristine, mitoxantrone and paclitaxel in FISS cell lines [41, 42]. However, the results of in vitro studies do not always correlate with those of in vivo studies.

Masitinib, which is a selective and efficient tyrosine kinase inhibitor due to binding at c-Kit, PDGFR and Lyn, has shown an anti-proliferative effect in two FISS cell lines [43]. Nevertheless, in further studies, when it was used together with radiotherapy, it has not enhanced sensitivity to radiation in FISS cells [44]. Further clinical studies to assess Masitinib effectiveness are needed, although studies on the other tyrosine kinase inhibitor Toceranib, which was registered for canine mast cell tumour treatment, on 18 cats failed to show efficacy for FISS treatment [45].

Liposomal doxorubicin (Caelyx), both in vitro and in vivo using a xenograft murine model, was found to be efficient in combination with radiotherapy for adjuvant treatment of FISS. Animals that received combined therapy (Caelyx 3 mg/kg and radiation 2 × 3.5 Gy or Caelyx 3 mg/kg and radiation 2 × 5 Gy) showed significantly smaller tumour sizes than the control groups [46].

Our results demonstrated that glutathione-stabilized gold nanoparticles non-covalently modified with doxorubicin (Au-GSH-Dox) could enhance the anti-tumour efficacy of free doxorubicin in FISS cell lines with high P-glycoprotein activity (the main efflux pump responsible for multidrug resistance and one of the reasons for ineffective chemotherapy treatment) [47]. The results of in vitro studies confirmed by *in ovo* studies were significant ($P < 0.001$), and the reduction in tumour size was visible after a single intra-tumoural injection of Au-GSH-Dox [48]. Furthermore, a chick embryo chorioallantoic membrane (CAM) model was established by our group to expand knowledge of the biological behaviour of FISS and to screen novel anticancer agents [48, 49].

However, to confirm the efficacy of Caelyx, Au-GSH-Dox or Masitinib, further in vivo studies should be performed.

### Immunotherapy

A recombinant canarypox virus (ALVAC) expressing feline interleukin-2 (IL-2) (an important T cell stimulatory cytokine approved as an exogenous anti-tumour agent) is approved for use as adjunctive immunotherapy after surgery and brachytherapy for primary FISS in cats without enlarged lymph nodes and lung metastasis. This treatment should be administered in five subcutaneous injections in the region of the sutures after tumour excision, which may cause some controversy due to the pathogenesis of the disease. However, the efficiency and safety of ALVAC (6 consecutive doses of less than $10^{6.5}$ $EAID_{50}$ ALVAC IL-2 in the low-dose group and up to $10^{8.9}$ $EAID_{50}$ ALVAC IL-2 in the high-dose group, which was initially given 6 times once a week and then every 2 weeks (e.g., days 0, 7, 14, 21, 35, and 49), with the first dose administered on the day before radiotherapy as an adjunct therapy for surgery and brachytherapy (4 fractions at 6.5 Gy on day 1, day 1 + 8 h, day 3, and day 3 + 8 h), has been demonstrated over a 1-year follow-up period. In a study performed on 71 cats with primary FISS, the authors demonstrated one of the highest DFI values (>765 days) reported thus far in FISS [50]. This veterinary medicinal product (Oncept IL-2, Merial) has been successfully registered in most European countries.

## Conclusions

The selection of treatment for FISS depends on the clinical staging of the disease. Performing CT or MRI is recommended as an additional diagnostic tool to assess the actual size of the tumour and exclude metastasis. The most effective method of FISS treatment includes combining radical surgery with pre- or postoperative radiotherapy. Histological margin determination is the most important predictive factor for FISS, and resecting tumours with clear margins significantly prolongs DFI. Chemotherapy may be used as a palliative method of treatment or may be considered, depending on the condition of the animal, as adjunctive therapy for surgery and radiotherapy. Doxorubicin seems to be the drug of choice, although there remains insufficient evidence regarding its efficacy. In cats with FISS without metastasis, the use of immunostimulant treatment with Oncept IL-2 as a complementary immunotherapy, in association with surgery and brachytherapy, may also be considered to reduce the risk of relapse and increase the time to relapse. However, this vaccine is not a classical vaccine and is not intended for prophylactic use or to stimulate specific active immunity.

Good co-operation between first-stage veterinary doctors, veterinary oncologists, veterinary surgeons from reference clinics and histopathologists, who assess for clear margins (the main prognostic factor), is essential for complete management of cats with FISS.

#### Abbreviations

ALVAC: recombinant canarypox virus; Au-GSH-Dox: glutathione-stabilized gold nanoparticles conjugated to doxorubicin; CAM: chorioallantoic membrane; CT: computed tomography; DFI: disease-free interval; FeLV: feline leukaemia virus; FISS: feline injection-site sarcoma; IL-2: interleukin-2; IV: intravenously; MRI: magnetic resonance imaging; SBRT: stereotactic body radiation therapy.

#### Authors' contributions

KZK performed the literature review and drafted the manuscript. AW and RL contributed to the final manuscript. All authors read and approved the final manuscript.

#### Authors' information

KZ-K is assistant professor and a veterinary specialist in feline and canine diseases. Her Ph.D. thesis and postdoctoral research focuses on a novel method of FISS treatment, specifically the use of gold nanoparticles as drug carriers, and she has overseen several grant projects within this area. AW is a Ph.D. student, and her studies focuses on FISS treatment and multidrug resistance in FISS. RL is a professor and a specialist in feline and canine diseases. He has published numerous studies on feline and canine internal diseases, especially in the field of veterinary oncology.

#### Acknowledgements

We acknowledge Cerys Evans for the English language support. We would also like to acknowledge the professional manuscript services of American Journal Experts. We would like to thank Dr. Izabella Dolka from the Warsaw University of Life Sciences for providing Fig. 1.

#### Competing interests

The authors declare that they have no competing interests.

#### Funding

We acknowledge the support of the National Science Centre (UMO-2015/17/D/NZ5/04241). The author's experiments cited in this paper were supported by the Polish National Science Centre Project DEC-2012/07/N/NZ4/02413.

#### References

1. Hartmann K, Day MJ, Thiry E, Lloret A, Frymus T, Addie D, et al. Feline injection-site sarcoma ABCD guidelines on prevention and management. J Feline Med Surg. 2015;17:606–13.
2. Hendrick MJ, Goldschmidt MH. Do injection site reactions induce fibrosarcomas in cats? J Am Vet Med Assoc. 1991;199:968.
3. Hendrick MJ, Goldschmidt MH, Shofer FS, Wang Y-Y, Somlyo AP. Postvaccinal sarcomas in the cat: epidemiology and electron probe microanalytical identification of aluminum1. Cancer Res. 1992;52:5391–4.
4. Hendrick MJ, Brooks JJ. Postvaccinal sarcomas in the cat: histology and immunohistochemistry. Vet Pathol. 1994;31:126–9.
5. Couto SS, Griffey SM, Duarte PC, Madewell BR. Feline vaccine-associated fibrosarcoma: morphologic distinctions. Vet Pathol. 2002;39:33–41.

6. Saba CF. Vaccine-associated feline sarcoma: current perspectives. Vet Med Res Rep. 2017;8:13–20.
7. Kass PH, Barnes WG, Spangler WL, Chomel BB, Culbertson MR. Epidemiologic evidence for a causal relation between vaccination and fibrosarcoma tumorigenesis in cats. J Am Vet Med Assoc. 1993;203:396–405.
8. Kass PH, Spangler WL, Hendrick MJ, McGill LD, Esplin DG, Lester S, et al. Multicenter case-control study of risk factors associated with development of vaccine-associated sarcomas in cats. J Am Vet Med Assoc. 2003;223:1283–92.
9. Macy DW. The potential role and mechanisms of FeLV vaccine-induced neoplasms. Semin Vet Med Surg (Small Anim). 1995;10:234–7.
10. Dean R, Adams V, Whitbread T, Scase T, Dunham S, Mellor D, et al. Study of feline injection site sarcomas. Vet Rec. 2006;159:641–2.
11. Munday JS, Banyay K, Aberdein D, French AF. Development of an injection site sarcoma shortly after meloxicam injection in an unvaccinated cat. J Feline Med Surg. 2011;13:988–91.
12. Martano M, Morello E, Iussich S, Buracco P. A case of feline injection-site sarcoma at the site of cisplatin injections. J Feline Med Surg. 2012;14:751–4.
13. Esplin DG, Bigelow M, McGill LD, Wilson SR. Fibrosarcoma at the site of a Lufenuron injection in a cat. Vet Cancer Soc Newsl. 1999;23:8–9.
14. Carminato A, Vascellari M, Marchioro W, Melchiotti E, Mutinelli F. Microchip-associated fibrosarcoma in a cat. Vet Dermatol. 2011. doi:10.1111/j.1365-3164.2011.00975.x.
15. Daly MK, Saba CF, Crochik SS, Howerth EW, Kosarek CE, Cornell KK, et al. Fibrosarcoma adjacent to the site of microchip implantation in a cat. J Feline Med Surg. 2008;10:202–5.
16. Buracco P, Martano M, Morello E, Ratto A. Vaccine-associated-like fibrosarcoma at the site of a deep nonabsorbable suture in a cat. Vet J. 2002;163:105–7.
17. Martano M, Morello E, Ughetto M, Iussich S, Petterino C, Cascio P, et al. Surgery alone versus surgery and doxorubicin for the treatment of feline injection-site sarcomas: a report on 69 cases. Vet J. 2005;170:84–90.
18. Romanelli G, Marconato L, Olivero D, Massari F, Zini E. Analysis of prognostic factors associated with injection-site sarcomas in cats: 57 cases (2001–2007). J Am Vet Med Assoc. 2008;232:1193–9.
19. Giudice C, Stefanello D, Sala M, Cantatore M, Russo F, Romussi S, et al. Feline injection-site sarcoma: recurrence, tumour grading and surgical margin status evaluated using the three-dimensional histological technique. Vet J. 2010;186:84–8.
20. Phelps HA, Kuntz CA, Milner RJ, Powers BE, Bacon NJ. Radical excision with five-centimeter margins for treatment of feline injection-site sarcomas: 91 cases (1998–2002). J Am Vet Med Assoc. 2011;239:97–106.
21. Travetti O, di Giancamillo M, Stefanello D, Ferrari R, Giudice C, Grieco V, et al. Computed tomography characteristics of fibrosarcoma—a histological subtype of feline injection-site sarcoma. J Feline Med Surg. 2013;15:488–93.
22. Cronin K, Page RL, Spodnick G, Dodge R, Hardie EN, Price GS, et al. Radiation therapy and surgery for fibrosarcoma in 33 cats. Vet Radiol Ultrasound. 1998;39:51–6.
23. Séguin B. Feline injection site sarcomas. Vet Clin N Am Small Anim Pract. 2002;32:983–95.
24. Ferrari R, Di Giancamillo M, Stefanello D, Giudice C, Grieco V, Longo M, et al. Clinical and computed tomography tumour dimension assessments for planning wide excision of injection site sarcomas in cats: How strong is the agreement? Vet Comp Oncol. 2015. doi:10.1111/vco.12173.
25. McEntee MC, Page RL. Feline Vaccine-Associated Sarcomas. J Vet Intern Med. 2001;15:176–82.
26. Davidson EB, Gregory CR, Kass PH. Surgical excision of soft tissue fibrosarcomas in cats. Vet Surg. 1997;26:265–9.
27. Hershey AE, Sorenmo KU, Hendrick MJ, Shofer FS, Vail DM. Prognosis for presumed feline vaccine-associated sarcoma after excision: 61 cases (1986–1996). J Am Vet Med Assoc. 2000;216:58–61.
28. Kobayashi T, Hauck ML, Dodge R, Page RL, Price GS, Williams LE, et al. Preoperative radiotherapy for vaccine associated sarcoma in 92 cats. Vet Radiol Ultrasound. 2002;43:473–9.
29. Mayer MN, Treuil PL, Larue SM. Radiotherapy and surgery for feline soft tissue sarcoma. Vet Radiol Ultrasound. 2009;50:669–72.
30. Eckstein C, Guscetti F, Roos M, de Las Martín Mulas J, Kaser-Hotz B, Rohrer Bley C. A retrospective analysis of radiation therapy for the treatment of feline vaccine-associated sarcoma. Vet Comp Oncol. 2009;7:54–68.
31. Cohen M, Wright JC, Brawner WR, Smith AN, Henderson R, Behrend EN. Use of surgery and electron beam irradiation, with or without chemotherapy, for treatment of vaccine-associated sarcomas in cats: 78 cases (1996–2000). J Am Vet Med Assoc. 2001;219:1582–9.
32. Nolan MW, Griffin LR, Custis JT, LaRue SM. Stereotactic body radiation therapy for treatment of injection-site sarcomas in cats: 11 cases (2008–2012). J Am Vet Med Assoc. 2013;243:526–31.
33. Bentzen SM. Preventing or reducing late side effects of radiation therapy: radiobiology meets molecular pathology. Nat Rev Cancer. 2006;6:702–13.
34. Rassnick KM, Rodrigues CO, Khanna C, Rosenberg MP, Kristal O, Chaffin K, et al. Results of a phase II clinical trial on the use of ifosfamide for treatment of cats with vaccine-associated sarcomas. Am J Vet Res. 2006;67:517–23.
35. Hahn KA, Endicott MM, King GK, Harris-King FD. Evaluation of radiotherapy alone or in combination with doxorubicin chemotherapy for the treatment of cats with incompletely excised soft tissue sarcomas: 71 cases (1989–1999). J Am Vet Med Assoc. 2007;231:742–5.
36. Poirier VJ, Thamm DH, Kurzman ID, Jeglum KA, Chun R, Obradovich JE, et al. Liposome-encapsulated doxorubicin (Doxil) and doxorubicin in the treatment of vaccine-associated sarcoma in cats. J Vet Intern Med. 2002;16:726–31.
37. Kleiter M, Tichy A, Willmann M, Pagitz M, Wolfesberger B. Concomitant liposomal doxorubicin and daily palliative radiotherapy in advanced feline soft tissue sarcomas. Vet Radiol Ultrasound. 2010;51:349–55.
38. Barber L, Sorenmo K, Cronin K, Shofer F. Combined doxorubicin and cyclophosphamide chemotherapy for nonresectable feline fibrosarcoma. J Am Anim Hosp Assoc. 2000;36:416–21.
39. Bray J, Polton G. Neoadjuvant and adjuvant chemotherapy combined with anatomical resection of feline injection-site sarcoma: results in 21 cats. Vet Comp Oncol. 2014. doi:10.1111/vco.12083.
40. Bregazzi VS, LaRue SM, McNiel E, Macy DW, Dernell WS, Powers BE, et al. Treatment with a combination of doxorubicin, surgery, and radiation versus surgery and radiation alone for cats with vaccine-associated sarcomas: 25 cases (1995–2000). J Am Vet Med Assoc. 2001;218:547–50.
41. Williams LE, Banerji N, Klausner JS, Kapur V, Kanjilal S. Establishment of two vaccine-associated feline sarcoma cell lines and determination of in vitro chemosensitivity to doxorubicin and mitoxantrone. Am J Vet Res. 2001;62:1354–7.
42. Banerji N, Li X, Klausner JS, Kapur V, Kanjilal S. Evaluation of in vitro chemosensitivity of vaccine-associated feline sarcoma cell lines to vincristine and paclitaxel. Am J Vet Res. 2002;63:728–32.
43. Lawrence J, Saba C, Gogal R, Lamberth O, Vandenplas ML, Hurley DJ, et al. Masitinib demonstrates anti-proliferative and pro-apoptotic activity in primary and metastatic feline injection-site sarcoma cells. Vet Comp Oncol. 2011;10:143–54.
44. Turek M, Gogal R, Saba C, Vandenplas ML, Hill J, Feldhausser B, et al. Masitinib mesylate does not enhance sensitivity to radiation in three feline injection-site sarcoma cell lines under normal growth conditions. Res Vet Sci. 2014;96:304–7.
45. Holtermann N, Kiupel M, Hirschberger J. The tyrosine kinase inhibitor toceranib in feline injection site sarcoma: efficacy and side effects. Vet Comp Oncol. 2016. doi:10.1111/vco.12207.
46. Petznek H, Kleiter M, Tichy A, Fuchs-Baumgartinger A, Hohenadl C. Murine xenograft model demonstrates significant radio-sensitising effect of liposomal doxorubicin in a combination therapy for feline injection site sarcoma. Res Vet Sci. 2014;97:386–90.
47. Wójcik M, Lewandowski W, Król M, Pawłowski K, Mieczkowski J, Lechowski R, et al. Enhancing anti-tumor efficacy of doxorubicin by non-covalent conjugation to gold nanoparticles—in vitro studies on feline fibrosarcoma cell lines. PLoS ONE. 2015;10:e0124955. doi:10.1371/journal.pone.0124955.

6

# The usefulness of uterine lavage and acute phase protein levels as a diagnostic tool for subclinical endometritis in Icelandic mares

Monika Sikora[1*], Jarosław Król[2], Marcin Nowak[2], Tadeusz Stefaniak[3], Gudmar Aubertsson[4] and Roland Kozdrowski[1]

**Abstract**

**Background:** Endometritis is a common problem in a broodmare practice, often leading to infertility. The diagnosis is based on several methods such as cytology, bacteriology and histopathology; however the outcome of these methods may be inconclusive even when used together. The objectives of this study were: (1) to investigate the usefulness of acute phase proteins as an additional diagnostic tool for diagnosis of subclinical endometritis in mares and (2) to evaluate the association between macroscopic changes in uterine flushes and inflammation of the uterus. Materials were collected from 53 Icelandic mares with subclinical endometritis. Endometrial swabs and uterine lavage for cytological and bacteriological examinations and two endometrial biopsies were taken. Blood samples were collected 12–24 h after ovulation to determine the concentrations of serum amyloid A and haptoglobin in the 53 subfertile mares and, for comparison, from 20 non-pregnant mares that later conceived.

**Results:** Twenty-five mares were classified as positive for endometritis based on endometrial biopsy, which was used as the 'gold standard'. We observed a correlation between cloudy efflux in the lavage and (1) polymorphonuclear cell (PMN) infiltration of the endometrium ($P = 0.031$), (2) positive cytology in samples obtained by cotton swabs ($P = 0.019$) and uterine lavage ($P = 0.011$), and (3) positive microbiology from samples obtained by cotton swabs ($P = 0.001$) and uterine lavage ($P = 0.047$). The degree of agreement between PMN infiltration and positive cytology from samples taken by cotton swabs and uterine lavage was fair to moderate. We found no association between the concentration of acute phase proteins and infiltration of the endometrium by PMNs, or with positive results of cytological and microbiological examinations.

**Conclusions:** Measurement of serum amyloid A and haptoglobin was not proven useful for diagnosis of subclinical endometritis in Icelandic mares. Macroscopic changes in the fluid collected by lavage were not consistently indicative of infection, but when present they indicate inflammation in the uterus with a high probability.

**Keywords:** Mare, Endometritis, Efflux, Acute phase proteins

## Background

Inflammation of the endometrium is one of the main causes of reduced fertility in the mare [1]. According to published data, it is the third most important clinical problem in horses after colic and respiratory diseases [2].

Traditionally, the diagnosis of endometritis is based on history, clinical findings and results of microbiological, cytological and histopathological examinations [3]. A detailed history of infertility can provide many important clues. LeBlanc and Causey reported that a short inter-estrus interval may already indicate the presence of

*Correspondence: monika.sikora88@gmail.com
[1] Department of Reproduction and Clinic of Farm Animals, Faculty of Veterinary Medicine, Wroclaw University of Environmental and Life Sciences, Plac Grunwaldzkistreet 49, 50366 Wroclaw, Poland

abnormalities in the uterus [3]. Detection of intrauterine fluid is an indicator for clinical endometritis, however this sign may be absent in subclinical cases of endometritis [3, 4]. Subclinical endometritis has been described as a 'hidden' endometritis in mares, which did not show the typical signs of endometritis such as accumulation of fluid in the uterus [3].

The breeding season of mares is regulated by photoperiod because lengthening of days activates their reproductive system. Conditions for the domestic maintenance of horses in Iceland are broadly very similar to the natural situation. Foaling takes place in the field and should happen in the early summer to allow foals to reach a reasonable size before winter. Therefore, the timely diagnosis and effective treatment of infertility are very important for successful breeding in Iceland.

Traditionally in Iceland, the mares are covered by a stallion in a harem, without human intervention. In recent times, artificial insemination and hand mating have become popular, allowing deeper observation of infertility in these mares; however, no report is available on the causes of infertility in Icelandic horses.

One of many methods used both for treatment of endometritis and to collect samples from the uterus for cytological and microbiological examinations is uterine lavage (UL). LeBlanc et al. [5] and Christoffersen et al. [6] used a low volume flush, infusing 60 and 250 ml of fluid, respectively, into the uterus. After centrifuging the recovered fluid, the supernatant was decanted and the pellets were used for cytological and microbiological examinations.

Endometrial biopsy is internationally recognized as a reliable, risk-free and meaningful method for diagnosing endometritis and for prognostic evaluation of endometrial conditions in the mare [7]. However, the long waiting time for test results makes it inappropriate for immediate treatments [4, 8, 9]. Routinely, in practice only one biopsy is collected, but results obtained from a single biopsy sample may be misleading. A study performed after slaughter showed that a single biopsy is not enough to determine the severity of degenerative changes in the mare uterus with sufficient accuracy [10]. Another post mortem study revealed that evaluation of inflammation using both cytological and histological techniques does not give the same results in different sampling sites [11].

In many cases, despite negative results obtained from cytology, microbiology and histopathology, the mare still could not become pregnant.

Acute phase proteins (APP) are sensitive, but not specific, systemic markers of inflammation [12]. Serum amyloid A (SAA) is a protein that increases rapidly, with larger amplitude (>100-fold) changes after tissue injury, infection or inflammation. The concentration of SAA in healthy horses is very low or undetectable and ranges from <0.5 to 20 mg/l [13, 14]. Haptoglobin (Hp) is already present in blood plasma of healthy horses (0.2–1 g/l) and its concentration increases only 1–10 times during inflammation [14]. Tuppits et al. [15] found no differences in the concentrations of APP before and after artificial insemination. However, Christoffersen et al. [16] observed a transient increase of SAA concentration after intrauterine infusion with a high dose of *Escherichia coli* during diestrus. In contrast to these results, Christoffersen et al. [1] found no changes in plasma concentrations of SAA after inoculation with lower doses of *E. coli* during estrus and these differences appear to be both dose-dependent and cycle-related. Krakowski et al. [17] suggested that high concentrations of SAA and Hp prior to ovulation and insemination may be an indicator of latent subclinical endometritis, which cannot be diagnosed by ultrasonography. This suggested to us the need to examine the usefulness of APP levels as an additional tool for diagnosing subclinical endometritis.

The aim of this study was to evaluate the usefulness of uterine lavage with 1 l physiological saline and measurement of APP as a diagnostic tool for subclinical endometritis in Icelandic mares. In this study, the concentrations of SAA and Hp in blood collected from barren and fertile mares were examined to evaluate the usefulness of this test.

## Methods

### Mares

All samples were collected from Icelandic Horse mares, in estrus, during one breeding season from May to August 2014 in Dýralæknir Sandhólaferja Veterinary Clinic, Hella in Iceland.

Our study group consisted of 53 mares, aged from 3 to 25 (12.34 ± 5.72) years, with a history of infertility. All these mares were suspected for subclinical endometritis. They were qualified for the study based on the following criteria: they had been bred three or more times unsuccessfully in the same breeding season, or had a history of a minimum of 1 year's reproductive failure. All the mares were in estrus, ultrasound examination of the reproductive tract showed no intrauterine fluid and no discharge from the vagina was observed. All were clinically healthy, they were kept under the same conditions and none was previously treated for endometritis.

### Control group

The control group comprised 20 fertile mares of the Icelandic Horse breed, which became pregnant after insemination or natural covering. All these mares were clinically healthy, kept under the same conditions and had no history of infertility. In this group, blood samples were collected to determine the concentrations of SAA and Hp in healthy, fertile mares that subsequently became pregnant after insemination. All of the mares were in estrus, with no intrauterine fluid observed in the ultrasound examination and no discharge from the vagina. All mares were evaluated by transrectal palpation and ultrasonography at intervals of 24 h to assess the time of ovulation. Blood samples were collected 12–24 h after ovulation. Fifteen days after ovulation, a pregnancy check was performed with ultrasound. From the material collected, only plasma samples that came from mares diagnosed positively for pregnancy were used for determination of SAA and Hp. Twenty mares were diagnosed as pregnant 15 days after ovulation, and in blood plasma from these mares the concentrations of SAA and Hp were determined. The concentrations of SAA and Hp taken from 53 barren mares were compared with their levels in 20 non-pregnant mares that later conceived. This comparison was used to investigate differences in the concentrations of APP in barren mares and in healthy, fertile mares that achieved pregnancy at the first attempt.

#### Sample collection

All mares were examined while restrained in stocks. The sample collections were performed after a complete reproductive assessment of the mares, including evaluation of the external genital tract and manual transrectal palpation as well ultrasonography examinations (using Ge Logiq Book XP, USA) of the reproductive tract to determine cycle stage and to exclude intrauterine fluid. During examination of the external genital tract, in all of these mares 80 % of the labia lengths were below the pelvic brim. Afterwards, the tail was bandaged, the vulva and the perineum were cleaned with povidone-iodine (Betadine®-Polyvidonum iodinatum, MEDA Pharma S.p.A., Milan, Italy) and dried with a paper towel and samples were always collected in the same order: swab, lavage and biopsies.

#### Cotton swabs

First, for cytological and bacteriological examinations, material from the uterus was collected using a double-guarded uterine cotton swab (CS; Minitube, Tiefenbach, Germany). The cotton swab was inserted into the uterus by manually passing it through the cervix. The tip of the swab was hidden in the hand and the labia were spread by additional staff to minimize infection by vaginal and vulvar skin flora. The procedure for sample collection by cotton swabs was carried out as described by Walter et al. [18].

#### Uterine lavage

Then, uterine lavage (UL) was performed using a commercial sterile uterus flushing tube (EQUIVET Uterine Flushing Tube Sterile; Kruuse, Denmark). The sterile catheter for UL was manually passed into the uterus and 1 l of sterile physiological saline warmed to 38 °C was infused from a bag into the uterus. The fluid was allowed to become distributed within the uterus and then collected into the same bag by gravity flow. The recovered fluid volume and color were recorded as described below and the bag was hung for sedimentation by gravity for at least 1 h. The clarity of the recovered fluid was recorded according to LeBlanc et al. [5] and was graded as clear, cloudy, efflux with debris (mucus stains) and efflux with blood (from pink to red coloration). Then, 50 ml of efflux was aspirated from the bottom of the bag, which was previously disinfected with alcohol, by puncturing it with a sterile needle into a 50 ml tube and centrifuged at ×400*g* for 10 min. The supernatant was decanted and the sediment was used for cytological and bacteriological examinations.

#### Endometrial biopsies

After lavage, two endometrial biopsies (EB) were taken from the dorsal wall of the base of each uterine horn (left and right) and fixed in 10 % formalin for histopathological examination. The biopsies were collected using a sterilized biopsy punch (Equi-Vet, Kruuse, Denmark) that was manually passed through the cervix and then directed into the left and right horns with a finger and through rectal manipulation with the other hand. The biopsies were always taken in the same order: first from the left and then from the right horn. The endometrial biopsies were immediately fixed and sent to the Department of Pathology at the Wroclaw University of Environmental and Life Sciences in Poland, where histopathological examination for inflammation of the endometrium was performed.

#### Blood sample collections

Blood samples were collected once from 12 to 24 h after ovulation from the external jugular vein into 10 ml heparinized tubes. From each mare, 10 ml of blood was collected into heparinized tubes and centrifuged at ×800*g* for 10 min. Then the serum was transferred to 2 ml microcentrifuge tubes, stored at −20 °C and sent on dry ice to the Department of Immunology, Pathophysiology and Veterinary Preventive Medicine at the Wroclaw University of Environmental and Life Sciences in Poland, where the concentration of APP was determined.

#### Examination of samples

Cytological smears were performed on cellular material collected using cotton swabs and from a sterile swab that was placed into the sediment obtained from uterine flushing. The swabs were rolled onto a sterile microscope glass and air-dried. The smears were stained using Diff-Quick stain (Medion Diagnostics AG, Duedinden, Switzerland) and examined with light microscopy under oil immersion (1000× magnification) for the presence of polymorphonuclear cell (PMN). We counted 300 cells in each sample. When PMN cells represented more than 2 % of all cells in the sample, it was considered positive for endometritis [11, 19–21]. The samples collected by CS and UL were evaluated according to the same criteria.

Next, the same samples that had been used for cytology were placed on a blood agar (bioMérieux, France, supplemented with 5 % defibrinated sheep blood), MacConkey Agar (bioMérieux) and Sabouraud Dextrose Agar (Oxoid, UK) for microbiological examination. The media were incubated aerobically at 37 °C for 24 h and the growth of microorganisms was recorded. Negative plates were incubated further and re-examined after 48 and 72 h for the presence of bacteria and yeasts. Then the plates were stored in a refrigerator and sent chilled to the Department of Pathology at the Wroclaw University of Environmental and Life Sciences, Poland, where microbiological examination was conducted. Isolated bacteria were preliminarily identified based on colony characteristics and cell morphology, Gram staining, hemolytic activity and a catalase test. Gram-positive and catalase-positive cocci were further examined using the ID 32 STAPH identification system (bioMérieux). Gram-positive rods were identified by means of the API CORYNE kit (bioMérieux), and Gram-negative ones using conventional biochemical reactions (acid production from glucose and lactose, and indole, urease and $H_2S$ tests).

If more than 90 % of the colonies on a given plate were identical, they were considered as a positive and pure culture [22]. Mixed cultures of three or more microorganisms were regarded as contaminations and recorded as a negative growth result [21, 23]. Non-pathogenic bacteria were recorded only if isolated in pure culture [5].

Formalin-fixed biopsies were cut into 4 μm sections and stained with eosin and hematoxylin. Evaluation was performed under light microscopy for infiltration by PMN and eosinophils of the endometrial luminal epithelium and the *stratum compactum*. Samples were considered positive for acute endometritis if three or more PMN per five fields (400× magnification, BX53 optical microscope Olympus, Tokyo, Japan) were found in at least one of the biopsies [5, 6, 24] and we also evaluated the infiltration of the *stratum compactum* and *stratum spongiosum* by eosinophils using similar criteria.

The concentrations of SAA were assessed using the Multispecies SAA ELISA Kit (Tridelta Development, TP 802, Ireland) according to the manufacturer's instructions. All samples were analyzed in duplicate. The absorbance was read at a wavelength of 450 nm using 630 nm as a reference with a Biotek μQuant reader (BioTek Instruments Inc., Winooski, VT, USA). The intra- and inter-assay CVs were 2.1 and 5.2 %, respectively. The concentration of Hp was determined by the guaiacol method according to Jones and Mould [25]. The intra-assay CV was 10.4 % and the inter-assay CV was 13.5 %.

#### Statistical analysis

For statistical analysis, we used Fisher's Exact test and the Chi square test. The significance level was set at $P < 0.05$. Sensitivity and specificity were calculated using the PMN infiltration in endometrial biopsies as the 'gold standard'. Sensitivity was calculated as the proportion of mares with PMN infiltration in biopsies and a positive result from the compared tests (CS and UL). Specificity was calculated as the proportion of mares with no PMN infiltration of the endometrium and a negative result from the compared tests (CS and UL). A positive predictive value was calculated from the proportion of mares with PMN infiltration of the endometrium among the positive results in the compared tests (CS and UL). A negative predictive value was calculated as the proportion of mares with negative histology among the negative results in the compared tests (CS and UL) [23]. Cohen's coefficient (*k*) was calculated to evaluate the agreement of PMN infiltration in biopsy samples taken from the left and the right horn and the positive results of cytology and bacteriology from samples obtained by CS and UL as well as changes in the appearance of the efflux. Agreement was designated as follows: poor if $k \leq 0.2$, fair if $0.21 < k < 0.41$, moderate if $0.41 < k < 0.6$, substantial if $0.61 < k < 0.8$; and good if $k > 0.8$ [11, 26].

### Results

#### Histopathology

A total of 106 endometrial biopsies obtained from two locations were examined and PMN infiltration of the endometrium was present in 25 of 53 mares (47.2 %). Only 10 of the 25 mares with PMN infiltration of the endometrium (40 %) exhibited an increase of PMN in both biopsies that were collected from the base of each horn. Fifteen mares (60 %) had infiltration of PMN in only one horn (12 mares—left horn, 3 mares—right horn). We also observed that 25 of the subfertile mares had an eosinophil infiltration (three or more eosinophils per five high magnification fields at ×400) in at least one biopsy but only in 14 mares was this correlated with PMN infiltration of endometrium. Eleven mares had eosinophilic infiltration of the endometrium, but without PMN infiltration.

### Cytology

Positive results of cytological examination were observed in nine of 53 samples collected by lavage (17 %) and in five of 53 obtained by swabs (9.4 %, Table 1). Six samples showing the presence of PMN on cytology slides were correlated with positive results of the bacteriological examination. We observed a statistically significant relationship between PMN infiltration of the endometrium and positive cytology in samples collected by cotton swab ($P = 0.02$) and those obtained from uterine lavage ($P = 0.0001$). The sensitivity, specificity, positive predictive values (PPV) and negative predictive values (NPV) and the agreement ($k$) between PMN infiltration of the endometrium in samples obtained from the left and right uterine horns are shown in Table 1. The agreement ($k$) between PMN infiltration and positive cytology in samples obtained from CS was fair and we did not find differences between biopsies taken from the left and right uterine horns. However, the agreement between positive cytology obtained from UL and PMN infiltration of the endometrium was moderate in biopsies taken from the right uterine horn and only fair in biopsies obtained from the left horn.

### Microbiology

Microorganisms were isolated from six of 53 uterine lavages (11.3 %) and from nine of 53 swabs (17 %, Table 1). In three mares, positive bacteriological results were confirmed in samples collected by both CS and UL: in two cases we found *Staphylococcus* spp. and in one case *E. coli.* The most frequently isolated bacteria in samples collected by endometrial swabs were β-hemolytic streptococci isolated from five of nine (55.5 %) and *Staphylococcus* spp. in three of nine (33.3 %). *E. coli* as well as *Micrococcus* spp. were isolated from one of nine uterine swabs. The most common micro-organisms isolated from uterine lavages were *Staphylococcus* spp. isolated from three of six lavages (50 %) and *E. coli* from two of six (33.3 %). These two organisms were isolated from 83.3 % of the positive flush cultures. In one lavage we isolated *Corynebacterium* spp. (one of six lavages). The presence of bacteria and its relationship to positive cytology and histology results are presented in Table 2. We observed no significant relationship between PMN infiltration of the endometrium and positive results of microbiological examination from samples obtained by CS and UL, but there was a statistically significant relationship between positive cytology and positive microbiology in samples collected by endometrial swabs ($P = 0.03$). The Cohen's ($k$) coefficient between positive bacteriology results from samples obtained by CS and UL and PMN infiltration of the endometrium in samples obtained from both the left and right uterine horns was usually only poor or fair, and we observed differences between the biopsy samples taken from the left and right uterine horns. The sensitivity, specificity, PPV, NPV and $k$ agreement are presented in Table 1.

**Table 1 Results of cytology and bacteriology in relation to PMN infiltration of the endometrium**

| Sampling technique | | Histo+ | Histo− | Total | Sens | Spec | PPV | NPV | $k$ left horn | $k$ right horn |
|---|---|---|---|---|---|---|---|---|---|---|
| CS | Cul+ | 6 | 3 | 9 | 0.24 | 0.893 | 0.667 | 0.568 | 0.192 | 0.204 |
| | Cul− | 19 | 25 | 44 | | | | | | |
| | Total | 25 | 28 | 53 | | | | | | |
| UL | Cul+ | 5 | 1 | 6 | 0.20 | 0.964 | 0.833 | 0.574 | 0.131 | 0.315 |
| | Cul− | 20 | 27 | 47 | | | | | | |
| | Total | 25 | 28 | 53 | | | | | | |
| CS | Cyt+ | 5 | 0 | 5 | 0.20 | 1.00 | 1.00 | 0.583 | 0.256 | 0.228 |
| | Cyt− | 20 | 28 | 48 | | | | | | |
| | Total | 25 | 28 | 53 | | | | | | |
| UL | Cyt+ | 9 | 0 | 9 | 0.360 | 1.00 | 1.00 | 0.636 | 0.277 | 0.431 |
| | Cyt− | 16 | 28 | 44 | | | | | | |
| | Total | 25 | 28 | 53 | | | | | | |

Positive cytological result from smears => 2 % PMNs of 300 cells (×1000); positive histological results from biopsies => 3 PMNs/5 fields (×400)

*PMN* polymorphonuclear cells, *Cul±* culture positive/negative, *Cyt±* cytology positive/negative, *Histo±* histopathology positive/negative (PMN infiltration in endometrium/no PMN infiltration in the endometrium), *CS* cotton swab, *UL* uterine lavage, *Sens* sensitivity, *Spec* specificity, *PPV* positive predictive values, *NPV* negative predictive values, *k* left/right horn- agreement between the number of PMN in biopsies samples taken from the left/right horn and the positive cytology and bacteriology in the compared tests (CS and UL)

**Table 2 Presence of bacteria according to results of cytological examination and PMN infiltration of the endometrium**

| Microorganisms | Cotton swab | | | | Uterine lavage | | | | Total |
|---|---|---|---|---|---|---|---|---|---|
| | Cyt+ | Cyt− | Histo+ | Histo− | Cyt+ | Cyt− | Histo+ | Histo− | |
| *Staphylococcus spp.* | 1 | 2 | 2 | 1 | 1 | 2 | 2 | 1 | 6 |
| β-hem. *Streptococcus* | 3 | 2 | 3 | 2 | 0 | 0 | 0 | 0 | 5 |
| *Escherichia coli* | 0 | 1 | 1 | 0 | 1 | 1 | 2 | 0 | 3 |
| *Micrococcus* spp. | 0 | 1 | 1 | 0 | 0 | 0 | 0 | 0 | 1 |
| *Corynebacterium* spp. | 0 | 0 | 0 | 0 | 1 | 0 | 1 | 0 | 1 |

*Cyt+/-* cytology positive/negative, *Histo±* histopathology positive/negative, *PMN* polymorphonuclear cells

Relationships among

(i) macroscopic evaluation of the efflux and
(ii) PMN infiltration of the endometrium, and
(iii) positive results of cytological and bacteriological examination.

The collected lavage fluid was assessed for its volume, color and transparency as described earlier. On average we recovered 960 ± 38 ml of fluid. We observed a statistically significant relationship between infiltration of the endometrium by PMN and cloudy efflux ($P = 0.031$), but there were no statistically significant relationships between clear efflux, efflux with blood or with debris and the presence of PMN in the endometrial biopsies. The sensitivity, specificity, positive and negative predictive values (PPV and NPV) and agreement (*k*) between the infiltration of PMN in endometrial biopsies taken from the left and right uterine horns are presented in Table 3.

### Acute phase proteins (serum amyloid A and haptoglobin)

SAA concentrations are shown in Fig. 1. In the subfertile group, the level of SAA varied widely, and in nine mares it reached very high concentrations (from 37.26 to 595.71 mg/l), whereas in the other subfertile mares it did not exceed 20 mg/l.

In the healthy mares from the control group, the concentration of SAA was uniform and in most cases, its level did not exceed the limit or was almost undetectable (on average 1.85 ± 2.04 mg/l, maximum 6.49 mg/l). As Fig. 2 shows, in the subfertile group 18.9 % of samples were above the norm, compared to the fertile mares in which no cases were reported.

The concentration of Hp was more constant than SAA in both groups. The Hp concentration on average was 1.27 ± 1.046 g/l in the subfertile mares and 1.13 ± 0.58 g/l in the fertile mares; these values were not significantly different.

Twelve out of 53 subfertile mares showed positive results in the bacteriological tests, but only in three mares was this associated with increased levels of SAA and Hp (*E. coli*, *Staphylococcus* spp., *Micrococcus* spp.).

## Discussion

Uterine lavage with 1 l of fluid or more is often performed for treatment of endometritis. LeBlanc et al. [5] and Christoffersen et al. [6] used a low-volume flush for diagnosing endometritis (60 and 250 ml, respectively), but the aim of our work was to demonstrate the usefulness of flushing with 1 l as a diagnostic method for endometritis.

In the present study, the sensitivity of cultures from uterine lavage was 0.20, much lower than the

**Table 3 Diagnostic evaluation of the efflux**

| Efflux | Sensitivity | Specificity | PPV | NPV | *k* left horn | *k* right horn |
|---|---|---|---|---|---|---|
| Clear | 0.160 | 0.643 | 0.286 | 0.462 | Negative values | |
| Cloudy | 0.440 | 0.857 | 0.733 | 0.632 | 0.307 | 0.322 |
| With debris | 0.680 | 0.607 | 0.607 | 0.680 | 0.327 | 0.156 |
| With blood | 0.400 | 0.536 | 0.435 | 0.500 | Negative values | |

Sensitivity, specificity, positive and negative predictive values (PPV and NPV) and the agreement (*k*) between the number of polymorphonuclear cells (PMN) infiltrated into the endometrial luminal epithelium and *stratum compactum* and type of efflux

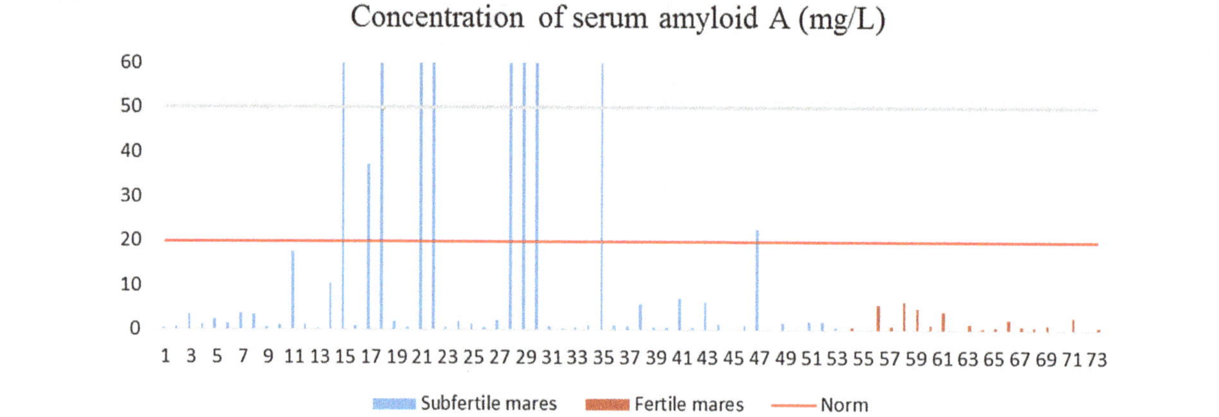


**Fig. 1** The concentration of SAA in the subfertile and fertile mares. The subfertile mares are numbered from 1 to 53 and the fertile mares are numbered from 54 to 73. Permissible norm of serum amyloid A (SAA) is from 0.5 to 20 mg/l

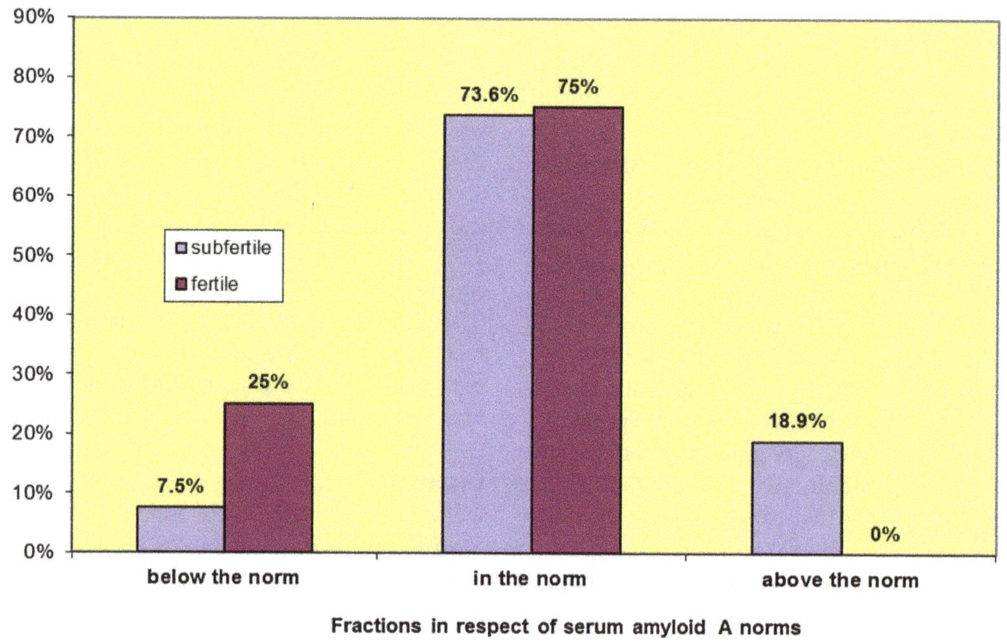


**Fig. 2** Fractions in respect of serum amyloid A norms. Below the norm (<0.5 mg/l), within the norm (0.5–20 mg/l), or above the norm (>20 mg/l), and as a group: subfertile and fertile mares

sensitivity levels reported by Christoffersen et al. [6] and LeBlanc et al. [5], which were 0.75 and 0.72, respectively. The lower sensitivity of the microbiology tests in our study compared to results of those reports could be due to the high dilution by fluid used for uterine lavage in our work. The low isolation of cultures may indicate either a natural resistance of Icelandic mares to uterine infections, or the good conditions for maintenance of these horses in a country involving very limited use of antibiotics in the treatment of reproductive disorders.

Christoffersen et al. [6] used a double-guarded lavage system and compared the sensitivity of samples obtained by CS, UL and biopsy. They found that the sensitivity from lavages was much higher than that from biopsies for microbiological evaluation but much lower for cytological examination. In our study, the sensitivity of cytology (0.36) obtained from UL was higher than the sensitivity (0.08) reported by Christoffersen et al. [6] using double-guarded lavage.

The bacteria most frequently isolated from UL in the study from LeBlanc et al. [5] were *E. coli* and beta-hemolytic streptococci, however, in our study the most common micro-organisms isolated from uterine flushes were *Staphylococcus* spp. followed by *E. coli.* LeBlanc et al. [5] reported that bacteria were isolated from about 45 % of the clear efflux samples and cloudy and mucoid effluxes were highly associated with isolation of bacteria. In our study, all of the clear effluxes had negative bacteriology and we did not find a correlation between the macroscopic evaluation of the recovered fluid and the type of microorganism. However, we found statistically significant relationships between a cloudy efflux and PMN infiltration of the endometrium, positive cytology and isolation of bacteria.

LeBlanc et al. [5] considered that the flushing should be regarded as contaminated if the bacteriological evaluation was positive, cytology was negative and no PMN infiltration in the endometrial biopsies was observed. In our study, all flushes from which bacteria were isolated had clarity changes and eleven of 15 cloudy effluxes (73.3 %) were associated with PMN infiltration of the endometrium. Usually, if three or more cultures are isolated, the sample is classified as having contamination [21, 23] and is recorded as a negative. In our study, mixed infections with beta-hemolytic *Streptococcus* and *Staphylococcus* spp. were found only in one CS. Overbeck et al. [11] compared five different sampling locations for collections with cytological brushes and observed that eight of 10 positive-scored uteri had both positive and negative locations for endometritis. When a large volume of liquid is infused into the uterus during lavage, it fills the entire interior of the uterus and becomes exposed to a larger surface area. Although we isolated more bacteria using CS than with lavages, the sensitivity of cytology from samples using UL was higher than from CS. Riddle et al. [27] reported that endometrial cytology identified twice as many mares with endometritis as did endometrial culture. In turn, Nielsen et al. [22] who compared cytological and bacteriological examination from two different laboratories, pointed out the importance of performing both bacteriological and cytological evaluation in diagnosis of endometritis. Moreover, Kozdrowski et al. [20] reported that the method used for cytological evaluation influences the results, and using criteria based on counting the numbers of PMN in relation to epithelial cells they found that the best cut-off point indicating endometritis is 2 % of PMN. The same criteria were also used by Overbeck et al. [11, 21].

Infiltration by PMN into the luminal epithelium and *stratum compactum* is used as the reference standard for diagnosis of endometritis [4, 5, 11, 20, 21, 23, 28]. Nielsen et al. [28] found that the infiltration of PMN into the endometrium was correlated with the 70-day pregnancy rates, in contrast to cytological evaluation, which was not correlated. Routinely in practice, only one biopsy sample is collected. Fiala et al. [10] in their study performed after slaughter concluded that only one biopsy is not enough to verify the quantity of degenerative changes in the uterus. Overbeck et al. [11], in a post mortem study using cytological brushes and endometrial biopsies, observed that the inflammation process is not the same in different uterine locations. In the present study, all of the mares were in estrus and only 10 of 25 mares with positive histology (40 %) showed increased PMN in both biopsies. Thus, fifteen of 25 mares with PMN infiltration (60 %) would not have been diagnosed as positive for endometritis if only one biopsy had been taken. The present authors agree with the opinion of Overbeck et al. [11] that it is critical to take more than one sample under clinical conditions.

Endometrial infiltration of eosinophils was found in biopsies of 25 infertile mares. Blumenthal et al. [29] in their study on endometriosis in women showed that eosinophils are involved in tissue remodeling and wound healing. They also pointed out that fibrosis is associated with eosinophil degranulation. Several older studies [30–33] affirmed that eosinophils are involved in tissue remodeling in the uterus of estrogen-treated rats and mice. Adegboyega et al. [34] observed a relationship between eosinophils and chronic endometritis in women. The authors showed that 73 % of endometrial biopsies with eosinophil infiltration should have been diagnosed as chronic endometritis, because immunohistochemical examination revealed the presence of plasma cells, which is consistent with chronic endometritis, but they did not find a statistically significant correlation between the number of eosinophils and the presence of plasma cells. In our opinion, eosinophilic infiltration is more in line with the assumptions from the studies of Adegboyega et al. [34] and Blumenthal et al. [29] than with the estrogen hypothesis, because all of the mares in our study were in estrus and only a few had increased eosinophils in the endometrium. The lack of control biopsies from fertile mares precludes us from explaining if the cycle stage and inflammation of the uterus have an influence on eosinophil infiltration in the mare endometrium.

In a study involving microscopic examination of endometrial biopsies from retired sports mares, Kilgenstein et al. [35] found only 3 % of 189 mares exhibited eosinophilic endometritis. Wehrend et al. [36] studied the distribution of eosinophils and mast cells in cervical tissue in mares and observed that eosinophils are present in the *lamina propria mucosa* and *tunica muscularis*. The authors concluded that eosinophils are part of the local cellular immune system of the equine cervix. We think that eosinophils may perform similar functions in the uterus as in the cervix. Kenney [37] and Schiemann et al.

[38] suspected that pneumovagina and some other irritation causes infiltration by eosinophils. However, abnormal formation of the vulva was not detected in mares in our study, so in our opinion, the presence of eosinophils in the mare endometrium is not always connected with pneumovagina or with irritation of the endometrium.

The utility of APP as systemic markers of inflammation in horses has been studied by many authors, in response to EED, in mares with experimentally induced ascending placentitis or influenza, or as prognostic indicators for horses with inflammatory disease [17, 39–41]. Jacobsen and Andersen [14] described diseases and disease states accompanied by increased blood levels of SAA in horses. In our study, SAA and Hp levels in blood samples were examined as a potential indicator of uterine health in mares with subclinical endometritis. Krakowski et al. [17] suggested that high levels of APP already present before ovulation may be an indication of infertility in mares and could be used as an early indicator of subclinical endometritis. In contrast to the above mentioned studies, Tuppits et al. [15] did not find differences in SAA, Hp and Fb concentrations over time before and after artificial insemination. Christoffersen et al. [1] showed that plasma concentration of SAA in response to intrauterine inoculation of *E. coli* appears to be dose-dependent. Moreover, Christoffersen et al. [16] observed that during diestrus all experimental mares had increased SAA in blood samples 24 h post inoculation (pi). In our study, *E. coli* was isolated from two mares but only one of these mares showed a large increase in SAA. Tuppits et al. [15] hypothesized that the ability of local inflammation in the uterus to cause a systemic APP reaction depends on the estrous cycle stage during the inflammation and on the influence of progesterone and estrogens. The different results of these studies may depend on different cycle stages of the mares or different post-inoculation times after which blood samples were collected. Brodzki et al. [42] found that levels of SAA and Hp were higher in cows with subclinical endometritis. Nash et al. [43] found no increase of SAA 24 h after treatment but there was a high level of SAA in two cases both before and after treatment, which may be an indicator for another ongoing disease in the mares.

In our study, the concentrations of SAA and Hp were measured in blood samples collected once from 12 to 24 h after ovulation in subfertile and fertile mares and we did not find an association between APP concentrations and infertility of mares. Just as Nash et al. [43] described, we also found high concentrations of SAA in a few mares, which may perhaps suggest another inflammatory process occurring in the mares that may or may not indirectly affect infertility.

## Conclusions

The usefulness of SAA and Hp concentrations as a markers for subclinical endometritis in mares could not be conclusively demonstrated. The high concentrations found in a few cases were not associated with subclinical endometritis. Probably, they are an indication of another ongoing disease in the mares.

The association of cloudy lavage efflux and isolation of bacteria may point to a practical aspect of uterine lavage. While changes in the fluids collected are not always indicative of infection, they can indicate inflammatory changes occurring within the uterus with a high probability. We conclude that if cloudy efflux or debris is seen in the lavage fluid, when 1 l of fluid is used, the mare has endometritis and requires treatment.

### Abbreviations

APP: acute phase proteins; CS: cotton swab; Cul±: microbiology positive/negative; CV: coefficient of variation; Cyt±: cytology positive/negative; EB: endometrial biopsy; EED: early embryonic death; Fb: fibrinogen; Histo±: histopathology positive/negative; Hp: haptoglobin; *k*: Cohen's coefficient agreement; NPV: negative predictive values; pi: post inoculation; PMN: polymorphonuclear cells; PPV: positive predictive values; SAA: serum amyloid A; Sens: sensitivity; Spec: specificity; UL: uterine lavage.

### Authors' contributions

All authors were involved in discussing and interpreting the data described in this study. MS contributed to sample collection, cytological analysis, analysis of the results and writing the manuscript. JK contributed by microbiological examination. MN contributed by histopathological examination. TS contributed by determination of SAA and Hp. GA provided the opportunity to conduct this research in his clinic, contributed to conceiving the study and sample collection, as well as assisting with paperwork. RK contributed in conceiving the study, sample collection, cytological analysis, analysis of the results and writing the manuscript. All authors read and approved the final manuscript.

### Author details

[1] Department of Reproduction and Clinic of Farm Animals, Faculty of Veterinary Medicine, Wroclaw University of Environmental and Life Sciences, Plac Grunwaldzkistreet 49, 50366 Wroclaw, Poland. [2] Department of Pathology, Faculty of Veterinary Medicine, Wroclaw University of Environmental and Life Sciences, C. K. Norwidastreet 31, 50375 Wroclaw, Poland. [3] Department of Immunology, Pathophysiology and Veterinary Preventive Medicine, Faculty of Veterinary Medicine, Wroclaw University of Environmental and Life Sciences, C. K. Norwidastreet 31, 50375 Wroclaw, Poland. [4] Dýralæknir Sandhólaferja, 851 Hella, Iceland.

### Acknowledgements

This research was supported by statutory research and development activity funds assigned to Faculty of Veterinary Medicine, Wroclaw University of Environmental and Life Sciences.

The authors are indebted to Dr. Barry Bavister for help with editing this manuscript.

### Competing interests

The authors declare that they have no competing interests.

**References**


1. Christoffersen M, Woodward E, Bojesen AM, Jacobsen S, Petersen MR, Troedsson MHT, Lehn-Jensen H. Inflammatory responses to induced infectious endometritis in mares resistant or susceptible to persistent endometritis. BMC Vet Res. 2012;8:41.
2. Traub-Dargatz JL, Salman MD, Voss JL. Medical problems of adult horses as ranked by equine practitioners. J Am Vet Res. 1991;198:1745–7.
3. LeBlanc MM, Causey RC. Clinical and subclinical endometritis in the mare: both threats to fertility. Reprod Domest Anim. 2009;44(Suppl 3):10–22.
4. Buczkowska J, Kozdrowski R, Nowak M, Raś A, Staroniewicz Z, Siemieniuch MJ. Comparison of the biopsy and cytobrush techniques for diagnosis of subclinical endometritis in mares. Reprod Biol Endocrinol. 2014;12:27.
5. LeBlanc MM, Magsig J, Stromberg AJ. Use of a low-volume uterine flush for diagnosing endometritis in chronically infertile mares. Theriogenology. 2007;68:403–12.
6. Christoffersen M, Brandis L, Samuelsson J, Bojesen AM, Troedsson MHT, Petersen MR. Diagnostic double-guarded low-volume uterine lavage in mares. Theriogenology. 2015;83:222–7.
7. Schoon HA, Schoon D, Klug E. Die Endometriumbiopsie bei der Stute im klinisch-gynaekologischen Kontext. Pferdeheilkunde. 1997;13:453–64.
8. Ricketts SW, Barrelet A. A retrospective review of the histopathological features seen in a series of 4241 endometrial biopsy samples collected from UK Thoroughbred mares over a 25 year period. Pferdeheilkunde. 1997;13:525–30.
9. Snider TA, Sepoy C, Holyoak GR. Equine endometrial biopsy reviewed: observation, interpretation and application of histopathologic data. Theriogenology. 2011;75:1567–81.
10. Fiala SM, Esmeraldino A, Jobim MIM, Garbade P, Wolf CA, Richter G, Gregory RM, Mattos RC. Endometrial fibrotic changes. Is one biopsy enough to diagnose degenerative changes? Anim Reprod Sci. 2010;121(Suppl):89–90.
11. Overbeck W, Jäger K, Schoon H-A, Witte TS. Comparison of cytological and histological examinations in different locations of the equine uterus-an in vitro study. Theriogenology. 2013;79:1262–8.
12. Cray C, Belgrave RL. Haptoglobin quantitation in serum samples from clinically normal and clinically abnormal horses. J Equine Vet Sci. 2014;34:337–40.
13. Crisman MV, Scarratt WK, Zimmerman KL. Blood proteins and inflammation in the horse. Vet Clin North Am Equine Pract. 2008;24:285–97.
14. Jacobsen S, Andersen PH. The acute phase protein serum amyloid A (SAA) as a marker of inflammation in horses. Equine Vet Educ. 2007;19:38–46.
15. Tuppits U, Orro T, Einarsson S, Kask K, Kavak A. Influence of the uterine inflammatory response after insemination with frozen-thawed semen on serum concentrations of acute phase proteins in mares. Anim Reprod Sci. 2014;146:182–6.
16. Christoffersen M, Baagoe CD, Jacobsen S, Bojesen AM, Petersen MR, Lehn-Jensen H. Evaluation of the systemic acute phase response and endometrial gene expression of serum amyloid A and pro- and anti-inflammatory cytokines in mares with experimentally induced endometritis. Vet Immunol Immunop. 2010;138:95–105.
17. Krakowski L, Krawczyk CH, Kostro K, Stefaniak T, Novotny F, Obara J. Serum levels of acute phase proteins: SAA, Hp and progesterone (P4) in mares with early embryonic death. Reprod Domest Anim. 2011;46:624–9.
18. Walter J, Neuberg KP, Failing K, Wehrend A. Cytological diagnosis of endometritis in the mare: investigations of sampling techniques and relation to bacteriological results. Anim Reprod Sci. 2012;132:178–86.
19. Ball BA, Shin SJ, Pattern VH, Lein DH, Woods GL. Use of a low-volume uterine flush for microbiologic and cytologic examination of the mare's endometrium. Theriogenology. 1988;29:1269–83.
20. Kozdrowski R, Sikora M, Buczkowska J, Nowak M, Raś A, Dzięcioł M. Effects of cycle stage and sampling procedure on interpretation of endometrial cytology in mares. Anim Reprod Sci. 2015;154:56–62.
21. Overbeck W, Witte TS, Heuwieser W. Comparison of three diagnostic methods to identify subclinical endometritis in mares. Theriogenology. 2011;75:1311–8.
22. Nielsen JM, Troedsson MH, Pedersen MR, Bojesen AM, Lehn-Jensen H, Zent WW. Diagnosis of endometritis in the mare based on bacteriological and cytological examinations of the endometrium: comparison of results obtained by swabs and biopsies. J Equine Vet Sci. 2010;30:27–30.
23. Nielsen JM. Endometritis in the mare: a diagnostic study comparing cultures from swab and biopsy. Theriogenology. 2005;64:510–8.
24. Ricketts SW, Alonso S. Assessment of the breeding prognosis of mares using paired endometrial biopsy techniques. Equine Vet J. 1991;23:185–8.
25. Jones GE, Mould DL. Adaptation of Guaiacol (peroxidase) test for haptoglobins to microtitration plate system. Res Vet Sci. 1984;37:87–92.
26. Cocchia N, Paciello O, Auletta L, Uccello V, Silvestro L, Mallardo K, Paraggio G, Pasolini MP. Comparison of cytobrush, cotton swab, and low-volume uterine flush techniques to evaluate endometrial cytology for diagnosing endometritis in chronically infertile mares. Theriogenology. 2012;77:89–98.
27. Riddle WT, LeBlanc MM, Stromberg AJ. Relationships between uterine culture, cytology and pregnancy rates in a Thoroughbred practice. Theriogenology. 2007;68:395–402.
28. Nielsen JM, Nielsen FH, Peersen MR. Diagnosis of equine endometritis—microbiology, cytology and histology of endometrial biopsies and correlation to fertility. Pferdeheilkunde. 2012;28:8–13.
29. Blumenthal RD, Samoszuk M, Taylor AP, Brown G, Alisauskas R, Goldenberg DM. Degranulating eosinophils in human endometriosis. Am J Pathol. 2000;156:1581–8.
30. Brokelmann J, Fawcett D. The localization of endogenous peroxidase in the rate uterus and its induction by estradiol. Biol Reprod. 1969;1:59–71.
31. Bassett E. Infiltration of eosinophils into the modified connective tissue of oestrus and pregnant animals. Nature. 1962;194:1259–61.
32. Bergman F, Damber M, Linden U, Paul K. Mast cells and eosinophil granulocytes in the oestrogen-stimulated mouse uterus. Acta Endocrinol. 1972;69:77–86.
33. King W, Alen T, DeSombre E. Localization of uterine peroxidase activity in estrogen-treated rats. Biol Reprod. 1981;25:859–70.
34. Adegboyega PA, Pei Y, McLarty J. Relationship between eosinophils and chronic endometritis. Hum Pathol. 2012;41:33–7.
35. Kilgenstein HJ, Schoeniger S, Schoon D, Schoon HA. Microscopic examination of endometrial biopsies of retired sports mares: an explanation for the clinically observed subfertility? Res Vet Sci. 2015;99:171–9.
36. Wehrend A, Huchzermeyer S, Bostedt H. Distribution of eosinophils and mast cells in the cervical tissue of non-gravid mares during dioestrus. Reprod Dom Anim. 2005;40:562–3.
37. Kenney RM. Cyclic and pathologic changes of the mare endometrium as detected by biopsy, with a note on early embryonic death. J Am Vet Med Assoc. 1978;172:241–62.
38. Schiemann V, Bartmann CP, Kirpal G, von Reiswitz A, Schoon H-A, Klug E. Diagnostic hysteroscopy in the mare- uterine contamination and endometrial reaction. Pferdeheilkunde. 2001;17:557–64.
39. Coutinho da Silva MA, Canisso IF, MacPherson ML, Johnson AEM, Divers TJ. Serum amyloid A concentration in healthy periparturient mares and mares with ascending placentitis. Equine Vet J. 2013;45:619–24.
40. Hulten C, Sandgren B, Skioldebrand E, Klingeborn B, Marhaug G, Forsberg M. The acute phase protein serum amyloid A (SAA) as an inflammatory marker in equine influenza virus infection. Acta Vet Scand. 1999;40:323–33.
41. Westerman TL, Tornquist SJ, Foster CM, Poulsen KP. Evaluation of serum amyloid A and haptoglobin concentrations as prognostic indicators for horses with inflammatory disease examined at a tertiary care hospital. Am J Vet Res. 2015;76:882–8.
42. Brodzki P, Kostro K, Krakowski L, Marczuk J. Inflammatory cytokine and acute phase protein concentrations in the peripheral blood and uterine washings of cows with subclinical endometritis in the late postpartum period. Vet Res Commun. 2015;39:143–9.
43. Nash DM, Sheldon IM, Herath S, Lane EA. Markers of uterine innate immune response of the mare. Anim Reprod Sci. 2010;119:31–9.

7

# Efficacy of rabies vaccines in dogs and cats and protection in a mouse model against European bat lyssavirus type 2

Tiina Nokireki[1*], Miia Jakava-Viljanen[1], Anna-Maija Virtala[2] and Liisa Sihvonen[1,2]

**Abstract**

**Background:** Rabies is preventable by pre- and/or post-exposure prophylaxis consisting of series of rabies vaccinations and in some cases the use of immunoglobulins. The success of vaccination can be estimated either by measuring virus neutralising antibodies or by challenge experiment. Vaccines based on rabies virus offer cross-protection against other lyssaviruses closely related to rabies virus. The aim was to assess the success of rabies vaccination measured by the antibody response in dogs (n = 10,071) and cats (n = 722), as well as to investigate the factors influencing the response to vaccination when animals failed to reach a rabies antibody titre of ≥ 0.5 IU/ml. Another aim was to assess the level of protection afforded by a commercial veterinary rabies vaccine against intracerebral challenge in mice with European bat lyssavirus type 2 (EBLV-2) and classical rabies virus (RABV), and to compare this with the protection offered by a vaccine for humans.

**Results:** A significantly higher proportion of dogs (10.7%, 95% confidence interval CI 10.1–11.3) than cats (3.5%; 95% CI 2.3–5.0) had a vaccination antibody titre of < 0.5 IU/ml. In dogs, vaccination with certain vaccines, vaccination over 6 months prior the time of antibody determination and vaccination of dogs with a size of > 60 cm or larger resulted in a higher risk of failing to reach an antibody level of at least 0.5 IU/ml. When challenged with EBLV-2 and RABV, 80 and 100% of mice vaccinated with the veterinary rabies vaccine survived, respectively. When mice were vaccinated with the human rabies vaccine and challenged with EBLV-2, 75–80% survived, depending on the booster. All vaccinated mice developed sufficient to high titres of virus-neutralising antibodies (VNA) against RABV 21–22 days post-vaccination, ranging from 0.5 to 128 IU/ml. However, there was significant difference between antibody titres after vaccinating once in comparison to vaccinating twice (P < 0.05).

**Conclusions:** There was a significant difference between dogs and cats in their ability to reach a post vaccination antibody titre of ≥ 0.5 IU/ml. Mice vaccinated with RABV-based rabies vaccines were partly cross-protected against EBLV-2, but there was no clear correlation between VNA titres and cross-protection against EBLV-2. Measurement of the RABV VNA titre can only be seen as a partial tool to estimate the cross-protection against other lyssaviruses. Booster vaccination is recommended for dogs and cats if exposed to infected bats.

**Keywords:** Antibody, EBLV-2, Lyssavirus, Protection, Rabies, Vaccination

## Background

Rabies is a fatal encephalomyelitis caused by lyssaviruses. Rabies virus (RABV) causes about 99% of all rabies cases in humans, mostly in Asia and Africa. Even though the case fatality is almost 100%, the disease can be prevented by pre-exposure vaccination and by post-exposure treatment shortly after exposure. Pre-exposure vaccination can prevent the disease, but booster vaccination upon exposure is required to ensure that the immune system responds optimally [1]. Thirteen other lyssavirus species have been accepted by the International Committee on Taxonomy of Viruses, and two additional species have

*Correspondence: tiina.nokireki@evira.fi
[1] Finnish Food Safety Authority Evira, Mustialankatu 3, 00790 Helsinki, Finland

been identified. Phylogenetic analysis and the virus–host relationship suggest that all 16 currently identified species of lyssaviruses can be divided into phylogroups. Phylogroup I comprises RABV, Duvenhage virus, European bat lyssavirus types 1 and 2 (EBLV-2), Australian bat lyssavirus, Aravan virus, Khujand virus, Irkut virus and Bokeloh bat lyssavirus, whereas Lagos bat virus, Mokola virus and Shimoni bat virus form phylogroup II [2, 3]. West Caucasian bat virus, Ikoma lyssavirus and Lleida bat lyssavirus may be representatives of possible new phylogroups [4–6]. Gannoruwa bat lyssavirus probably belongs to phylogroup I [7].

Human infections usually result from the bite of a rabid dog infected with RABV [1]. However, in a small number of cases, the infection results from contact with bats [8]. Two confirmed human cases caused by European bat lyssavirus type 2 (EBLV-2), one in Finland in 1985 [9, 10] and one in the UK in 2002 [11] have been reported. EBLV-2 is known to associate with two closely related *Myotis* bat species, Daubenton's (*Myotis daubentonii*) and pond bats (*M. dascyneme*). EBLV-2 has sporadically been isolated from Daubenton's bats in the Netherlands [12], Switzerland [13], the UK [14], Finland [15, 16], Germany [17], Denmark [18] and Norway [19]. Finland was declared a rabies-free country by the OIE in 1991. Nevertheless, rabies can remain a residual risk to public health due to the natural circulation of EBLV-2 [15, 16]. Spillovers from chiropters to carnivores are not unusual, and at least two spillovers of RABV from bats to carnivore hosts have occurred, which have succeeded in being maintained through time [20, 21]. No spillover infections to other mammals than humans have been detected for EBLV-2. In experimental infections, EBLV-2 has been shown to cause fatal disease in foxes [22], sheep [23] and mice [24, 25]. European bat lyssavirus type 1 (EBLV-1), however, has been detected in natural infections of stone martens (*Martes foina*) [26], sheep [27] and domestic cats [28].

The assessment of rabies vaccine efficacy [1, 29, 30] is usually undertaken by immunisation and virus challenge using laboratory animals (potency test). The efficacy of vaccination can be indirectly assessed by measuring antibodies from serum. Cellular immunity, however, is also important in clearing a virus infection [31]. Virus-neutralising antibody assays are used to verify that an immune response has occurred. An internationally accepted threshold titre of 0.5 IU/ml has been adopted [1]. However, it has been shown that vaccinated animals with low antibody levels have survived RABV challenge, indicating that other immune mechanisms also protect against rabies infection. On the other hand, according to Aubert [32], the presence of detectable neutralising antibodies against rabies at the time of challenge does not indicate protection for all animals. Nevertheless, animals with neutralising antibodies at the time of challenge are significantly better protected against RABV than those without detectable virus neutralizing antibodies (VNA) [32, 33]. Information on the protection and cross-protection efficacy of rabies vaccines against all other lyssaviruses under field conditions is still limited. Protection is inversely related to the genetic distance of the lyssavirus from RABV [34, 35].

The type of vaccine used, number of vaccinations, interval between vaccination and blood sampling, age at vaccination, sex, reproductive status, size and breed can all influence the antibody response of animals vaccinated against rabies [36–39]. In post-vaccination serological studies, the percentage of animals with inadequate titres has been 3.1–8.1% for dogs [36, 38, 40] and 2.85% for cats [36]. As many as 53% (95% CI 41–65%) of imported rescue dogs from Eastern Europe have been found to have inadequate titres after rabies vaccination [41].

Pre-exposure vaccination is recommended for people potentially at risk of rabies, such as veterinarians, laboratory workers and bat handlers. People who work with rabies viruses in laboratories or vaccination production facilities should have VNA tested every 6 months [1]. According to WHO recommendations, 0.5 IU/ml is a sufficient antibody level, considered to be proof of an adequate vaccination response, and a booster vaccination is recommended for levels lower than this. A series of booster vaccinations is also required after exposure to lyssavirus [1]. The same threshold titre is applied in dogs and cats to confirm a satisfactory response to vaccination prior to international travel. All vaccines currently available are based on RABV. According to studies conducted to investigate the cross-neutralisation of sera and cross-protection in a mouse model against different lyssaviruses, they offer variable cross-protection against other lyssaviruses [34, 35, 42–46]. However, there are no official recommendations by WHO concerning whether the current procedure of pre-and post-exposure treatment would need to be modified for people who are exposed to other lyssaviruses than RABV.

The aim of this study was to assess the success of rabies vaccination measured by the antibody response in dogs and cats, as well as to study the factors influencing the inability of animals to produce a sufficient antibody response. In addition, the aim was to assess how well an RABV-based rabies vaccine, selected based on the ability to induce an antibody response in dogs and cats, affords protection in a mouse model against intracerebral challenge with EBLV-2 isolated from a Finnish bat (FI-EBLV-2), as well as against challenge with RABV isolated from a Finnish raccoon dog (FIRD-RABV). We also examined the protection offered by a rabies vaccine for humans and the correlation between VNA titres and cross-protection against EBLV-2 in mice.

## Methods

### Viruses

A Finnish EBLV-2 (FI-EBLV-2) isolate obtained from a Daubenton's bat in 2009 (GenBank Accession Number JX129233) was used as the challenge virus. The original bat brain suspension was intracerebrally inoculated into eight newborn mice (ScaNmri suckling mice) with each mouse receiving 20 μl of the suspension. The brain suspension from these eight newborn mice was subsequently inoculated into 4-week-old mice to amplify the virus and obtain the required quantity of virus stock to be used as the challenge virus in this study. RABV isolated from a Finnish raccoon dog (FIRD-RABV) (R1470/88) in 1988 was also used in this study. The original archived brain passage had been kept at − 70 °C since 1990, and for this challenge study it was grown in the brain of 4-week-old mice to amplify the virus and obtain the required quantity of virus stock.

### Vaccination and virus challenge of mice

Three- to four-week-old NMRI mice (Harlan, NL; n = 20 per challenge virus and n = 5 vaccine only) were vaccinated intra-peritoneally with 0.1 ml of vaccine diluted 1:10 in physiological saline solution with a 16-mm needle. When the human vaccine (Rabies-Imovax®; Sanofi-Pasteur MSD, France, batch G1391-4) was used, the mice were vaccinated either once (group a) or twice (group b) with a 2-week interval between the initial and the booster vaccination. When the animal vaccine (Rabisin® vet; Merial, France, batch L374051) was used, the mice were vaccinated once. Vaccines were purchased from Helsinki University Pharmacy. The protocol was modified from the European Pharmacopoiea protocol [29]: the minimum lethal dose ($MLD_{50}$) for the intra-cranial challenge was determined according to protocol of European Pharmacopoeia [29] and 50 $MLD_{50}$ was used. The mice were challenged intra-cranially with 30 μl of virus suspension according to the procedure described by WHO [47] 28 days after vaccination. The mice were anesthetized by inhalation anaesthesia using isoflurane, and they were given 0.05–0.1 mg/kg buprenorphine hydrochloride subcutaneously at the time of intra-cranial challenge. The back titration of five mice per group was set up with 50 $MLD_{50}$, 5 $MLD_{50}$ and 0.5 $MLD_{50}$ of each virus. Five mice per vaccine were not challenged. The mice were monitored twice per day for any clinical signs of rabies, and to minimize suffering they were killed when signs of rabies infection were obvious (weight loss, behavioural changes, neurological signs and paralysis) or when the observation period of 6 weeks had ended.

Serum was collected from the vaccinated mice prior to the challenge 21 or 22 days after the vaccination. The serum was collected from the lateral tail vein by appropriately trained personnel. The tail was first warmed and blood was collected with a 23-gauge needle. The target volume was 100 μl. At the end of the trial, the mice were euthanized either by the time they were showing clinical signs or after the monitoring period. To confirm the presence of rabies infection, the brains of the mice were collected and a fluorescent antibody test (FAT) [30] was performed on the brain. Smears prepared from a sample of brain tissue were fixed in high-grade cold acetone, air dried and then stained with specific conjugate (FITC Anti-Rabies Monoclonal Globulin, Fujirebio Diagnostics and Rabies Antinucleocapsid conjugate, Bio-Rad). FAT slides were then examined for specific fluorescence using a fluorescence microscope. The seroconversion of the vaccinated mice was analysed using the rapid fluorescent focus inhibition test RFFIT [30]. Five microlitres of sample was diluted 1:10. Serial dilutions of test sera were mixed with the challenge virus (CVS-11, ATCC VR-959) preparation and BHK-21 cells. Samples were fixed and stained with specific conjugate (FITC Anti-Rabies Monoclonal Globulin, Fujirebio Diagnostics). Residual virus was detected using a standard fluorescence microscope. The serum neutralisation end-point titre was defined as the dilution factor of the highest serum dilution at which 50% of the observed microscopic fields contained one or more infected cells. OIE/WHO human reference serum was used to convert the end point titre into IU/ml.

### Serological analysis of dogs and cats

The antibody responses of dogs and cats were determined using the FAVN test [48]. This test involves the neutralisation of a constant amount of rabies virus CVS-11 strain adapted to cell culture before inoculating cells susceptible to rabies virus (BHK-21 C13). The serum titre was the dilution at which 100% of the virus was neutralised in 50% of the wells. This titre was expressed in IU/ml by comparing it with the neutralising dilution of OIE serum of dog origin under the same test conditions.

### Selection of dog and cat samples

This was a case–control study with a duration of 5 years. During 2009–2013, 10,793 serum samples from dogs (n = 10 071) and cats (n = 722) were sent to the Finnish Food Safety Authority Evira for post-vaccination efficacy tests. Of these samples, 1055 dogs that had an antibody titre of < 0.5 IU/ml and for which submission data were available comprised the case group for dogs. An approximately similar number of dogs with submission data that had an antibody titre of ≥ 0.5 IU/ml were randomly assigned to the control group (n = 1626). In cats, only 25 had an antibody titre of < 0.5 IU/ml (cases), and a much larger number of cats that had antibody titre of ≥ 0.5 IU/ml were randomly assigned to the control group (n = 241). Submission forms for these samples were evaluated. Three inactivated rabies vaccines were used for dogs and cats in Finland during 2009–2013: Wistar-G52 strain vaccine, BHK-21cell vaccine with Pasteur RIV strain and Flury LEP strain vaccine.

### Statistical analysis

The 95% confidence intervals (CI) for valid percentages (excluding missing values) were calculated with Jeffrey's method [49] using EpiTools [50]. Statistical analyses were performed using the statistical software SPSS 22.0 (IBM SPSS Statistical Package version 22, USA). The outcome variable was failure to reach the required antibody level (0 for antibody level ≥ 0.5 IU/ml, denoting the ability to reach the required antibody level, and 1 for < 0.5 IU/ml, denoting failure). Independent variables collated in the dataset were the vaccine used, age at vaccination, breed and size (only for dogs), gender, the number of vaccinations and the time from vaccination to sampling. Dogs were categorised into five different breed size groups based on their height (< 30 cm, 30–45 cm, 46–60 cm, > 60 cm and unknown). Furthermore, 277 different dog breeds were originally categorized into 10 groups by the Fédération Cynologique Internationale. Animals were divided into two age groups: up to 1 year and over 1 year old. Based on the time interval between vaccination and sampling, three groups were created: sampling less than 3 months after vaccination, 3–6 months after vaccination and more than 6 months after vaccination. First, Fisher's exact test and crude logistic regression analyses were performed to examine the pairwise associations between the outcome and each independent variable separately. Variables with $P \leq 0.2$ were included in the multivariable logistic regression analysis, with separate models for cats and dogs, and variables with Wald's $P < 0.05$ were included in the final model. Correlations between independent variables were calculated with the Phi test (no important ones were found). A causal diagram was used to assess potential confounders; their impacts on the other variables in the model were verified, but none needed to be included in the models. Pairwise interactions were assessed. Since a significant interaction was found in dogs between the vaccine used and the age of the dog, two separate models were created: one for dogs up to 1 year old and another for older dogs. Additionally, for younger dogs, the time interval between vaccination and sampling was categorized into two groups: up to or more than 6 months. The goodness of fit of the final model was assessed with the Omnibus test, Nagelkerke's $R^2$ and the Hosmer and Lemeshow test, and by calculating the area under the curve (AUC).

## Results

### Results of the vaccine potency test

When challenged with FIRD-RABV, all of the vaccinated mice survived. When challenged with FI-EBLV-2, 80% of the vaccinated mice survived after vaccination with the veterinary vaccine. When mice were vaccinated with the human vaccine, 75–80% of the mice survived, depending on the booster (Table 1). All vaccinated mice developed sufficient to high VNA titres against RABV, ranging from 0.5 to 128 IU/ml. The signs of rabies appeared 7–8 days post-infection with EBLV-2 and 6–7 days post-infection with RABV. Mice that succumbed after challenge with FI-EBLV-2 virus had a VNA titre of 2–64 IU/ml against RABV (individual results not shown). There were no statistically significant differences between the VNA titres of the mice that survived the challenge in comparison to those that succumbed after the challenge with EBLV-2 (Fig. 1). Mice vaccinated twice with Rabies-Imovax® or once with Rabisin® vet had significantly higher antibody titres than those vaccinated once with Rabies-Imovax® ($P < 0.05$) (Fig. 2).

### Results of the serological analysis of vaccinated dogs and cats

Of the 10,071 dog samples analysed during 2009–2013, 1073 (10.7%; 95% confidence interval CI 10.1–11.3) had

**Table 1 Rabies vaccination protection following an intracranial challenge in mice**

| | Total number of mice | Survival after challenge with | |
|---|---|---|---|
| | | FIRD-RABV n (%) | FI-EBLV-2 n (%) |
| Rabies Imovax, vaccinated twice | 20 | 20 (100) | 16 (80) |
| P value[1] | | 0.000 | 0.002 |
| Rabies Imovax, vaccinated once | 20 | ND | 15 (75) |
| P value[1] | | | 0.005 |
| Virus control 50 $MLD_{50}$ | 5 | 0 (0) | 0 (0) |
| Virus control 5 $MLD_{50}$ | 5 | 2 (40) | 2 (40) |
| Virus control 0.5 $MLD_{50}$ | 5 | 4 (80) | 4 (80) |
| Rabisin, vaccinated once | 20 | 20 (100) | 16 (80) |
| P value[1] | | | 0.002 |
| Virus control 50 $MLD_{50}$ | 5 | 0 (0) | 0 (0) |
| Virus control 5 $MLD_{50}$ | 5 | 2 (40) | 2 (40) |
| Virus control 0.5 $MLD_{50}$ | 5 | 3 (60) | 4 (80) |

[1] P value derived using Fisher's exact test for the number of vaccinated and challenged mice that survived relative to the total and compared with the 50 $MLD_{50}$ virus control mice

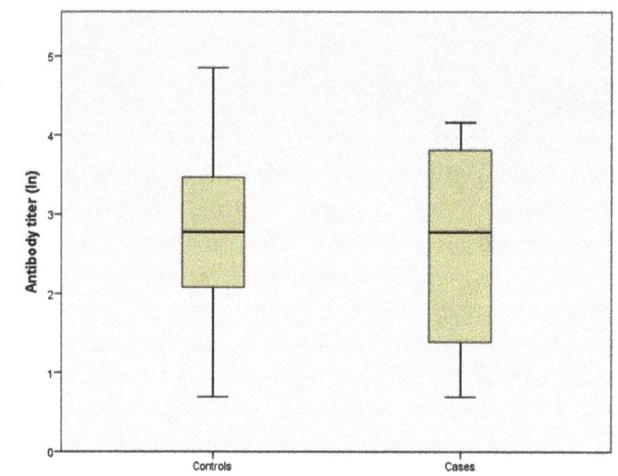


**Fig. 1** Comparison of VNA titers (ln) of the mice that survived the challenge (controls) and of the mice that succumbed after the challenge with EBLV-2 (cases). The interquartile range is the difference between the 75th and 25th percentiles and corresponds to the length of the box. The lines in the boxes represent the medians, the whiskers represent the minimum and maximum, unless there are values more than 1.5 times the interquartile range above 75th percentile, in which case it is the third quartile plus 1.5 times the interquartile range

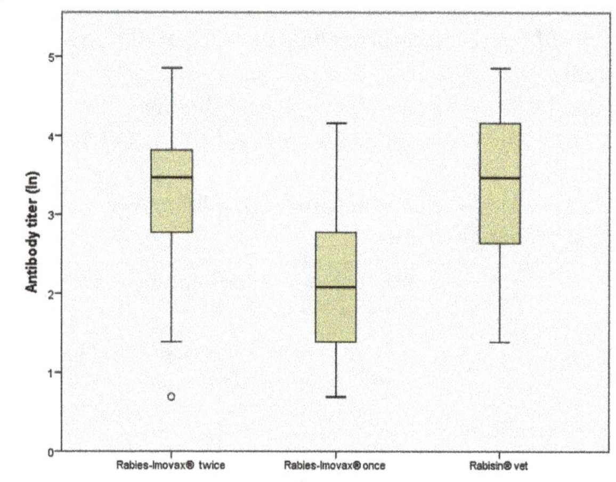


**Fig. 2** Comparison of VNA titers (ln) in three groups of mice vaccinated with different vaccines or vaccination schemes. The interquartile range is the difference between the 75th and 25th percentiles and corresponds to the length of the box. The lines in the boxes represent the medians, the whiskers represent the minimum and maximum, unless there are values more than 1.5 times the interquartile range above 75th percentile, in which case it is the third quartile plus 1.5 times the interquartile range. Circles represent outliers that are > 2 box lengths below the 25th percentile

a VNA titre of < 0.5 IU/ml. Of the 722 cats analysed, only 25 (3.5%; 95% CI 2.3–5.0) had a VNA titre of < 0.5 IU/ml.

**Risk factors for failure to produce sufficient antibody levels in dogs and cats**

Descriptive data for the dogs and cats in the case–control study are provided in Tables 2 and 3. Younger dogs were associated with lower antibody titres ($P < 0.05$, data not shown). Since there was a significant interaction between the variables dog age and the vaccine used, two multivariable logistic regression models for dogs were constructed: one for dogs up to 1 year old and another for older dogs. For younger dogs, the Flury LEP vaccine was used significantly more often than for older dogs ($P < 0.05$, data not shown). For both age groups, dogs vaccinated with the Flury LEP vaccine only and dogs vaccinated with the Pasteur RIV vaccine only had a significantly higher risk of failing to reach an antibody level of 0.5 IU/ml in comparison to dogs vaccinated with the Wistar-G52 vaccine only (Tables 4, 5). Additionally, for both age groups, vaccination with the Flury LEP vaccine only had the highest risk of failing to reach an antibody level of 0.5 IU/ml. In younger dogs, these risks were higher than in older dogs. In younger dogs, if the time between vaccination and sampling was over 3 months, the risk of failing to reach an antibody level of 0.5 IU/ml was significantly higher than if the time span was shorter. In older dogs, the risk was higher if the time was over 6 months. For older dogs (over 1 year) of a larger size (> 30 cm), the risk of failing to reach an antibody level of 0.5 IU/ml was greater. In younger dogs, those over 60 cm had a higher risk compared to smaller dogs.

In cats, we observed no statistically significant differences between the vaccines used (Table 6). However, there was a similar tendency towards a higher risk of failing to reach an antibody level of 0.5 IU/ml for vaccination with the Flury LEP vaccine only compared to vaccination with the Wistar-G52 vaccine only. Cats that were vaccinated at the age of up to 1 year old had a significantly higher risk of failing to reach an antibody level of 0.5 IU/ml than cats vaccinated at an older age. Similarly to dogs, cats that were sampled for testing 3–6 months or over 6 months after vaccination had a significantly higher risk of failing to reach an antibody level of 0.5 IU/ml than cats that had been sampled less than 3 months after vaccination.

## Discussion

New lyssaviruses related to RABV have been discovered, and it is possible that there may still be undetected bat lyssaviruses in many parts of the world. Bats do not often interact with people, but transmission of lyssaviruses to humans and pets has been documented. Finland experienced a human death from EBLV-2 in 1985 [9, 10], and better knowledge of the effectiveness of cross-protection is therefore needed to predict the impact of

**Table 2 Descriptive data on samples included in the statistical analysis of dog sera (n = 2681) tested for rabies antibody response after vaccination in Finland during 2009–2013**

| Variable | Levels | Antibody response < 0.5 IU/ml (n = 1055) | | Antibody response ≥ 0.5 IU/ml (n = 1626) | |
|---|---|---|---|---|---|
| | | n | % (95% CI) | n | % (95% CI) |
| Age at vaccination (year) | | | | | |
| ≤ 1 | | 544 | 52.2 (49.2–55.2) | 328 | 20.3 (18.4–22.3) |
| > 1 | | 498 | 47.8 (44.8–50.8) | 1289 | 79.3 (77.7–81.6) |
| Gender | | | | | |
| Female | | 500 | 54.7 (51.5–57.9) | 750 | 52.7 (50.1–55.3) |
| Male | | 414 | 45.3 (42.1–48.5) | 672 | 47.3 (44.7–49.9) |
| Number of vaccinations | | | | | |
| Once | | 941 | 89.2 (87.2–91.0) | 1071 | 65.9 (63.5–68.1) |
| Twice | | 99 | 9.4 (7.7–11.3) | 433 | 26.6 (24.5–28.8) |
| More than twice | | 15 | 1.4 (0.8–2.3) | 122 | 7.5 (6.3–8.9) |
| Time btw vaccination and sampling (months) | | | | | |
| < 3 | | 21 | 2.3 (1.5–3.4) | 158 | 11.1 (9.6–12.9) |
| 3–6 | | 335 | 36.8 (33.7–39.9) | 459 | 32.3 (30.0–34.8) |
| > 6 | | 555 | 60.9 (57.7–64.1) | 802 | 56.5 (53.9–59.1) |
| Vaccine used | | | | | |
| Only vaccine Wistar-G52 | | 53 | 7.3 (5.6–9.4) | 229 | 22.1 (19.7–24.7) |
| Only vaccine Pasteur RIV | | 298 | 41.3 (37.7–44.9) | 387 | 37.4 (34.5–40.4) |
| Only vaccine Flury LEP | | 315 | 43.6 (40.0–47.3) | 233 | 22.5 (20.0–25.1) |
| Other | | 56 | 7.8 (6.0–9.9) | 186 | 18.0 (15.7–20.4) |
| FCI group | | | | | |
| FCI1 | | 142 | 15.0 (12.8–17.4) | 186 | 13.4 (11.7–15.2) |
| FCI2 | | 114 | 12.1 (10.1–14.2) | 146 | 10.5 (9.0–12.2) |
| FCI3 | | 106 | 11.2 (9.3–13.3) | 191 | 13.7 (12.0–15.6) |
| FCI4 | | 33 | 3.5 (2.5–4.8) | 47 | 3.4 (2.5–4.4) |
| FCI5 | | 138 | 14.6 (12.4–16.9) | 183 | 13.2 (11.5–15.0) |
| FCI6 | | 43 | 4.5 (3.4–6.0) | 46 | 3.3 (2.5–4.3) |
| FCI7 | | 75 | 7.9 (6.3–9.8) | 77 | 5.5 (4.4–6.8) |
| FCI8 | | 133 | 14.1 (12.0–16.4) | 158 | 11.4 (9.8–13.1) |
| FCI9 | | 109 | 11.5 (9.6–13.7) | 266 | 19.1 (17.1–21.3) |
| FCI10 | | 31 | 3.3 (2.3–4.6) | 36 | 2.6 (1.8–3.5) |
| No FCI group | | 22 | 2.3 (1.5–3.4) | 55 | 4.0 (3.0–5.1) |
| Breed size (cm) | | | | | |
| < 30 | | 178 | 19.2 (16.8–21.9) | 434 | 32.3 (29.9–34.9) |
| 30–45 | | 295 | 31.9 (28.9–34.9) | 408 | 20.4 (28.0–32.9) |
| 46–60 | | 208 | 22.5 (19.9–25.2) | 267 | 19.9 (17.8–22.1) |
| > 60 | | 245 | 26.5 (23.7–29.4) | 233 | 17.4 (15.4–19.5) |

FCI group 1: Sheepdogs and Cattledogs (except Swiss Cattledogs), FCI group 2: Pinscher and Schnauzer—Molossoid and Swiss Mountain and Cattledogs, FCI group 3: Terriers, FCI group 4: Dachshunds, FCI group 5: Spitz and primitive types, FCI group 6: Scent hounds and related breeds, FCI group 7: Pointing Dogs, FCI group 8: Retrievers—Flushing Dogs—Water Dogs, FCI group 9: Companion and Toy Dogs, FCI group 10: Sighthounds

*CI* confidence interval, *n* number of cases

rabies vaccination if exposed to infected bats, as EBLV-2 appears to be enzootic at least in some areas in Finland [15, 16]. The immune response elicited by RABV-based rabies vaccines has been shown to be capable of cross-protection against those lyssaviruses in phylogroup I, but not for those that do not belong to this phylogroup [42–45]. However, even though EBLV-2 belongs to the same phylogroup I as RABV, the protection induced by rabies vaccines has only been limited in an experimental virus challenge study in mice, even with the production of VNAs [34].

**Table 3 Descriptive data on samples included in the statistical analysis of cat sera (n = 266) tested for the rabies antibody response after vaccination in Finland during 2009–2013**

| Variable | Levels | Antibody response < 0.5 IU/ml (n = 25) | | Antibody response ≥ 0.5 IU/ml (n = 241) | |
|---|---|---|---|---|---|
| | | n | % (95% CI) | n | % (95% CI) |
| Age at vaccination (year) | | | | | |
| | ≤ 1 | 12 | 48.0 (29.5–66.9) | 47 | 19.6 (14.9–25.0) |
| | > 1 | 13 | 52.0 (33.1–70.5) | 193 | 80.4 (75.0–85.1) |
| Gender | | | | | |
| | Female | 5 | 20.0 (8.1–38.4) | 89 | 58.6 (50.6–66.2) |
| | Male | 8 | 32.0 (16.4–51.5) | 63 | 26.1 (20.9–31.9) |
| Number of vaccinations | | | | | |
| | Once | 24 | 96.0 (82.8–99.6) | 194 | 80.5 (75.5–85.5) |
| | Twice | 1 | 4.0 (0.4–17.2) | 42 | 17.4 (13.0–22.6) |
| | More than twice | 0 | 0.0 (0–9.5) | 5 | 2.1 (0.8–4.5) |
| Time btw vaccination and sampling (months) | | | | | |
| | < 3 | 1 | 5.3 (0.6–22.1) | 78 | 42.2 (35.2–49.4) |
| | 3–6 | 8 | 42.1 (22.3–64.1) | 70 | 37.8 (31.1–45.0) |
| | > 6 | 10 | 52.6 (31.2–73.4) | 37 | 20.0 (14.7–26.2) |
| Vaccine used | | | | | |
| | Only vaccine Wistar-G52 | 3 | 25.0 (7.6–52.9) | 39 | 25.7 (19.2–33.0) |
| | Only vaccine Pasteur RIV | 1 | 8.3 (0.9–32.8) | 63 | 41.4 (33.8–49.4) |
| | Only vaccine Flury LEP | 6 | 50.0 (24.3–75.7) | 25 | 16.4 (11.2–22.9) |
| | Other | 2 | 16.7 (3.6–43.6) | 25 | 16.4 (11.2–22.9) |

*CI* confidence interval, *n* number of cases

VNAs are the main method of protection during rabies infection, and the role of cell-mediated and innate immunity is poorly understood. Measuring the VNA titre is currently the most common way to assess the success of vaccination, and an internationally accepted threshold of 0.5 IU/ml has therefore been adopted as an adequate titre. In our study, all mice developed a sufficient VNA titre against RABV after vaccination, but mice that had VNA titres of 2–64 IU/ml, which is higher than the accepted threshold, succumbed after challenge with FI-EBLV-2 virus, whereas all mice survived the challenge with FIRD-RABV. Due to this discrepancy between the VNA titres and cross-protection from the disease, people and animals need a post-exposure vaccination, regardless of their prior pre-exposure vaccination and antibody measurement result, if they are exposed to lyssaviruses. The intracranial route of infection was used because of the guidelines in the European Pharmacopoeia's protocol. Pharmacopoeial methods are reference methods and the suitability of the method has been demonstrated. However, it should be noted that the intracranial exposure route used in our study is not the natural infection route.

Possible exposure to other lyssaviruses than RABV has especially raised concerns over whether RABV-based vaccines offer sufficient cross-protection and whether a higher cut-off for protection against EBLV-2 would be required. Studies have suggested that either higher serum VNA titres [34] or higher doses of rabies immunoglobulins are required [45] in humans. There is marked individual variation in the comparative neutralisation patterns

**Table 4 Multivariable logistic regression results of risk factors for not reaching the antibody level of 0.5 IU/ml after vaccination against rabies in dogs up to 1 year old (n = 872) in Finland during 2009–2013**

| Independent variable | Logistic regression coefficient B | Wald's *P* value | Odds ratio (95% CI) |
|---|---|---|---|
| Vaccine | | | |
| Wistar-G52 only | Na | Na | 1 |
| Pasteur RIV only | 2.049 | 0.000 | 7.8 (4.1–14.5) |
| Flury LEP only | 2.608 | 0.000 | 13.6 (7.0–26.2) |
| D other | 0.466 | 0.406 | 1.6 (0.5–4.8) |
| Breed size (cm) | | | |
| < 30 | Na | Na | 1 |
| 30–60 | 0.308 | 0.221 | 1.4 (0.8–2.2) |
| > 60 | 1.159 | 0.000 | 3.2 (1.7–5.9) |
| Time btw vaccination and sampling (months) | | | |
| < 3 | Na | Na | 1 |
| 3 6 | 1.100 | 0.001 | 4.1 (1.8–9.1) |
| > 6 | 1.508 | 0.000 | 4.5 (2.0–10.4) |
| Constant | −2.907 | 0.000 | 0.055 |

*Na* not applicable, *CI* confidence interval, *other* dogs vaccinated abroad with vaccines not available in Finland or with a combination of different vaccines

**Table 5 Multivariable logistic regression results of risk factors for not reaching the antibody level of 0.5 IU/ml after vaccination against rabies in dogs older than 1 year (n = 1787) in Finland during 2009–2013**

| Independent variable | Logistic regression coefficient B | Wald's P value | Odds ratio (95% CI) |
|---|---|---|---|
| Vaccine | | | |
| Wistar-G52 only | Na | Na | 1 |
| Pasteur RIV only | 0.926 | 0.000 | 2.5 (1.5–4.1) |
| Flury LEP only | 1.271 | 0.000 | 3.6 (2.2–5.9) |
| Other | 0.243 | 0.418 | 1.3 (0.7–2.3) |
| Breed size (cm) | | | |
| < 30 | Na | Na | 1 |
| 30–60 | 0.464 | 0.013 | 1.6 (1.1–2.3) |
| > 60 | 0.823 | 0.000 | 2.3 (1.5–3.5) |
| Time btw vaccination and sampling (months) | | | |
| < 6 | Na | Na | 1 |
| > 6 | 1.432 | 0.000 | 4.2 (2.8–6.3) |
| Constant | −3.180 | 0.000 | 0.042 |

*Na* not applicable, *CI* confidence interval, *other* dogs vaccinated abroad with vaccines not available in Finland or with a combination of different vaccines

**Table 6 Crude and multivariable logistics regression results of risk factors for not reaching the antibody level of 0.5 IU/ml after vaccination against rabies in cats in Finland during 2009–2013**

| Independent variable | Logistic regression coefficient B | Wald's P value | Odds ratio (95% CI) |
|---|---|---|---|
| In crude logistic regressions | | | |
| Vaccine (n = 164) | | | |
| Wistar-G52 only | Na | 1 | Na |
| Pasteur RIV only | −1.578 | 0.178 | 0.2 (0.0–2.1) |
| Flury LEP only | 1.138 | 0.130 | 3.1 (0.7–13.6) |
| Other | 0.039 | 0.967 | 1.0 (0.2–6.7) |
| Age at vaccination (n = 265) | | | |
| < 1 year vs ≥ 1 year | 1.332 | 0.002 | 3.8 (1.6–8.9) |
| Time btw vaccination and sampling (n = 204) (months) | | | |
| < 3 | Na | 1 | Na |
| 3–6 | 2.188 | 0.042 | 8.9 (1.1–73.1) |
| > 6 | 3.048 | 0.004 | 21.1 (2.6–170.9) |
| In multivariable logistic regression (n = 159) | | | |
| Vaccine | | | |
| Wistar-G52 only | Na | 1 | Na |
| Pasteur RIV only | −1.090 | 0.378 | 0.3 (0.03–3.8) |
| Flury LEP only | 1.475 | 0.085 | 4.4 (0.8–23.5) |
| Other | 0.827 | 0.439 | 2.3 (0.3–16.6) |
| Age at vaccination | | | |
| < 1 year vs ≥ 1 year | 2.282 | 0.006 | 9.8 (1.9–48.8) |
| Time btw vaccination and sampling (months) | | | |
| < 3 | Na | 1 | Na |
| 3–6 | 1.615 | 0.19 | 5.0 (0.5–56.2) |
| > 6 | 2.906 | 0.026 | 18.3 (1.4–235.3) |
| Constant | −5.439 | 0.000 | 0.004 |

*Na* not applicable, *CI* confidence interval, *other* cats vaccinated abroad with vaccines not available in Finland or with a combination of different vaccines of human sera against different lyssaviruses [34, 42]. Our studies indicated that the RABV antibody level does not clearly correlate with protection against EBLV-2. Therefore, laboratory personnel working with EBLV-2 should be regularly vaccinated and their antibody level should be monitored every 6 months, but it is still unclear what RABV antibody level would be protective. Therefore, booster vaccinations are recommended after possible exposure to lyssaviruses, and particular attention should be paid to the wound care after exposure. No laboratory accidents with other lyssaviruses than RABV have so far been reported.

Several factors influence the antibody level reached in an animal after vaccination, including the vaccine used, vaccine administration and the animal receiving the vaccine. Based on our studies, it is advisable that dogs that need a sufficient antibody test result due to international travel should be vaccinated twice with a rabies vaccine and then regularly receive a booster. Sihvonen et al. [40] demonstrated that a single vaccination of dogs with rabies vaccine induced moderate but short-term seroconversion in 96.9% of dogs, but in 17% of dogs the antibody titre did not last for a whole year in a population that had not previously been vaccinated. If vaccinations are only performed by veterinarians in veterinary clinics and vaccines are stored according to the manufacturer's instructions, this might have a positive effect on the outcome. Factors such as the consistency (virus strain, cell culture and adjuvants) of the vaccine influence the vaccination response.

The difference between the proportions of dogs (around 11%) and cats (around 3%) that failed to reach the antibody level of 0.5 IU/ml might be caused by differences in genetic variation within the two species, as pedigree dogs are purebred, whereas the majority of cats in our study material were mixed breeds. The key genetic elements of immune responsiveness lie within the genes of the major histocompatibility complex (MHC). It has been suspected that cats have more limited diversity in immune response genes than dogs, but recent research has demonstrated similar variation in the MHC in cats to that found in dogs [51]. In our study, there was a significant difference in the ability of different vaccines to induce the antibody level of 0.5 IU/ml in dogs. This has also been reported in earlier studies [36–39], and may be due to differences in the immunogenicity of the vaccines or the potency of the vaccine batches. Moreover, veterinarians should note that there are significant differences between vaccines in their ability to induce an immune response. This difference between the vaccines was not statistically significant in cats, perhaps due to the type two error of an insufficient sample size, since there were so few (n = 25) failures to reach the threshold of 0.5 IU/ml in cats.

The time between vaccination and sampling was a significant risk factor for both dogs and cats failing to reach the threshold of 0.5 IU/ml. The antibody level peaks at slightly different times after vaccination with different vaccines, and the level starts to decline afterwards [37]. Larger dogs had a greater risk of failing to reach the required antibody level. Increasing the dose would not probably be a solution, since it has been shown that if there is a sufficient antigen to create a response, larger doses will not increase antibody production. Kennedy et al. [37] suggested that larger breeds might have deeper sub-cutaneous fat, which could reduce the level of the antibody response. The breed might also be a factor, not just the size of the dog, since even though most failures to reach the anticipated antibody level occurred in larger breeds, some smaller breeds had significant test failure rates [52]. Specific dog breeds have a genetically determined immune function, and a study has confirmed breed-specific serological response patterns to vaccination. The high interbreed and relatively low intrabreed variation in MHC alleles and haplotypes could provide an explanation for the reports of interbreed variation in immune responses to vaccines [53]. The higher risk of failing to reach 0.5 IU/ml for dogs and cats aged up to 1 year old could be due to the administration of vaccines before the animals had reached full immunocompetency, or due to maternal antibodies [36, 39].

In rabies-free countries, the rabies vaccination coverage of cats and dogs is likely to be lower than in rabies enzootic countries. Cats, especially in the countryside, often freely roam outside and are therefore able to encounter wildlife, consequently being at greater risk of exposure to rabid animals, and especially to bats, than dogs. Host switching of lyssaviruses from bats to mammals has successfully occurred in history [20, 21]. Natural spillover of EBLV-2 to other mammals than humans has not been demonstrated. Only a small proportion of cats failed to reach the required antibody level in our study, but the vaccination coverage of cats against rabies is assumed to be low in many rabies-free countries, at least in Finland. Based on the number of vaccination doses sold, we estimated that about 10–20% of 700,000 Finnish cats have been vaccinated against rabies. The rabies vaccination coverage is higher for dogs, estimated at around 40–65% based on the rabies vaccine sales in Finland.

We demonstrated in the mouse model challenge that an RABV-based animal vaccine offers cross-protection against challenge with the FI-EBLV-2 strain isolated from a bat. Therefore, it is recommended that even in rabies-free countries, dogs and cats that come into contact with lyssavirus and infected bats should be vaccinated against rabies. Booster vaccination is recommended for dogs, especially of large breeds. Moreover, veterinarians should pay attention to the choice of vaccine used.

## Conclusions

A veterinary RABV-based rabies vaccine, selected based on the ability to induce the best antibody response of the vaccines compared for dogs and cats in this study, offered cross-protection against EBLV-2 challenge in a mouse model in comparison with a challenge with RABV. Our mouse model provided an indication that the RABV antibody level and protection against EBLV-2 are not clearly correlated, and this most probably reflects the situation in other mammals and humans. There was a statistically significant difference in VNA titres between three groups of mice vaccinated with different vaccines or vaccination schemes. Approximately 11% of vaccinated dogs tested from the field failed to have an antibody titre of 0.5 IU/ml or more. By comparison, only a small proportion of cats failed to reach the required antibody level. Booster vaccination and vaccinating dogs and cats encountering bats is recommended, since vaccination also offers cross-protection against EBLV-2.

### Authors' contributions

TN participated in the study design, conducted the challenge experiment, performed the serological and virological analysis and drafted the manuscript. MJV and LS participated in the study design and critically revised the draft for important intellectual content. AMV supervised the statistical analysis and critically revised the draft for important intellectual content. All authors read and approved the final manuscript.

### Author details

[1] Finnish Food Safety Authority Evira, Mustialankatu 3, 00790 Helsinki, Finland. [2] Department of Veterinary Biosciences, Faculty of Veterinary Medicine, University of Helsinki, P.O. Box 66, 00014 Helsinki, Finland.

### Acknowledgements

Thanks to Raili Heinonen, Sanna Karumaa and Tiina Peltonen, and other technicians at Evira, for their technical assistance. Thanks to Veera Karkamo, DVM, for the autopsies of mice.

### Competing interests

The authors declare that they have no competing interests.

### Funding

This study was funded by the Ministry of Agriculture and Forestry (Grant MMM 2682/311/2009) and the Finnish Food Safety Authority Evira.

### References


1. WHO expert consultation on rabies 2013. http://apps.who.int/iris/bitstream/10665/85346/1/9789240690943_eng.pdf. Accessed 12 Nov 2016.
2. Badrane H, Bahloul C, Perrin P, Tordo N. Evidence of two lyssavirus phylogroups with distinct pathogenicity and immunogenicity. J Virol. 2001;75:3268–76.
3. Kuzmin IV, Mayer AE, Niezgoda M, Markotter W, Agwanda B, Breiman RF, et al. Shimoni bat virus, a new representative of the *Lyssavirus* genus. Virus Res. 2010;149:197–210.
4. Kuzmin IV, Hughes GJ, Botvinkin AD, Orciari LA. Rupprecht CE phylogenetic relationships of Irkut and West Caucasian bat viruses within the *Lyssavirus* genus and suggested quantitative criteria based on the N gene sequence for lyssavirus genotype definition. Virus Res. 2005;111:28–43.
5. Marston DA, Horton DL, Ngeleja C, Hampson K, McElhinney LM, Banyard AC, et al. Ikoma lyssavirus, highly divergent novel lyssavirus in an African civet. Emerg Infect Dis. 2012;18:664–7.
6. Ceballos NA, Morón SV, Berciano JM, Nicolás O, López CA, Juste J, et al. Novel lyssavirus in bat, Spain. Emerg Infect Dis. 2013;19:793–5.
7. Gunawardena P, Marston D, Ellis R, Wise E, Karawita A, Breed A, et al. *Lyssavirus* in Indian flying foxes, Sri Lanka. Emerg Infect Dis. 2016;22:1456–8.
8. Johnson N, Vos A, Freuling C, Tordo N, Fooks AR, Müller T. Human rabies due to lyssavirus infection of bat origin. Vet Microbiol. 2010;142:151–9.
9. Lumio J, Hillbom M, Roine R, Ketonen L, Haltia M, Valle M, et al. Human rabies of bat origin in Europe. Lancet. 1986;15:378.
10. Roine RO, Hillbom M, Valle M, Haltia M, Ketonen L, Neuvonen E, et al. Fatal encephalitis caused by a bat-borne rabies-related virus: clinical findings. Brain. 1988;111:1505–16.
11. Fooks AR, McElhinney LM, Pounder DJ, Finnegan CJ, Mansfield K, Johnson N, et al. Case report: isolation of a European bat lyssavirus type 2a from a fatal human case of rabies encephalitis. J Med Virol. 2003;71:281–9.
12. Van der Poel WHM, Van der Heide R, Verstraten E, Takumi K, Lina PHC, Kramps JA. European bat lyssaviruses, the Netherlands. Emerg Infect Dis. 2005;11:1854–9.
13. Kappeler A. First case of rabies in a bat in Switzerland. Rabies Bull Eur. 2002;16:11.
14. Whitby JE, Heaton PR, Black EM, Wooldridge M, McElhinney LM, Johnstone P. First isolation of a rabies-related virus from a Daubenton's bat in the United Kingdom. Vet Rec. 2000;147:385–8.
15. Jakava-Viljanen M, Lilley T, Kyheröinen E-M, Huovilainen A. First encounter of European bat lyssavirus type 2 (EBLV-2) in a bat in Finland. Epidemiol Infect. 2010;138:1581–5.
16. Nokireki T, Huovilainen A, Lilley T, Kyheröinen EM, Ek-Kommonen C, Sihvonen L, Jakava-Viljanen M. Bat rabies surveillance in Finland. BMC Vet Res. 2013;9:174.
17. Freuling C, Grossmann E, Conraths FJ, Schameitat A, Kliemt J, Auer E, et al. First isolation of EBLV-2 in Germany. Vet Microbiol. 2008;131:26–34.
18. Rasmussen TB, Chriél M, Baagøe HJ, Fjederholt E, Kooi EA, Belsham GJ, Bøtner A. Detection of European bat lyssavirus type 2 in Danish Daubenton's bats using a molecular diagnostic strategy. In: Proceedings of 8th Annual EPIZONE Meeting, 23–25.9.2014, Copenhagen, Denmark.
19. Moldal T, Vikøren T, Cliquet F, Marston DA, van der Kooij J, Madslien K, Ørpetveit I. First detection of European bat lyssavirus type 2 (EBLV-2) in Norway. BMC Vet Res. 2017;13:216.
20. Leslie MJ, Messenger S, Rohde RE, Smith J, Cheshier R, Hanlon C, Rupprecht CE. Bat-associated rabies virus in skunks. Emerg Infect Dis. 2006;12:1274–7.
21. Daoust PY, Wandeler AI, Casey GA. Cluster of rabies cases of probable bat origin among red foxes in Prince Edward Island, Canada. J Wildl Dis. 1996;32:403–6.
22. Cliquet F, Picard-Meyer E, Barrat J, Brookes SM, Healy DM, Wasniewski M, Litaize E, Biarnais M, Johnson L, Fooks AR. Experimental infection of foxes with European bat lyssaviruses type-1 and 2. BMC Vet Res. 2009;5:19.
23. Brookes SM, Klopfleisch R, Müller T, Healy DM, Teifke JP, Lange E, Kliemt J, Johnson N, Johnson L, Kaden V, Vos A, Fooks AR. Susceptibility of sheep to European bat lyssavirus type-1 and -2 infection: a clinical pathogenesis study. Vet Microbiol. 2007;125:210–23.
24. Banyard AC, Healy DM, Brookes SM, Voller K, Hicks DJ, Núñez A, Fooks AR. *Lyssavirus* infection: 'low dose, multiple exposure' in the mouse model. Virus Res. 2014;181:35–42.
25. Healy DM, Brookes SM, Banyard AC, Núñez A, Cosby SL, Fooks AR. Pathobiology of rabies virus and the European bat lyssaviruses in experimentally infected mice. Virus Res. 2013;172:46–53.
26. Müller T, Cox J, Schafer R, Johnson N, McElhinney LM, Geue JL, Tjørnehøj K, Fooks AR. Spill-over of European bat lyssavirus type 1 into a stone marten (*Martes foina*) in Germany. J Vet Med B Infect Dis Vet Public Health. 2004;51:49–54.
27. Tjørnehøj K, Fooks AR, Agerholm JS, Rønsholt L. Natural and experimental infection of sheep with European bat lyssavirus type-1 of Danish bat origin. J Comp Pathol. 2006;134:190–201.

28. Tjørnehøj K, Rønsholt L, Fooks AR. Antibodies to EBLV-1 in a domestic cat in Denmark. Vet Rec. 2004;155:571–2.
29. European Pharmacopoeia 6.0. (2008). Monograph 0451: Rabies vaccine (inactivated) for veterinary use. European Directorate for the quality of medicines and healthcare [EDQM], Council of Europe, Strasbourg, France.
30. OIE manual of diagnostic tests and vaccines for terrestrial animals 2015. http://www.oie.int/en/international-standard-setting/terrestrial-manual/access-online/. Accessed 12 Nov 2016.
31. Moore SM, Wilkerson MJ, Davis RD, Wyatt CR, Briggs DJ. Detection of cellular immunity to rabies antigens in human vaccines. J Clin Immunol. 2006;26:533–45.
32. Aubert MF. Practical significance of rabies antibodies in cats and dogs. Rev Sci Tech. 1992;3:735–60.
33. Hooper DC, Morimoto K, Bette M, Weihe E, Koprowski H, Dietzschold B. Collaboration of antibody and inflammation in clearance of rabies virus from the central nervous system. J Virol. 1998;72:3711–9.
34. Brookes SM, Parsons G, Johnson N, McElhinney LM, Fooks AR. Rabies human diploid cell vaccine elicits cross-neutralising and cross-protecting immune responses against European and Australian bat lyssaviruses. Vaccine. 2005;23:4101–9.
35. Malerczyk C, Selhorst T, Tordo N, Moore S, Müller T. Antibodies induced by vaccination with purified chick embryo cell culture vaccine (PCECV) cross-neutralize non-classical bat lyssavirus strains. Vaccine. 2009;27:5320–5.
36. Mansfield KL, Burr PD, Snodgrass DR, Sayers R, Fooks AR. Factors affecting the serological response of dogs and cats to rabies vaccination. Vet Rec. 2004;154:423–6.
37. Kennedy LJ, Lunt M, Barnes A, McElhinney L, Fooks AR, Baxter DN, et al. Factors influencing the antibody response of dogs vaccinated against rabies. Vaccine. 2007;25:8500–7.
38. Minke JM, Bouvet J, Cliquet F, Wasniewski M, Guiot AL, Lemaitre L, et al. Comparison of antibody responses after vaccination with two inactivated rabies vaccines. Vet Microbiol. 2008;133:283–6.
39. Berndtsson LT, Nyman A-K, Rivera E, Klingeborn B. Factors associated with the success of rabies vaccination of dogs in Sweden. Acta Vet Scand. 2011;53:22.
40. Sihvonen L, Kulonen K, Neuvonen E, Pekkanen K. Rabies antibody in vaccinated dogs. Acta Vet Scand. 1995;36:87–91.
41. Klevar S, Høgåsen HR, Davidson RK, Hamnes IS, Berndtsson LT, Lund A. Cross-border transport of rescue dogs may spread rabies in Europe.
42. Horton DL, McElhinney LM, Marston DA, Wood JL, Russell CA, Lewis N, Kuzmin IV, Fouchier RA, Osterhaus AD, Fooks AR, Smith DJ. Quantifying antigenic relationships among the lyssaviruses. J Virol. 2010;84:11841–8.
43. Malerczyk C, Freuling C, Gniel D, Giesen A, Selhorst T, Müller T. Cross-neutralization of antibodies induced by vaccination with purified chick embryo cell vaccine (PCECV) against different *Lyssavirus* species. Hum Vaccin Immunother. 2014;10:2799–804.
44. Hanlon CA, Kuzmin IV, Blanton JD, Weldon WC, Manangan JS, Rupprecht CE. Efficacy of rabies biologics against new lyssaviruses from Eurasia. Virus Res. 2005;111:44–54.
45. Liu Y, Chen Q, Zhang F, Zhang S, Li N, Lian H, Wang Y, Zhang J, Hu R. Evaluation of rabies biologics against Irkut virus isolated in China. J Clin Microbiol. 2013;51:3499–504.
46. Fekadu M, Shaddock JH, Sanderlin DW, Smith JS. Efficacy of rabies vaccines against Duvenhage virus isolated from European house bats (*Eptesicus serotinus*), classic rabies and rabies-related viruses. Vaccine. 1988;6:533–9.
47. Koprowski H. The mouse inoculation test in: laboratory techniques in rabies. 4th ed. Geneva: World Health Organization; 1996.
48. Cliquet F, Aubert MFA, Sagné L. Development of a fluorescent antibody virus neutralizing test (FAVN test) for the quantitation of rabies-neutralising antibody. J Immunol Methods. 1998;212:79–87.
49. Brown L, Cai T, DasGupta A. Interval estimation for a binominal proportion. Stat Sci. 2001;16:101–33.
50. Sergeant ESG. Epitools epidemiological calculators. AusVet Animal Health Services and Australian Biosecurity Cooperative Research Centre for Emerging Infectious Disease. 2015. http://epitools.ausvet.com.au/content.php?page=home. Accessed 22 Apr 2015.
51. Day MJ. Immune system development in the dog and cat. J Comp Pathol. 2007;137(Suppl 1):S10–5.
52. Kennedy LJ, Lunt M, Barnes A, McElhinney LM, Fooks AR, Ollier WER. Do dogs vary in their response to rabies vaccination?. In: Proceedings of the 48th annual congress of the british small animal veterinary association. 2005. p. 550.
53. Kennedy LJ, Barnes A, Happ GM, Quinnell RJ, Bennett D, Angles JM, Day MJ, Carmichael N, Innes JF, Isherwood D, Carter SD, Thomson W, Ollier WE. Extensive interbreed, but minimal intrabreed, variation of DLA class II alleles and haplotypes in dogs. Tissue Antigens. 2002;59:194–204.

# 8

# Survey of interdigital phlegmon outbreaks and their risk factors in free stall dairy herds in Finland

Miia Kontturi[1*], Minna Kujala[1], Reijo Junni[1], Erja Malinen[2], Eija Seuna[2], Sinikka Pelkonen[3], Timo Soveri[1] and Heli Simojoki[1]

**Abstract**

**Background:** Severe outbreaks of interdigital phlegmon (IP) associated with a high morbidity and major economic losses have occurred in Finland in the past decade. A survey was performed to indicate the current occurrence of infectious hoof diseases and to identify herd level risk factors predisposing to an outbreak of IP.

**Results:** Responses to a questionnaire revealed that an outbreak of IP defined as morbidity ≥5% within the 1st month of the outbreak, had occurred in 18.0% of the respondent study farms. Risk factors for an outbreak included animal transport between herds, i.e. either animal purchase or contract heifer rearing, enlargement or renovation of the barn, and if the fields of the farm had been organically cultivated. Having any kind of mechanical ventilation in comparison to natural ventilation seemed to lower the risk of IP. Additionally, the farms that had experienced an outbreak of IP often had other infectious hoof diseases. However, it was unclear which disease appeared first.

**Conclusions:** More attention is needed before and during enlargement or renovation of the barn and substantial planning is crucial for every part of the enlargement process in dairy farms.

**Keywords:** Interdigital phlegmon, Outbreak, Risk factors, Infectious hoof diseases, Foot rot, Foul in the foot, Interdigital necrobacillosis

## Background

Recently, several dairy herds in Finland experienced a sudden outbreak of interdigital phlegmon (IP). These outbreaks mainly occurred in recently built or renewed free stall barns and caused major economic losses due to high morbidity, antibiotic treatment of the affected cows and discarded milk [1]. No preceding trauma to the interdigital cleft of the affected cows has been reported. Previously, only a few cases of infectious hoof diseases were detected in Finnish dairy farms.

At the same time, the structure of dairy industry in Finland has changed, based on the statistics of National Resources Institute Finland the average number of lactating cows per herd has more than doubled during last 15 years, and the change from tie stalls to free stalls have also occurred simultaneously. In addition, several new techniques have been introduced in the farms, like mixed ration feeding and automatic milking system.

A lot of research has been done on the aetiology and possible risk factors of IP. *Fusobacterium necrophorum* is considered a major pathogen in IP [2, 3] although several other bacteria and environmental factors influence the development of disease [4, 5]. Typically, the first sign of IP is slight lameness, which becomes more apparent when the infection progresses. A swelling of the interdigital area and the bulbs of the heels together with a fetid odour are regarded as characteristic. Soon a fissure forms with swollen protruding edges along the interdigital cleft. In severe cases, systemic signs may appear, which include fever, recumbency, anorexia and decrease in milk production [6]. IP reduces milk yield [7] and can result in an early culling of the affected cow [7, 8].

*Correspondence: miia.kontturi@helsinki.fi
[1] Department of Production Animal Medicine, Faculty of Veterinary Medicine, University of Helsinki, Paroninkuja 20, 04920 Saarentaus, Finland

In general, IP occurs as a sporadic disease in cattle. The frequency or prevalence of IP has been reported being 0.2–5% in herds in North America [9–11], but some other reports of earlier outbreaks of IP exist where the incidence may be as high as 17–25% [12, 13].

As long ago as 1945, Johnson [14] reported that the increase in the incidence of IP is associated with increased animal traffic between herds and cases occur when cattle are introduced to a pasture with alfa–alfa hay or clover. A trauma to the interdigital skin and muddy conditions were mentioned as predisposing factors for the disease. Other studies have also investigated a preceding trauma and muddy or moist conditions underneath the hooves as predisposing factors [4, 6]. In addition, Gupta et al. [6] mentioned seasonality, intensive farm practice, concrete flooring and coarse sand. A Danish study reported cow-level risk factors that included calving, first parity and free stall housing in comparison to tie stall housing [15].

However, most of this research on IP is quite old or does not focus on the actual outbreaks. In response to numerous outbreaks of IP in dairy herds in Finland, we wanted to investigate the possible herd level risk factors and furthermore, to describe the current situation of infectious hoof diseases in Finland.

## Methods

### Study population

In the spring of 2013, a questionnaire regarding infectious hoof diseases was sent to all Finnish dairy farms in a dairy herd recording database that had ≥50 cows in 2012 (n = 1134). The total number of comparable dairy herds in Finland in the spring of 2013 was 1245 [16] and therefore, our initial target population covered 91.1% of the herds of similar size in Finland. The contact data was received from ProAgria agricultural data processing center. Only free stall herds were included in the study.

### Study questionnaire

The final draft of the five-page questionnaire contained 35 questions of general herd data, which included herd size, mean milk yield and region, and questions about the barn characteristics and herd management details. The key items asked are listed in Table 1. The number of the cow compartments meant the number of barns or separate sections of a barn for milking cows. Some farmers separate their milking cows for example based on udder health or milk yield. The flooring choices in the questionnaire were slatted or solid with or without rubber, where the choice 'with rubber' included rubber everywhere or only partly in the alleys or manure pack flooring in non-insulated free stall barns. The ventilation system choices contained natural or mechanical systems with or without an additional precision ventilation of the manure drain.

**Table 1 Summary of the herd and barn characteristics and management practices included in the questionnaire**

| Herd and barn characteristics | Management practices |
|---|---|
| Herd size | Mixed ration feeding |
| Mean milk yield | Outdoor access during summer |
| Region | Outdoor access during winter |
| Number of cow compartments | Hoof trimming frequency |
| Stall type (freestall or tiestall) | Stocking density |
| Free stall type (insulated, partly insulated, non-insulated) | Enlargement or renovation of the barn |
| Flooring (slatted or concrete and with or without rubber) | Animal purchase |
| Milking in a parlour or an automatic milking system | Contract heifer rearing |
| Ventilation system | Fields in organic farming |

The mixed ration feeding included total or partial mixed ration. One question covered any possible enlargement or renovation of the barn in 3-year period prior to the outbreak of IP or 3 year period prior to answering the questionnaire. Two questions inquired about the animal transport between herds i.e. the animal purchase during the past year and information about where the heifers of the herd are kept. Some farms in Finland do not raise their own heifers and instead their calves are sent to another herd, where they are kept until the animals return to the home herd before the first calving. In general, Finnish contract heifer rearing units have animals from several independent farms. Another question inquired about whether the fields of the farm were cultivated organically.

Additionally, the dairy farmers were asked several questions about the leg and claw health in their herd. First, they had to clarify whether they had experienced (1) an outbreak of IP in the last 10 years, in other words had several cases of IP in a short period, or (2) had only a few cases of IP, or (3) had no cases of IP at all. The common signs of IP were described as a list. They included fever, lameness, swelling above a hoof, shaking of a leg, bad odour in the hoof region, and lesions in between the hooves or in the heel. The farmers had to choose the signs exhibited by their affected animals and record the number of the affected cows within first 2 weeks of the outbreak.

Second, we inquired about the signs of interdigital dermatitis (ID), digital dermatitis (DD), interdigital hyperplasia (IH) and verrucous dermatitis. Similarly, the signs of ID and DD were listed and included lesions between the hooves or in the heel and reddish, painful lesions in the hoof region. Third, we asked for the dairy farmer's observations about whether the herd had occurrences in excess of 5% white line lesions that needed a hoof blocking for treatment and any visual signs of calf diphtheria i.e. buccal abscesses in suckling calves.

Most of the cases of IP in Finland are diagnosed and treated by veterinarians, because of a strict national antibiotic policy. In the outbreaks, the correct diagnosis is achieved relatively straightforward. Therefore, we expected the IP status given in the questionnaire to be accurate. On the other hand, ID and DD are rarer and their signs are confusing, so we predicted more variation with these answers. Because of this unpredictability and possible confusion of the farm staff in making the correct diagnosis of ID and DD we considered the existence of any of their listed signs as other infectious hoof disease than IP.

The questionnaire was pilot tested with two dairy veterinarians and producers and modified based on their feedback. The final drafts of the questionnaire were mailed to dairy farmers with an enclosed paid return envelope. An alternative option was to answer the same questionnaire online. Furthermore, all dairy veterinarians in Finland were informed about the survey and asked to remind their dairy farmer clients. No separate reminders were sent to farmers themselves. After the return of the questionnaires, some of the farms were called to clarify certain answers.

### Statistical analyses

We collated and inserted the data from the original paper document questionnaire into Excel spreadsheets and used Stata IC version 14 (Stata Corporation, Texas, USA) for statistical analyses. Only free stall barns with a complete information on the IP status of the herd were included in the analyses. A $P$ value <0.05 was considered statistically significant. The descriptive data are presented as percentages. The possible outbreak of IP associated putative disorders were tested using the Chi squared test.

Our study herds were categorized into three groups according to the IP status of the herd, thus: (1) outbreak of IP, (2) few cases of IP, and (3) no IP in the herd. The herds with no IP are hereafter referred to as the control herds. An outbreak of IP was defined as morbidity due to IP being ≥5% during the 1st month of the outbreak.

The predictors included herd size, milk yield, region and all variables listed in Table 2. Herd size was a continuous variable. Data on herd size were not normally distributed, thus they were divided into three herd size classes: (1) 50–65, (2) 66–99, and (3) ≥100 cows per herd. Milk yield was a normally distributed continuous variable and was presented as 1000 kg in analyses. The geographical location of the herd was categorized into four groups based on counties in Finland; (1) southern, (2) western, (3) eastern, and (4) northern region. The flooring variable was categorized into (1) slatted concrete, (2) solid concrete, (3) slatted floor with rubber, and (4) solid floor with rubber. The ventilation system was divided in two groups; (0) natural ventilation, (1) natural ventilation with an additional precision ventilation of the manure drain or mechanical ventilation with or without an additional precision ventilation of the manure drain. This latter option is later referred as a mechanical ventilation system.

The enlargement or renovation of the barn was a dichotomous variable, where (0) no enlargement or renovation in 3 years prior to the outbreak in outbreak herds or no enlargement or renovation in 3 years' prior replying to the survey in control herds and (1) enlargement or renovation in 3 year period prior to the outbreak in outbreak herds or enlargement or renovation during the 3 year period prior to replying to the survey in control herds. The open or closed herd variable discriminated between two groups; (0) closed herd i.e. no purchase of cattle and no contract heifer rearing, (1) open herd i.e. purchase of cattle or contract heifer rearing or both.

The sample size in the model was 294 herds with an occurrence of an outbreak of IP 19%. An odds ratio (OR) 2.7 with a power of 0.9 for predictors was determined as significant for this sample size, assuming the proportion of exposed controls for this predictor was 25%.

### Statistical model

We excluded the herds with few cases of IP from the statistical analysis of the risk factors of an IP outbreak. Associations between all predictors and the outcome were computed using simple logistic regression. The predictors with association ≤0.2 were included in the full model. A manual stepwise backwards procedure was used to build the nested model. Removed variables were evaluated at each step for confounding effects by checking if the coefficients for remaining variables had changed over 20%. The region, herd size and the milk yield were considered to be confounding variables and therefore, were kept in the model. Moreover, full and nested models were compared with the logistic likelihood ratio test.

We tested all biologically plausible interactions, but detected no significant association. We also evaluated the model by sensitivity and specificity test and roc-curve of the model. The assumptions of the model were controlled by normality and scatter plots of the model residuals. One herd was found to be an outlier, but because it did not change the results essentially, it was kept in the model.

## Results

A total of 390 questionnaires were returned resulting in a response rate of 34.4%. Of these responses, 355 free stall herds had complete information on their IP status and therefore were included in the study.

**Table 2 Descriptive statistics of the study herds (n = 355)**

| Variable | Replies (n)[1] | Control (%) | Few cases of IP (%) | Outbreak of IP (%) | Total (%) |
|---|---|---|---|---|---|
| Study herds (n) | *355* | *259 (73.0%)* | *32 (9.0%)* | *64 (18.0%)* | *355 (100%)* |
| Region | 353 | | | | |
| Southern | | 37 (14.4%) | 2 (6.2%) | 5 (7.8%) | 44 (12.4%) |
| Western | | 116 (45.1%) | 14 (43.8%) | 33 (51.6%) | 163 (46.2%) |
| Eastern | | 55 (21.4%) | 8 (25.0%) | 12 (18.7%) | 75 (21.3%) |
| Northern | | 49 (19.1%) | 8 (25.0%) | 14 (21.9%) | 71 (20.1%) |
| Barn characteristics | | | | | |
| Number of cow compartments in the barn | 355 | | | | |
| 1 | | 218 (84.2%) | 24 (75.0%) | 36 (56.3%) | 278 (78.3%) |
| ≥2 | | 41 (15.8%) | 8 (25.0%) | 28 (43.7%) | 77 (21.7%) |
| Free stall type | 345 | | | | |
| Insulated | | 198 (78.6%) | 19 (61.3%) | 36 (58.1%) | 253 (73.3%) |
| Partly insulated | | 42 (16.7%) | 11 (35.5%) | 23 (37.1%) | 76 (22.0%) |
| Non-insulated | | 12 (4.7%) | 1 (3.2%) | 3 (4.8%) | 16 (4.7%) |
| Flooring | 341 | | | | |
| Slatted concrete | | 120 (48.2%) | 13 (41.9%) | 28 (45.9%) | 161 (47.2%) |
| Solid concrete | | 62 (24.9%) | 10 (32.3%) | 17 (27.9%) | 89 (26.1%) |
| Slatted rubber | | 17 (6.8%) | 1 (3.2%) | 4 (6.5%) | 22 (6.5%) |
| Solid rubber | | 50 (20.1%) | 7 (22.6%) | 12 (19.7%) | 69 (20.2%) |
| Milking system | 345 | | | | |
| Milking parlour | | 121 (48.0%) | 11 (35.5%) | 22 (35.5%) | 154 (44.6%) |
| Automatic milking system | | 131 (52.0%) | 20 (64.5%) | 40 (64.5%) | 191 (55.4%) |
| Ventilation system | 343 | | | | |
| Natural | | 56 (22.2%) | 10 (32.3%) | 30 (50.0%) | 96 (28.0%) |
| Mechanical[2] | | 196 (77.8%) | 21 (67.7%) | 30 (50.0%) | 247 (72.0%) |
| Management practices | | | | | |
| Total or partial mixed ration feeding | 355 | | | | |
| No | | 140 (54.1%) | 7 (21.9%) | 13 (20.3%) | 160 (45.1%) |
| Yes | | 119 (45.9%) | 25 (78.1%) | 51 (79.7%) | 195 (54.9%) |
| Outdoor access during summer | 355 | | | | |
| No | | 154 (59.5%) | 17 (53.1%) | 47 (73.4%) | 218 (61.4%) |
| Yes | | 105 (40.5%) | 15 (46.9%) | 17 (26.6%) | 137 (38.6%) |
| Outdoor access during winter | 353 | | | | |
| No | | 214 (82.6%) | 23 (76.7%) | 55 (85.9%) | 292 (82.7%) |
| Yes | | 45 (17.4%) | 7 (23.3%) | 9 (14.1%) | 61 (17.3%) |
| Hoof trimming frequency | 355 | | | | |
| 0–1 | | 80 (30.9%) | 8 (25.0%) | 20 (31.2%) | 108 (30.4%) |
| ≥2 | | 179 (69.1%) | 24 (75.0%) | 44 (68.8%) | 247 (69.6%) |
| Stocking density (cows/stall) | 345 | | | | |
| <1 | | 90 (35.9%) | 10 (32.2%) | 34 (54.0%) | 134 (38.8%) |
| 1 | | 132 (52.6%) | 14 (45.2%) | 23 (36.5%) | 169 (49.0%) |
| >1 | | 29 (11.5%) | 7 (22.6%) | 6 (9.5%) | 42 (12.2%) |
| Enlargement[3] within 3 years | 349 | | | | |
| No | | 180 (69.8%) | 14 (50.0%) | 21 (33.3%) | 215 (61.6%) |
| Yes | | 78 (30.2%) | 14 (50.0%) | 42 (66.7%) | 134 (38.4%) |
| Open or closed herd | 353 | | | | |
| Closed herd | | 189 (73.3%) | 17 (53.1%) | 24 (38.1%) | 230 (65.2%) |
| Open herd | | 69 (26.7%) | 15 (46.9%) | 39 (61.9%) | 123 (34.8%) |

**Table 2 continued**

| Variable | Replies (n)[1] | Control (%) | Few cases of IP (%) | Outbreak of IP (%) | Total (%) |
|---|---|---|---|---|---|
| Fields in organic farming | 355 | | | | |
| No | | 242 (93.4%) | 27 (84.4%) | 55 (85.9%) | 324 (91.3%) |
| Yes | | 17 (6.6%) | 5 (15.6%) | 9 (14.1%) | 31 (8.7%) |

*IP* interdigital phlegmon

[1] The column 'Replies (n)' describes the number of replies given to each question

[2] Natural with additional precision ventilation of the manure drain or mechanical with or without additional precision ventilation of the manure drain

[3] Enlargement or renovation of the barn

The mean herd size was 79.8 dairy cows (range 50–293.7) and the mean yearly milk yield of the herds was 9364 kg (6800–12,500 kg). Table 2 summarizes the barn characteristics and management practices of the study herds.

Sixty-four out of 355 herds (18.0%) had had an outbreak of IP with morbidity ≥5% within the 1st month of the outbreak. All reported outbreaks had occurred in the year 2004 or later and a majority (68.8%) within the 2009–2013 period (Fig. 1). Furthermore, 32 (9.0%) respondents reported few cases of IP in the herd. Out of 64 IP herds 14 (21.9%) reported cases of IP in heifers and 11 (17.2%) in calves. A year after the outbreak, in 21 out of 47 outbreak herds (44.7%) still had sporadic cases of IP in cows, in 4 herds (8.5%) in heifers, and in 1 herd (2.1%) in calves. Signs of IP cases in the 64 outbreak herds were as follows: 33 (51.6%) herds reported fever, 62 (96.9%) lameness, 62 (96.9%) swelling above a hoof, 36 (56.3%) shaking of a leg, 34 (53.1%) bad odour in the hoof region, 50 (78.1%) lesions in between the hooves and 25 (39.1%) lesions in the heel.

#### Risk factors for an outbreak of IP

We compared control farms (n = 239) and farms with an outbreak of IP (n = 55) and analyzed the associations of various predictors. Out of 323 herds, we included 294 herds with a complete dataset in the analysis. Table 3 presents the results of a logistic regression model.

#### Occurrence of an outbreak of IP associated putative diseases

We studied the association of an outbreak of IP with the occurrence of various other hoof diseases and visual signs of calf diphtheria such as buccal abscesses. Interdigital hyperplasia, verrucous dermatitis and other infectious hoof diseases, like ID and DD, were detected more frequently (Pearson's $Chi^2$ 28.6, 10.4, and 46.4 respectively, in all $P < 0.01$) among the herds with an outbreak of IP

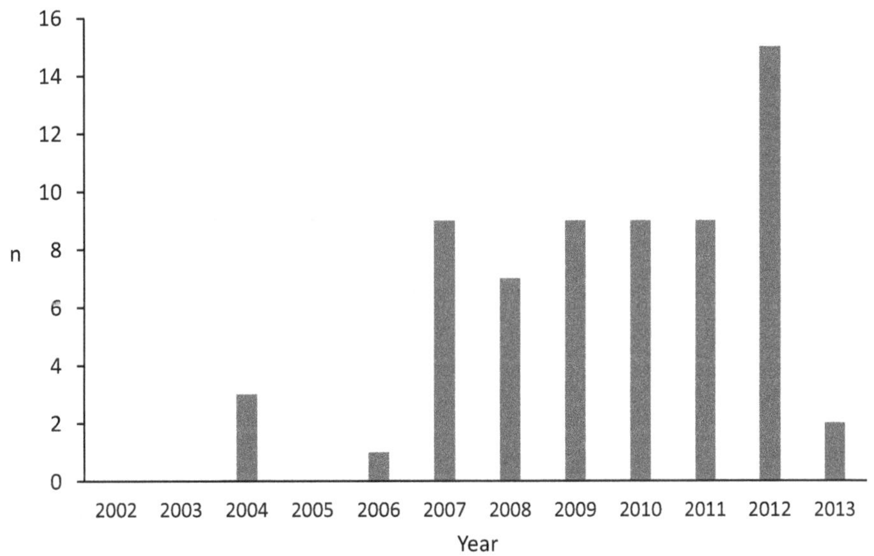


**Fig. 1** Number of the herds with an outbreak of interdigital phlegmon (IP) per year. The number (n = 64) of the herds with an outbreak of IP based on the replies to our survey. The survey was performed in May 2013 and therefore, the last year in this chart is incomplete

**Table 3 Final logistic regression model for an outbreak of interdigital phlegmon (IP)**

| Variable | n | Odds ratio | *P* value | 95% CI[1] | Wald[2] |
|---|---|---|---|---|---|
| Free stall type | | | | | |
| Insulated | 221 | Referent | | | 0.09 |
| Partly insulated | 60 | 0.31 | 0.06 | 0.09–1.05 | |
| Non-insulated | 13 | 0.14 | 0.07 | 0.02–1.20 | |
| Ventilation | | | | | |
| Natural | 84 | Referent | | | |
| Mechanical[3] | 210 | 0.18 | <0.01 | 0.06–0.54 | |
| Herd size | | | | | |
| 50–65 | 125 | Referent | | | 0.07 |
| 66–99 | 115 | 0.97 | 0.94 | 0.41–2.26 | |
| ≥100 | 54 | 2.60 | 0.04 | 1.03–6.58 | |
| Enlargement[4] within 3 years | | | | | |
| No | 184 | Referent | | | |
| Yes | 110 | 3.32 | <0.01 | 1.58–6.98 | |
| Open or closed herd | | | | | |
| Closed herd | 194 | Referent | | | |
| Open herd | 100 | 4.91 | <0.01 | 2.32–10.37 | |
| Fields in organic farming | | | | | |
| No | 270 | Referent | | | |
| Yes | 24 | 3.75 | 0.02 | 1.21–11.66 | |
| Milk yield[5] | 294 | 0.73 | 0.18 | 0.45–1.16 | |
| Region | | | | | |
| Southern | 38 | Referent | | | 0.56 |
| Western | 138 | 1.75 | 0.40 | 0.48–6.37 | |
| Eastern | 62 | 2.10 | 0.30 | 0.51–8.65 | |
| Northern | 56 | 2.77 | 0.17 | 0.65–11.82 | |
| _Constant | | 1.88 | 0.80 | 0.02–218.92 | |

The associations of various herd level variables and an outbreak of IP. The number of the outbreak herds in the model is 55 and control herds 239 (n = 294)

[1] 95% CI = 95% confidence interval

[2] Wald-test was used to test the overall *P* value of the variable

[3] Natural with additional precision ventilation of the manure drain or mechanical with or without additional precision ventilation of the manure drain

[4] Enlargement or renovation of the barn

[5] Milk yield is in 1000 kg

(Fig. 2). Similarly, buccal abscesses in suckling calves were observed more often (Pearson's Chi$^2$ 65.3, $P < 0.01$).

## Discussion

We determined the current situation regarding infectious hoof diseases in Finland. Eighteen percent of the herds who responded to the questionnaire in our study were diagnosed as having an outbreak of IP with morbidity ≥5% within the 1st month of the outbreak, whereas 9.0% of the herds who reported having sporadic cases of IP did not fulfill our definition of an outbreak. Interestingly, those farms that had experienced an outbreak of IP, often had other infectious hoof diseases. However, it was impossible to deduce from our study design and survey data, which disease appeared first in the herd. Likewise, a study from the Netherlands reported that the presence of other infectious hoof disorders, such as interdigital dermatitis and heel horn erosion (IDHE) and IP, increased the risk for DD, and IP appeared to be strongly associated with DD (OR = 4.4) [17]. Other reports of correlations between other infectious hoof diseases than IP also exist [18–20]. Recently, veterinary practitioners in Finland have observed an increase in the number of buccal abscesses in young dairy calves in herds with a previous outbreak of IP. Our survey data supports this observation. A buccal abscess may characterize a sign of calf diphtheria; a respiratory tract disease where *F. necrophorum* plays a part in the pathogenesis [21, 22].

We investigated the possible herd level risk factors for an outbreak of IP to occur. Our study determined recent enlargement or renovation of the barn to be a risk factor for an outbreak of IP. During the enlargement process, both the cattle and the dairy producers suffer from stress; they must adapt to a new building, and management regime that differ from the old system. Before the introduction of the new free stall, some overstocking may occur in the old building, which would plausibly increase the infection pressure. Occasionally, when the cattle are compelled to move into new free stall, the facility can still be a construction site, which might increase the risk for injuries and is an additional burden and stress factor to farmers. As part of the restructuring and the enlargement, the tradition of the family managed farm may end, and the cattle in the enlarged herds will be managed by employed staff. If the management is not of sufficient quality or there are fewer stockmen to look after more cows, the risk of mistakes and unnoticed signs of ill-health may increase.

We also determined the animal transport between herds to be a risk factor for an outbreak of IP. This was not surprising, because of the infectious nature of the disease [3, 6]. Moreover, the purchase of new animals occurs more frequently during the enlargement of a herd, and contract heifer rearing is also more common before or after the enlargement when producers try to adapt to different management strategies to deal with the increasing herd size. Buying in new heifers from other farms has been reported as a risk for DD [23–25]. On the other hand, a new animal in a herd always meets different environment and management, which may affect its immunology. The possible causality of the animal purchase and the IP outbreak in our study was unclear in the questionnaire data and therefore, purchase of heifers may not be a causal factor in the IP outbreak but simply be a simultaneous management course of action in the farm.

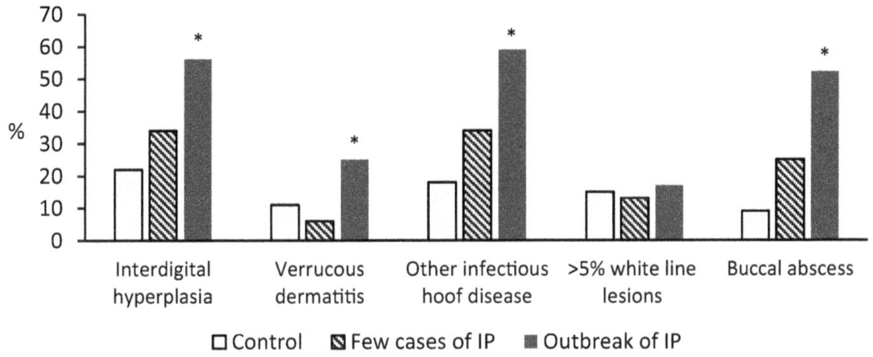


**Fig. 2** Interdigital phlegmon (IP) associated putative diseases and occurrence (%) in various disease groups. The occurrence of various diseases in group with no outbreak of IP i.e. control herds (n = 259), group with few cases of IP (n = 32) and group with an outbreak of IP (the morbidity of IP ≥5% during the 1st month of the outbreak, n = 64). The definition of the other infectious hoof diseases includes lesions in between the hooves or in the heel and reddish, painful lesions in the hoof region. The >5% white line lesions describes lesions that needed a hoof blocking for treatment, and buccal abscesses characterize visual signs of calf diphtheria in suckling calves. The Chi squared test was used between control and outbreak herds and significant difference is marked with $*P < 0.01$

We also found that organically cultivated fields were a risk factor. Even though the number of the herds with organically cultivated fields (n = 24) was small in our model, the post hoc power analysis (0.88) showed that the group was big enough to detect the possible risk. In Finland, the soil lacks selenium (Se), and in conventional farming the use of fertilizers with Se supplement is standard. However, the regulations of organic farming limit the use of fertilizers and if Se supplement is not added in the feed, a deficiency might occur. Low blood Se level might alter the immunological status of the cows and increase disease susceptibility. For example, some studies have detected an association with low Se and vitamin E deficiency and udder health [26, 27]. Another possible underlying cause in organic farming may be the excessive use of clover in the silage. Johnson [14] speculated as long ago as 1945 that clover might be a reason for an increased incidence of IP. Moreover, due to the EU regulations of organic farming (Council regulation 2007/834/EC) animal purchase is more likely to happen between other organic herds. The risk of IP spreading from one organic farm to another is increased if the IP is more common in organic farms than conventional ones. None of these possible factors listed above could be ascertained by only one question in this survey. More details about the grazing conditions, trace element status and grass and clover species content of fields would be needed in future studies to investigate such possible factors.

Any form of mechanical ventilation was found to decrease the risk of an outbreak of IP. We presume that the better the ventilation the drier the indoor air and less ammonia in the free stall. Furthermore, the drier the indoor air the cleaner the cows are. Two Norwegian studies reported that barns with low air humidity had cleaner animals [28] and for each 10% increase in relative air humidity, the risk of dirty thighs increased [29]. In the past, moist conditions underneath the hooves have been associated with IP [4, 6]. Several studies have also found associations between other infectious hoof diseases and dirty claws or legs or dirty alleys [20, 25, 30, 31]. The flooring type had no effect on the outbreaks of IP in our study in contrast to studies of DD from the UK and USA. Solid flooring of grooved concrete was identified as a risk factor for DD in the UK [32] and in the USA [24] when compared to textured concrete floors.

In this study, an overstocking was not a risk for an outbreak of IP. However, the animal protection law in Finland prohibits an overstocking and one stall per cow is compulsory. This may have affected the responses of farmers. Additionally, the stocking situation in the barn varies constantly.

Replies to our survey represented the regional differences in dairy farming in Finland quite well; all areas were represented and replies from areas with more dairy cows, like provinces Pohjanmaa and Savo, were a greater number. Additionally, the mean milk yield of the study herds related appropriately to free stall herds of similar size. However, some bias may exist in our results. Presumably the farms that had problems with infectious hoof diseases were more prone to answer the survey and therefore, our results may be moderately skewed. Although we could detect several possible risk factors for an outbreak of IP, we were not able to specify why there has been so many of these outbreaks in Finland. One reason could be that other countries had experienced similar outbreaks much earlier [12, 13, 33], and due to Finland's relative isolation Finnish dairy herds are still immunologically quite naïve and therefore more susceptible to IP.

## Conclusions

This study revealed risk factors that were associated with the outbreaks of IP in Finland. These risk factors were animal transport between herds, enlargement or renovation of the barn and organic cultivation of the fields. However, having a forced ventilation system in the free stall barn lowered the risk. These results suggest that more attention is needed before and during the enlargement process and substantial planning is crucial in every part of that undertaking. Since the farms that had experienced an outbreak of IP, often had other infectious hoof diseases as well we speculated that this strategic approach would additionally reduce the incidence of these further diseases.

### Authors' contributions

All authors participated in planning the study, MKo, MKu, RJ, TS, and HS designed the questionnaire, MKo collected the data, MKo, MKu and HS performed the statistical analyses and MKo drafted the manuscript. All authors read and approved the final manuscript.


### Author details

[1] Department of Production Animal Medicine, Faculty of Veterinary Medicine, University of Helsinki, Paroninkuja 20, 04920 Saarentaus, Finland. [2] Veterinary Bacteriology Research Unit, Finnish Food Safety Authority Evira, Mustialankatu 3, 00790 Helsinki, Finland. [3] Veterinary Bacteriology Research Unit, Finnish Food Safety Authority Evira, Neulaniementie 4, 70210 Kuopio, Finland.



### Acknowledgements

We thank Anne Mikkola and Maarit Mäki from University of Helsinki, Saari unit for the technical assistance with the mailing of the questionnaires and we also thank all the dairy farmers who replied to our survey.


### Competing interests

The authors declare that they have no competing interests. TS is a deputy editor of Acta Veterinaria Scandinavica but has not in any way been involved in the editorial handling of the manuscript or decision making.


### Funding

This study was funded by the Ministry of Agriculture and Forestry project (2066/312/2011) for infectious hoof diseases in new free stalls in Finland, Valio Ltd and the Mercedes Zachariassen Foundation.


### References


1. Häggman J, Junni R, Simojoki H, Juga J, Soveri T. The costs of interdigital phlegmon in four loose-housed Finnish dairy herds. Acta Vet Scand. 2015;57:90.
2. Flint JC, Jensen R. Pathology of necrobacillosis of the bovine foot. Am J Vet Res. 1951;12:5–13.
3. Clark BL, Stewart DJ, Emery DL. The role of *Fusobacterium necrophorum* and *Bacteroides melaninogenicus* in the aetiology of interdigital necrobacillosis in cattle. Aust Vet J. 1985;62:47–9.
4. Johnson DW, Dommert AR, Kiger DG. Clinical investigations of infectious foot rot of cattle. J Am Vet Med Assoc. 1969;155:1886–91.
5. Berg JN, Loan RW. *Fusobacterium necrophorum* and *Bacteroides melaninogenicus* as etiologic agents of foot rot in cattle. Am J Vet Res. 1975;36:1115–22.
6. Gupta RB, Fincher MG, Bruner DW. A study of the etiology of foot-rot in cattle. Cornell Vet. 1964;54:66–77.
7. Hernandez J, Shearer JK, Webb DW. Effect of lameness on milk yield in dairy cows. J Am Vet Med Assoc. 2002;220:640–4.
8. Booth CJ, Warnick LD, Gröhn YT, Maizon DO, Guard CL, Janssen D. Effect of lameness on culling in dairy cows. J Dairy Sci. 2004;87:4115–22.
9. DeFrain JM, Socha MT, Tomlinson DJ. Analysis of foot health records from 17 confinement dairies. J Dairy Sci. 2013;96:7329–39.
10. Cramer G, Lissemore KD, Guard CL, Leslie KE, Kelton DF. Herd- and cow-level prevalence of foot lesions in Ontario dairy cattle. J Dairy Sci. 2008;91:3888–95.
11. Oberbauer AM, Berry SL, Belanger JM, McGoldrick RM, Pinos-Rodriquez JM, Famula TR. Determining the heritable component of dairy cattle foot lesions. J Dairy Sci. 2013;96:605–13.
12. David GP. Severe foul-in-the-foot in dairy cattle. Vet Rec. 1993;132:567–8.
13. Doherty M, Bassett H, Markey B, Healy A, Sammin D. Severe foot lameness in cattle associated with invasive spirochaetes. Ir Vet J. 1998;1:195–8.
14. Johnson KL. Infectious pododermatitis in dairy cattle. N Am Vet. 1945;26:665–7.
15. Alban L, Lawson LG, Agger JF. Foul in the foot (interdigital necrobacillosis) in Danish dairy cows—frequency and possible risk factors. Prev Vet Med. 1995;24:73–82.
16. National Resources Institute Finland: number of dairy cows in various herd sizes 1.5.2012. http://stat.luke.fi/en/number-bovine-animals-1-may-2012_en. Accessed 20 Apr 2017.
17. Holzhauer M, Hardenberg C, Bartels C, Frankena K. Herd- and cow-level prevalence of digital dermatitis in the Netherlands and associated risk factors. J Dairy Sci. 2006;89:580–8.
18. Manske T, Hultgren J, Bergsten C. Prevalence and interrelationships of hoof lesions and lameness in Swedish dairy cows. Prev Vet Med. 2002;54:247–63.
19. Capion N, Thamsborg SM, Enevoldsen C. Prevalence and severity of foot lesions in Danish Holstein heifers through first lactation. Vet J. 2009;182:50–8.
20. Knappe-Poindecker M, Gilhuus M, Jensen TK, Klitgaard K, Larssen RB, Fjeldaas T. Interdigital dermatitis, heel horn erosion, and digital dermatitis in 14 Norwegian dairy herds. J Dairy Sci. 2013;96:7617–29.
21. Ryff JF, Lee AM. The etiology of calf diphtheria. Am J Vet Res. 1946;7:41–4.
22. Panciera RJ, Perino LJ, Baldwin CA, Morton RJ, Swanson JE. Observations of calf diphtheria in the commercial feedlot. Agri-practice. 1989;10:12–7.
23. Rodriguez-Lainz A, Melendez-Retamal P, Hird DW, Read DH, Walker RL. Farm- and host-level risk factors for papillomatous digital dermatitis in Chilean dairy cattle. Prev Vet Med. 1999;42:87–97.
24. Wells SJ, Garber LP, Wagner BA. Papillomatous digital dermatitis and associated risk factors in US dairy herds. Prev Vet Med. 1999;38:11–24.
25. Rodríguez-Lainz A, Hird DW, Carpenter TE, Read DH. Case-control study of papillomatous digital dermatitis in Southern California dairy farms. Prev Vet Med. 1996;28:117–31.
26. Smith KL, Harrison JH, Hancock DD, Todhunter DA, Conrad HR. Effect of vitamin E and selenium supplementation on incidence of clinical mastitis and duration of clinical symptoms. J Dairy Sci. 1984;67:1293–300.
27. Jukola E, Hakkarainen J, Saloniemi H, Sankari S. Blood Selenium, vitamin E, vitamin A, and β-carotene concentrations and udder health, fertility treatments, and fertility. J Dairy Sci. 1996;79:838–45.
28. Hauge SJ, Kielland C, Ringdal G, Skjerve E, Nafstad O. Factors associated with cattle cleanliness on Norwegian dairy farms. J Dairy Sci. 2012;95:2485–96.
29. Ruud LE, Bøe KE, Østerås O. Risk factors for dirty dairy cows in Norwegian freestall systems. J Dairy Sci. 2010;93:5216–24.
30. Somers JGCJ, Frankena K, Noordhuizen-Stassen EN, Metz JHM. Prevalence of claw disorders in Dutch dairy cows exposed to several floor systems. J Dairy Sci. 2003;86:2082–93.
31. Relun A, Lehebel A, Bruggink M, Bareille N, Guatteo R. Estimation of the relative impact of treatment and herd management practices on prevention of digital dermatitis in French dairy herds. Prev Vet Med. 2013;110:558–62.
32. Barker ZE, Amory JR, Wright JL, Mason SA, Blowey RW, Green LE. Risk factors for increased rates of sole ulcers, white line disease, and digital dermatitis in dairy cattle from twenty-seven farms in England and Wales. J Dairy Sci. 2009;92:1971–8.

# Analytical validation of bovine plasma ceruloplasmin measurement by *p*-phenylenediamine oxidation and effect of storage time and freezing temperature

Hussein Awad Hussein[1*] and Rudolf Staufenbiel[2]

**Abstract**

**Background:** Determination of ceruloplasmin (Cp) activity in plasma can provide an objective measure of the health of dairy cows as well as it can be used for various diagnostic purposes. The current study was designed to perform an analytical validation of a method for the determination of plasma Cp activity in dairy cows and to evaluate the influences of plasma storage times and temperatures as well as freeze–thaw cycles on the activity of this enzyme. This cohort was carried out on ten cows. For each cow, 24 aliquots of plasma, which were stored at different temperature regimes, were prepared. Both intra- and interassay coefficients of variation (CVs) were determined. The linearity was evaluated using bovine plasma Cp standard.

**Results:** The mean values of intra- and interassay CVs were 1.08 and 2.12%, respectively. Results of linearity testing showed a high correlation coefficient ($r = 0.998$, $P < 0.001$). After 3 days of storage at room temperature and refrigeration, the plasma activity of Cp was significantly lowered ($P < 0.05$). Plasma samples kept at freezing for 3 months revealed insignificant changes in the activity of Cp. Repeated freeze–thaw cycles for three times had no significant influence on the activity of Cp.

**Conclusions:** The method is easy and may be valid at values of Cp ranging from 100 to 1000 mg/L. It seems that keeping of plasma samples at room temperature and refrigeration longer than 3 days is unsuitable for Cp measurement. In addition, Cp remains stable in plasma samples stored at freezing as well as repeat freeze–thaw cycles.

**Keywords:** Biochemistry, Cows, Refrigeration, Thawing

## Background

Ceruloplasmin (Cp), a copper containing protein in plasma, was first identified in 1948 by Holmberg and Laurell [1]. It is a α2-glycoprotein synthesized in the liver containing six atoms of copper in its structure [2, 3]. In addition, Cp contains hexosamine, hexose, and neuraminic acid [4]. It has a ferroxidase activity and contains more than 95% of the copper present in plasma [5]. Cp has several functions. It is essential for iron homeostasis [6] and is involved in cellular prooxidant [7] and antioxidant [8] processes, as well as antibacterial host defense [9].

From the clinical point of view, Cp determination could provide information about the health status of cattle [10]. Cp is a mild to moderate acute phase protein that increases in concentration in association with inflammation [11–13]. Furthermore, it undergoes physiological changes during different lactation stages of dairy cows [14]. In addition, Cp has a potentiality for evaluation of copper status in dairy cows [15, 16].

Many quantitative methods had been used for Cp measurement in plasma or serum [4]. In veterinary clinical laboratories, most assays for estimation of Cp are based on oxidation of compounds such as

*Correspondence: hhussein@aun.edu.eg

[1] Internal Veterinary Medicine, Department of Animal Medicine, Faculty of Veterinary Medicine, Assiut University, Assiut 71526, Egypt

*p*-phenylenediamine (PPD) or its *N*-dimethyl derivative and *O*-dianisidine dihydrochloride [17–19].

For multiple experimental time points, plasma samples may be subjected to different periods of storage before analysis [20]. From the practical point of view, the stored plasma samples may be reanalyzed to confirm the previous results or to perform additional analysis. Therefore, the stability of the analytes must be assured before giving results, or before establishing new investigations [21].

The objectives of the current study were to perform an analytical validation of a manual method for measurement of plasma Cp in Holstein dairy cows and to evaluate the influences of some methodological aspects related to plasma storage times and temperatures as well as freeze–thaw cycles on the activity of this enzyme.

## Methods

### Animals

Ten Holstein dairy cows (age range 3–6 years) at their mid lactation (15–18 weeks postpartum) were included in this study. All animals were between 2nd or 5th lactation seasons. All cows originated from a herd of State of Brandenburg, Germany, were housed in a free stall, and fed a diet of grass and maize silage and concentrate as a totally mixed ration (TMR). All cows were randomly chosen and were clinically healthy. On the basis of clinical examinations [22] made before sample collection, cows that had diseases which might have provoked an acute phase reaction were excluded from the study.

### Blood sampling and study design

From each cow, 30 mL of blood were sampled from a coccygeal vein into three heparinized vacutainer tubes. After centrifugation (3000 rpm, 15 min), plasma samples of each cow were harvested and pooled, and subsequently divided into aliquots. Twenty-four aliquots for each cow were prepared each aliquot containing 0.4 mL plasma. Two aliquots were used immediately for the assay (T0 measurements), and five and three aliquots were frozen at − 20 °C for studying the influence of freezing and repeated freeze–thaw cycles, respectively on the activity of Cp. Seven aliquots were kept at refrigerator temperature (4 °C) and the last seven aliquots were stored at room temperature (around 20 °C) (Fig. 1).

The three aliquots (1–3) that were kept at − 20 °C for studying the influence of freeze–thaw cycles on the activity of Cp were analyzed at three different days as the following: After 24 h, aliquots 1, 2, and 3 from each cow were thawed at room temperature (20 °C) for 30 min. Aliquot 1 was used for the assay (and then discarded), and aliquots 2 and 3 were refrozen. At 48 h, according to the same procedure, aliquot 2 was assayed and aliquot 3 was refrozen. At 72 h, aliquot 3 was thawed and assayed. The five aliquots from each cow stored at − 20 °C were analyzed after storage of 1, 2, 4, 8, and 12 weeks. The last 14 aliquots from each cow that were kept at room temperature and 4 °C were assayed at day 1, 2, 3, 4, 5, 7, and 10 after the beginning of storage.

### Biochemical assays

The activity of Cp was measured by *p*-phenylenediamine oxidation [14, 23]: 100 μL of plasma sample was diluted with 2 mL 0.1 M acetate buffer (adjusted to pH 5.45) and added to 1 mL freshly prepared buffered *p*-phenylenediamine solution (27.6 mmol/L) (Sigma-Aldrich, Germany) (adjusted to pH 5.45 using sodium bicarbonate), and then incubated at 37 °C. The absorbance reflecting the intensity of the purple coloured product was measured by a spectrometer at 530 nm, after 5 min (A5) and 30 min (A30) using sodium azide 1.5 M (Sigma-Aldrich, Germany) for stopping the enzyme reaction. The oxidase activity of Cp that was indicated by the absorbance was expressed in mg/L according to the following equation: Cp (mg/L) = (A30 − A5) × 752. The rate of formation of the coloured product of the enzymatic reaction is proportional to the concentration of plasma Cp; this is why the enzymatic activity is expressed as milligrams of Cp by liter of plasma instead of commonly used enzymatic units. There were 240 assays in total (10 cows, 24 aliquots, and 1 constituent).

### Analytical validation

#### *Precision*

Intra-assay coefficients of variations (CVs) were calculated after analysis of two plasma samples and analyzed ten times in a single assay run. Interassay coefficients of variations were determined by analyzing the same two samples in ten separate runs carried out on different days. All these samples were stored frozen at − 20 °C in aliquots.

#### *Linearity*

Linearity was evaluated directly by analyzing serial dilutions (1/2, 1/4, 1/8, 1/16, 1/32, 1/64, 1/128, and 1/256) of bovine plasma ceruloplasmin standard (BIO-VAR Ltd, Armenia). To determine the range of ceruloplasmin at which the relationship is linear, other dilutions (68, 61, 54, 47, 40, 33, 27, 20, 13, and 6%) of the dilution 1/4 of ceruloplasmin standard were prepared and analyzed. Furthermore, the limit of detection (LOD) of the assay was determined as the lowest concentration of an analyte (ceruloplasmin) in a sample that can be detected but not necessarily quantified, under the stated condition of the test [24]. In addition, the limit of quantitation (LOQ) was calculated as the lowest concentration of an analyte (Cp) in the sample that can be determined with acceptable

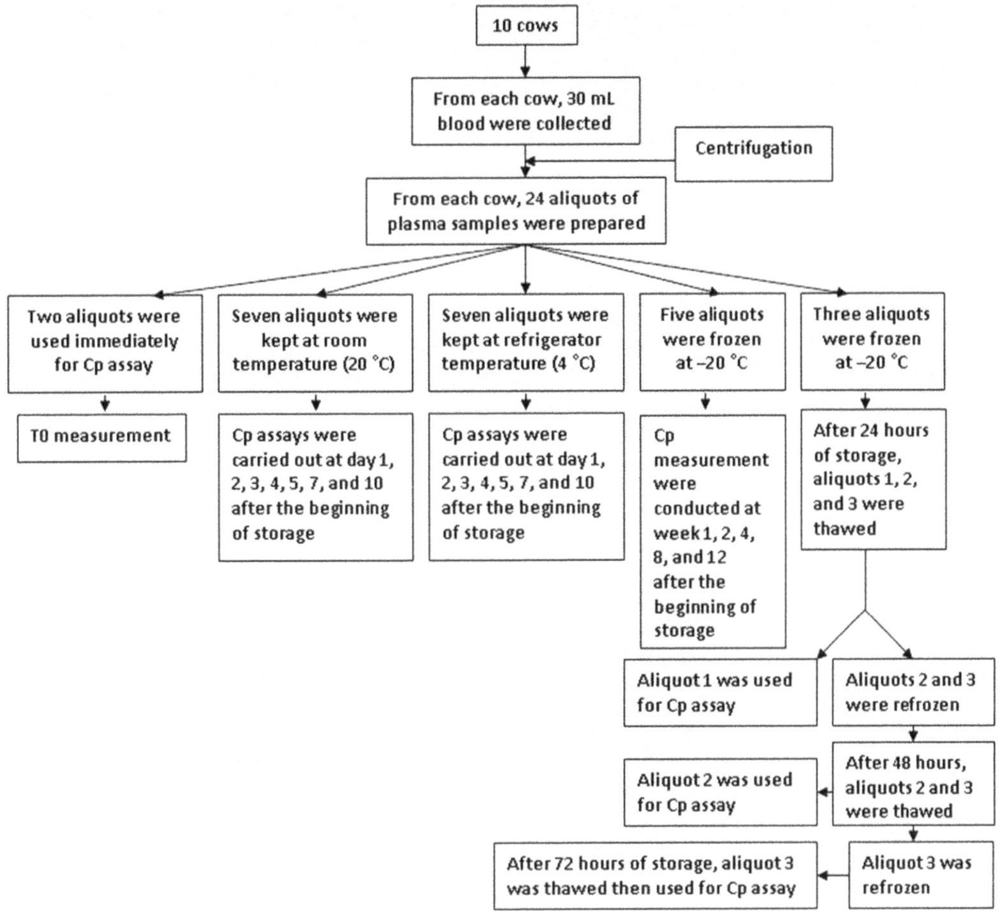


**Fig. 1** Schematic diagram representing study design and storage temperatures

precision and accuracy under the stated condition of the test [25]. Both LOD and LOQ were calculated from the linear regression using the following equation [24]:

$$\text{LOD or LOQ} = (\text{F} \times \text{SD}) \div \text{b}$$

where F is a factor of 3.3 in the case of LOD or a factor of 10 in the case of LOQ, SD: standard deviation of the intercept, b: slope of the regression line.

### Statistical analysis

Data were analyzed statistically using SPSS software (SPSS statistical program, SPSS Inc., Version 16, Chicago, IL, USA). Intra- and interassay CVs were calculated using routine descriptive statistical procedures. Ordinary regression analysis was performed to investigate the linearity under dilutions. The heteroscedasticity was tested using Breusch–Pagan test. Repeated measurements of the general linear model using Bonferroni multiple comparison test were used to investigate the influence of storage time on the plasma activity of Cp. Paired T test was used for statistical analysis of the differences between samples stored at room temperatures and refrigeration. For all statistical examinations, results were considered significant at $P < 0.05$. All data are presented as mean ± SD.

## Results

Table 1 shows the results of the precision study of Cp. Intra-assay CVs of plasma series 1 and 2 were 1.25 and 0.91%, respectively. In addition, interassay CVs of series 1 and 2 were 2.37 and 1.87%, respectively. It seemed that the between-run CVs were higher than the within-run, but all CVs were lower than 10%.

Figure 2 illustrates the relationships between Cp determined by the method and the different dilutions of Cp standard. Dilutions of the stock of Cp standard revealed quadratic regression equation with a correlation coefficient of $r = 0.921$ (Fig. 2a). A linear relationship was found using different dilutions of diluted Cp standard with a correlation coefficient of $r = 0.998$ (Fig. 2b). Linearity ranged from 100 to 1000 mg/L. Limit of detection (LOD) and limit of quantitation (LOQ) of Cp were

**Table 1 Precision analysis of ceruloplasmin (Cp) using *p*-phenylenediamine assay**

| | Intra-assay | | | Interassay | | |
|---|---|---|---|---|---|---|
| | Mean | Standard deviation | Coefficient of variation (%) | Mean | Standard deviation | Coefficient of variation (%) |
| Series 1 Cp (mg/L) (n = 10) | 233 | 2.91 | 1.25 | 228 | 5.41 | 2.37 |
| Series 2 Cp (mg/L) (n = 10) | 276 | 2.50 | 0.91 | 275 | 5.15 | 1.87 |

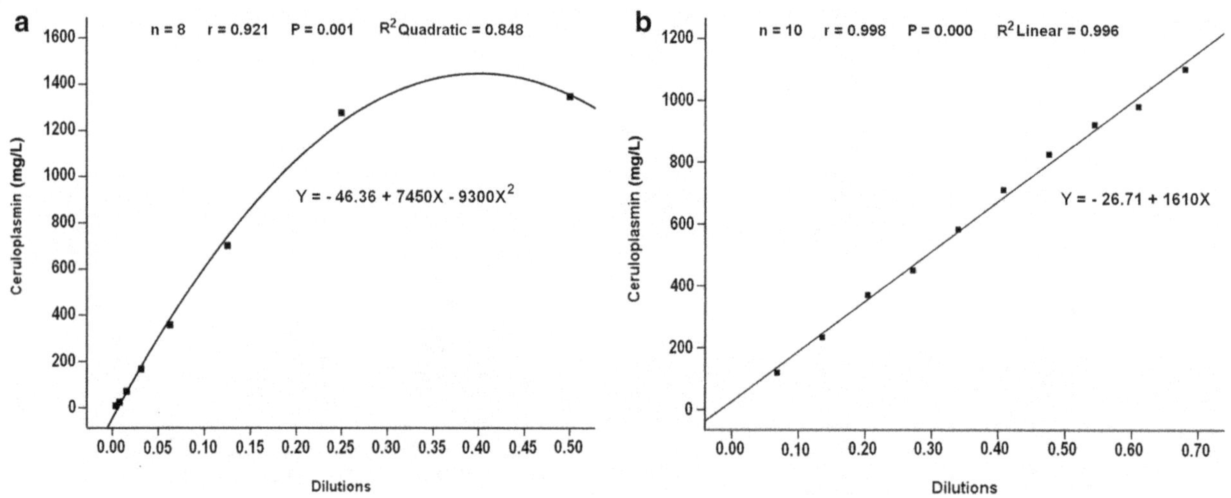


**Fig. 2 a** Quadratic regression of ceruloplasmin standard. **b** Linear regression of diluted ceruloplasmin standard

0.1 and 0.3 mg/L, respectively. The variance of residuals was constant with fitted values of the response variable. Furthermore, the residual analysis between the dependent variable (Cp, at different storage temperatures) and the regression of standardized residuals was linear and the distance from the fitted line and errors tended to be consistent (Fig. 3), indicating the residuals were homoscedastic.

The plasma activity of Cp over time showed a highly significant decrease in samples stored at room temperature and at refrigeration at 4 °C ($P < 0.001$, Table 2). The plasma samples stored at room temperature and refrigeration had more markedly reduced Cp activity from day 4 onward, with the significantly lowest activity on day 10 of storage compared with the initial values ($P < 0.05$). Furthermore, on days 5, 7, and 10 of storage, the activity of Cp was significantly higher in samples stored at refrigeration than at room temperature ($P < 0.05$), ($P < 0.05$), and ($P < 0.01$), respectively (Fig. 4). In addition, Cp activity dropped by 20 and 12% on day 10 after plasma storage at room temperature and refrigeration, respectively.

For 3 months of plasma storage at freezing, the Bonferroni multiple-comparison test revealed insignificant changes ($P > 0.05$) in the activity of Cp (Table 3). On the other hand, three cycles of freezing and thawing had almost no effect on the activity of Cp (Table 4).

## Discussion

Ceruloplasmin has been studied in dairy cows, and it is considered an important and useful indicator for evaluation of copper status in these animals [15, 16]. In addition, Cp has mild to moderate acute phase reaction in dairy cows with subclinical mastitis [26] and dairy calves with diarrhea [27]. No reports are available discussing the analytical validation or the influence of certain methodological aspects of the activity of Cp in dairy cows, but two studies have discussed the validation of automated methods for measuring this protein in canine serum [19] and pigs [28]. Therefore, it was of interest to perform an analytical validation of Cp assays as well as studying the influence of some methodological aspects, related to plasma storage times and temperatures, on the activity of this protein in Holstein dairy cows.

The results revealed a good assay precision with intra- and interassay CVs lower than 10%. These CVs were lower than those obtained using a manual method [29] or an automated method [19] for canine serum samples. Such variation in CVs may be attributed to the sample or

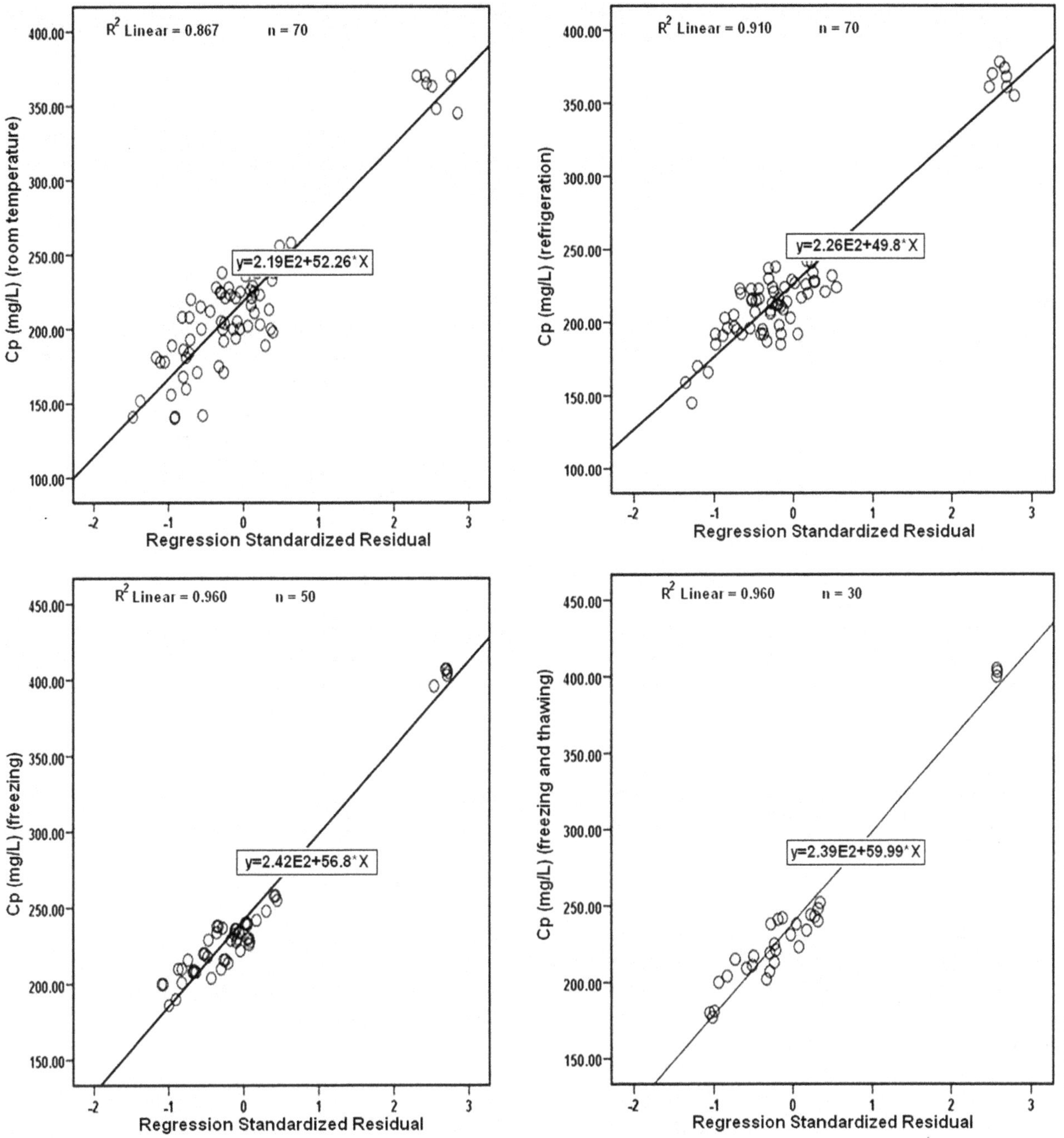


**Fig. 3** Linear regression between ceruloplasmin level (the dependent variable) and the regression standardized residuals at different storage temperatures

**Table 2 Influence of plasma storage at room and refrigeration temperatures on the activity of ceruloplasmin**

| | Storage temperature | Storage days | | | | | | | |
|---|---|---|---|---|---|---|---|---|---|
| | | 0 | 1 | 2 | 3 | 4 | 5 | 7 | 10 |
| Ceruloplasmin (mg/L) (n = 10) | Room temperature (20–25 °C) | $241 \pm 59^a$ | $240 \pm 50^a$ | $238 \pm 51^a$ | $236 \pm 47^a$ | $217 \pm 57^b$ | $206 \pm 62^{bc}$ | $201 \pm 57^{bc}$ | $193 \pm 57^c$ |
| Ceruloplasmin (mg/L) (n = 10) | Refrigeration (+ 4 °C) | $241 \pm 59^a$ | $241 \pm 50^a$ | $238 \pm 49^a$ | $237 \pm 51^a$ | $223 \pm 52^b$ | $218 \pm 56^{bc}$ | $216 \pm 54^{bc}$ | $211 \pm 55^c$ |

[abc] Values of different superscript letters in the same row differ significantly $P < 0.05$

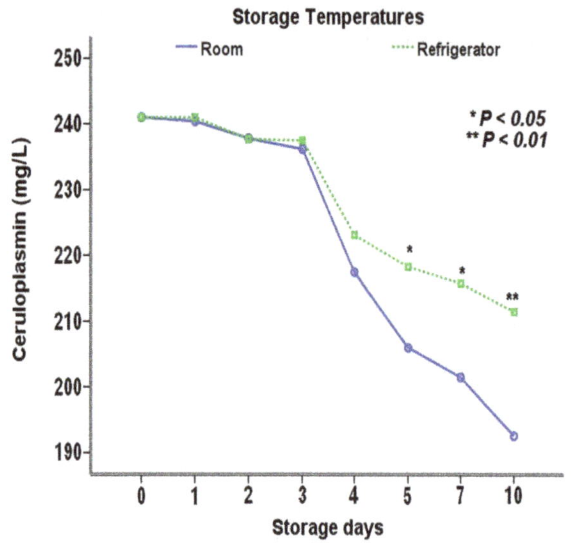


**Fig. 4** Influence of storage for 10 days at room temperature and refrigeration on the activity of ceruloplasmin

animal species differences. As reported elsewhere [14], Cp activity in serum samples was approximately 30% lower relative to heparinized plasma.

The analytical accuracy was directly estimated by linearity assays. The linearity under dilution showed high regression coefficients, indicating that the assay measured Cp in a linear manner with a detection limit of 0.1 mg/L. These results were supported by previous studies in dogs [19] and pigs [28]. In the current study, the linearity ranged from 100 to 1000 mg/L, demonstrating that Cp correlated strongly with the dilutions; therefore, the method may give good results in this range.

Certain clinical trials and research studies may require delayed analyses of collected plasma samples. To accomplish these analyses, blood samples are separated by centrifugation, and then the harvested plasma is quickly frozen [30]. Furthermore, often researchers need to reanalyze a few or all of the plasma analytes to confirm conclusions or previous results. Under such circumstances, plasma samples may need to be frozen and thawed repeatedly. On the other hand, data on storage stability of Cp, and the effect of the temperature and duration of storage on its activity in veterinary medicine are still limited. Therefore, it is important to collect information about the effect of storage on its activity, as one of the pre-analytical factors that may affect the results of the assay.

The diminished activities of Cp in the plasma samples stored at room temperature and refrigeration may be related to the liability and degradation of this protein resulting from the changes in its molecular configuration during storage. Although the activities of Cp were lowered, its values were within the reference range (143–459 mg/L) as previously reported [14]. In previous studies, it was indicated that the stability of protein might be changed with the temperature storage [31, 32]. In the present study, the activity of Cp was higher in the plasma samples stored at refrigeration as compared to room temperature after 10 days of storage, indicating that the stability of Cp was higher at refrigeration than room temperature. In this study, it seems that storage of plasma samples at freezing for 3 months did not have a significant influence on the activity of Cp. Similarly, in another study, where human plasma samples were stored at – 20 °C over a period of 1 year, no significant changes in Cp activity was noted [33]. In the current study, three cycles of freezing and thawing had almost no effect on the activity of Cp, which may indicate a stable plasma Cp during repeated freeze–thaw cycles. However, the effect of repeated freeze–thaw cycles of plasma samples may need more than three cycles to be noticed, indicating further research work may be required in this regard.

## Conclusions

The evaluated method for Cp measurement could be successfully applied in Holstein dairy cows and may contribute to a wide use of Cp assays in bovine medicine. Furthermore, the method is easy, cheap, and may be

**Table 4 Influence of repeated freeze–thaw cycles on the activity of ceruloplasmin**

| | Freeze–thaw cycles | | | |
|---|---|---|---|---|
| | 0 | 1 | 2 | 3 |
| Ceruloplasmin (mg/L) (n = 10) | 241 ± 59[a] | 242 ± 61[a] | 238 ± 62[a] | 237 ± 61[a] |

[a] No significant difference $P > 0.05$

**Table 3 Influence of plasma storage at deep-freezing on the activity of ceruloplasmin**

| | Storage temperature | Weeks of storage | | | | | |
|---|---|---|---|---|---|---|---|
| | | 0 | 1 | 2 | 4 | 8 | 12 |
| Ceruloplasmin (mg/L) (n = 10) | Freezing (– 20 °C) | 241 ± 59[a] | 241 ± 59[a] | 239 ± 61[a] | 238 ± 57[a] | 245 ± 59[a] | 241 ± 59[a] |

[a] No significant difference $P > 0.05$

valid at values of Cp ranging from 100 to 1000 mg/L. It seems that keeping of plasma samples at room temperature and refrigeration is unsuitable for Cp measurement. In addition, Cp remains stable in plasma samples stored at freezing as well as in samples subjected to repeated freeze–thaw cycles.

## Abbreviations

Cp: ceruloplasmin; CV: confidence intervals; LOD: limit of detection; LOQ: limit of quantification; PPD: *p*-phenylenediamine; SPSS: statistical package for the social sciences; TMR: totally mixed ration.

## Authors' contributions

HAH collected the samples and conducted the experiment. HAH performed statistical analysis and manuscript preparation. RS performed the study design and concept as well as assisted in manuscript review. Both authors read and approved the final manuscript.

## Author details

[1] Internal Veterinary Medicine, Department of Animal Medicine, Faculty of Veterinary Medicine, Assiut University, Assiut 71526, Egypt. [2] Klinik für Klauentiere, Freie Universität Berlin, 14163 Berlin, Germany.

## Acknowledgements

The authors gratefully acknowledge the manager and staff of the study farm for their valuable support. Without their kind cooperation, this study would have been impossible to conduct. The authors acknowledge Dr. Anja Müller, Vet Med Labor, Ludwigsburg, for manuscript revision.

## Competing interests

The authors declare that they have no competing interests.

## Funding

Not applicable.

## References

1. Holmberg G, Laurell C. Investigations in serum copper. II. Isolation of the copper containing protein, and a description of its properties. Acta Chem Scand. 1948;2:550–6.
2. Martinez-Subiela S, Tecles F, Parra M, Ceron J. Acute phase proteins: general concepts and main clinical applications in veterinary medicine. In: Anales de Veterinaria de Murcia. vol. 17. 2001. p. 99–116.
3. O'Brien P, Bruce R. Endogenous toxins: targets for disease treatment and prevention, vol. 2. Weinheim: Wiley; 2009. p. 405–6.
4. Rice EW. Ceruloplasmin assay in serum: standardization of ceruloplasmin activity in terms of international enzyme units. Stand Meth Clin Chem. 1963;4:39–46.
5. Hellman NE, Giltin JD. Ceruloplasmin metabolism and function. Annu Rev Nutr. 2002;2002(22):439–58.
6. Harris ZL, Takashi Y, Miyajima H, Serizawa M, Macgillivary RT, Giltin JD. Aceruloplasminemia: molecular characterization of this disorder of iron metabolism. Proc Natl Acad Sci USA. 1995;92:2539–43.
7. Ehrenwald E, Fox P. Role of endogenous ceruloplasmin in low density lipoprotein oxidation by human U937 monocytic cells. J Clin Investig. 1996;97:884–90.
8. Al-Timimi D, Dormandy T. The inhibition of lipid autoxidation by human ceruloplasmin. Biochem J. 1977;168:283–8.
9. Klebanoff S. Bactericidal effect of $Fe^{2+}$, ceruloplasmin, and phosphate. Arch Biochem Biophys. 1992;295:302–38.
10. Skinner JG. Special report. International standardization of acute phase proteins. Vet Clin Pathol. 2001;30:2–7.
11. Sheldon IM, Noakes DE, Rycroft A, Dobson H. Acute phase protein responses to uterine bacterial contamination in cattle after calving. Vet Rec. 2001;148:172–5.
12. Szczubiał M, Dąbrowski R, Kankofer M, Bochniarz M, Albera E. Concentration of serum amyloid A and activity of ceruloplasmin in milk from cows with clinical and subclinical mastitis. Bull Vet Inst Pulawy. 2008;52:391–5.
13. Cerón JJ, Eckersall PD, Martínez-Subiela S. Acute phase proteins in dogs and cats: current knowledge and future perspectives. Vet Clin Pathol. 2005;34:85–99.
14. Hussein HA, Staufenbiel R, Müller AE, El-Sebaie A, Abd-El-Salam M. Ceruloplasmin activity in Holstein dairy cows: effects of lactation stages and anticoagulants. Comp Clin Pathol. 2012;21:705–10.
15. Laven RA, Lawrence KE, Livesey CT. The assessment of blood copper status in cattle: a comparison of measurements of caeruloplasmin and elemental copper in serum and plasma. N Z Vet J. 2007;55:171–6.
16. Hussein HA, Staufenbiel R. Variations in copper concentration and ceruloplasmin activity of dairy cows in relation to lactation stages with regard to ceruloplasmin to copper ratios. Biol Trace Elem Res. 2012;146:47–52.
17. Regassa F, Noakes DE. Acute phase protein response of ewes and the release of PGFM in relation to uterine involution and the presence of intrauterine bacteria. Vet Rec. 1999;144:502–6.
18. Lewis EJ, Bishop J, Cashin CH. Automated quantification of rat plasma acute phase reactants in experimental inflammation. J Pharmacol Methods. 1989;21:183–94.
19. Cerón JJ, Martínez-Subiela S. An automated spectrophotometric method for measuring canine ceruloplasmin in serum. Vet Res. 2004;35:671–9.
20. Cray C, Rodriguez M, Zaias J, Altman N. Effects of storage temperature and time on clinical biochemical parameters from rat serum. J Am Assoc Lab Anim Sci. 2009;48:202–4.
21. Cuhadar S, Koseoglu M, Atay A, Dirican A. The effect of storage time and freeze–thaw cycles on the stability of serum samples. Biochem Med. 2013;23:70–7.
22. Jackson PG, Cockcroft PD. Clinical examination of farm animals. Hoboken: Blackwell Science Ltd; 2002. p. 9–140.
23. Sunderman F, Nomoto S. Measurement of human serum ceruloplasmin by its *p*-phenylenediamine oxidase activity. Clin Chem. 1970;16:903–10.
24. Shrivastava A, Gupta V. Methods for the determination of limit of detection and limit of quantitation of the analytical methods. Chron Young Sci. 2011;2:21–5.
25. Armbruster D, Pry T. Limit of blank, limit of detection and limit of quantitation. Clin Biochem Rev. 2008;29:S49–52.
26. Szczubiał M, Dabrowski R, Kankofer M, Bochniarz M, Komar M. Concentration of serum amyloid A and ceruloplasmin activity in milk from cows with subclinical mastitis caused by different pathogens. Pol J Vet Sci. 2012;15:291–6.
27. Hajimohammadi A, Nazifi S, Ansari-Lari M, Khoshmanzar M, Bigdeli S. Identifying relationships among acute phase proteins (haptoglobin, serum amyloid A, fibrinogen, ceruloplasmin) and clinical findings in dairy calf diarrhea. Comp Clin Pathol. 2013;22:227–32.
28. Martínez-Subiela S, Tecles F, Ceron J. Comparison of two automated spectrophotometric methods for ceruloplasmin measurement in pigs. Res Vet Sci. 2007;83:12–9.
29. Solter PF, Hoffmann WE, Hungerford LL, Siegel JP, St Denis SH, Dorner JL. Haptoglobin and ceruloplasmin as determinants of inflammation in dogs. Am J Vet Res. 1991;52:1738–42.
30. Ridker PM, Rifai N, Pfeffer MA, Sacks F, Braunwald E. Long-term effects of pravastatin on plasma concentration of C-reactive protein. Circulation. 1999;100:230–5.
31. Jaenicke R. Protein structure and function at low temperatures. Philos Trans R Soc Lond B Biol Sci. 1990;1990(326):535–51.
32. Kumar S, Tsai CJ, Nussinov R. Thermodynamic differences among homologous thermophilic and mesophilic proteins. Biochemistry. 2001;40:14152–65.
33. Jansen EH, Beekhof PK, Schenk E. Long-term stability of biomarkers of the iron status in human serum and plasma. Biomarkers. 2013;18:365–8.

# 10

# Comparison of acute phase reaction and postoperative stress in pigs undergoing video-assisted thoracoscopic versus thoracotomy pneumonectomy

Hai-Feng Liu[1], Li Gao[1], Tao Liu[1], Yan-Jiang[2] and Hong-Bin Wang[1*]

**Abstract**

**Background:** Video-assisted thoracoscopic surgery (VATS) has been used for many thoracic diseases as an alternate approach to thoracotomy. The aim of this study was to compare the surgical outcome of pneumonectomy using VATS with that using thoracotomy pneumonectomy in pigs. Fourteen pigs were equally divided into two groups; one group underwent VATS and the other group underwent transthoracic pneumonectomy. We monitored pre-, intra-, and post-operative physiologic parameters, along with blood cell count, serum C-reactive protein (CRP), serum amyloid A (SAA), interleukin-6 (IL-6) and cortisol. The differences between the two approaches were analyzed.

**Results:** Mean surgical time in the VATS group (160.6 ± 16.2 min) was significantly longer than that in the thoracotomy group (123.7 ± 13.2 min). In both groups, CRP and IL-6 concentrations were significantly increased at postoperative 4 h, and then gradually decreased to preoperative levels. CRP and IL-6 at postoperative day 1 were significant lower in the VATS group compared with the thoracotomy group. SAA was significantly increased at postoperative days 1 and 3 in both groups compared with preoperative levels. Cortisol was significantly increased immediately after surgery in both groups compared with preoperative levels, and was significantly higher in the thoracotomy group than the VATS group at postoperative 4 h and 1 day.

**Conclusions:** There was no difference between the two groups in physiologic parameters and blood cell count. However, the results indicate that VATS resulted in a smaller incision, less acute-phase reaction, less stress and less pain compared with thoracotomy pneumonectomy.

**Keywords:** VATS, Pneumonectomy, Acute-phase reaction, Body stress, Postoperative pain

## Background

Video-assisted thoracoscopic surgery (VATS) has been used as a diagnostic and therapeutic platform to perform a wide variety of thoracic cavity surgical procedures [1], including surgical lung biopsy, cancer staging, treatment of pneumothorax, pericardiotomy, and pericardial window creation [2]. It is clinically well accepted that VATS is less painful and results in less stress than traditional thoracotomy procedures. Recent reports have also confirmed the safety and benefits of VATS [3, 4].

Surgical procedures are commonly performed on animals as a model for humans. Experimental pneumonectomy has been performed in pigs [5], and the short-term outcome of thoracoscopic lung lobectomy for primary lung tumors has been performed in dogs [6]. Several studies on VATS procedures in animals have evaluated stress parameters and postoperative outcomes [7, 8]; there have also been studies into the outcomes of VATS lobectomy [9].

To thoroughly assess the impact of minimally invasive surgical techniques on acute-phase reactions, stress

*Correspondence: hbwang1940@163.com
[1] Department of Veterinary Surgery, College of Veterinary Medicine, Northeast Agricultural University, No. 59 Mucai Street, Gongbin Road, Xiangfang District, Harbin 150030, People's Republic of China

responses, and postoperative pain, we designed a clinical study comparing such factors in pigs undergoing pneumonectomy via the VATS approach versus thoracotomy to determine the feasibility and safety of both approaches.

## Methods

### Animals

Fourteen healthy Bama miniature pigs with an average bodyweight of 22.57 ± 1.5 kg were used for this study. The pigs were obtained from Bama miniature pigs Farm of College of Life Sciences (Harbin, China). The pigs were housed individually under steady temperature (around 20 °C) and lighting conditions (12 h light/dark cycle), and fed free piglet diet (Shenzhen Jinxinnong Feed, China) and tap water ad libitum. All animals were preoperatively assessed as healthy after physical examination and complete blood count. Animals were randomized and equally divided into two groups: Group I underwent VATS pneumonectomy, and Group II underwent thoracotomy pneumonectomy.

### Surgical preparation

Baseline physiologic parameters were determined just before surgery (t = 0), including routine blood testing, heart rate (HR), rectal temperature, and serum concentrations of C-reactive protein (CRP), serum amyloid A (SAA), interleukin-6 (IL-6), and cortisol.

After a 24 h feeding fast and a 2 h drinking fast, all pigs were administered the same general anesthesia and were monitored and managed similarly. Each pig was premedicated with subcutaneous atropine sulfate (0.04 mg/kg) and intramuscular cefazolin (20 mg/kg). General anesthesia was induced with intramuscular xylazine (1 mg/kg) and ketamine hydrochloride (10 mg/kg), and maintained with 1.5–3% isoflurane in oxygen after intubation. Respiration was maintained via mechanical ventilation with the anesthetic gas machine (respiratory frequency 12 breaths per min, tidal volume 15–20 ml/kg, inspiratory: expiratory ratio = 1:2). Sterile instruments were used for all procedures. Physiological parameters were monitored using an invigilator (MP30; Philips, The Netherlands).

The animal was placed in the supine position. The surgical site (left chest from the clavicle to the last rib and from the sternum to the spine) was shaved, aseptically prepared, and draped for surgery. A heating blanket was placed between the animal and the operating table. All surgical procedures were performed by the same trained veterinary surgeons in the same environment.

Sterile instruments were used for all thoracotomy and VATS procedures. For the VATS procedures, the endoscopes and other equipment underwent high-level disinfection.

### VATS procedure

Two portals were created: the endoscope portal (portal 1) and the surgical portal (portal 2). Portal 1 (1 cm diameter) was created by a trocar inside a metal tube, and was located between the eighth and the ninth rib. Portal 2 (2–3 cm diameter) was created using a scalpel and an endotherm knife, and was located between the fifth and the sixth rib. A 10/11 mm trocar-cannula unit (Optcla Medical Instrument Co. Ltd., Hangzhou, P. R. China) was inserted through the chest wall at portal 1. An endoscope (0°, 10 mm diameter, 330 mm long; Olympus, Hamburg, Germany) attached to a video endoscopic camera and light source (Olympus) was then advanced through this tube into the chest cavity. The margin of portal 2 was treated with an electric coagulation knife for hemostasis.

Lung-grasping forceps were used to lift the lung lobe and expose the hilum of the lung. The pulmonary artery, pulmonary vein, and the bronchus were carefully separated using hemostatic forceps and a homemade tool (peanuts). Electrocautery was used to separate the redundant tissue. The pulmonary artery and pulmonary veins were clipped and transected, and the bronchus was transected after double ligation. The bronchus ligation needed an extra transfixion ligation. All lung lobes in the left chest were excised in the following order: the middle lobe, the upper lobe, and the sub-adjacent lobe. Physiological saline (200 ml at approximately 40 °C) was used to check the bronchus ligation and syringe the thoracic cavity; this liquid was then extracted through a vacuum absorber.

### Thoracotomy procedure

An 8–10 cm incision was created using a scalpel and an electric coagulation knife between the seventh and the eighth rib. The eighth rib was sawed-off to provide a better operating space and view. An endotherm knife was used for blood coagulation. The surgical field was expanded using a wound spreader. The surgical procedure was the same as in the VATS group.

### Monitoring and postoperative care

All animals were reared and monitored in the same environment. The clinical appearance of the pigs, including mental status, movements, appetite, fecal appearance and wound healing, including presence of hemorrhage and inflammation, was evaluated daily for 15 days. Animals were placed in a warm room after anesthesia and transferred to a hog house 6 h later. Freely available water was provided 6 h postoperatively, and pig feed was provided 18 h postoperatively.

A 5 mg fentanyl patch (Duragesic; Janssen Pharmaceutical, China) was applied after surgery, and renewed every 3 for 6 days. Antibiotic prophylaxis consisted of intramuscular cefazolin sodium (50 mg/kg; Harbin Pharmaceutical Group Co., Ltd., General Pharm. Factory, China) twice a day for 2 days.

The following parameters were recorded: HR, rectal temperature, operating time, incision size, postoperative complications, and time of standing up. Hematology examination including white blood cell (WBC), erythrocyte count (EC), lymphocyte (LY), and granulocyte (Gran) count was performed preoperatively and 1, 2, 3, 5, 7, and 14 days after surgery.

Blood samples were collected (preoperatively and 4 h, 1, 3, 5, 7 and 14 days postoperatively,) through the precaval vein, and were centrifuged for 15 min at 1000 g. Serum for biomarkers analysis was stored at −80 °C, and was assayed using commercially available ELISA kits with specific monoclonal antibodies (PharMingen, BD Biosciences, San Diego, CA, USA) according to the manufacturer's instructions. CRP, SAA, IL-6, and cortisol were measured preoperatively and postoperatively at 4 h, day 1, 3, 5, 7, and 14.

At postoperative day 15, the pigs were euthanized. Pigs were induced with xylazine and ketamine hydrochloride before 300 mg xylocaine was injected intravenously. Necropsy was performed to examine the thoracic cavity condition and postoperative compliance.

### Statistical analysis

Standard statistical methods were used to analyze data. Data were reported as the mean ± SD. Statistical differences within each group were determined by two-way analysis of variance. The paired-sample t test was used to compare the two groups. Significance level was established at $P < 0.05$. Statistical analyses were performed with SPSS software (SPSS Inc., Chicago, IL, USA).

## Results

All animals survived the follow-up period of 14 days. Total pneumonectomy was successfully performed via both VATS and thoracotomy, with complete removal of all left lobes in 14 animals. The operating time for the VATS procedure was significantly longer than for the thoracotomy procedure (VATS 160.6 ± 16.2 min *vs* thoracotomy 123.7 ± 13.2 min, $P < 0.05$).

No animal in either group had intra- or peri-operative complications. There was no evidence of hemorrhage, and no areas of iatrogenic trauma from introduction of surgical instruments. The total length of all skin incisions was 4.5–5.5 cm in the VATS group and 8–10 cm in the thoracotomy group. No other abnormalities were found in either group. All pigs were considered to have returned to their normal activity levels by 24 h after surgery.

Rectal temperature was measured before surgery (baseline) and at the designated intra- and post-operative time points (Fig. 1b). Rectal temperature was decreased in all animals intraoperatively and there was no significant difference between the two groups at any time point. Two pigs in the VATS group and four pigs in the thoracotomy group experienced hyperpyrexia on postoperative day 1 and 2, and returned to baseline 5 days after surgery.

The WBC count in both groups was significantly increased at postoperative days 1, 2, and 3 compared with preoperatively (all $P < 0.05$), and returned to normal level 2 weeks after surgery (Fig. 2a). There was no significant change in erythrocyte count values after the procedure in either group (Fig. 2b). The LY count and the Gran count were significantly increased 1 day after surgery in both groups ($P < 0.05$) (Fig. 2c, d). The LY count had returned

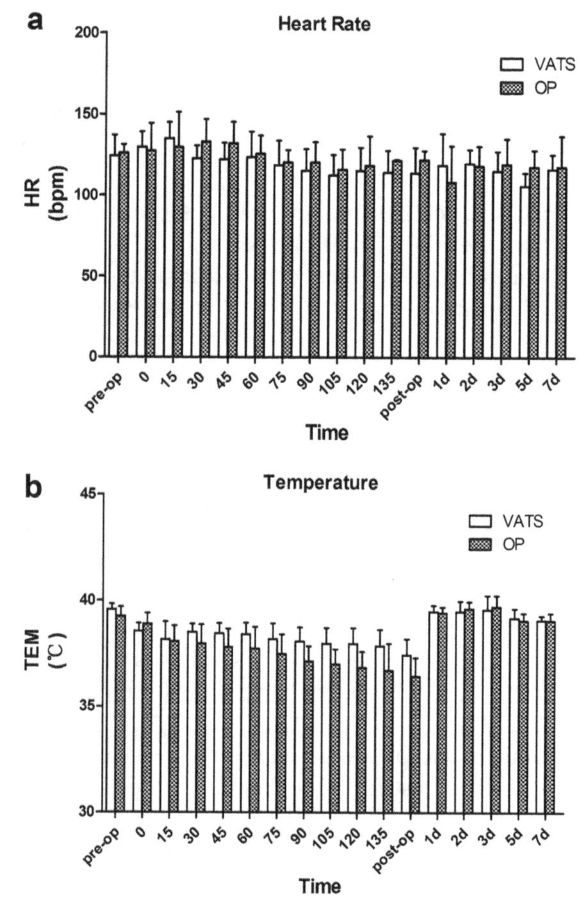


**Fig. 1** Heart rate (**a**) and temperature (**b**) in 14 pigs that underwent pneumonectomy ($n = 7$ for VATS and $n = 7$ for open thoracotomy). *$P < 0.05$ compared with preoperative value (baseline). $^{\#}P < 0.05$ for VATS vs transthoracic approach at the same time point. *VATS* video-assisted thoracoscopic surgery, *bpm* beats per minute

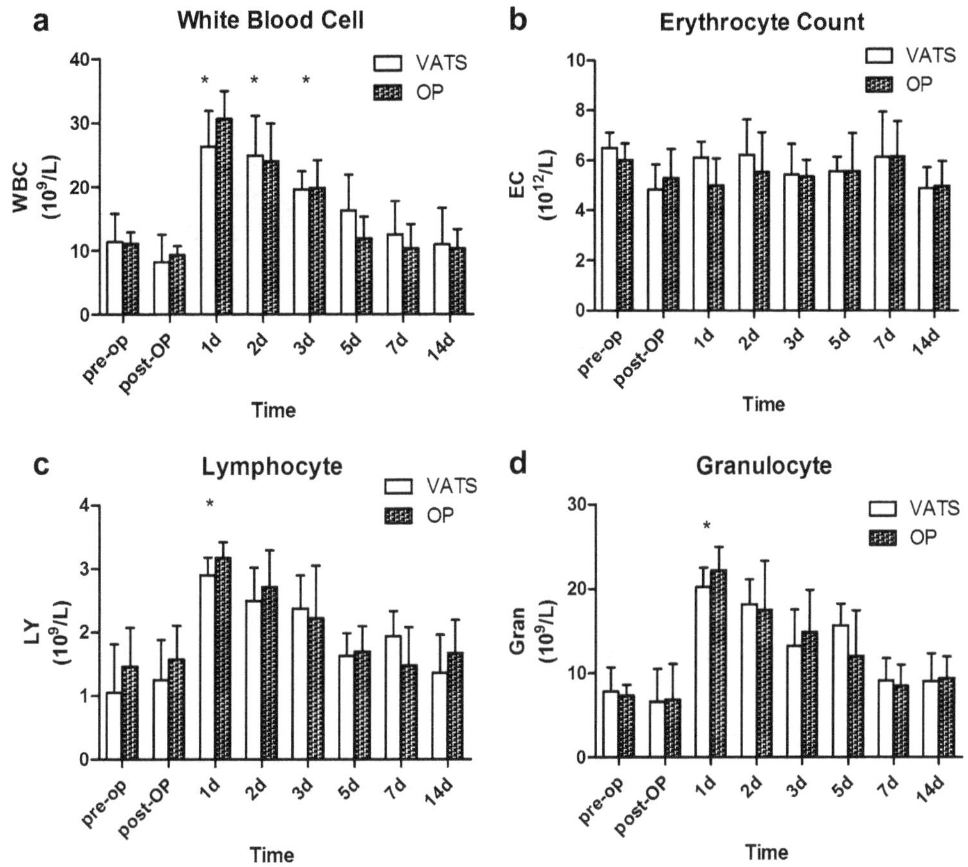


**Fig. 2** White blood cell count (**a**), erythrocyte count (**b**), lymphocyte count (**c**), and granulocyte count (**d**) in 14 pigs that underwent pneumonectomy ($n = 7$ for VATS and $n = 7$ for open thoracotomy). *$P < 0.05$ compared with preoperative value (baseline). $^{\#}P < 0.05$ for VATS vs transthoracic approach at the same time point. *VATS* video-assisted thoracoscopic surgery

to normal level at postoperative day 5 and the Gran count had returned to normal level at postoperative day 7.

The serum concentrations of CRP in both groups were significantly increased at postoperative 4 h, day 1 and day 3 compared with preoperative levels ($P < 0.05$), and then decreased gradually back to baseline by 7 days postoperatively (Fig. 3a). CRP at postoperative day 1 in the VATS group was significantly lower than that in the thoracotomy group ($P < 0.05$).

The serum concentrations of SAA in both groups were significantly increased at postoperative day 1 and day 3 ($P < 0.05$), and then decreased gradually back to baseline by 7 days postoperatively (Fig. 3b). SAA in the thoracotomy group tended to be higher than that in the VATS group, although this difference was not significant ($P > 0.05$). There was no significant difference in SAA between the two groups at any time point.

The serum concentration of IL-6 in both groups was significantly higher at postoperative 4 h, day 1 and day 3 compared with preoperative levels ($P < 0.05$), and then decreased gradually back to baseline by 5 days postoperatively (Fig. 3c). IL-6 at postoperative day 1 in the VATS group was significantly lower than that in the thoracotomy group ($P < 0.05$), with no difference between groups at any other time point.

The serum concentration of cortisol was increased significantly immediately postoperatively compared with preoperative levels in both groups ($P < 0.05$), and then decreased gradually back to baseline by 5 days postoperatively (Fig. 3d). Cortisol at postoperative 4 h and day 1 was significantly higher than preoperative levels in both groups ($P < 0.05$). The cortisol level was significantly lower in the VATS group than in the thoracotomy group at postoperative 4 h and day 1. No significant difference in cortisol was observed between the two groups at any other time point.

## Discussion

We successfully performed pneumonectomy in the hemithorax via VATS and thoracotomy without major intra- or post-operative complications. Thus, both VATS and the transthoracic approach are viable alternative techniques to total pneumonectomy.

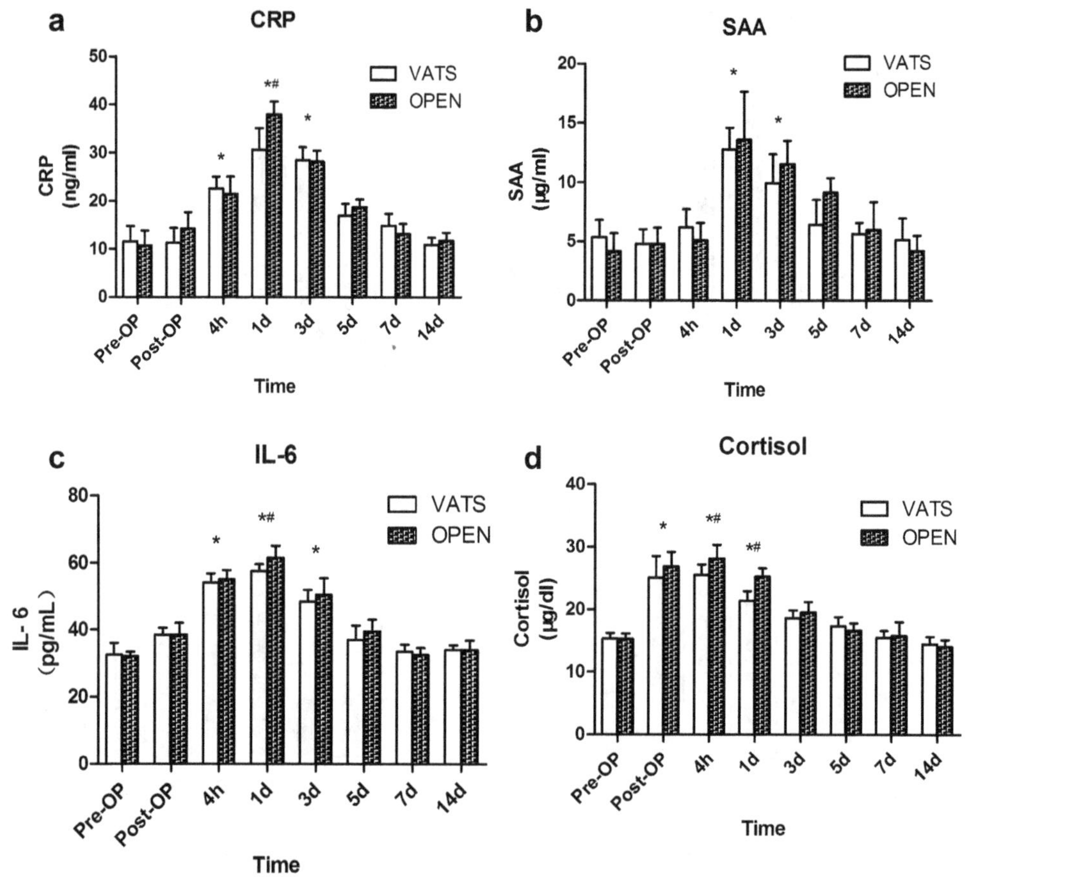


**Fig. 3** Serum concentrations of CRP (**a**), SAA (**b**), IL-6 (**c**) and cortisol (**d**) in 14 pigs that underwent pneumonectomy ($n = 7$ for VATS and $n = 7$ for open thoracotomy). *$P < 0.05$ compared with preoperative value (baseline). #$P < 0.05$ for VATS vs transthoracic approach at the same time point. *VATS* video-assisted thoracoscopic surgery, *CRP* C-reactive protein, *SAA* serum amyloid A

Pneumonectomy is a lung resection technique used in humans and animals to remove all lung lobes when bilobectomy or lobectomy techniques are inadequate to remove the pathology in the hemithorax. Pneumonectomy procedures are performed under some pathological conditions such as lung tumors, congenital lung anomalies, chronic lung collapse, chronic progressive lung inflammation, post-traumatic diffuse parenchymal laceration, and bronchial rupture. Lung lobes can be excised through either thoracotomy or VATS.

Since the first pioneering lobectomy was carried out by VATS [10, 11], the method is now well established as an alternative to thoracotomy for major resections of lung cancer and benign disease [12, 13]. Recent studies have shown that VATS results in a lower concentration of inflammatory cytokines [14], lower risk of developing chest infection, reduced pain, and better lung function than thoracotomy [15, 16].

In the present study, there was a decrease in rectal temperature postoperatively. The central nervous system is restrained in animals undergoing general anesthesia, which results in a decrease in body temperature, HR, respiratory rate and blood pressure. The longer the duration of general anesthesia, the greater the decrease. So the longer surgical time in the VATS group compared with the thoracotomy group led to the lower postoperative body temperature, HR, respiratory rate and blood pressure.

The concentration of CRP and IL-6 in the VATS group was significantly lower than that in the thoracotomy group. The same trend has been found previously in VATS lobectomy [14]. CRP increases rapidly after surgery and indicates the degree of injury [17]. The severe trauma caused by surgery and anesthesia were the reasons for the significant postoperative increases in WBC, CRP and IL-6; however, in pigs, the longer incision in the thoracotomy group seemed to cause more inflammatory reaction than the longer operating time in the VATS group. Although the VATS group had a longer operating time, suturing the incision took more time in the thoracotomy group. Cortisol was significantly lower postoperatively in the VATS group compared with the thoracotomy group. Similarly, cortisol in patients who experienced VATS is reportedly lower than in those undergoing traditional thoracic surgery [18, 19]. It is therefore suggested that thoracotomy causes more postoperative pain and body stress than VATS.

Standard pleural drainage was not used in our study. We did not observe leakage or pneumothorax in any pig. Chest drain use is still controversial, as thoracotomy incisions could damage the intercostal nerves and lead to chronic neuropathy [20]. Satherley et al. [21] reported that the use of an intercostal chest drain after lung biopsy increased the period of hospitalization, and Nakashima et al. [22] reported that postoperative morbidity did not increase after thoracoscopic lung wedge resection without a chest tube. Luckraz et al. [23] reported that an intercostal chest drain was not needed in patients that had received VATS lung resection if no air leakage was noted at surgery. Intraoperative blood loss was not recorded in the current study, as there was very minimal intraoperative bleeding in both groups; however, the blood loss observed in the VATS group was subjectively less than in the thoracotomy group. The reason for this may be the better visual field and accuracy of operation because of the magnified image provided by the endoscope in VATS.

## Conclusions

The use of a minimally invasive surgical technique (VATS) in pigs reduced the acute-phase response, surgical stress and postoperative pain. The VATS approach is the optimal option for thoracic surgery in pigs.

### Abbreviations

CRP: C-reaction protein; EC: erythrocyte count; Gran: neutrophilic granulocyte; HR: heart rate; IL-6: interleukin- 6; LY: lymphocyte; SAA: serum amyloid A; VATS: video-assisted thoracoscopic surgery; WBC: white blood cell.

### Authors' contributions

HBW and LG designed this experiment. HFL wrote the manuscript and analysed the data. HBW revised the manuscript. TL and YJ performed the surgery and sample collection. All authors read and approved the final manuscript.

### Author details

[1] Department of Veterinary Surgery, College of Veterinary Medicine, Northeast Agricultural University, No. 59 Mucai Street, Gongbin Road, Xiangfang District, Harbin 150030, People's Republic of China. [2] College of Veterinary Medicine, Northeast Agricultural University, Harbin 150030, People's Republic of China.

### Acknowledgements

Thanks to Kelly Zammit of Liwen Bianji (Edanz Group China) for the assistance on my manuscript writing.

### Competing interests

The authors declare that they have no competing interests.

### Funding

This study was supported by the National Natural Science Foundation of China (Grant Nos. 31272617, 31472245).

### References

1. Peng J, An S, Wang HP, Che XL, Ning XG, Liu J, et al. Video-assisted thoracoscopic surgery lobectomy for lung cancer versus thoracotomy: a less decrease in sVEGFR2 level after surgery. J Thorac Dis. 2016;8:323–8.
2. Neragimiandoab S, Linden PA, Ducko CT, Bueno R, Richards WG, Sugarbaker DJ, et al. VATS pericardiotomy for patients with known malignancy and pericardial effusion: survival and prognosis of positive cytology and metastatic involvement of the pericardium: a case control study. Int J Surg. 2008;6:110–4.
3. Falcoz PE, Puyraveau M, Thomas PA, Decaluwe H, Hurtgen M, Petersen RH, et al. Video-assisted thoracoscopic surgery versus open lobectomy for primary non-small-cell lung cancer: a propensity-matched analysis of outcome from the European Society of Thoracic Surgeon database. Eur J Cardiothorac Surg. 2016;49:602–9.
4. Wu N, Wu L, Qiu C, Yu Z, Xiang Y, Wang M, et al. A comparison of video-assisted thoracoscopic surgery with open thoracotomy for the management of chest trauma: a systematic review and meta-analysis. World J Surg. 2015;39:940–52.
5. Bufalari A, Monte VD, Pecoriello R, Donati L, Ceccarelli S, Cagini L, et al. Experimental left pneumonectomy in pigs: procedure and management. J Surg Res. 2015;198:208–16.
6. Bleakley S, Duncan CG, Monnet E. Thoracoscopic lung lobectomy for primary lung tumors in 13 dogs. Vet Surg. 2015;44:1029–35.
7. Mayhew PD, Friedberg JS. Video-assisted thoracoscopic resection of noninvasive thymomas using one-lung ventilation in two dogs. Vet Surg. 2008;37:756–62.
8. Steffey MA, Daniel L, Mayhew PD, Affolter VK, Soares JH, Smith A. Video-assisted thoracoscopic extirpation of the tracheobronchial lymph nodes in dogs. Vet Surg. 2015;44(Suppl 1):50–8.
9. Mayhew PD, Hunt GB, Steffey MA, Culp WT, Mayhew KN, Fuller M, et al. Evaluation of short-term outcome after lung lobectomy for resection of primary lung tumors via video-assisted thoracoscopic surgery or open thoracotomy in medium- to large-breed dogs. J Am Vet Med Assoc. 2013;243:681–8.
10. Lewis RJ, Sisler GE, Caccavale RJ. Imaged thoracic lobectomy: should it be done? Ann Thorac Surg. 1992;54:80–3.
11. Kirby TJ, Rice TW. Thoracoscopic lobectomy. Ann Thorac Surg. 1993;56:784–6.
12. Liu C, Pu Q, Guo C, Xiao Z, Mei J, Lin M, et al. Non-grasping en bloc mediastinal lymph node dissection for video-assisted thoracoscopic lung cancer surgery. BMC Surg. 2015;15:38.
13. Harris CG, James RS, Tian DH, Yan TD, Doyle MP, Gonzalez-Rivas D, et al. Systematic review and meta-analysis of uniportal versus multiportal video-assisted thoracoscopic lobectomy for lung cancer. Ann Cardiothorac Surg. 2016;5:76–84.
14. Yim AP, Wan S, Lee TW, Arifi AA. VATS lobectomy reduces cytokine responses compared with conventional surgery. Ann Thorac Surg. 2000;70:243–7.
15. Phan K, Yan TD. VATS segmentectomy for pulmonary metastasis. Ann Cardiothorac Surg. 2014;3:192–3.
16. Cao C, Manganas C, Ang SC, Peeceeyen S, Yan TD. Video-assisted thoracic surgery versus open thoracotomy for non-small cell lung cancer: a meta analysis of propensity score-matched patients. Interact Cardiovasc Thorac Surg. 2013;16:244–9.
17. Zhang SX, Zhang JT, Zhang N, Shi J, Wang HB. Comparison of laparoscopic-assisted and open colopexy in dogs. Bull Vet Inst Pulawy. 2012;56:415–7.
18. Yin Y. Comparative analysis of efficacy of VATs treatment and traditional thoracic surgery for the mediastinal tumor. Chin J Clin Oncol Rehabil. 2014;10:1164–6.
19. Asteriou C, Lazopoulos A, Rallis T, Gogakos AS, Paliouras D, Tsakiridis K, et al. Video-assisted thoracic surgery reduces early postoperative stress. A single-institutional prospective randomized study. Ther Clin Risk Manag. 2015;12:59–65.

# 11

# Effect of propofol and remifentanil on cerebral perfusion and oxygenation in pigs

Mai Louise Grandsgaard Mikkelsen[1*], Rikard Ambrus[2], James Edward Miles[1], Helle Harding Poulsen[1], Finn Borgbjerg Moltke[3,4] and Thomas Eriksen[1]

**Abstract**

The objective of this review is to evaluate the existing literature with regard to the influence of propofol and remifentanil total intravenous anaesthesia (TIVA) on cerebral perfusion and oxygenation in healthy pigs. Anaesthesia has influence on cerebral haemodynamics and it is important not only in human but also in veterinary anaesthesia to preserve optimal regulation of cerebral haemodynamics. Propofol and remifentanil are widely used in neuroanaesthesia and are increasingly used in experimental animal studies. In translational models, the pig has advantages compared to small laboratory animals because of brain anatomy, metabolism, neurophysiological maturation, and cerebral haemodynamics. However, reported effects of propofol and remifentanil on cerebral perfusion and oxygenation in pigs have not been reviewed. An electronic search identified 99 articles in English. Title and abstract screening selected 29 articles for full-text evaluation of which 19 were excluded with reasons. Of the 10 peer-reviewed articles included for review, only three had propofol or remifentanil anaesthesia as the primary study objective and only two directly investigated the effect of anaesthesia on cerebral perfusion and oxygenation (CPO). The evidence evaluated in this systematic review is limited, not focused on propofol and remifentanil and possibly influenced by factors of potential importance for CPO assessment. In one study of healthy pigs, CPO measures were within normal ranges following propofol-remifentanil anaesthesia, and addition of a single remifentanil bolus did not affect regional cerebral oxygen saturation ($rSO_2$). Even though the pool of evidence suggests that propofol and remifentanil alone or in combination have limited effects on CPO in healthy pigs, confirmative evidence is lacking.

**Keywords:** Animal model, Brain, Oxygenation, Perfusion, Pig, Propofol, Remifentanil, Neuroanaesthesia

## Background

Preservation of optimal cerebral perfusion and oxygenation (CPO) is the primary concern in assessing neurocritical patients undergoing surgery or sedation in the intensive care unit or for diagnostic procedures, and is equally important in both human and veterinary anaesthesia [1, 2]. Animal models have been used increasingly over the last decade to study the significance of influential factors on cerebral haemodynamics and to achieve better understanding of mechanisms regulating CPO. Rodents and primates are widely used in neuroscience but recently the interest for use of pigs in neuroscience has increased. The pig is readily available through commercial sources and the gyrencephalic porcine brain resembles the human brain in several areas of gross anatomy, growth, and development [3]. The pig brain shows similarities in gyral pattern, distribution of grey and white matter, cerebral blood flow, and metabolism to the human brain. In addition, similarities in neurophysiological development and post-natal maturation with human brains are of value in human neuro-embryology and paediatric neuro-science [3–5]. Various porcine models have been described with the objective of CPO evaluation, but mostly they have been developed in the context of neurological trauma or diseases, such as traumatic brain injury

*Correspondence: mailo@sund.ku.dk
[1] Department of Veterinary Clinical and Animal Sciences, University of Copenhagen, 16 Dyrlægevej, 1870 Frederiksberg C, Denmark

[6, 7], subdural haematoma [8], intracranial hypertension [9, 10], as well as epilepsy [11] and stroke [12].

Cerebral perfusion and cerebral oxygenation are two separate measures that are often used simultaneously and sometimes interchangeably as clinical assessment measures to evaluate the physiological status of the brain. Both measures are used to assess the risk of ischemic brain damage and thus to predict clinical outcome and prognosis of the patient. The cerebral perfusion is often clinically assessed by evaluation of changes in the cerebral blood flow (CBF). Cerebral blood flow is controlled by homeostatic regulation of the cerebral perfusion pressure (CPP) and cerebral vascular resistance (CVR). Mean arterial blood pressure (MAP) and the intracranial pressure (ICP) are determinants of CPP giving CPP = MAP−ICP, and CBF may therefore be assumed as CBF = MAP−ICP/CVR [13–16]. Overall, several physiological or pathological conditions therefore may influence cerebral perfusion. Physiological alterations in blood pressure, cerebral metabolic rate, temperature, arterial carbon dioxide or oxygen contents, blood viscosity and pathological conditions such as hypertension, vascular disease, trauma or seizures all may influence perfusion [2, 13–16]. Mean arterial pressure can under normal conditions, and for patients in supine position, adequately represent the CPP for evaluation of CBF [16]. Clinically, CPP is used as an indirect index for CBF [17]. The maintenance of constant and stable CBF is essential for optimal cerebral metabolism and function, and is under normal physiological conditions secured by intrinsic cerebral autoregulatory mechanisms [16]. Cerebral autoregulation is the haemodynamic ability of the cerebral vasculature to maintain a constant CBF despite changes in blood pressure and consequently changes in MAP [18]. The limit of this preservative regulatory mechanism is generally observed in the MAP range of 50–150 mmHg. When MAP is above or below these values, CBF varies markedly with MAP, because the ability of the individual vessels to change in diameter has been exhausted [19].

Cerebral oxygenation represents a measure for the amount of oxygen actually available for consumption and energy metabolism in the cerebral tissue, and can be defined as either the brain tissue partial pressure of oxygen ($brPO_2$) [20], or as regional cerebral oxygen saturation ($rSO_2$) [21]. Venous jugular oxygen saturation ($SvjO_2$) normally provides an indirect measure for cerebral oxygen utilization, and thereby gives a qualitative assessment of CBF, but it is also used as a measure for global cerebral oxygen saturation. These parameters represent the oxygen content available within the tissue or in the vascular circuit, and are therefore dependent on CBF [1, 14, 22, 23].

Different methods and technologies have been established for the quantification and evaluation of cerebral haemodynamics, but no gold standard method has been fully validated to date, which makes comparison between the results of different studies challenging [1, 24, 25]. Historically, CBF has been studied by technically advanced methods like the nitrous oxide method [26], the krypton uptake method [27] or xenon 133 injection method [28, 29], but can be evaluated by modern techniques such as transcranial Doppler ultrasonography, laser Doppler flowmetry (LDF), positron emission tomography scanning, functional magnetic resonance imaging [14, 15, 20] or laser speckle contrast imaging [30, 31].

Target ranges for cerebral monitoring have been defined for healthy humans (Table 1), but are less well defined for pigs, which should be considered when assessing CPO in porcine models. CBF in pigs has been reported to decrease with age, being approximately 48, 44 and 27 ml/min/100 g in newborn, juvenile and adult pigs respectively [32], and thus may be comparable to the values identified in humans (Table 1).

Normal target values for $SvjO_2$ during anaesthesia have not been defined in pigs but Mutch et al. [33] and two studies included in this review reported mean values between 74.3 and 82.7 % (Table 6), and CPP has been found to vary with anaesthesia [34]. For $brPO_2$, normal values in pigs have been found to be 25–30 mm Hg [35], which is similar to the range defined in humans (Table 1). Regional cerebral oxygen saturation measured by near infrared spectroscopy (NIRS) is simple, continuous and non-invasive and widely used in human neuroanaesthesia. Thus, it has been suggested that NIRS has potential as a central modality in the cerebral monitoring strategy [21]. NIRS has also been investigated in pigs and a

**Table 1 Target ranges for anaesthesia related cerebral perfusion and oxygenation measures in humans**

| Target | Measure | Limits | Reference |
|---|---|---|---|
| CerAutoReg[a] | mm Hg | 50–150 | [18] |
| MAP | mm Hg | >80 | [18, 93] |
| CPP | mm Hg | 50–70 | [14, 17] |
| $rSO_2$ | % | 60–80 | [22, 90] |
| $SvjO_2$ | % | 50–75 | [15, 22] |
| $brPO_2$ | mm Hg | 25–50 | [17, 90] |
| CBF | ml/min/100 g | 25–50 | [94] |
| CarotidBF | ml/min | 275 ± 52 | [95] |

*MAP*: mean arterial pressure; *ICP*: intracranial pressure; *CPP*: cerebral perfusion pressure; *$rSO_2$*: regional cerebral oxygen saturation; *$SvjO_2$*: jugular venous oxygen saturation; *$brPO_2$*: brain tissue partial pressure of oxygen; *CBF*: cerebral blood flow; *CarotidBF*: carotid blood flow

[a] Upper and lower limits for cerebral autoregulation—highest in newborn lowest in adults

normal value of 65 %, has been suggested [36], ranging from 57 to 72 %. In piglets, an ischaemic threshold of 35 % has also been suggested [37].

Most studies investigating CPO in porcine models are carried out in anaesthetized animals. General anaesthesia aims at depressing consciousness and cerebral activity. General anaesthesia influences systemic cardiovascular function and consequently will affect CPO. However, when properly monitored and managed, general anaesthesia should not alter CPO significantly in the healthy brain [38, 39]. The choice of anaesthesia should be evaluated when assessing studies evaluating CPO. Consideration should be given both to the isolated effect of single anaesthetic drugs, drug combinations as well as systemic physiologic status [39].

Inhalation anaesthesia elicits a dose-related suppressive effect of cerebral metabolism, but also has a direct dilating effect on the cerebral vessels that potentially will increase CBF. The net effect on CBF will be determined by dominating force of these competing and opposing effects [14, 40]. The general assumption is that most intravenous anaesthetic drugs will cause an indirect and dose-dependent decrease in CBF by decreasing cerebral metabolism [18, 41–44]. Only ketamine seems to be an exception to this, by expressing the opposite effect on cerebral metabolism, and thereby increasing CBF [43, 45]. Opioids in general are believed to have minimal effect on CBF in clinical doses, but their effect on cerebral haemodynamics may vary depending on patient status and anaesthetic drugs used [14].

The choice between inhalation and intravenous anaesthesia in neurosurgery is debated and even though no single anaesthetic drug or regimen appears absolutely superior to others [39], an increasing tendency to use intravenous protocols as the basic regimen for neurosurgical anaesthesia, has been reported [46–49]. Significant differences in baseline measurement of MAP and CPP between inhalation anaesthesia and total intravenous anaesthesia (TIVA) in piglets have been reported, but no differences in CBF or $PbrO_2$ were however evident between the anaesthesia regimens [34].

Total intravenous anaesthesia (TIVA) with a combination of propofol and remifentanil is an anaesthetic regimen that is widely used in neuroanaesthesia, and has advantages over inhalation anaesthesia (sevoflurane and isoflurane) with regard to desirable traits like fast recovery, a low incidence of nausea and vomiting, anticonvulsive potential, preservation of cerebral autoregulation and neuroprotection [40, 49–51]. Propofol is the most widely used intravenous anaesthetic agent in both human and veterinary medicine [49, 52–54]. Due to its global depressant properties in the central nervous system, it acts as a very potent hypnotic agent, which can be used for both induction and maintenance of general anaesthesia, and for sedation. Its favourable pharmacokinetic profile ensures a fast onset of action and rapid recovery even after prolonged administration [55]. Propofol may indirectly reduce CBF mainly due to depression of the systemic blood pressure [53, 55]. The hypotensive effect is caused by a decrease in sympathetic activity and intracellular calcium flux resulting in vasodilation [55]. In pigs, the vasodilation caused by propofol has also been related to release of nitric oxide by the vascular endothelium [55]. Propofol has little or no effect on the conductive system of the heart and does not cause myocardial depression, but inhibits the tachycardiac response to hypotension by inhibition of the baroreceptor reflex [53, 55]. The overall cerebral effect of propofol has been demonstrated to reduce CBF, cerebral metabolic rate of oxygen and intracranial pressure, but it also acts as an antioxidant and has neuroprotective properties [53, 56, 57]. Remifentanil is an ultra-short-acting opioid with very potent and selective μ-receptor agonist activity. It is preferred to fentanyl or other opioids due to its non-organ specific metabolism by blood and tissue esterases, which consequently results in a faster clearance and thereby faster recovery independent of infusion duration [58]. The main cardiovascular impact of remifentanil is dominated by moderate bradycardia and a marked decrease in systemic blood pressure. The use of remifentanil in humans thus, has an increased incidence of hypotensive periods in comparison with other opioids [58, 59]. In contrast to this and compared to fentanyl-sevoflurane, remifentanil-propofol anaesthesia is in human clinical studies also reported to increase the incidence of arterial hypertension, hence the influence of remifentanil on CPO is somewhat unpredictable and may depend on the anaesthetic agent used [59]. In humans low and moderate dose remifentanil caused increase in regional CBF while remifentanil in high, supra-clinical doses caused a decrease in regional CBF [59], and no impairment of the cerebrovascular carbon dioxide reactivity [60]. It has been suggested that remifentanil in general decreases the cerebral metabolic rate of oxygen and only has minimal effect on intra cranial pressure [59, 61] and that the combined use of propofol and remifentanil preserves and improves cerebral autoregulation [59]. The overall effects of propofol and remifentanil on CBF and cerebral autoregulation in selected animal species are summarised in Table 2. Since the pig is increasingly of interest as a translational model in neurocritical research, it is important to reveal whether propofol and remifentanil influence CPO differently in pigs compared to humans. The objective of this review is to evaluate the existing literature with regard to the influence of propofol and remifentanil TIVA on cerebral perfusion and oxygenation in healthy pigs.

**Table 2 Summary of the effects of propofol and remifentanil on cerebral blood flow and cerebral autoregulation in selected animal species used in experimental neuroscience**

| Species | CBF | | | CA | | References |
|---|---|---|---|---|---|---|
| | P | R | PR | P | PR | |
| Humans | ↓ | ↑↓* | ↓ | Preserved | Preserved | [18, 52, 55, 56, 58] |
| Dog | ↓ | ↓ | • | Preserved | • | [96, 97] |
| Rabbit | ↓ | • | • | • | • | [98] |
| Rat | ↓ | • | • | Preserved | • | [99] |

*CBF*: cerebral blood flow; *CA*: cerebral autoregulation; *P*: propofol; *R*: remifentanil; *PR*: propofol-remifentanil combination; ↑: increased; ↓: decreased; •: uncertain; *: dose dependant

## Search strategy

On May 10th 2016, an electronic database search was made in Agricola 1970 to April 2016, Agris 1975 to March 2016, Biosis Previews 1969–2009, CAB Abstracts 1910–2016 week 17, Embase 1974–2016 May 9th, International Pharmaceutical Abstracts 1970–April 2016, Zoological Record 1978–2009, Epub ahead of print, In-process and Other non-indexed citations, MEDLINE daily and MEDLINE 1946 to present. The specific terms used for the different search components were: (1) cerebral or brain or central nervous system (CNS), (2) CNS, (3) 1 OR 2, (4) pig or pigs or piglet or piglets or swine or swines or landrace or porcine or minipig or minipigs, (5) 3 and 4, (6) propofol or remifentanil or TIVA, (7) TIVA, (8) TIVA, (9) 6 or 7 or 8, (10) 5 and 9, (11) guinea or guineapig or guineapigs or guinea-pig or guinea-pigs, (12) 10 not 11. The only filter applied was English, and the reference lists of relevant articles and recent reviews were hand-searched for additional studies. Three authors did the screening individually and any disagreement in selection were settled by mutual agreement.

Studies that evaluated CPO and used propofol or remifentanil for TIVA in healthy pigs of all ages and breeds were included in the systematic review. This also included studies that only indirectly assessed the effect of propofol or remifentanil on CPO. Studies where additional anaesthetic drugs were given for maintenance of anaesthesia were excluded. Eligible records (Fig. 1) were retrieved in full text and screened for relevant anaesthesia protocols and outcome data.

## Data extraction

This systematic review is based on the principles recommended by the SYRCLE collaboration [62] and O´Connors and Sargeant [63]. Primary outcome data relevant to this systematic review were any CPO parameter. Secondary outcome data extracted were publication year, study type, number of animals, breed, bodyweight, age, gender, doses of preanaesthetic and other medications, doses of propofol and remifentanil, and MAP.

Synthesis of the CPO-data was made on the basis of means, standard deviations and 95 % confidence intervals and is discussed with regard to secondary outcome data. Standard errors of means were transformed to standard deviations. If not reported, animal age was estimated based on weight [64–66].

## Review

### Search results

The electronic search identified 99 articles in english, of which 29 were eligible after title and abstract screening. Of these, 19 studies were excluded after full text examination (Fig. 1). Of the10 peer-reviewed articles included in this review, only three had propofol or remifentanil anaesthesia as the primary study objective, and only two investigated the effect of anaesthesia on CPO (Table 3). The studies were published between 2001 and 2014, and all but one, were non-survival studies. Post-intervention data from the survival study were not included in this review.

### *Animals*

Data from a total of 133 animals are included in this review. All studies used farm pigs. Eight of the studies used animals with a bodyweight between 16 and 33 kg, while one used animals between 7.5 and 14.5 kg and another between 21.5 and 92.8 kg. Seven studies used female and three used male pigs: none of the studies used both (Table 4).

### *Anaesthesia*

Three studies used a combination of propofol and remifentanil, and seven studies used propofol alone (Table 3). In all studies, anaesthesia was induced with propofol intravenously (iv) (1–4 mg/kg) and maintained with propofol (3–15 mg/kg/h). In 3 studies remifentanil was given in a dose range of 0.2–0.35 μg/kg/min. In addition to propofol and remifentanil infusion, Silva et al. [67] investigated the effect of a single intravenous bolus of 5 μg/kg remifentanil. Intramuscularly (im)

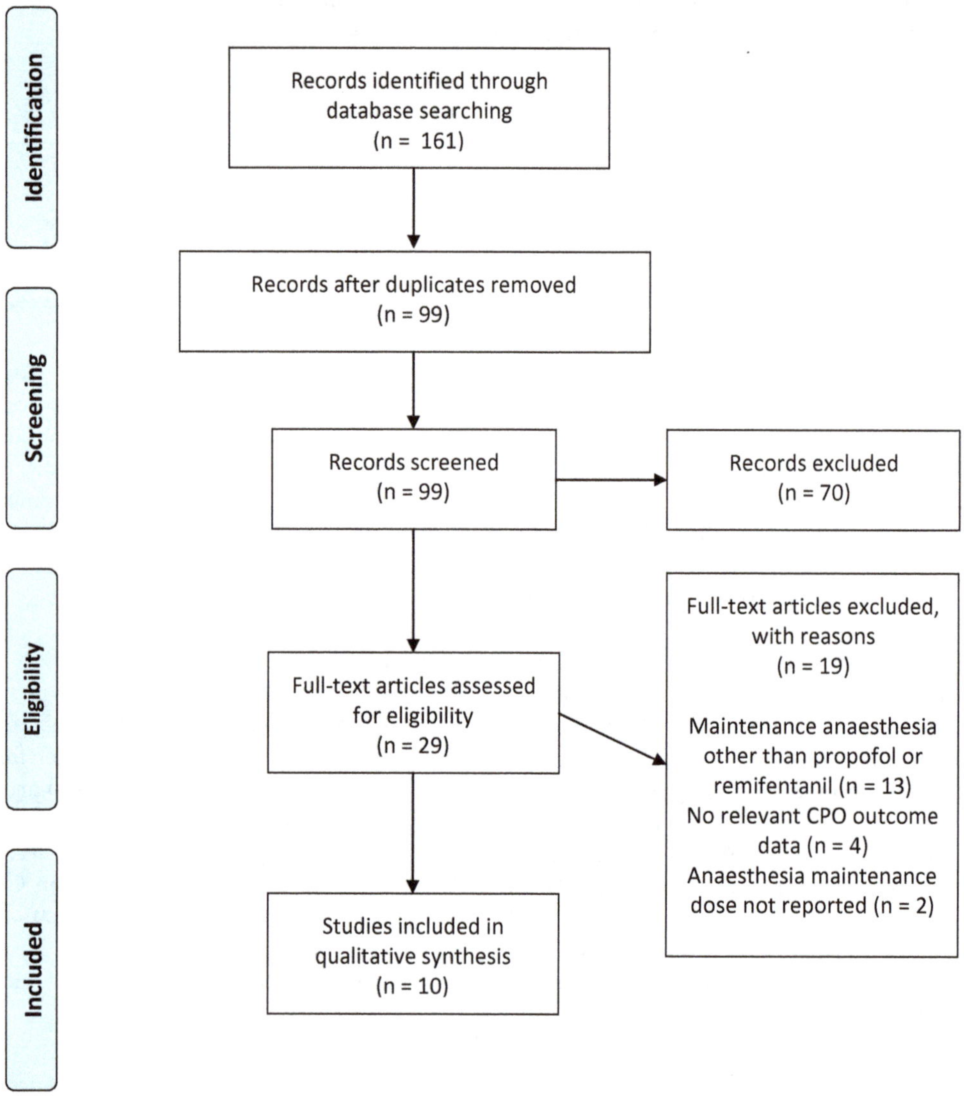


**Fig. 1** PRISMA flow chart, Based on [102]

azaperone 4 mg/kg was used in two studies while ketamine, 10–33 mg/kg im, was used for premedication in eight of the studies. Six of these studies used ketamine alone, one added xylazine and one added xylazine, tiletamine and zolazepam. Single bolus pancuronium was used for muscle relaxation in one study [68], and flunixin, 2.2 mg/kg im was used pre-emptively for postoperative analgesia in one single survival study [69].

### *Study design*

The included studies were animal intervention studies. Four studies used a 1-group design with pre-post-test assessment. Six 6 studies used a 2-group design of which 4 used random sequence allocation. Only Silva et al. [67] studied the effects of propofol-remifentanil anaesthesia on CPO as the primary objective. The remaining 9 studies did not have CPO in relation to anaesthesia as their primary objective. However, all were clear in their description of objectives and possible factors of influence are discussed below.

### Extracted data

Predefined respiratory baseline limits were similar across studies, with target limits set at a respiratory rate of 10–14/min, tidal volume of 10–20 ml/kg, arterial $CO_2$ ($PaCO_2$) or end tidal $CO_2$ ($EtCO_2$) between 35 and 45 mmHg, arterial oxygen ($PaO_2$) >80 mm Hg and oxygen saturation ($SpO_2$) >90 %. However, not all parameters were reported in all studies. Predefined haemodynamic baseline limits were not reported in detail in any of the studies, but Boezaart [68], Navarro et al. [70], Silva et al. [71] and Srinivasan et al. [72], reported that

**Tabel 3 Anaesthesia relevant data**

| Study ID [reference] | Premedication. drug (dose[a]) | Propofol dose[b] (induction/maintenance) | Remifentanil dose |
|---|---|---|---|
| Boezaart [68] | Ketamine (10 mg/kg im) Pancuronium (0.1 mg/kg) | 2.0 mg/kg/3.0 mg/kg/h | 0.35 mikrogram/kg/min |
| Kajimoto et al. [82] | Ketamine (33 mg/kg im) xylazine (2 mg/kg im) | 1.0–2.0 mg/kg/15.0 mg/kg/h for 15 min then 12.0/mg/h for 45 min then 9.0 mg/kg/h for 60 min then 7.5 mg/kg for 120 min | Not used |
| Lurie et al. [73] | Ketamine (21.9–25.0 mg/kg im) | 2.3 mg/kg + 1.0 mg/kg/9.6 mg/kg/h | Not used |
| Navarro et al. [70] | Ketamine/Telazol/xylazine im (not reported) | 1.5 mg/kg/9.0 mg/kg/h | Not used |
| Silva et al. [71] | Azaperone (4 mg/kg im) | 4.0 mg/kg/15.0 mg/kg/h | 0.3 mikrogram/kg/min followed by 0.2 mikrogram/kg/min |
| Silva et al. [67] | Azaperone (4 mg/kg im) | 4.0 mg/kg/15.0 mg/kg/h | 0.3 mikrogram/kg/min + 5 mikrogram/kg bolus |
| Srinivasan et al. [72] | Ketamine (21.2–31.3 mg/kg im)[c] | 2.0–3.0 mg/kg/9.6 mg/kg | Not used |
| Yannopoulos et al. [100] | Ketamine (23.0–23.7 mg/kg im) | 1.0 mg/kg/9.6 mg/kg/h | Not used |
| Yannopoulos et al. [101] | Ketamine (21.7–23.5 mg/kg im) | 2.0 mg/kg/9.6 mg/kg/h | Not used |
| Yannopoulos et al. [69] | Ketamine (25.6–30.3 mg/kg im) | 2.3 mg/kg/9.6 mg/kg/h | Not used |

[a] Doses are calculated based on animal weight

[b] Doses reported as mikrogram/kg/min are converted to mg/kg/h for easier comparison

[c] Calculated under the assumption that lowest dose was given to animals with lowest weight

**Tabel 4 Animal and publication relevant data**

| Study ID [reference] | Animal intervention study | Random sequence allocation | n | Gender/pig breed | Weight (kg)[a] | Age in weeks |
|---|---|---|---|---|---|---|
| Boezaart [68] | 1 group | NA | 10 | Female/pigs | 22–28 | 8–9[b] |
| Kajimoto et al. [82] | 2 groups | No | 14 | Male/yorkshire | 7.8–14.5 | 4–6[c] |
| Lurie et al. [73] | 2 groups | Yes | 22 | Female/farm pigs | 30.4 ± 1.3 | 9–11[b] |
| Navarro et al. [70] | 1 group | NA | 6 | Female/swine | 21.5–92.8 | 8–21[b] |
| Silva et al. [71] | 2 groups | Yes | 12 | Male/large white | 27.0 ± 3.6 | 12[d] |
| Silva et al. [67] | 1 group | NA | 12 | Male/Large white | 26.2 ± 3.6 | 12[d] |
| Srinivasan et al. [72] | 1 group | NA | 13 | Female/domestic farm pigs | 16–33 | 12–16 |
| Yannopoulos et al. [100] | 2 groups | Yes | 16 | Female/farm pigs | 30 ± 0.5 | 10–11[b] |
| Yannopoulos et al. [101] | 2 groups | No | 12 | Female/yorkshire-farm cross | 31 ± 1.2 | 10–11[b] |
| Yannopoulos et al. [69] | 2 groups | Yes | 16 | Female/farm pigs | 25.2 ± 2.1 | 8–9[b] |

*n*: number of animals; *NA*: not applicable

[a] Mean ± SD or upper and lower limits

[b] Age in weeks estimated from weight post hoc if not reported

[c] Reported as 27–41 days

[d] Reported as 3 months

haemodynamic baseline recordings had to be stable prior to intervention. MAP and the 95 % confidence interval of all studies were within the limits of cerebral autoregulation (Table 5).

Cerebral blood flow was reported on the basis of directly measured transdural flow in tissue perfusion units, indirectly measured carotid artery blood flow in ml/min or jugular venous oxygen saturation ($SvjO_2$) in % or as cerebral perfusion pressure (CPP) in mm Hg. Mean CPP was reported in four studies and ranged from 68 to 74.8 mm Hg (Table 6).

Cerebral oxygenation was reported on the basis of direct measurement of brain tissue partial pressure of oxygen ($brPO_2$) in mm Hg or indirect transcranial measurement of regional cerebral oxygen saturation ($rSO_2$) in %. Data for $brPO_2$ from one study [73] was not reported in absolute values, but were extracted from a graph. Values for $rSO_2$ between 51 and 65 % were reported in three

**Table 5 Means and 95 % confidence intervals of reported MAP**

| Study ID [reference] | n | Outcome | Measure | Mean | CI 95 % (LL) | CI 95 % (UL) |
|---|---|---|---|---|---|---|
| Boezaart [68] | 10 | MAP | mm Hg | 89.0 | 82.6 | 95.4 |
| Kajimoto et al. [82] | 7 | MAP | mm Hg | 69.0 | 63.1 | 74.9 |
| Lurie et al. [73] | 22 | MAP | mm Hg | 91.8 | 85.3 | 98.2 |
| Navarro et al. [70] | 6 | MAP | mm Hg | Range | 70.0 | 110.0 |
| Silva et al. [67] | 12 | MAP | mm Hg | 72.7 | 67.4 | 78.0 |
| Silva et al. [71] | 12 | MAP | mm Hg | 73.0 | 67.3 | 78.7 |
| Yannopoulos et al. [100] | 16 | MAP | mm Hg | 81.0 | 73.9 | 88.1 |
| Yannopoulos et al. [101] | 12 | MAP | mm Hg | 90.0 | 81.2 | 98.8 |
| Yannopoulos et al. [69] | 16 | MAP[a] | mm Hg | 90.1 | 83.8 | 96.4 |

*n*: number of animals; *MAP*: mean arterial pressure; *CI*: confidence interval; *LL*: lower limit; *UL*: upper limit

[a] Calculated from systolic and diastolic blood pressure

**Table 6 Means and 95 % confidence levels of reported cerebral perfusion measures**

| Study ID [reference] | n | Outcome | Measure | Mean | CI 95 % (LL) | CI 95 % (UL) |
|---|---|---|---|---|---|---|
| Boezaart [68] | 10 | CBF | TPU | 44.7 | 29.2 | 60.2 |
| Lurie et al. [73] | 22 | CarotidBF | ml/min | 119.4 | 101.8 | 136.9 |
| Silva et al. [67] | 12 | SvjO2 | % | 82.7 | 77.0 | 88.3 |
| Silva et al. [71] | 12 | SvjO2 | % | 79.0 | 73.9 | 84.1 |
| Srinivasan et al. [72] | 13 | CPP | mm Hg | 73.6 | 67.0 | 80.2 |
| Yannopoulos et al. [69] | 16 | CarotidBF | ml/min | 174.8 | 153.6 | 196.0 |
| Yannopoulos et al. [100] | 16 | CPP | mm Hg | 68.0 | 61.6 | 74.4 |
| Yannopoulos et al. [101] | 12 | CPP | mm Hg | 74.0 | 64.6 | 83.4 |
| Yannopoulos et al. [69] | 16 | CPP | mm Hg | 74.8 | 67.2 | 82.3 |

*n*: number of animals; *CI*: confidence interval; *LL*: lower limit; *UL*: upper limit; *CBF*: cerebral blood blow; *CarotidBF*: carotid blood flow; *SvjO2*: jugular venous haemoglobinoxygen saturation; *CPP*: cerebral perfusion pressure

studies while one study reported an $rSO_2$ range from 65 to 80 % (Table 7).

**Evaluation of the effects of propofol and remifentanil**

This systematic review was not able to identify studies with the primary objective to investigate the combined effects of propofol and remifentanil TIVA on cerebral perfusion and oxygenation in pigs. Thus, the question of how propofol and remifentanil affects CPO in healthy pigs remains uncertain. Silva et al. [67] investigated the effect of a single high dose remifentanil bolus (5 μg/kg iv) on cerebral oxygenation during TIVA with propofol and remifentanil. They reported CPO outcome measures during propofol-remifentanil infusion (Tables 5, 6, 7), that were within the normal target limits, while a single bolus of remifentanil significantly lowered cerebral oxygenation, yet still within normal limits (Table 1). Silva et al. [67] suggest that this decrease may be associated with a decrease in cardiac output rather than altered cerebral metabolism. The primary aim of the remaining nine articles was not to

**Table 7 Means and 95 % confidence intervals of reported cerebral oxygenation measures**

| Study ID [reference] | n | Outcome | Measure | Mean | CI 95 % (LL) | CI 95 % (UL) |
|---|---|---|---|---|---|---|
| Kajimoto et al. [82] | 7 | rSO2 | % | 51.0 | 47.1 | 54.9 |
| Lurie et al. [73] | 22 | brPO2[a] | mm Hg | 13.2 | 9.9 | 16.5 |
| Navarro et al. [70] | 6 | rSO2 | % | Range | 65.0 | 80.0 |
| Silva et al. [67] | 12 | rSO2 | % | 62.3 | 58.6 | 65.9 |
| Silva et al. [71] | 12 | rSO2 | % | 65.0 | 61.6 | 68.4 |

*n*: number of animals; *CI*: confidence interval; *LL*: lower limit; *UL*: upper limit; *rSO2*: regional cerebral oxygene saturation; *brPO2*: brain tissue partial pressure of oxygen

[a] Extrapolated from graph

investigate the effects of propofol or propofol-remifentanil anaesthesia on CPO. Hence, data from these studies may have been influenced by factors other than anaesthesia with propofol or remifentanil. Beydon et al. [74] who studied bispectral index stability in response to haemodynamic instability, suggested that a propofol-remifentanil TIVA with a lower dose propofol (8.4 mg/kg/h) and a higher dose of remifentanil (0.54 μg/kg/min) provides a more stable anaesthetic depth compared to propofol-remifentanil TIVA with a higher dose of propofol (26.7 mg/kg/h) and lower dose of remifentanil (0.34 μg/kg/min). Relative to the findings made by Beydon et al. [74], Boezaart et al. [68] used a very low dose of propofol for maintenance (3 mg/kg/h) and a low dose of remifentanil, while the remainder of articles reviewed here, used a low–mid range propofol dose and a low remifentanil dose (Table 3). Silva et al. [71] defined a stable level of anaesthesia as total muscle relaxation, absence of palpebral reflex, and absence of hemodynamic response to interdigital space clamping. Srinivasan et al. [72] titrated anaesthesia on the basis of heart rate, blood pressure, tail and hoof response and spontaneous breathing. The depth of anaesthesia and consequently the stress response to surgical stimulation thus may differ between studies, which makes comparison difficult. None of the studies however, reported concerns about insufficient anaesthetic depth.

### *Choice of model*

The studies included used farm pigs of different breeds that were only specified in 4 of the studies (Table 4). Farm pig breeding standards vary from country to country resulting in pig breeds of varying anatomy and physiology. When used in scientific studies thus, detailed consideration should be given to the choice of pig breed [3, 75]. None of the studies reviewed here used mini or micro pig breeds but different farm pig breeds only, hence we find it acceptable to consider results as relatively comparable provided that age is taken into consideration. Based on the relationship between bodyweight and age, the animals included were approximately between 1 and 6 months old [64, 65]. For neurodevelopmental comparison to the human brain, it has been estimated that 1 week of life in the piglet approximates 1 month of life in humans [66]. Therefore, these animals could be considered equivalent to infants between 4 months and 2 years of age and may be the basis for a translational model of this paediatric subpopulation, while it seems less advisable to use this model in studies aiming at the human adult or geriatric subpopulation [76]. Cerebral autoregulation has been shown to be impaired more extensively in newborn than in juvenile pigs in response to traumatic brain injury [4], which indicates an age-dependent maturation of the cerebral autoregulatory response. Consequently, the youngest animals would be more sensitive to periods of hypotension (e.g. in response to anaesthetic induction) and potentially result in an over-interpretation of differing CPO responses between animals at both ends of the age span. This may explain the relatively broad range of $rSO_2$ values in the study by Navarro et al. [70], since this study was conducted on few animals (n = 6) with body weights ranging from 21.5 to 92.8 kg and estimated ages of approximately 8–21 weeks. In parallel, the relatively wide range in MAP observed may also be a result of an uneven sensitivity to the propofol doses between animals with different age. As a result, an inter-animal comparison could be biased due to unequal physiological prerequisites, even if cerebral oxygenation was still within target limits for pigs.

Gender has been described as a factor influencing cerebral autoregulation in piglets [77, 78]. None of the selected studies discussed the choice of animal gender.

### *Anaesthesia and drug contamination*

Anaesthesia related discussion was brief and not given in all of the selected publications and main motivators for the choice of anaesthesia were animal welfare and analgesia while less attention was given to the potential influence of anaesthesia on their main outcome measures. Premedication was an integrated part of the anaesthetic protocol in all 10 studies and might influence outcome data, possibly in a dose dependent manner. Ketamine, which was used in eight out of the ten studies included in this review, is recommended for premedication-induction and reduction of stress response in pigs [39]. Ketamine has also been reported to increase CBF, ICP, and cerebral metabolic rate at high doses in pigs [40, 45, 79–81]. None of the studies addressed the risk of drug contamination bias or length of washout periods, even though doses $\geq$30 mg/kg of ketamine were used for premedication in some of the studies [69, 72, 82]. However, from the trial descriptions we believe that the preparatory periods were long enough to reduce the risk of drug contamination bias in the assessed studies [83]. If this also is the case for the two studies [70, 82] that combined ketamine premedication with either xylazine alone or ketamine with tiletamine, zolazepam and xylazine, is unclear. However another $\alpha_2$-agonist, medetomidine, has been reported to have a more prolonged effect on heart rate in minipigs [84] and xylazine has been reported to reduce local cerebral CBF in rats [85]. Azaperone, which was used for sedation in two studies (Table 3) has been reported to influence both cerebral and systemic haemodynamics, but is in general believed to have little influence on haemodynamics [86].

Boezaart [68] used pancuronium for muscle relaxation. High-dose pancuronium has been reported to widen the cerebral autoregulatory range in newborn piglets, but the single bolus of 0.1 mg/kg, which was given at time of premedication is not expected to have influenced cerebral haemodynamics [87].

In one survival study [69] the nonsteroidal anti-inflammatory drug flunixin was given for post-operative analgesia intramuscularly, 1 h before surgical intervention. Flunixin has a relatively fast onset, and a long half-life of approximately 7 h in pigs [88]. The acute effect of flunixin on the haemodynamics of the normal pig brain has not been investigated, but other cyclooxygenase inhibitors have been reported to affect CBF when administered intravenously. Prostaglandin synthesis is cyclooxygenase dependent and plays a central role in maintaining CBF and cerebral autoregulation. It may be speculated that inhibition of prostaglandin synthesis by flunixin may influence CBF and consequently cerebral oxygenation [89]. The potential influence of flunixin on CPO assessment was not discussed by Yannopoulos et al. [69].

Premedication, in terms of dose, time from administration to the beginning of CPO measurement, and expected serum concentration of drugs and active metabolites is relevant to assessing the risk of drug related outcome contamination. Even though this is considered insignificant for primary outcome assessment, this was not addressed in any of the 10 articles reviewed.

#### *Methods of CPO measurements*

Monitoring CPO is a complex assessment of principally different variables such as systemic blood pressure, intra cranial pressure, tissue oxygen tension or haemoglobin saturation—all of which may be influenced by choice of monitoring technique [1, 20, 31, 90].

It is difficult to compare the cerebral perfusion measures reported in the selected articles. CBF was reported in 4 studies (Table 6). Lurie et al. [73] and Yannopoulos et al. [69] quantified a global measure of CBF by identical techniques of LDF over the exposed left common carotid artery. Lurie et al. [73] reported significantly lower values than Yannopoulos et al. [69] despite similar animal weight, gender and anaesthetic protocols. Yannopoulos et al. [69] additionally used 2.2 mg/kg flunixin im prior to surgery, which would be expected to reveal the opposite relationship, since flunixin in theory may have a CBF lowering effect. However, wide carotid blood flow limits have been reported earlier. Boezaart [68] also used LDF, but measured CBF locally through a drilled craniotomy, and reported it as relative tissue perfusion units, where the other studies reported it as absolute ml/min. Comparison of the CBF from the three studies is difficult because of the difference in measuring techniques, brain area of interest and wide normal flow limits [32, 91].

CPP was reported in four studies with a range between 68 and 74.8 mmHg, which is similar to previously reported CPP in healthy pigs anaesthetized with midazolam and fentanyl after ketamine and xylazine sedation [34]. More studies are required to verify this, and to determine a more exact range for CPP in pigs during different types of anaesthesia. Collectively however, none of the reported cerebral perfusion measures (Table 6) were outside the normal ranges for humans that are available in the literature (Table 1).

Cerebral oxygenation is a measure of oxygen available for consumption and energy metabolism in the brain. Lurie et al. [73] reported a mean $brPO_2$ baseline value of 13.2 mm Hg, 95 % CI [9.9–16.5 mm Hg]. This $brPO_2$ is well outside the target ranges available in healthy swine of 25–30 mm Hg [35] and further, is within the ischaemic range of <15 mm Hg in humans [1, 22, 92]. Lurie et al. [73] used the baseline as a relative comparison to post-interventional measures, however the relatively low $brPO_2$ is not discussed in the article.

Non-invasive measurement of $rSO_2$ with near infrared spectroscopy was performed in 4 studies and baseline values were reported for both propofol studies and for propofol and remifentanil studies (Table 7). Navarro et al. [70] reported an $rSO_2$ range between 65 and 80 % with the upper range slightly above the target range of 57–72 % [36]. Kajimoto et al. [82] reported an $rSO_2$ mean of 51 %, 95 % CI (47.1; 54.9). This lower oxygenation measure could be related to the use of younger animals in this study and the high-dose ketamine and xylazine in the premedication used in this experiment. The earlier stage of neurodevelopment could render the animals more susceptible to sedative agents, which would lead to a more extensive metabolic cerebral depression and therefore lower oxygen demand.

## Conclusions

Even though the very limited pool of evidence reviewed here, it suggests that propofol and remifentanil alone or in combination have limited effects on CPO in healthy pigs, confirmative evidence is lacking. In one study baseline CPO measures were within normal target ranges in healthy pigs during propofol-remifentanil TIVA. Addition of a single remifentanil dose significantly reduced $rSO_2$ but not beyond normal target ranges.

There is a need for standardised porcine studies with the primary objective of studying the influence of anaesthetic drugs on CPO in non-diseased animals.

#### Abbreviations

$brPO_2$: brain tissue partial pressure of oxygen; CBF: cerebral blood flow; CPO: cerebral perfusion and oxygenation; CPP: cerebral perfusion pressure; LDF: laser Doppler flow; MAP: mean arterial pressure; $rSO_2$: regional cerebral oxygen saturation; $SvjO_2$: jugular venous oxygen saturation; TIVA: total intravenous anaesthesia.

**Authors' contributions**

MLGM and TE conceived the overall objective, design and preliminary protocol for this systematic review. MLGM was responsible for building and conducting the primary literature search and drafting the manuscript. Record screening, secondary literature searches, extraction and interpretation of data were conducted in close collaboration with TE and RA. Data analysis and statistical revision was done in collaboration with JEM. FBM and HHP contributed with substantial intellectual guidance and interpretations of data, as well as critical revision of the manuscript in the topics of human and veterinary anaesthesia, respectively. All authors read and approved the final manuscript.

**Author details**

[1] Department of Veterinary Clinical and Animal Sciences, University of Copenhagen, 16 Dyrlægevej, 1870 Frederiksberg C, Denmark. [2] Department of Surgical Gastroenterology C, Rigshospitalet, University of Copenhagen, 9 Blegdamsvej, 2100 Copenhagen Ø, Denmark. [3] Department of Neuroanaesthesia, Rigshospitalet, University of Copenhagen, 9 Blegdamsvej, 2100 Copenhagen Ø, Denmark. [4] Department of Anaesthesia, Sealand Hospital, University of Copenhagen, 1 Lykkebækvej, 4600 Køge, Denmark.

**Acknowledgements**

We would like to thank Rune Rasmussen for constructive discussion of the revised manuscript.

**Competing interests**

The authors declare that they have no competing interests.

**References**

1. Grocott HP, Davie S, Fedorow C. Monitoring of brain function in anesthesia and intensive care. Curr Opin Anesthesio. 2010;23:759–64.
2. Otto KA. Physiology, pathophysiology, and anesthetic management of patients with neurological disease. In: Grimm KA, Lamont LA, Tranquilli WJ, Greene SA, Robertson SA, editors. Veterinary Anesthesia and Analgesia – The fifth edition of Lumb and Jones. Ames Iowa: Wiley; 2015. p. 559–83.
3. Lind NM, Moustgaard A, Jelsing J, Vajta G, Cumming P, Hansen AK. The use of pigs in neuroscience: modeling brain disorders. Neurosci Biobehav R. 2007;31:728–51.
4. Armstead WM. Age-dependent cerebral hemodynamic effects of traumatic brain injury in newborn and juvenile pigs. Microcirculation. 2000;7:225–35.
5. Swindle MM, Makin A, Herron AJ, Clubb FJ, Frazier KS. Swine as models in biomedical research and toxicology testing. Vet Pathol. 2012;49:344–56.
6. Malhotra AK, Schweitzer JB, Fox JL, Fabian TC, Proctor KG. Cerebral perfusion pressure directed therapy following traumatic brain injury and hypotension in swine. J Neurotraum. 2003;20:827–39.
7. Friess SH, Ralston J, Eucker SA, Helfaer MA, Smith C, Margulies SS. Neurocritical care monitoring correlates with neuropathology in a swine model of pediatric traumatic brain injury. Neurosurgery. 2011;69:1139–47.
8. Timaru-Kast R, Meissner A, Heimann A, Hoelper B, Kempski O, Alessandri B. Acute subdural hematoma in pigs: role of volume on multiparametric neuromonitoring and histology. J Neurotraum. 2008;25:1107–19.
9. Nilsson F, Akeson J, Messeter K, Ryding E, Rosen I, Nordstrom CH. A porcine model for evaluation of cerebral haemodynamics and metabolism during increased intracranial pressure. Acta Anaesth Scand. 1995;39:827–34.
10. Andrade AF, Soares MS, Patriota GC, Belon AR, Paiva WS, Bor-Seng-Shu E, et al. Experimental model of intracranial hypertension with continuous multiparametric monitoring in swine. Arq Neuro-Psiquiat. 2013;71:802–6.
11. Van Gompel JJ, Bower MR, Worrell GA, Stead M, Meier TR, Goerss SJ, et al. Swine model for translational research of invasive intracranial monitoring. Epilepsia. 2011;52:E49–53.
12. Kuluz JW, Prado R, He D, Zhao W, Dietrich WD, Watson B. New pediatric model of ischemic stroke in infant piglets by photothrombosis: acute changes in cerebral blood flow, microvasculature, and early histopathology. Stroke. 2007;38:1932–7.
13. Lucas SJ, Tzeng YC, Galvin SD, Thomas KN, Ogoh S, Ainslie PN. Influence of changes in blood pressure on cerebral perfusion and oxygenation. Hypertension. 2010;55:698–705.
14. Mishra LD. Cerebral blood flow and anaesthesia: a review. Indian J Anaesth. 2002;46:87–95.
15. Gupta AK, Azami J. Update of neuromonitoring. Curr Anaesth Crit Care. 2002;13:120–8.
16. Lassen NA. Cerebral blood flow and oxygen consumption in man. Physiol Rev. 1959;39:183–238.
17. Prabhakar H, Sandhu K, Bhagat H, Durga P, Chawla R. Current concepts of optimal cerebral perfusion pressure in traumatic brain injury. J Anaesthesiol Clin Pharmacol. 2014;30:318–27.
18. Dagal A, Lam AM. Cerebral autoregulation and anesthesia. Curr Opin Anesthesio. 2009;22:547–52.
19. Smith AL, Neigh JL, Hoffman JC, Wollman H. Effects of general anesthesia on autoregulation of cerebral blood flow in man. J Appl Physio. 1970;29:665–9.
20. Smythe PR, Samra SK. Monitors of cerebral oxygenation. Anesthesiol Clin N A. 2002;20:293–313.
21. Moerman A, Hert S. Cerebral oximetry. The standard monitor of the future? Curr Opin Anesthesio. 2015;28:703–9.
22. Mahajan C, Rath GP, Bithal PK. Advances in neuro-monitoring. Anesth Essays Res. 2013;7:312–8.
23. Barone DG, Czosnyka M. Brain monitoring: do we need a hole? An update on invasive and noninvasive brain monitoring modalities. Sci World J. 2014. doi:10.1155/2014/795762 **(eCollection 2014)**.
24. Le Roux P, Menon DK, Citerio G, Vespa P, Bader MK, Brophy GM, et al. Consensus summary statement of the International Multidisciplinary Consensus Conference on Multimodality Monitoring in Neurocritical Care: a statement for healthcare professionals from the Neurocritical Care Society and the European Society of Intensive Care Medicine. Neurocrit Care. 2014;21(Suppl 2):S1–26.
25. Benedik PS. Monitoring tissue blood flow and oxygenation: a brief review of emerging techniques. Crit Care Nurs Clin North Am. 2014;26:345–56.
26. Kety SS, Schmidt CF. The nitrous oxide method for the quantitative determination of cerebral blood flow in man: theory, procedure and normal values. J Clin Invest. 1948;27:476–83.
27. Lassen NA, Munck O. The cerebral blood flow in man determined by the use of radioactive krypton. Acta Physiol Scand. 1955;33:30–49.
28. Ingvar DH, Cronqvist S, Ekberg R, Risberg J, Hoedt-Rasmussen K. Normal values of regional cerebral blood flow in man, including flow and weight estimates of gray and white matter. A preliminary summary. Acta Neurol Scand Suppl. 1965;14:72–8.
29. Ingvar DH, Lassen NA. Methods for cerebral bloodflow measurements in man. Br J Anaesth. 1965;37:216–24.
30. Parthasarathy AB, Weber EL, Richards LM, Fox DJ, Dunn AK. Laser speckle contrast imaging of cerebral blood flow in humans during neurosurgery. a pilot clinical study. J Biomed Opt. 2010;15:1–8.
31. Briers D, Duncan DD, Hirst E, Kirkpatrick SJ, Larsson M, Steenbergen W, et al. Laser speckle contrast imaging: theoretical and practical limitations. J Biomed Opt. 2013. doi:10.1117/1.Jbo.18.6.066018.
32. Harada J, Takaku A, Endo S, Kuwayama N, Fukuda O. Differences in critical cerebral blood flow with age in swine. J Neurosurg. 1991;75:103–7.
33. Mutch WAC, Lefevre GR, Thiessen DB, Girling LG, Warrian RK. Computer-controlled cardiopulmonary bypass increases jugular venous oxygen saturation during rewarmin. Ann Thorac Surg. 1998;65:59–65.
34. Bruins B, Kilbaugh TJ, Margulies SS, Friess SH. The anesthetic effects on vasopressor modulation of cerebral blood flow in an immature swine model. Anesth Analg. 2013;116:838–44.
35. Maas AI, Fleckenstein W, de Jong DA, van Santbrink H. Monitoring cerebral oxygenation: experimental studies and preliminary clinical results of continuous monitoring of cerebrospinal fluid and brain tissue oxygen tension. Acta Neurochir Suppl (Wien). 1993;59:50–7.
36. Xanthos T, Bassiakou E, Koudouna E, Tsirikos-Karapanos N, Lelovas P, Papadimitriou D, et al. Baseline hemodynamics in anesthetized Landrace-Large White swine: reference values for research in cardiac

arrest and cardiopulmonary resuscitation models. J Am Assoc Lab Anim Sci. 2007;46:21–5.
37. Kurth CD, Levy WJ, McCann J. Near-infrared spectroscopy cerebral oxygen saturation thresholds for hypoxia-ischemia in piglets. J Cereb Blood Flow Metab. 2002;22:335–41.
38. Wenzel V, Padosch SA, Voelckel WG, Idris AH, Krismer AC, Bettschart-Wolfensberger R, Lindner KH. Survey of effects of anesthesia protocols on hemodynamic variables in porcine cardiopulmonary resuscitation laboratory models before induction of cardiac arrest. Comp Med. 2000;50:644–8.
39. Alstrup AKO, Smith DF. Anaesthesia for positron emission tomography scanning of animal brains. Lab Anim. 2013;47:12–8.
40. Cole CD, Gottfried ON, Gupta DK, Couldwell WT. Total intravenous anesthesia: advantages for intracranial surgery. Neurosurgery. 2007;59(Suppl 2):369–77.
41. Lagerkranser M, Stange K, Sollevi A. Effects of propofol on cerebral blood flow, metabolism, and cerebral autoregulation in the anesthetized pig. J Neurosurg Anesth. 1997;9:188–93.
42. Veselis RA, Reinsel RA, Beattie BJ, Mawlawi OR, Feshchenko VA, DiResta GR, et al. Midazolam changes cerebral blood flow in discrete brain regions: an H2(15)O positron emission tomography study. Anesthesiology. 1997;87:1106–17.
43. Kaisti KK, Langsjo JW, Aalto S, Oikonen V, Sipila H, Teras M, et al. Effects of sevoflurane, propofol, and adjunct nitrous oxide on regional cerebral blood flow, oxygen consumption, and blood volume in humans. Anesthesiology. 2003;99:603–13.
44. Bonhomme V, Boveroux P, Hans P, Brichant JF, Vanhaudenhuyse A, Boly M, et al. Influence of anesthesia on cerebral blood flow, cerebral metabolic rate, and brain functional connectivity. Curr Opin Anaesthesio. 2011;24:474–9.
45. Langsjo JW, Maksimow A, Salmi E, Kaisti K, Aalto S, Oikonen V, et al. S-ketamine anesthesia increases cerebral blood flow in excess of the metabolic needs in humans. Anesthesiology. 2005;103:258–68.
46. Hans P, Bonhomme V. Why we still use intravenous drugs as the basic regimen for neurosurgical anaesthesia. Curr Opin Anaesthesio. 2006;19:498–503.
47. Schifilliti D, Grasso G, Conti A, Fodale V. Anaesthetic-related neuroprotection. intravenous or inhalational agents? CNS Drugs. 2010;24:893–907.
48. Chui J, Mariappan R, Mehta J, Manninen P, Venkatraghavan L. Comparison of propofol and volatile agents for maintenance of anesthesia during elective craniotomy procedures: systematic review and meta-analysis. Can J Anaesth. 2014;61:347–56.
49. Lauder GR. Total intravenous anesthesia will supercede inhalational anesthesia in pediatric anesthetic practice. Paediatr Anaesth. 2015;25:52–64.
50. Engelhard K, Werner C, Mollenberg O, Kochs E. Effects of remifentanil/propofol in comparison with isoflurane on dynamic cerebrovascular autoregulation in humans. Acta Anaesth Scand. 2001;45:971–6.
51. Conti A, Iacopino DG, Fodale V, Micalizzi S, Penna O, Santamaria LB. Cerebral haemodynamic changes during propofol-remifentanil or sevoflurane anaesthesia: transcranial Doppler study under bispectral index monitoring. Br J Anaesth. 2006;97:333–9.
52. Kay B, Rolly G. I.C.I. 35868, a new intravenous induction agent. Acta Anaesthesiol Belgica. 1977;28:303–16.
53. Berry SH. Injectable anesthetics. In: Grimm KA, Lamont LA, Tranquilli WJ, Greene SA, Robertson SA, editors. Veterinary anesthesia and analgesia—the fifth edition of Lumb and Jones. Ames Iowa: Wiley; 2015. p. 559–83.
54. Eikaas H, Raeder J. Total intravenous anaesthesia techniques for ambulatory surgery. Curr Opin Anaesthesio. 2009;22:725–9.
55. Marik PE. Propofol: therapeutic indications and side-effects. Curr Pharm Des. 2004;10:3639–49.
56. Adembri C, Venturi L, Pellegrini-Giampietro DE. Neuroprotective effects of propofol in acute cerebral injury. CNS Drug Rev. 2007;13:333–51.
57. Kotani Y, Shimazawa M, Yoshimura S, Iwama T, Hara H. The experimental and clinical pharmacology of propofol, an anesthetic agent with neuroprotective properties. CNS Neurosci Ther. 2008;14:95–106.
58. Servin FS, Billard V. Remifentanil and other opioids. Hand Exp Pharmacol. 2008;182:283–311.
59. Fodale V, Schifilliti D, Praticò C, Santamaria LB. Remifentanil and the brain. Acta Anaesth Scand. 2008;52:319–26.
60. Klimscha W, Ullrich R, Nasel C, Dietrich W, Illievich UM, Wildling E, et al. High-dose remifentanil does not impair cerebrovascular carbon dioxide reactivity in healthy male volunteers. Anesthesiology. 2003;99:834–40.
61. Baker KZ, Ostapkovich N, Sisti MB, Warner DS, Young WL. Intact cerebral blood flow reactivity during remifentanil/nitrous oxide anesthesia. J Neurosurg Anesth. 1997;9:134–40.
62. Hooijmans CR, Rovers MM, de Vries RB, Leenaars M, Ritskes-Hoitinga M, Langendam MW. SYRCLE's risk of bias tool for animal studies. BMC Med Res Methodol. 2014;14:43. doi:10.1186/1471-2288-14-43.
63. O'Connor AM, Sargeant JM. Critical appraisal of studies using laboratory animal models. ILAR J. 2014;55:405–17.
64. Pond WG. Biology of the domestic pig. Ithaca: Comstock Publishing Associates; 2001.
65. Swindle MM. Swine in the laboratory: surgery, anesthesia, imaging, and experimental techniques. 2nd ed. Boca Raton: CRC Press; 2007.
66. Conrad MS, Johnson RW. The domestic piglet: an important model for investigating the neurodevelopmental consequences of early life insults. Annu Rev Anim Biosci. 2015;3:245–64.
67. Silva A, Venancio C, Ortiz AL, Souza AP, Amorim P, Ferreira DA. The effect of high doses of remifentanil in brain near-infrared spectroscopy and in electroencephalographic parameters in pigs. Vet Anaesth Analg. 2014;41:153–62.
68. Boezaart AP. Effects of cerebrospinal fluid loss and epidural blood patch on cerebral blood flow in swine. Region Anesth Pain M. 2001;26:401–6.
69. Yannopoulos D, Matsuura T, McKnite S, Goodman N, Idris A, Tang WC, et al. No assisted ventilation cardiopulmonary resuscitation and 24-hour neurological outcomes in a porcine model of cardiac arrest. Crit Care Med. 2010;38:254–60.
70. Navarro LH, Lima RM, Khan M, Dominguez WG, Voigt RB. Kinsky MP et cardiovascular status during hemorrhagic shock in a swine model. J Trauma Acute Care Surg. 2012;73(Suppl 1):S140–6.
71. Silva A, Ortiz AL, Venancio C, Souza AP, Ferreira LM, Branco PS, et al. Effects of acute bleeding followed by hydroxyethyl starch 130/0.4 or a crystalloid on propofol concentrations, cerebral oxygenation, and electroencephalographic and haemodynamic variables in pigs. Vet. Med Int. 2014. doi:10.1155/2014/710394.
72. Srinivasan V, Nadkarni VM, Yannopoulos D, Marino BS, Sigurdsson G, McKnite SH, et al. Spontaneous gasping decreases intracranial pressure and improves cerebral perfusion in a pig model of ventricular fibrillation. Resuscitation. 2006;69:329–34.
73. Lurie KG, Yannopoulos D, McKnite SH, Herman ML, Dris AH, Nadkarni VM, et al. Comparison of a 10-breaths-per-minute versus a 2-breaths-per-minute strategy during cardiopulmonary resuscitation in a porcine model of cardiac arrest. Resp Care. 2008;53:862–70.
74. Beydon L, Desfontis JC, Ganster F, Petres J, Gautier F, Ferec S, et al. BIS response to tamponade and dobutamine in swine varies with hypnotic/opiate ratio. Ann Fr Anesth. 2009;28:650–7.
75. Bollen PJA, Hansen AK, Alstrup AKO. The Laboratory Swine. 2nd ed. Boca Raton: CRC Press; 2010.
76. Zisowsky J, Krause A, Dingemanse J. drug development for pediatric populations: regulatory aspects. Pharmaceutics. 2010;2:364–88.
77. Armstead WM, Kiessling JW, Kofke WA, Vavilala MS. Impaired cerebral blood flow autoregulation during posttraumatic arterial hypotension after fluid percussion brain injury is prevented by phenylephrine in female but exacerbated in male piglets by extracellular signal-related kinase mitogen-activated protein kinase upregulation. Crit Care Med. 2010;38:1868–74.
78. Armstead WM, Kiessling JW, Riley J, Kofke WA, Vavilala MS. Phenylephrine infusion prevents impairment of ATP- and calcium-sensitive potassium channel-mediated cerebrovasodilation after brain injury in female, but aggravates impairment in male, piglets through modulation of ERK MAPK upregulation. J Neurotraum. 2011;28:105–11.
79. Akeson J, Bjorkman S, Messeter K, Rosen I, Helfer M. Cerebral pharmacodynamics of anaesthetic and subanaesthetic doses of ketamine in the normoventilated pig. Acta Anaesth Scand. 1993;37:211–8.
80. Schmidt A, Ryding E, Akeson J. Racemic ketamine does not abolish cerebrovascular autoregulation in the pig. Acta Anaesth Scand. 2003;47:569–75.

81. Schmidt A, Oye I, Akeson J. Cerebral physiological responses to bolus injection of racemic, S(+)- or R(-)-ketamine in the pig. Acta Anaesth Scand. 2005;49:1436–42.
82. Kajimoto M, Atkinson DB, Ledee DR, Kayser EB, Morgan PG, Sedensky MM, et al. Propofol compared with isoflurane inhibits mitochondrial metabolism in immature swine cerebral cortex. J Cereb Blood Flow Met. 2014;34:514–21.
83. Bjorkman S, Akeson J, Nilsson F, Messeter K, Roth B. Ketamine and midazolam decrease cerebral blood flow and consequently their own rate of transport to the brain: an application of mass balance pharmacokinetics with a changing regional blood flow. J Pharmacokinet Biop. 1992;20:637–52.
84. Authier S, Gervais J, Fournier S, Gauvin D, Maghezzi S, Troncy E. Cardiovascular and respiratory safety pharmacology in Göttingen minipigs. Pharmacological characterization. J Pharmacol Toxicol. 2011;64:53–9.
85. Lei H, Grinberg O, Nwaigwe CI, Hou HG, Williams H, Swartz HM, et al. The effects of ketamine-xylazine anesthesia on cerebral blood flow and oxygenation observed using nuclear magnetic resonance perfusion imaging and electron paramagnetic resonance oximetry. Brain Res. 2001;913:174–9.
86. van Woerkens LJ, Duncker DJ, Huigen RJ, van der Giessen WJ, Verdouw PD. Redistribution of cardiac output caused by opening of arteriovenous anastomoses by a combination of azaperone and metomidate. Br J Anaesth. 1990;65:393–9.
87. Chemtob S, Barna T, Beharry K, Aranda JV. Enhanced cerebral blood flow autoregulation in the newborn piglet by d-tubocurarine and pancuronium but not by vecuronium. Anesthesiology. 1992;76:236–44.
88. Pairis-Garcia MD, Karriker LA, Johnson AK, Kukanich B, Wulf L, Sander S, et al. Pharmacokinetics of flunixin meglumine in mature swine after intravenous, intramuscular and oral administration. BMC Vet Res. 2013. doi:10.1186/1746-6148-9-165.
89. Schiefecker AJ, Pfausler B, Beer R, Sohm F, Sabo J, Knauseder V, et al. Parenteral diclofenac infusion significantly decreases brain-tissue oxygen tension in patients with poor-grade aneurysmal subarachnoid hemorrhage. Crit Care. 2013. doi:10.1186/cc12714.
90. Nathanson M, Moppett IK, Wiles M. Neuroanaesthesia. Oxford: Oxford University Press; 2011.
91. Udassi JP, Udassi S, Shih A, Lamb MA, Porvasnik SL, Zaritsky AL, et al. Novel adhesive glove device (AGD) for active compression-decompression (ACD) CPR results in improved carotid blood flow and coronary perfusion pressure in piglet model of cardiac arrest. Resuscitation. 2012;83:750–4.
92. Brain Trauma Foundation. Guidelines for the management of severe traumatic brain injury. J Neurotraum. 2007;24(Suppl 1):S3–6.
93. El Beheiry H. Protecting the brain during neurosurgical procedures: strategies that can work. Curr Opin Anaesthesio. 2012;25:548–55.
94. Veenith T, Menon DK. The cerebral circulation. In: Matta BF, Menon DK, Smith M, editors. Core topics in neuroanaesthesia and neurointensive care. Cambridge: Cambridge University Press; 2011. p. 17–21.
95. Ford MD, Alperin N, Lee SH, Holdsworth DW, Steinman DA. Characterization of volumetric flow rate waveforms in the normal internal carotid and vertebral arteries. Physiol Meas. 2005;26:477–88.
96. Artru AA, Shapira Y, Bowdle TA. Electroencephalogram, cerebral metabolic, and vascular responses to propofol anesthesia in dogs. J Neurosurg. Anesth. 1992;4:99–109.
97. Hoffman WE, Cunningham F, James MK, Baughman VL, Albrecht RF. Effects of remifentanil, a new short-acting opiod, on cerebral blood flow, brain electric activity, and intracranial pressure in dogs anesthetized with isoflurane and nitrous oxide. Anesthesiology. 1993;79:107–13.
98. Ramani R, Todd MM, Warner DS. A dose response study of the influence of propofol on cerebral blood flow, metabolism and the electroencephalogram in the rabbit. J Neurosurg Anesth. 1992;4:110–9.
99. Werner C, Hoffman WE, Kochs E. Schulte am Esch J, Albrecht RF. The effects of propofol on cerebral spinal cord blood flow in rats. Anesth Analg. 1993;76:971–5.
100. Yannopoulos D, Aufderheide TP, McKnite S, Kotsifas K, Charris R, Nadkarni V, et al. Hemodynamic and respiratory effects of negative tracheal pressure during CPR in pigs. Resuscitation. 2006;69:487–94.
101. Yannopoulos D, Metzger A, McKnite S, Nadkarni V, Aufderheide TP, Idris A, et al. Intrathoracic pressure regulation improves vital organ perfusion pressures in normovolemic and hypovolemic pigs. Resuscitation. 2006;70:445–53.
102. Moher D, Liberati A, Tetzlaff J, Altman DG. The PRISMA Group. Preferred Reporting Items for Systematic Reviews and Meta-Analyses: the PRISMA Statement. PLoS Med. 2009. doi:10.1371/journal.pmed1000097.

# A comparison of unheated loose housing with stables on the respiratory health of weaned-foals in cold winter conditions

Reija Junkkari[1*], Heli Simojoki[2], Minna-Liisa Heiskanen[3], Sinikka Pelkonen[4], Satu Sankari[1], Riitta-Mari Tulamo[1] and Anna Mykkänen[1]

**Abstract**

**Background:** Newly weaned horses in Finland are often moved to unheated loose housing systems in which the weanlings have free access to a paddock and a shelter. This practice is considered to be good for the development of young horses. The daily temperatures can stay below − 20 °C in Finland for several consecutive weeks during the winter season. However, the effect of unheated housing in a cold climatic environment on the respiratory health of weanlings under field conditions has not been studied before. This investigation was an observational field-study comprising 60 weanlings among 11 different voluntary participant rearing farms in Finland. Weanlings were either kept in unheated loose housing systems (n = 36) or in stables (n = 24) and were clinically examined on two separate occasions 58 days apart in cold winter conditions.

**Results:** The odds of clinical respiratory disease were lower in the older foals ($\log_e$ days); OR = 0.009, P = 0.044). The plasma fibrinogen concentration was higher when the available space ($m^2$/weanling) in the sleeping hall was smaller (P = 0.014) and it was lower when the sleeping hall was not insulated (P = 0.010). The plasma fibrinogen concentrations at the second examination were lower with a body condition score above 3 (P = 0.070). Standardbreds kept in loose housing systems had a lower body condition score than Finnhorses or Standardbreds kept in stables at both examinations (P = 0.026 and P = 0.007, respectively). Haemoglobin level was lower in weanlings in loose housing systems compared to their counterparts at the first examination (P = 0.037). Finnhorses had higher white blood cell count than Standardbreds at first (P = 0.002) and at the second examination (P = 0.001).

**Conclusions:** Keeping weanling horses in cold loose housing systems does not seem to increase the occurrence of respiratory disease, but special attention should be focused on ventilation, air quality and feeding-practices. Our field study data suggest it might be advantageous to keep Standardbred foals born late in the season in a stable over the Finnish winter.

**Keywords:** Cold-winter loose-housing, Respiratory disease, Stables, Weaned-foals

## Background

In a loose housing system, horses are kept in groups and where they can freely move between the paddock and the shelter. The loose housing practice is considered to be good for the development of young horses and foals because of the social contacts between individuals, fresh air and free movement [1–3]. The daily temperatures in winter in Finland and some other Nordic countries, fluctuate from − 14 to 0 °C and in certain areas of Finland they can fall below − 20 °C for several consecutive weeks [4]. After weaning at 5–6 months of age, the foals are moved to loose housing. This is done from October

*Correspondence: reija.junkkari@helsinki.fi
[1] Department of Equine and Small Animal Medicine, University of Helsinki, Helsinki 00014, Finland

to December. We estimate that the proportion of foals kept in loose housing systems in Finland is around 30%. The cold housing environment increases the energy consumption of weanlings in early winter but not in late winter and weanlings gain weight at the expected rates when the energy consumed meets the increased demand caused by cold ambient temperature [5, 6].

Weaning [7, 8], transport [9, 10] and the inclusion into a new herd [11] causes substantial stress for foals. Stress, in turn, causes immunosuppression in young horses and increases the risk of respiratory disease [12]. Weanlings from several different farms are moved to central loose housing systems, and it is therefore highly likely that the whole group of weanlings in a centralised rearing facility will have encountered different pathogens earlier in life. Several viruses can cause respiratory infections in horses [13–18]. There is, however, increasing evidence that bacteria, especially *Streptococcus zooepidemicus*, can be a primary pathogen in respiratory tract infections in horses [19–21].

Certain laboratory tests can be useful in detecting equine respiratory disease or differentiating between non-infectious inflammation and viral or bacterial infection. A determination of blood white blood cell count (WBC) alone, may not be helpful in clinical cases because WBCs show quite substantial variation in healthy horses [22] and also between horses of different breeds [23]. On the other hand, low serum iron concentration is a good indicator for infection especially when combined with analysis for acute phase proteins such as serum amyloid A (SAA) and fibrinogen [24, 25]. The amount of SAA is negligible in a healthy horse but it increases rapidly in tissue trauma or in non-infectious or infectious inflammation cases and then it returns to baseline within 11–22 days [26, 27]. Plasma fibrinogen concentrations have a relatively wide normal range in the adult horse (2–4 g/L) [23]. The fibrinogen concentration increases over 24–72 h after the onset of inflammation and has a relatively long half-life of approximately 5 days [28]. Therefore, fibrinogen concentration is not as effective as SAA concentration is in detecting acute changes in disease progression but it does indicate a recent or ongoing infection. The plasma fibrinogen concentration of young horses seems to be higher than that of adult horses, and values can exceed 5 mg/L in healthy, 4–5-month-old horses [29, 30]. Both fibrinogen and SAA concentrations in foals with bacterial infections are higher than in foals with non-bacterial or uncertain diagnoses [31]. Reduced blood haemoglobin (Hb) concentration may indicate presence of a chronic infection [32]. Differentiating local infections from systemic infections in the horse is, however, challenging. This is also the case for respiratory diseases, which can be classified as occurring as a local event or as part of a systemic condition [33].

In addition to infectious agents, management and housing conditions influence the respiratory health of horses [34–36]. Pasture is considered to be a better environment than a stable [37–39]. The quality of air in a stable is affected by the bedding material, the feed and the ventilation [40–42]. The quality of the hay is the most important factor that affects the particulate concentration in air within the breathing zone of an adult horse, and placing hay on the floor is better than hanging the hay in a hay-net [40–43]. Horses need shelter during the winter months in northern latitudes. Horses in loose housing systems have access to a sleeping hall where the temperature is usually slightly higher than outside ambient temperatures. Little information is available on the effects of living in cold temperatures on respiratory disease in horses and in weanlings. Exercise in cold air can induce bronchoconstriction and inflammatory changes in the lower airways for 48 h after exercise [44, 45] and extended exposure to cold conditions has been reported to increase the risk of mucus accumulation in the trachea of adult horses [36]. However, there is no evidence that cold ambient temperature is associated with clinical respiratory disease in adult horses. Moreover, as far as the authors are aware the effect of cold housing environment on the respiratory health of weanlings has not been studied before.

The first aim of this study was to compare two management systems of cold loose housing and conventional stabling, in terms of the incidence of respiratory disease of weanling horses. We hypothesized that the incidence of respiratory disease would not differ between the management systems. The secondary aim was to determine whether certain environmental factors in loose housing systems or the breed of the horse affect the risk of clinical respiratory disease and any changes in inflammatory markers.

## Methods

This study was an observational field study of weanling horses in two different types of housing units that consists of two examinations taken 58 days apart.

### Horses, housing and management

A total of 60 newly weaned horses that were housed on 11 separate farms were examined (Table 1). The farms were selected by the owners' willingness to participate and all weanling horses in these farms were included in the study. The weanlings were 139–232 days old (mean 187; SD 21) at the time of the first examination. Five of the farms had loose housing systems and six had conventional stables. The conditions in the loose housing farms (A–E) are presented in Table 2. Weanlings of the loose housing farms were kept in a group and were able to move freely

**Table 1 The breed, age and sex of the weanlings kept in different housing systems**

| Breed | n | Age/days | Loose housing | Stable | Colt | Filly |
|---|---|---|---|---|---|---|
| Standardbred | 42 | 190 (148–232) | 26 | 16 | 22 | 20 |
| Finnhorse | 18 | 179 (151–213) | 10 | 8 | 9 | 9 |

The number, sex and mean (range) age at the first examination of the weanlings kept in loose housing systems and stables

**Table 2 The conditions in loose housing systems**

| | A | B | C1 | C2 | D | E |
|---|---|---|---|---|---|---|
| Bedding | P | S | P + S | P + S | S | S |
| Insulation | x | x | | | x | x |
| Number of foals | 3 | 10 | 10 | 4 | 4 | 5 |
| Sleeping area/foal in $m^2$ | 15 | 3 | 5 | 3 | 10 | 19 |

The structure and conditions in the five loose housing farms (A–E). On farm C there were two separate sleeping halls, C1 and C2

*P* peat, *S* straw, *P* + *S* straw on top of a peat base

to and from the shelter. The loose housing farms A and C had an entrance shelter, wind box and plastic sheets, farm B had an entrance shelter, farm D had plastic sheets suspended that covered the entrance and farm E had an entrance shelter and plastic sheets. An entrance shelter is a two-sided roofed shelter in front of the sleeping hall opening. A wind box is an entrance shelter that has plastic sheets over the outer door opening. Plastic sheets were 30–50 cm-wide strips that hung in the door opening to block the wind but allowed the weanlings to walk through. There were no adult horses in the same shelters or paddocks with the weanlings in the loose housing farms. There were only Finnhorses in the loose housing farm E. Other farms had both Standardbreds and Finnhorses. In the stables, weanlings were kept in individual stalls inside a barn and the stall doors opened to the barn aisle and adult horses were housed in the same corridor with the weanlings. Humidity and air particulate content were not measured. The weanlings spent the nights in the stables and were turned out into a paddock in a group during the daytime. All weanlings were fed haylage ad libitum outdoors and concentrate in the stable or the sleeping hall. The weanlings where tethered beside the feeding buckets during feeding. The haylage was analysed (Seilab Oy, Seinäjoki, Finland) and the quality was fairly similar among the farms. The farms were located in Eastern Finland, and the daily temperatures in the area ranged from − 17.7 to + 2.2 °C (mean − 3.5 °C) in December 2014 and − 21.3 to − 2.1 °C (mean − 7.1 °C) in January 2015 (Finnish Meteorological Institute).

### Clinical examination

The horses were examined on the farms at the beginning of the study in November–December 2014 and again 58 days later, in January 2015. Foals had been kept on the study farms for 2–50 (median 23; SD 16) days before the first visit. Special attention was paid to any signs of respiratory disease. The horses were considered to have a clinical respiratory disease based on the following criteria: temperature $\geq$ 38.3 °C and one or more of the following signs: cough, nasal/ocular discharge or increased respiratory sounds [14, 18]. The body condition (1: thin, 2: fair, 3: good, 4: fat, 5: very fat) was scored according to Carroll and Huntington [46].

### Blood analyses

Blood was drawn from the jugular vein into ethylenediaminetetraacetic acid (EDTA)-anticoagulated tubes for centrifugation and subsequent plasma analysis and also into plain tubes for coagulation and subsequent serum analysis during both farm visits. Samples were stored at room temperature for 6–8 h and then at + 4 °C until the samples were analysed within 48 h. Blood samples were taken from 60/60 weanlings during the first visit. Blood samples were obtained from 59/60 weanlings during the second visit, because one of the weanlings strongly resisted the sampling. Complete blood cell counts were analysed using an ADVIA 2120i Hematology System with multispecies software (Siemens Healthcare Diagnostics, Tarrytown, NY, USA) and using the cyanmethaemoglobin method for haemoglobin determination. Plasma fibrinogen was measured with the heat precipitation method [35]. An immunoturbidometric assay (Eiken SAA LZ, Eiken Chemical, Tokio, Japan) was carried out for serum amyloid A (SAA) and a colorimetric method for serum iron (Fe). The serum analyses were performed with an automatic clinical chemistry analyser (Konelab 30i, Thermo Fisher Scientific, Vantaa, Finland).

### Statistical analyses

After validation checks for data inconsistencies and missing entries, statistical analyses were carried out using Stata Intercooler version 11.0 (Stata Corporation, College Station, Texas, USA). Factors that affected clinical respiratory disease (0/1) at the first examination were analysed with a logistic mixed model. At the second examination, the proportion of clinically affected horses (6/60) was too low for statistical analysis. Factors that affected WBC, Hb, plasma fibrinogen and serum iron (Fe) at the first and second examinations were analysed by a linear mixed model. The plasma fibrinogen concentration was transformed using the natural logarithm in order to meet the assumption of a normal distribution.

Predictors in all models were the recumbency area available per weanling, body condition score ($\leq$ 2.5, 3, $\geq$ 3.5), conditions of the stable (1–3), bedding (1–4), breed (Standardbred/Finnhorse), sex (colt/filly), type of stable (loose housing system/stall) and age of the foal (continuous predictor). Age was transformed to a natural logarithm to achieve a normal distribution. The recumbency area available per weanling was categorized into a dichotomous variable: below 8 $m^2$ and over 8 $m^2$. The conditions of the housing were categorized 1–3 as follows: 1: weanlings in a stable, 2: loose house stalls with insulation and 3: loose house stalls without insulation. The bedding types were 1: peat, 2: straw, 3: a mixture of straw and peat, 4: pelleted materials. The breed and sex of the foal were treated as confounders, so they were forced in all models. The age of the foal when it was moved to a loose housing system was available only for 36 foals, so this predictor could not be used in the models. Associations between all predictors in first and second examination and the outcomes were computed using simple logistic regression (clinical respiratory disease) or univariable regression analysis (fibrinogen, Hb, WBC, Fe). The predictors with association $P \leq 0.2$ were included in the final models.

The full and final logistic model of clinical respiratory disease included age, conditions of the stable, bedding, sex and breed. The model fit was assessed using the assumptions of normality and homogeneity of variances, which were evaluated by checking the residuals. The final linear mixed model of fibrinogen at the first examination also included age, conditions of the stable, sex and breed. The final linear mixed model of fibrinogen at the second examination included the body condition score, conditions of the stable, sex and breed. Additionally, there was an interaction between the lying area and conditions of the stable, therefore the interaction term and lying area were also included in these models. The final linear mixed model of Hb at the first examination included type of stable, recumbency area available per horse, body condition score, sex and breed. The final linear mixed model of Hb at the second examination included age, sex and breed. The final linear mixed model of WBC at the first examination included age and breed. The final linear mixed model of WBC at the second examination included the breed. The final linear mixed model of Fe at the first examination included bedding, conditions of the stable, sex and breed. The final linear mixed model of Fe at the second examination included conditions of the stable, sex and breed. The farm was used as a random effect in all the models. Assumptions of the model were controlled using normality and scatter plots of the model residuals.

The association of the clinical respiratory disease with fibrinogen at the first examination was analysed by the Student's t test. Test $P \leq 0.05$ were considered to be statistically significant.

## Results

### Clinical respiratory disease

Assessment of the incidence of clinical respiratory disease was the principal objective. Clinical respiratory disease at the first examination was diagnosed in 28% (17/60) of the weanlings and 11 of these had a purulent nasal discharge. As much as 39% (14/36) of the loose housed weanlings compared 13% (3/24) stabled weanlings had a clinical respiratory disease at the first examination. The percentages at the second examination were 10% (6/60) for the whole study population, 11% (4/36) for loose housed weanlings and 8% (2/24) stabled. Three weanlings had purulent nasal discharge at the second examination. One weanling of the six with clinical respiratory disease had acute disease at the second examination and the other five had already manifested respiratory signs at the first examination. The greater age ($\log_e$ days) of the weanling decreased the odds ratio (OR) for having clinical respiratory disease (OR = 0.009, P = 0.044) at the first examination. As an interpretation, 2 weeks increase of age cause lower OR for clinical respiratory disease (OR = 0.56). The conditions in loose housing systems did not influence the occurrence of clinical disease. There was no statistical difference between the horses kept in stables or in loose housing systems. The breed or sex of the horse did not influence the occurrence of clinical disease.

### Plasma fibrinogen and haematology (secondary results)

The plasma fibrinogen concentrations are presented in Tables 3 and 4. The fibrinogen concentration at the first examination was higher in younger horses (coeff = – 0.41, P = 0.033, Fig. 1) and in loose housing stalls where the lying area available per weanling was less than 8 $m^2$ (coeff = 0.17, P = 0.014). Plasma fibrinogen concentrations were lower if the sleeping hall was

**Table 3 The mean haematological values of Standardbred weanlings**

| | 1st visit stable | 1st visit Lh | 2nd visit stable | 2nd visit Lh |
|---|---|---|---|---|
| Serum SAA (mg/L) | 0.9 [± 0.5] | 1.2 [± 1.6] | 0.7 [± 0.4] | 4.8 [± 17.8] |
| Plasma fibrinogen (g/L) | 5.0 [± 0.6] | 5.4 [± 1.1] | 4.6 [± 0.6] | 5.1 [± 0.7] |
| WBC ($10^9$/L)[a] | 12.0 [± 2.4] | 12.2 [± 2.3] | 10.4 [± 1.8] | 11.7 [± 2.6] |
| Fe (µmol/L) | 24 [± 9.4] | 29 [± 7.9] | 23 [± 4.7] | 27 [± 7.0] |
| Hb (g/L) | 141 [± 11.4] | 145 [± 11.5] | 134 [± 8.9] | 130 [0 ± 10.8] |

The mean haematological values [± SD] of Standardbred weanlings kept in loose housing (Lh), n = 26, and in stables, n = 16

*SAA* serum amyloid A, *WBC* white blood cell count, *Hb* haemoglobin

[a] Signifies being statistically different from the Finnhorse

**Table 4 The mean haematological values of Finnhorse weanlings**

| | 1st visit stable | 1st visit Lh | 2nd visit stable | 2nd visit Lh |
|---|---|---|---|---|
| Serum SAA (mg/L) | 0.4 [± 0.5] | 12 [± 24.2] | 1.3 [± 2.9] | 0.8 [± 0.5] |
| Plasma fibrinogen (g/L) | 4.8 [± 0.9] | 5.0 [± 0.9] | 4.2 [± 0.9] | 4.2 [± 1.0] |
| WBC ($10^9$/L)[a] | 14.8 [± 3.9] | 14.2 [± 2.0] | 14.3 [± 4.0] | 15.1 [± 2.8] |
| Fe (µmol/L) | 23 [± 6.8] | 24 [± 9.7] | 24 [± 7.7] | 21 [± 7.5] |
| Hb (g/L) | 132 [± 16.7] | 123 [± 10.8] | 120 [± 9.5] | 117 [± 5.1] |

The mean haematological values [± SD] in serum and plasma of Finnhorse weanlings kept in loose housing (Lh), n = 9, and in stables, n = 8

*SAA* serum amyloid A, *WBC* white blood cell count, *Hb* haemoglobin

[a] Signifies being statistically different from the Standardbred

not insulated (coeff = − 0.22, P = 0.01) compared to fibrinogen concentrations of stabled weanlings. The weanlings with clinical respiratory disease had a higher plasma fibrinogen concentration at the first examination (P < 0.001). The fibrinogen concentration at the second examination was higher in weanlings that had a body condition score under 3 compared to weanlings that had a body condition score of 3 (coeff = − 0.60, P = 0.022) or above 3 (coeff = − 0.75, P = 0.015) (Fig. 2). Neither the sex nor the breed of the foal had an effect on the fibrinogen concentration at either examination.

At both examination times, Finnhorse weanlings had a higher WBC count than Standardbreds; coeff = 2.22, P = 0.002 and coeff = 3.61, P < 0.001, respectively. By contrast, Hb was lower in Finnhorse than in Standarsbreds at the first (coeff = − 12.60, P < 0.001) and second (coeff = − 12.66, P < 0.001) examination. The horses kept in loose housing systems had lower Hb at the first examination (coeff = 8.41, P = 0.037) but not at the second examination.

Fe did not differ between the two breeds (Tables 3, 4). There was no association between a high WBC count and clinical respiratory disease. There was no statistically significant difference in Fe or SAA values between healthy and clinically affected horses. There was no difference in Fe values between loose housing system and stable but the values at the first examination were lower in those farms where mixture of peat and straw was used as bedding material (coeff = 9.26, P = 0.001) compared to peat bedding. Serum SAA exceeded the laboratory reference value in two horses at the first examination and one at the second examination.

### Body condition score

The body condition scores at both examinations are presented in Table 5. The Standardbred weanlings housed in a stable had a higher body condition score than those kept in loose housing systems at both examinations (P = 0.026 and P = 0.007, respectively). Mean (± SD) body condition score in Standardbreds in loose housing systems at the first examination was 2.7 (± 0.5) and 3.1 (± 0.4) for the stable weanlings. The mean scores at the second examination were 2.8 (± 0.3) and 3.2 (± 0.2), respectively. The mean body condition score in the Finnhorse weanlings in loose housing systems at the first examination was 3.7 (± 0.5) and 3.3 (± 0.7) those housed in the stables. The mean scores at the second examination were 3.6 (± 0.5) and 3.3 (± 0.4), respectively.

## Discussion

To our knowledge, this is the first study on respiratory disease in weanlings living in a cold climate. We found that, a young age of the weanling was the most important factor associated with the occurrence of clinical respiratory disease. There was no difference in the occurrence of clinical respiratory disease in weanlings housed in stables compared to loose housing systems. Heleski et al. [2] reported that regardless of the method of weaning, the blood cortisol levels of foals peak at 4 weeks post-weaning. The time from weaning to the first examination was not recorded in this present study. Therefore, it cannot be concluded whether this stress peak affected the risk of clinical disease. No differences were detected in relation to the breed or sex of the weanling in terms of clinical disease.

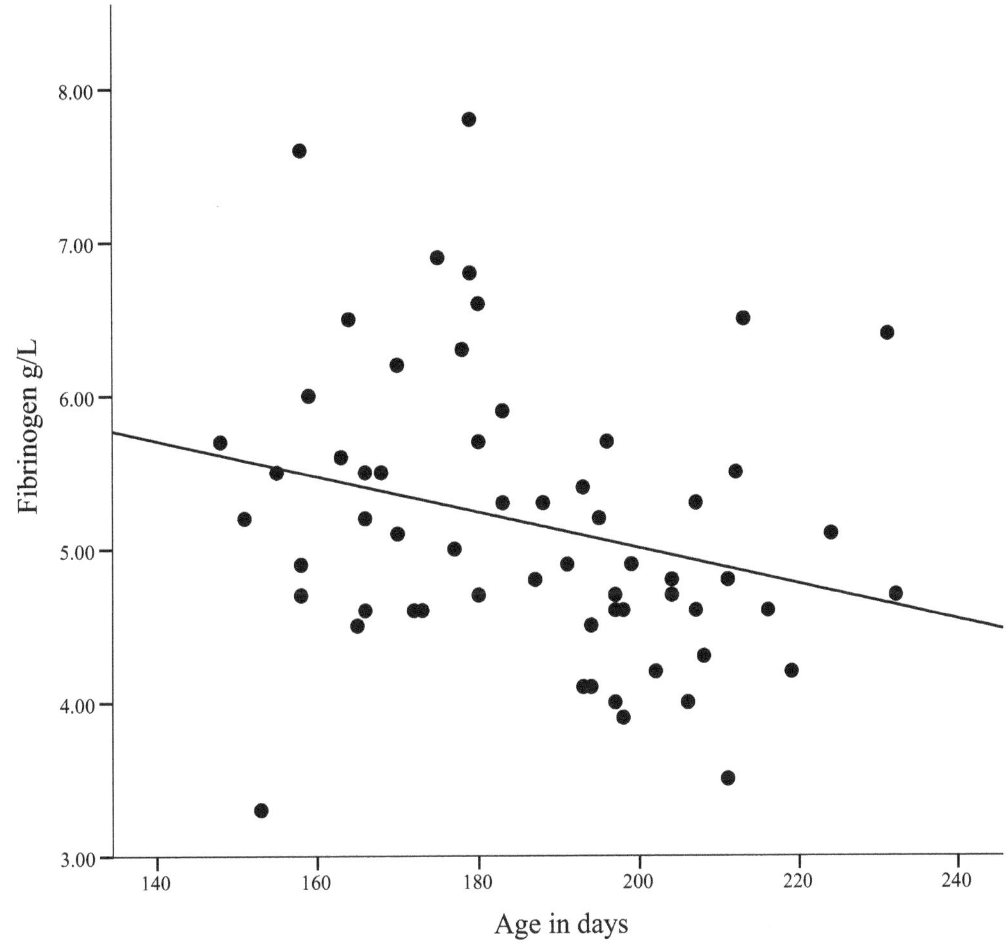


**Fig. 1** The plasma fibrinogen concentration (g/L) and age in days at the first examination of weanling horses, n = 60

High particulate and endotoxin concentrations in the breathing zone of a horse are known to induce inflammatory changes in the airways [43, 47]. Bedding [40, 48, 49], ventilation [50] and the quality and feeding method of the hay [40, 43] affect the air quality in animal shelters. In the loose housing farms the haylage was provided outside and in the stable farms also inside in the night time. The quality of the bedding was hence emphasized in the loose housing farms compared to stables when it comes to air particulate content inside the shelter because it was only potentially dusty material in sleeping halls. The humidity or air particulate concentration were not measured but air quality was estimated to be good in all stables and sleeping halls. We found that the bedding material or other differences in conditions did not affect the risk of clinical disease in cold loose housing. However, serum iron was found to be significantly lower when the bedding used in the sleeping hall was a mixture of peat and straw. This bedding combination was used in only one of the loose housing farms so it is possible that low iron concentration was associated with other factors on this farm and not the type of the bedding used.

The WBC count was higher and Hb values were lower in Finnhorses compared with Standardbreds at both examinations. This was an unexpected finding because the WBC reference values are lower for adult cold-blooded horses [23]. During the blood sampling, there was no difference in behaviour between the breeds that could explain the result. Blood haemoglobin concentration was lower in horses in loose housing systems at the first examination. Low haemoglobin concentration can be a sign of chronic infection or inadequate nutrition. The mean body condition score of the Standardbred weanlings kept in loose housing systems was significantly lower than those kept in a stable and Finnhorses in either management system (Table 2). There were both Standardbred and Finnhorse weanlings together in all but one loose housing farm that had only Finnhorses and the quality of the haylage did not differ among the farms. The weanlings on the loose housing farms were

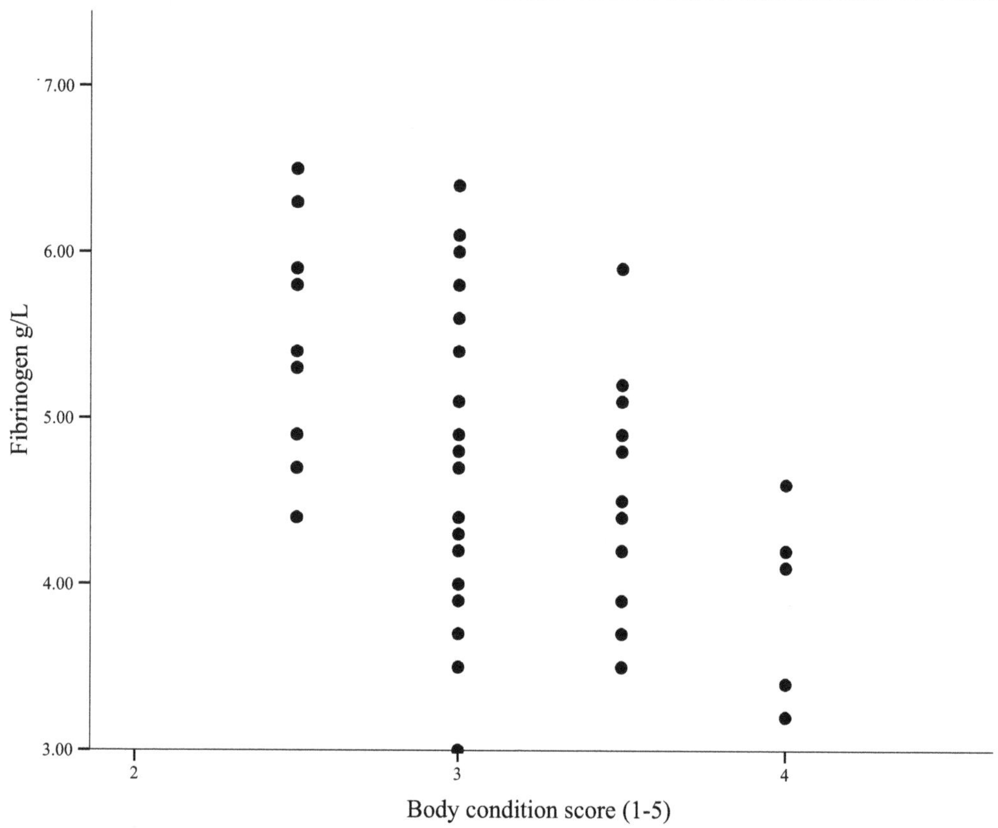


**Fig. 2** The plasma fibrinogen concentration (g/L) and body condition score at the second examination of weanling horses, n = 59

**Table 5 Body condition scores**

| | ≤ 2.5 | 3 | ≥ 3.5 |
|---|---|---|---|
| Standardbred Lh (n = 26) | 14[a]/10[a] | 10/14 | 2/2 |
| Standardbred stable (n = 16) | 2[a]/0[a] | 11/11 | 3/5 |
| Finnhorse Lh (n = 10) | 0/1 | 2/0 | 8/9 |
| Finnhorse stable (n = 8) | 2/0 | 2/4 | 4/4 |

The number of horses categorized by the body condition score (1: thin, 2: fair, 3: good, 4: fat, 5: very fat)

*Lh* loose housing, *n* number of horses in each group, *x/y* number of horses in each category at the first/second examination

[a] Signifies being statistically different between stable and loose housing systems

tied to the wall beside the feeding bucket when eating the concentrate feed. Standardbred weanlings hence had equal opportunities as the Finnhorse weanlings to access the concentrate feed and the haylage. Jørgensen et al. [51] reported that the adult Warmblood horses chose heated shelter more often than the Coldblood horses when weather was rainy and windy [51]. Since haylage was only available outside the shelter, it is possible that the Standardbred weanlings might have spent more time in the shelter and therefore ate less than their Finnhorse counterparts. This was not however the case in a study by Autio et al. [6], who showed that there was no difference between Standardbred and Finnhorse weanlings in respect of the time spent in the shelter/paddock. Although the energy consumed was not recorded in this study, it is also plausible that Standardbred weanlings might require more energy in cold temperatures than Finnhorses and feeding should be planned according to the breed.

Plasma fibrinogen concentrations were higher in cramped sleeping halls and when the sleeping hall was insulated. The air quality was not recorded in this study. In an earlier study made in the previous year (Airaksinen et al., not published), air humidity in these same, insulated sleeping halls was recorded to be higher than outside and in one sleeping hall ammonia was also detected. In that same study, the quality of the straw used in the loose housing farms varied and there were also mouldy straw bales among the ones used. During our visits, the air quality was good but the ambient temperature, quality of bedding material and the handling of the bedding in the shelter can vary on a daily basis and there might have been some prevailing air quality problems that were not detectable during the short time of our two visits. It is possible that the weanlings ranking lower in the hierarchy were unable to utilize fully the more cramped sleeping halls, as is also the situation among adult horses when the recumbency area is too small in relation to the group size [52]. Haylage was provided ad libitum from round bales on every loose housing farm involved in this study. Weanlings on the stable farms were fed haylage on the ground. Eating hay from round bales has been associated with an increased number of neutrophils in the airways of fully grown adult horses [36]. Environmental factors could also partly explain why inflammatory markers did not correlate with the clinical symptoms at the second examination. A study on calves showed that a poor group housing environment might enhance the risk of respiratory disease without changes in the blood leukocyte response [53].

The plasma fibrinogen concentration had a negative correlation with age. This finding is in accordance with the study by Harvey et al. [29] and Santos et al. [30], both of which reported the plasma fibrinogen concentration to be highest at the age of 3–5 months after which it decreases gradually until the age of 6–12 months. The mean age of the weanlings in the present study was 6.2 months at the time of the first examination. The plasma fibrinogen concentration in healthy Thoroughbreds in the same age group as used in this study was reported to be less than 4.5 g/L [29, 30]. At the first examination, the mean fibrinogen concentration in this study in clinically healthy horses (4.9 g/L) was higher than in previous reports but the range was wide (3.5–7.8 g/L). The fibrinogen concentration was associated with clinical disease at the first ($P = 0.004$) but not at the second examination. It seems that the younger weanlings especially, caught respiratory infections when moved to new herd but they recovered during the study period. The weanlings that had a high fibrinogen concentration at the first examination were however likely to have a higher fibrinogen concentration and a low body condition score at the end of the study period.

The definition of clinical disease was determined in the present study by combining the definitions from two previous studies on equine respiratory health [14, 18]. Due to the long distances to the farms, the weanlings could only be examined twice and plasma fibrinogen was chosen as a marker of infection because of its long half-life [54]. The plasma fibrinogen concentration is a significant but unspecific predictor of inflammatory disease and is often combined with serum iron and SAA concentration in clinical practice [24, 25, 33]. In this study neither the serum SAA nor hypoferremia was associated with clinical respiratory disease. This was unexpected because serum SAA and iron have been shown to be more sensitive and rapid inflammatory markers than the WBC count or plasma fibrinogen concentration [25, 26, 31, 33, 55]. The sample storage and analysis method used in the present study should not have influenced the serum SAA concentration [52, 53]. It is possible that there was no specific infectious agent that caused the respiratory symptoms. One weakness of our study is that mild clinical symptoms might not have been noticed if they had appeared occasionally. Respiratory disease can also be local and hence not induce the systemic signs of inflammation in the blood. The time the weanlings had spent in a new herd and housing facility before the first examination was not constant in this field study, which could have affected the results. However, the time the weanling had spent on the farm was indeed evaluated but had missing values and therefore was not included. The number of horses in the study was quite small ($n = 60$). For these reasons, the power of the study is low, which might have impacted on the results and thus some important factors could be underestimated. The region of Eastern Finland was chosen because of its low winter temperatures, which was an essential predisposing factor in this study, but this choice also limited the geographical area, which in turn limited the actual number of foal rearing farms that could be contacted. Moreover, only a proportion of the foal rearing farms in this limited geographical area volunteered to be participants. Nevertheless, this study was conducted under field conditions, which are the same as those encountered by veterinary practitioners in this region. A full evaluation of the influence of certain environmental factors requires a study design with a larger population of horses in more precisely defined conditions is required.

It would also be worthwhile to make a nationwide survey for weanling owners to evaluate the occurrence of respiratory disease in different management systems because veterinarians only detect cases that require medical attention.

## Conclusions

The occurrence of respiratory disease and fibrinogen concentrations were higher as the weanlings were younger in this study. Contrary to our expectations, fibrinogen concentrations were higher in animals living in the loose housing systems that had an insulated sleeping hall compared to those that live in systems with noninsulated sleeping hall or in the stable. Standardbred weanlings kept in loose housing had lower body condition scores than Finnhorses or those kept in a stable. Standardbreds in loose housing systems also had lower blood haemoglobin concentration at the first examination. According to our results Standardbred weanlings seem to have a higher energy demand in a cold environment compared to that of their Finnhorse counterparts. Keeping weanlings in cold loose housing systems does not seem to increase the occurrence of respiratory disease, but special attention should be focused on ventilation, air quality and feeding practices. Our data suggest it might be advantageous to keep Standardbred foals born late in the season in a stable over the winter. Further studies with more weanlings and farms are warranted to define the optimal loose housing conditions for weanlings under cold climate conditions.

#### Abbreviations

EDTA: ethylenediaminetetraacetic acid; Fe: iron; Hb: haemoglobin; Lh: loose housing; P: peat; P + S: a mixture of peat and straw; S: straw; SAA: serum amyloid A; WBC: white blood cell count.

#### Authors' contributions

RJ and AM performed the clinical examinations and blood sampling, SP and SS performed the bacterial culture and laboratory analysis, HS performed the statistical analyses, MLH and RT were involved writing the manuscript. All authors read and approved the final manuscript.

#### Author details

[1] Department of Equine and Small Animal Medicine, University of Helsinki, Helsinki 00014, Finland. [2] Department of Production Animal Medicine, University of Helsinki, Helsinki 00014, Finland. [3] Equine Information Centre, Neulaniementie 5, Kuopio 70210, Finland. [4] Research and Laboratory Department, Veterinary Bacteriology Research Unit, Finnish Food Safety Authority Evira, Neulaniementie 4, Kuopio 70701, Finland.

#### Acknowledgements

The authors thank the horse breeders and stable personnel for providing the opportunity to visit the farms and for their considerable help in handling the weanlings.

#### Competing interests

The authors declare that they have no competing interests.

#### Funding

This study was funded by the European Agricultural Fund for Rural Development: Europe investing in rural areas, the Finnish Veterinary Foundation, the Finnish Foundation of Veterinary Research, the Erkki Rajakoski Foundation and the Veterinary Society of Häme-Satakunta.

#### References

1. Zeep K, Schintzer U. Housing and training of horses according to their species-specific behavior. Livest Prod Sci. 1997;49:181–9.
2. Heleski CR, Shelle AC, Nielsen BD, Zanella AJ. Influence of housing on weanling horse behavior and subsequent welfare. Appl Anim Behav Sci. 2002;78:291–302.
3. Søndergaard E, Ladewig J. Group housing exerts a positive effect on the behaviour of young horses during training. Appl Anim Behav Sci. 2004;87:105–18.
4. Finnish Meteorologigal institute, Swedish Meteorologigal and hydrologigal institute.
5. Cymbaluk NF, Christison GI. Effects of diet and climate on growing horses. J Anim Sci. 1998;67:48–59.
6. Autio E, Heiskanen ML. Foal behaviour in loose housing/paddock environment during winter. Appl Anim Behav Sci. 2005;91:277–88.
7. Erber R, Wulf M, Rose-Meierhoefer S, Becker-Birck M, Moestl E, Aurich J, et al. Behavioral and physiological responses of young horses to different weaning protocols: a pilot study. Stress. 2012;15:184–94.
8. Henry S, Zanella AJ, Sankey C, Richard-Yris MA, Marko A, Hausberger M. Adults may be used to alleviate weaning stress in domestic foals (*Equus caballus*). Physiol Behav. 2012;106:428–38.
9. Smith BL, Jones JH, Hornof WJ, Miles JA, Longworth KE, Willits NH. Effects of road transport on indices of stress in horses. Equine Vet J. 1996;28:446–54.
10. Schmidt A, Hödl S, Möstl E, Aurich J, Müller J, Aurich C. Cortisol release, heart rate, and heart rate variability in transport-naive horses during repeated road transport. Domest Anim Endocrinol. 2010;39:205–13.
11. Alexander SL, Irvine CH. The effect of social stress on adrenal axis activity in horses: the importance of monitoring corticosteroid-binding globulin capacity. J Endocrinol. 1998;157:425–32.
12. Seung-Ho R, Koo HC, Park YK, Jung KW, Davis WC, Park YH, et al. Etiologic and immunologic characteristics of thoroughbred horses with bacterial infectious upper respiratory disease at the Seoul race park. J Microbiol Biotechnol. 2009;19:1041–50.
13. Dunowska M, Wilks CR, Studdert MJ, Meers J. Equine respiratory viruses in foals in New Zealand. N Z Vet J. 2002;50:140–7.
14. Newton JR, Wood JLN, Chanter N. A case control study of factors and infections associated with clinically apparent respiratory disease in UK Thoroughbred racehorses. Prev Vet Med. 2003;60:107–32.
15. Vairo S, Vandekerckhove A, Steukers L, Glorieux S, Van den Broeck W, Nauwynck H. Clinical and virological outcome of an infection with the Belgian equine arteritis virus strain 08P178. Vet Microbiol. 2012;157:333–44.
16. Horsington J, Hartley CA, Gilkerson JR. Seroprevalence study of Equine rhinitis B virus (ERBV) in Australian weanling horses using serotype-specific ERBV enzyme-linked immunosorbent assays. J Vet Diagn Invest. 2015;25:641–4.
17. Diaz-Mendez A, Viel L, Hewson J, Doig P, Carman S, Chambers T, Tiwari A, Dewey C. Surveillance of equine respiratory viruses in Ontario. Can J Vet Res. 2010;74:271–8.
18. Back H, Ullman K, Berntson TL, Riihimäki M, Penell J, Ståhl K, et al. Viral load of equine herpesviruses 2 and 5 in nasal swabs of actively racing standardbred trotters: temporal relationship of shedding to clinical findings and poor performance. Vet Microbiol. 2015;179:142–8.
19. Erol E, Locke SJ, Donahoe JK, Mackin MA, Carter CN. Beta-hemolytic *Streptococcus* spp. from horses: a retrospective study (2000–2010). J Vet Diagn Invest. 2012;24:142–7.
20. Lindahl SB, Aspán A, Båverud V, Paillot R, Pringle J, Rash NL, et al. Outbreak of upper respiratory disease in horses caused by *Streptococcus equi* subsp. *zooepidemicus* ST-24. Vet Microbiol. 2013;166:281–5.
21. Velineni S, Desoutter D, Perchec AM, Timoney JF. Characterization of a mucoid clone of *Streptococcus zooepidemicus* from an epizootic of equine respiratory disease in New Caledonia. Vet J. 2014;200:82–7.
22. Anhold H, Candon R, Chan DS, Amos W. A comparison of elevated blood parameter values in a population of thoroughbred racehorses. J Equine Vet Sci. 2014;34:651–5.
23. Jain CN. The horse: normal hematology with comments on response to disease. In: Schalm's veterinary hematology 4th edition. Philadelphia: Lea & Febiger; 1986. p. 154–5.
24. Borges AS, Divers TJ, Stokol T, Mohammed OH. Serum iron and plasma fibrinogen concentrations as indicators of systemic inflammatory diseases in horses. J Vet Intern Med. 2007;21:489–94.
25. Corradini I, Armengou L, Viu J, Rodríguez-Pozo ML, Cesarini C, Jose-Cunilleras E. Parallel testing of plasma iron and fibrinogen concentrations to detect systemic inflammation in hospitalized horses. J Vet Emerg Crit Care. 2014;24:414–20.
26. Hultén C, Sandgren B, Skiöldebrand E, Klingeborn B, Marhaug G, Forsberg M. The acute phase protein serum amyloid A (SAA) as an inflammatory marker in equine influenza virus infection. Acta Vet Scand. 1999;40:323–33.
27. Belgrave RL, Dickey MM, Arheart KL, Cray C. Assessment of serum amyloid A testing of horses and its clinical application in a specialized equine practice. J Am Vet Med Assoc. 2013;243:113–9.
28. Coyne CP, Hornof WJ, Kelly AB, O'Brien TR, DeNardo SJ. Rapid extraction, radioiodination, and in vivo catabolism of 125I-labeled fibrinogen in the horse. Am J Vet Res. 1985;46:2578–81.
29. Harvey JW, Asquith RL, McNulty PK, Kivipelto J, Bauer JE. Haematology of foals up to one year old. Equine Vet J. 1984;16:347–53.
30. Santos FCC, Feijó LS, Kasinger S, Junior FF, Curcio BR, Nogueira CEW. Hematologic values of Thoroughbred foals from birth to six months of age. Ciencia Anim Bras. 2014;15:307–12.
31. Hultén C, Demmers S. Serum amyloid A (SAA) as an aid in the management of infectious disease in the foal: comparison with total leucocyte count, neutrophil count and fibrinogen. Equine Vet J. 2002;34:693–8.

32. Reed SM, Bayly WM, Sellon DC. Disorders of specific body systems. In: Equine internal medicine 3 rd edition. St. Louis: Saunders; 2010. p. 736-40.
33. Hooijberg EH, van den Hoven R, Tichy A, Schwendenwein I. Diagnostic and predictive capability of routine laboratory tests for the diagnosis and staging of equine inflammatory disease. J Vet Intern Med. 2014;28:1587–93.
34. Burrell MH, Wood JL, Whitwell KE, Chanter N, Mackintosh ME, Mumford JA. Respiratory disease in thoroughbred horses in training: the relationships between disease and viruses, bacteria and environment. Vet Rec. 1996;139:308–13.
35. Ivester KM, Smith K, Moore GE, Zimmerman NJ, Couëtilt LL. Variability in particulate concentrations in a horse training barn over time. Equine Vet J Suppl. 2012;43:51–6.
36. Robinson NE, Karmaus W, Holcombe SJ, Carr EA, Derksen FJ. Airway inflammation in Michigan pleasure horses: prevalence and risk factors. Equine Vet J. 2006;38:293–9.
37. Holcombe SJ, Jackson C, Gerber V, Jefcoat A, Berney C, Eberhardt S, et al. Stabling is associated with airway inflammation in young Arabian horses. Equine Vet J. 2001;33:244–9.
38. Whittaker AG, Love S, Parkin TD, Duz M, Hughes KJ. Stabling causes a significant increase in the pH of the equine airway. Equine Vet J. 2009;4:940–3.
39. Berndt A, Derksen FJ, Edward Robinson N. Endotoxin concentrations within the breathing zone of horses are higher in stables than on pasture. Vet J. 2010;183:54–7.
40. Vandenput S, Istasse L, Nicks B, Lekeux P. Airborne dust and aeroallergen concentrations in different sources of feed and bedding for horses. Vet Q. 1997;19:154–8.
41. Clements JM, Pirie RS. Respirable dust concentrations in equine stables. Part 1: validation of equipment and effect of various management systems. Res Vet Sci. 2007;83:256–62.
42. Hessel EF, Garlipp F, Van den Weghe HFA. Generation of airborne particles from horse feeds depending on type and processing. J Equine Vet Sci. 2009;29:665–74.
43. Ivester KM, Couëtil LL, Moore GE, Zimmerman NJ, Raskin RE. Environmental exposures and airway inflammation in young thoroughbred horses. J Vet Intern Med. 2014;28:918–24.
44. Davis MS, Royer CM, McKenzie EC, Williamson KK, Payton M, Marlin D. Cold air-induced late-phase bronchoconstriction in horses. Equine Vet J Suppl. 2006;36:535–9.
45. Davis MS, Williams CC, Meinkoth JH, Malayer JR, Royer CM, Williamson KK, McKenzie EC. Influx of neutrophils and persistence of cytokine expression in airways of horses after performing exercise while breathing cold air. Am J Vet Res. 2007;68:185–9.
46. Carroll CL, Huntington PJ. Body condition scoring and weight estimation of horses. Equine Vet J. 1998;20:41–5.
47. Millerick-May ML, Karmaus W, Derksen FJ, Berthold B, Holcombe SJ, Robinson NE. Local airborne particulate concentration is associated with visible tracheal mucus in thoroughbred racehorses. Equine Vet J. 2013;45:85–90.
48. Airaksinen S, Heiskanen ML, Heinonen-Tanski H, Laitinen J, Laitinen S, Linnainmaa M, et al. Variety in dustiness and hygiene quality of peat bedding. Ann Agric Environ Med. 2005;12:53–9.
49. Saastamoinen M, Särkijärvi S, Hyyppä S. Reducing respiratory health risks to horses and workers: a comparison of two stall bedding materials. Animals. 2015;5:965–77.
50. Wålinder R, Riihimäki M, Bohlin S, Hogstedt C, Nordquist T, Raine A, et al. Installation of mechanical ventilation in a horse stable: effects on air quality and human and equine airways. Environ Health Prev Med. 2011;16:264–72.
51. Jørgensen GH, Aanensen L, Mejdell CM, Bøe KE. Preference for shelter and additional heat in horses exposed to Nordic winter conditions. Equine Vet J. 2016;48:720–6.
52. Baumgartner M, Zeitler-Feicht MH, Wohr AC, Wohling H, Erhard MH. Lying behaviour of group-housed horses in different designed areas with rubber mats, shavings and sand bedding. Pferdeheilkunde. 2015;31:211–20.
53. Cobb CJ, Obeidat BS, Sellers MD, Pepper-Yowell AR, Ballou MA. Group housing of Holstein calves in a poor indoor environment increases respiratory disease but does not influence performance or leukocyte responses. J Dairy Sci. 2014;97:3099–109.
54. Crisman MV, Scarrat WK, Zimmerman KL. Blood proteins and inflammation in the horse. Vet Clin N Am Equine Pract. 2008;24:285–97.
55. Hultén C, Grönlund U, Hirvonen J, Tulamo RM, Suominen MM, Marhaug G, et al. Dynamics in serum of the inflammatory markers serum amyloid A (SAA), haptoglobin, fibrinogen and alpha2-globulins during induced noninfectious arthritis in the horse. Equine Vet J. 2002;34:699–704.

13

# A longitudinal cohort study of acute puerperal metritis cases in Swedish dairy cows

Anna Ordell[1], Helle Ericsson Unnerstad[2], Ann Nyman[2], Hans Gustafsson[1,3] and Renée Båge[1,3*]

**Abstract**

**Background:** Acute puerperal metritis affects cows during the early postpartum period and causes fever, fetid vaginal discharge and general depression. The disease is severe and treatment with antimicrobials is often required. This study followed 79 Swedish dairy cows with acute puerperal metritis with registered treatment and outcome in terms of recovery. Bacteria isolated from the uterus and their susceptibility to penicillin were studied. Clinical cases were assigned by participating practitioners who examined the cows, performed uterine swab sampling, decided treatment and provided information about cow health and calving conditions. Fertility and culling data were collected from the official Swedish milk and health recording scheme. Recovery from disease was defined in four levels; as a cow that survived 1 or 4 months, was inseminated and subsequently became pregnant. Intervals from dates of first and latest calving to insemination date were studied.

**Results:** The most common bacterial findings were a mixed culture of *Escherichia coli* and bacteria such as Gram positive cocci, *Fusobacterium necrophorum*, *Clostridium* spp. or *Trueperella pyogenes*. The Gram positive cocci, *Pasteurella* spp. and *F. necrophorum* were generally susceptible to penicillin. The majority of cows (70%) were treated with penicillin in accordance with the Swedish policy on treatment of metritis while 19% were treated with tetracycline and 8% were not treated with antimicrobials. Recovery rates were similar between treatments. Besides "calving to last insemination" interval (CLI) that was 5 days shorter than the national mean, fertility was slightly reduced compared to national means. "Calving to first insemination" interval (CFI) was 4 days longer than national mean and number of inseminations/cow increased from 1.9 to 2.1. *Escherichia coli* culture positive cows did not become pregnant to the same extent as cows without *E. coli* in the uterus ($P = 0.046$). Twin births resulted in a longer CFI ($P = 0.034$). The culling rate was generally high (42% within 300 days after occurrence of metritis), though death associated with acute disease was low (6%).

**Conclusions:** *Escherichia coli* was the most common bacterial pathogen isolated from cases of acute puerperal metritis in the present study. This bacterium is inherently resistant to penicillin, but although most cows were treated with penicillin, death due to acute disease was low and recovery and final fertility results were acceptable. In times of emerging antimicrobial resistance and demand for prudent antimicrobial use, we suggest that penicillin is a "good enough" choice if antimicrobial treatment of acute puerperal metritis is needed.

**Keywords:** Reproductive health, Postpartum, Involution, Antimicrobial treatment, Antimicrobial resistance, Fertility, Culling, Recovery, Broad spectrum

## Background

It is well documented that reproductive diseases have a negative effect on herd reproductive performance [1, 2]. However, the long term effect of acute puerperal metritis (APM) has not been fully investigated and recent literature is not conclusive regarding its consequences for fertility [3, 4]. After parturition, the physical barrier of the uterus is broken, the vulva is slack and the cervix dilated, which allow bacteria to invade the uterine lumen. Bacterial contamination can be detected in 50–90% of dairy

*Correspondence: renee.bage@slu.se
[1] Department of Clinical Sciences, Swedish University of Agricultural Sciences, SE-750 07 Uppsala, Sweden

cows during the first two weeks postpartum (pp) [5, 6]. In a recent Danish study, comprising 125 pp cows from five different herds, bacteria were found in all cows using a DNA-fingerprinting method [7]. In most cases, the contaminated uterus will cleanse during involution without any clinical signs [8], although occasionally, due to heavy bacterial load, failure of the immune system or other factors, bacteria remain in the uterus and cause inflammation [9]. Acute puerperal metritis affects cows up to 3 weeks pp due to profound inflammation of the uterine wall associated with fever (rectal temperature ≥39.5 °C), fetid vaginal discharge and systemic illness [10]. Common bacterial findings, in conventional culture studies, in the uterus of metritic cows are *Escherichia coli*, *Trueperella pyogenes*, and *Fusobacterium necrophorum* according to several studies [11–15].

Cows diagnosed with APM are in most cases treated with antimicrobial drugs such as penicillin, oxytetracycline, ampicillin or ceftiofur [16, 17]. The APM treatment prevalence reported in the international literature is high and varies from 15% up to 69% [18]. In Sweden, the APM treatment incidence is 0.7% according to statistics from the Swedish official milk and health recording scheme (SOMRS). However, the definition of APM varies between studies, which complicate comparisons. Systemic illness is commonly mentioned in the disease definition [3, 18, 19], but not always used as an inclusion criterion [3, 17–19].

Antimicrobials are used worldwide to treat bacterial disorders in both animals and humans but the effect has started to falter due to diminished antimicrobial susceptibility. Ceftiofur is a broad spectrum antibiotic belonging to the cephalosporins and has no withdrawal time for milk from the treated animal. It has been reported to be effective for treatment of uterine infection [19]. However, the third-generation cephalosporins are listed by the World Health Organisation (WHO) as being critically important for human medicine [20]. Each use of antimicrobial drugs contributes to the emerging resistance [21] and an association is seen between veterinary antimicrobial use and antimicrobial resistance in livestock animals [22]. The increasing resistance in zoonotic bacteria among food-producing animals has been proposed to be a potential threat to public health [21]. Thus the increased popularity of this type of drug among veterinary practitioners and farmers constitutes a risk for increasing microbial resistance.

Treatment data from Swedish practitioners' records show that cases of APM account for 64% of the total amount of antimicrobials used in the treatment of reproductive disorders. Penicillin is used in 59% and tetracycline in 34% of all APM cases in Sweden according to the SOMRS. The Swedish Veterinary Association has stated a policy for antimicrobial use in farm animals [23]. The policy states that the use of quinolones and third and fourth-generation cephalosporins should be restricted, and that antibiotic therapy should be preceded by a diagnosis with the need for antimicrobials being evaluated in each case. According to this policy, the first-line antimicrobial therapy for most diseases in cattle is penicillin. The aim of the policy is to reduce the selective pressure on, and emergence of, resistant bacteria. It is based on literature reports of the efficacy of different treatment routines and the experience from practice that penicillin in most cases is sufficient as an antibacterial drug.

Uterine bacteria and their susceptibility to antibiotics in Swedish dairy cows with APM have not been investigated previously. The efficacy of different treatment routines in terms of how treated cows survive and remain in the herd, and whether they are inseminated and become pregnant are also unknown. The aim of this study was to investigate bacteria isolated from the uterus and their susceptibility to penicillin in cows diagnosed with APM by veterinary practitioners in Sweden, and to survey treatments used and assess the outcome in terms of survival and fertility.

## Methods

### Animal material and sampling method

Twenty practitioners from geographic areas with high number of dairy cows were instructed to sample cows with signs of APM for a longitudinal prospective cohort study. The sampling was approved by the Uppsala Animal Experiment Ethics Board (C303/11). Inclusion criteria were a fetid vaginal discharge, rectal temperature ≥39.5 °C and signs of systemic illness during the first week pp. No selection for breed, parity, housing or season was made, but cows that had already been treated with antibiotics since parturition were excluded. No treatment recommendations or instructions were given to the practitioners but they were asked to report which, if any, antibiotic substance was used, the duration of treatment, and other pharmaceutical drugs administered. The practitioners performed a clinical examination and recorded the cows' health status at the visit, and obtained information from the farmer concerning the calving history (Table 1).

A total of 79 cows from 55 herds were sampled during a study period from November 2011 to April 2014, with most cases collected in 2012 (87%). Acute puerperal metritis cases were recorded every month of the year with most cases in November–December and February (in total 43% of the cases) and fewest cases in June–August (8%). The mean herd size was 113 cows (range 15–554) and the herds' mean annually production was 9830 kg energy corrected milk (range 8014–11,433 kg). Among

**Table 1 Questions for the farmer about the calving history**

| Question | Possible answers |
|---|---|
| Calving location? | Individual calving box |
| | Group calving box |
| | On pasture |
| | Tied up in a pen |
| | In loose housing |
| | Other |
| Time for expulsion of foetal membranes? | Within 12 h pp |
| | 12–24 h pp |
| | More than 24 h pp |
| | Still retained at visit |
| Calving process? | Normal without assistance |
| | Assistance needed |
| | Other |

sampled cows, 28% were primiparous. The breed distribution was 53% Swedish Holstein, 43% Swedish Red and 4% crossbreed. Cows were sampled on average 4 days pp (range 1–8 days) and a retained placenta (not expelled within 24 h pp) was present in 78% of cases. According to the information given by the farmers, 67% of the cows had normal parturition (easy calving without or with slight assistance, according to codes used in reports to SOMRS), 16% twin birth, 9% abortion or premature parturition and 8% stillborn calves. Parturition took place in a group calving box (40%), in an individual calving pen (26%), tied up in a pen (23%) or in other areas (11%).

The practitioners were provided with both oral and written instructions for the sampling method, together with the sampling equipment. They were instructed to clean the external genital structures thoroughly prior to sampling with a uterine swab (Equi-Vet Uterine Culture Swab, Kruuse, Marslev, Denmark) and then take the sample according to the manufacturer's instructions: The swab was inserted via the vulva and cervix in a sheathed tube to avoid contamination. In the uterus the sheath was withdrawn, the sample was taken from the uterine mucosa and the swab was retracted into the protective tube before withdrawal. The long swab was cut and stored in Amie's medium (Sarstedt, Copan Italia S.p.A, Brescia, Italy) during transport by mail to the Department of Bacteriology, National Veterinary Institute, Uppsala, Sweden.

### Bacteriological culturing and antimicrobial susceptibility testing

All samples were cultured under both aerobic and anaerobic conditions and identified according to accredited conventional phenotypic methods at the Department of Bacteriology, National Veterinary Institute, Uppsala, Sweden.

The susceptibility to penicillin of isolates of Gram positive bacteria, *Pasteurella* spp. and *F. necrophorum* was tested by determination of minimum inhibitory concentration (MIC) according to the standards of the Clinical and Laboratory Standards Institute (CLSI) [24] using broth microdilution. Due to inherently low susceptibility to penicillin, Gram negative bacteria (other than *Pasteurella* spp. and *F. necrophorum*) and enterococci were not tested. For some bacterial species, changes were made compared to the CLSI standard, as described below.

Testing was performed using the panels VetMIC GP-mo (ver. 2) for Gram positive bacteria and *F. necrophorum* and VetMIC Large Animals for *Pasteurella* spp. (National Veterinary Institute, Uppsala, Sweden). The reference strain *Staphylococcus aureus* CCUG 15,915 was used as a quality control and results were within acceptable ranges. For susceptibility testing of *T. pyogenes*, colony material was suspended in 2 ml NaCl to 0.5–1 on the McFarland scale and then 10 μl were diluted in 5 ml Müller-Hinton Broth. From this dilution, 2–5 μl was inoculated on 5% horse blood agar in microdilution wells in GP-mo panels. The panels were incubated for 17–24 h at 37 °C in 5% $CO_2$. For susceptibility testing of *Pasteurella* spp., 5% horse serum was added to the Müller-Hinton Broth. For susceptibility testing of *F. necrophorum*, 100 μl of a bacterial suspension with $1–5 \times 10^6$ colony forming units (CFU)/ml was inoculated in each well. Susceptibility testing of other anaerobic bacteria than *F. necrophorum* was not performed.

### Survival and fertility data

Information about the sampled cows and their reproductive performance was obtained from the SOMRS, and the cows were followed from enrollment up to 18 months pp. The data obtained consisted of breed (Swedish Red/Swedish Holstein/crossbreed), parity, course of parturition (normal or assisted calving/stillbirth/twins), treatments for APM, fertility (number of inseminations, calving to first insemination interval (CFI), calving to last insemination interval (CLI), established pregnancy, fertility treatments) and culling (date, cause, euthanized/slaughter). The reasons for culling was provided by the farmer and recorded in the SOMRS.

### Statistical analyzis

Clinical records, results from bacterial culturing and antimicrobial susceptibility testing and database records on survival and fertility were statistically evaluated. Four findings indicating recovery from APM were used: (1) survival for 1 month pp (yes/no), (2) survival for four months pp (yes/no), (3) having been inseminated (yes/no) and (4) pregnancy established (yes/no). Furthermore, the two fertility variables CFI and CLI were analyzed.

The studied cows' CFI and CLI were categorized into CFI < 88 days and CFI ≥ 88 days and CLI < 130 days and CLI ≥ 130 days, respectively. The choices of 88–130 days were selected as the national means CFI and CLI in 2012 were 88–130 days, respectively [25]. Descriptive statistics were used to present the results of the distribution of the dependent (four signs of recovery and CFI ≥ 88 days and CLI ≥ 130 days) and independent variables. The independent variables were: presence of bacteria (yes/no), parity, breed, parturition (normal or assisted), twins (yes/no), retained placenta (yes/no), calving area (individual pen/group pen/tie stall/other), stillbirth (yes/no), rectal temperature >40 °C of an APM case (yes/no), treatment (only penicillin with or without non-steroidal anti-inflammatory drugs (NSAID)/only tetracycline with or without NSAID/nothing or only NSAID). Associations between the dependent variables and the independent variables were investigated using Fisher's exact-test, univariable and multivariable logistic regression models. For the multivariable models collinearity between the independent variables was assessed pair-wise by calculation of Spearman rank correlations. If there was proof of collinearity ($r \leq 0.70$) the variable with lowest $P$ value in the univariable analyzis was selected. Moreover, in all the multivariable model biologically plausible two-way interactions between the main effects were tested. The model fit of the multivariable analyzes was tested by visual examination of diagnostic plots according to [26]. A $P$ value of <0.05 was considered statistically significant. All statistical analyzes were performed using Stata Statistical Software (Release 11.2: College Station, TX, USA: StataCorp LP).

## Results

### Bacterial findings and antimicrobial susceptibility

Bacteria were isolated from 76 of the 79 samples (99% of the cultured samples, one had no bacterial growth and two samples were lost). Mixed growth was found in 68% of cultured samples (Table 2). Gram negative bacteria were found in 90% of the samples, and 45% contained at least one Gram positive bacterial species. Anaerobic bacteria were found in 31 samples (39%). Bacterial findings were dominated by *E. coli* often in combination with Gram positive cocci, *F. necrophorum*, and *Clostridium* spp. or *T. pyogenes*. Of the 65 *E. coli* isolates, 18% had haemolytic properties.

A total of 48 isolates were tested for penicillin susceptibility. Breakpoints for resistance are not available for all bacterial species; however, MICs were low in all tested isolates (Table 3).

### Treatment

The majority of cows were treated with penicillin, often in combination with NSAID (Table 4). Tetracycline was used, by either intramuscular or intrauterine administration, in 19% of cases. Two cows were treated with both penicillin and tetracycline and one cow was treated with enrofloxacin. The mean duration of antimicrobial treatment was 5 days (range 3–6 days) regardless of substance used. No antibiotic treatment was used in six cases. NSAID was given to 68 cows (86% of all cows), while 61, six and three were given meloxicam, ketoprofen and flunixin meglumin, respectively. One cow was treated with both meloxicam and ketoprofen.

No significant association was found between antibiotic treatment and the four recovery parameters or the two fertility variables. There was no significant association between antibiotic treatment and parity, breed, course of calving, retained placenta or bacterial findings. The only clinical sign the veterinarians registered was rectal temperature, which was not associated with treatment. No significant association between NSAID treatment and recovery could be found.

**Table 2 Distribution of isolates from 76 uterine bacterial samples in pure and mixed culture**

| Bacteria | Isolate | | Mono-culture | Mixed culture with n other bacteria | | | |
|---|---|---|---|---|---|---|---|
| | n | (%) | | *1* | 2 | 3 | 4 |
| *Escherichia coli* | 65 | (86) | 19 | 16 | 17 | 12 | 1 |
| Grampositive cocci[a] | 25 | (33) | 1 | 7 | 4 | 12 | 1 |
| *Fusobacterium necrophorum* | 18 | (24) | 0 | 0 | 10 | 8 | 0 |
| *Clostridium* spp. | 14 | (18) | 0 | 0 | 4 | 9 | 1 |
| *Trueperella pyogenes* | 16 | (21) | 1 | 6 | 5 | 3 | 1 |
| Other Gram-negative[b] | 9 | (12) | 2 | 3 | 3 | 1 | 0 |
| *Pasturella* spp. | 4 | (5) | 1 | 0 | 1 | 2 | 0 |

[a] Gram-positive cocci include various species of streptococci and enterococci

[b] Other Gram-negative bacteria include *Enterobacter* spp., *Acinetobacter* spp., *Proteus mirabilis*, *Proteus vulgaris*, *Providencia rettgeri* and *Aeromonas hydrophila*

**Table 3 Minimum inhibitory concentrations of penicillin for tested bacterial species**

| Bacterial species | MIC (mg/l) |
|---|---|
| *Trueperella pyogenes* | 0. 015–0.12 |
| *Fusobacterium necrophorum* | 0.03–0.06 |
| *Streptococcus* spp. | 0.03–0.06 |
| *Pasteurella* spp. | 0.12–0.25 |

### Fertility

Insemination was initiated for 44 cows (56%) and 31 (70%) of these subsequently became pregnant. Mean and median CFIs for these cows were 92 days (range 44–249 days) and 74.5 days (50% central range (CR): 66.5–103.5 days), respectively. In total, 26 cows had a CFI < 88 days and 18 cows had a CFI ≥ 88 days. The mean and median number of inseminations required for pregnancy was 2.1/cow (range 1–7) and 2.0 (50% CR: 1–3), respectively. Mean and median CLI was 125 days (range 65–291 days) and 112 days (50% CR: 86–146 days), respectively, for the 32 cows that became pregnant. In total, 18 cows had a CLI < 130 days and 14 cows had a CLI ≥ 130 days.

Cows with uterine *E. coli* infection had a tendency towards reduced likelihood for being inseminated compared to cows with other bacterial infections (OR = 0.24, 95% CI 0.04–1.22, *P* = 0.09) and for cows with *E. coli* infection, infection with haemolytic *E. coli* seemed to have a greater negative impact on the chance of being inseminated than for infections with non-haemolytic *E. coli* (OR = 0.32, 95% CI 0.09–1.18, *P* = 0.09). There was no significant association between the recovery parameters or fertility variables and other bacterial findings than *E. coli*, and no significant differences in treatment, culling, inseminations or pregnancy between cows with *E. coli* in either mixed culture, pure culture or negative cultures.

We found no significant association between the fertility variables and parity, breed, place of calving, retained placenta, abortion or premature parturition, stillbirth or course of calving. Cows giving birth to twins had significantly higher risk (OR = 9.6, CI 1.01–91.2, *P* = 0.05) of prolonged CFI than those with singletons. Moreover, having fever ≥40 °C on the day of examination tended to decreased the odds for subsequent pregnancy (OR = 0.32, CI 0.09–1.18, *P* = 0.09).

### Survival

In total, 43 cows (57%) were culled during the follow-up period. The mean number of days between calving and culling was 194 days (range 1–597 days). The proportion of cows culled within one month was 7/79 (9%), within four months it was 14/79 (18%) and after 18 months it was 42/79 (53%). The reported reason for culling/death was: unknown (36%), low milk production (25%), mastitis (17%), hoof/leg disorders (11%) and decreased fertility (11%).

The majority of culled cows were slaughtered, but 14 cows were euthanized or were found dead, of which half of the cases occurred within the first month pp. A significantly higher proportion of culled cows were multiparous (82%) than primiparous (18%) (*P* = 0.04 (Fisher's exact test, could not be run using logistic regression due to too few observations in some cells). All the cows culled in the first month pp were multiparous. The risk of culling within 4 months pp tended to be higher among cows that had aborted or had a premature parturition than cows that calved at term (OR = 5.0, 95% CI 0.90–27.9, *P* = 0.07). Moreover, the risk of culling within 4 months was significantly lower among cows calving in a group calving box compared to cows calving in a single cow calving pen (OR = 0.17, 95% CI 0.03–0.93, *P* = 0.04).

A distribution table presenting associations between the recovery variables and bacterial findings, antimicrobial treatment and risk factors, bacterial findings,

**Table 4 Recovery related to antimicrobial and non-steroidal anti-inflammatory drugs (NSAID) treatment in number (n) and percent (%) according to four definitions of recovery**

| Treatment group | n | Survived 1 month | | Survived 4 months | | Inseminated | | Pregnant | |
|---|---|---|---|---|---|---|---|---|---|
| | | n | (%) | n | (%) | n | (%) | n | (%) |
| Penicillin | 55 | 51 | (93) | 44 | (80) | 30 | (55) | 21 | (38) |
| With NSAID | 51 | 47 | (92) | 41 | (80) | 27 | (53) | 18 | (35) |
| Tetracycline | 15 | 12 | (80) | 12 | (80) | 9 | (60) | 6 | (40) |
| With NSAID | 11 | 9 | (82) | 9 | (82) | 7 | (64) | 5 | (45) |
| No antimicrobials | 6 | 5 | (83) | 5 | (83) | 3 | (50) | 2 | (33) |
| With NSAID | 4 | 4 | (100) | 4 | (100) | 3 | (75) | 2 | (50) |

Cows treated with both penicillin and tetracycline (n = 2) or treated with enrofloxacin (n = 1) were excluded antimicrobial treatment and risk factors for four recovery variables and two fertility variables (survived for 1 month and 4 months, inseminated, confirmed pregnant again, CFI and CLI), including results of the statistical analyzes is included as Additional file 1: Table S1.

## Discussion

In this observational study of Swedish dairy cows with APM, *E. coli* was the most common bacterial finding and often found in combination with one or more other bacterial species (Table 2), in agreement with other reports [10, 14, 15]. These bacteria are common in the uterus after calving both in diseased and non-diseased cows. However, specific bacterial pathogens are not associated with an increased risk for developing APM [10, 11, 14]. Bacterial findings in the present study were similar to those of other studies thus implicating that bacterial species per se are an unimportant factor for the large difference observed between the prevalence of APM in Swedish statistics (<1%) and in surveys from other countries (~20%) [17, 27].

As expected, the studied cows were exposed to the known risk factors for developing APM [28], i.e. 33, 16 and 78% had a history of difficult calving, twin birth and retained placenta, respectively although the incidences were higher than in the national statistics (being 2, 3 and 1%, respectively).

The majority of cows in the study (70%) were treated with penicillin which is in accordance with the Swedish policy on the use of antibiotics recommending penicillin as first choice treatment of APM. Consequently, the use of broad-spectrum antimicrobials such as tetracycline was low (19%), and ceftiofur was not used at all. The reason behind some veterinarians' choice not to use the recommended penicillin therapy in some cases of APM is unknown but may involve habit or clinical considerations such as herd specific historical therapy responses. The common use of broad-spectrum antimicrobials in the treatment of APM in studies from other countries may reflect treatment targeting *E. coli* as well as the availability of new broad-spectrum antibiotics (e.g. cephalosporin) without withdrawal time and reports of significant improvement in cure rates after their use [19]. However, a critical review of treating APM with ceftiofur concludes that lack of negative control groups and small samples sizes for some of the studies limits the scientific basis for this treatment [29]. One study found no significant effect of treatment with ceftiofur vs. animals treated with procaine penicillin G [16]. Another study provided some evidence that cows treated with ampicillin resulted in a more rapid clinical cure compared with cows treated with ceftiofur [30].

In the present study, all bacterial species (Gram-positive bacteria, *Pasteurella* spp. and *F. necrophorum*) that were tested for susceptibility to penicillin had low MICs, indicating clinical susceptibility (Table 3). It is known that *E. coli* is inherently resistant to penicillin, and consequently, we did not test *E. coli* isolates for susceptibility to penicillin.

The practitioners' choice of antimicrobial treatment did not influence the recovery variables in our cohort. No significant association was found between the treatment and parity, breed, risk factors, clinical condition or bacterial findings, which may be due to the low number of observations and a low statistical power. Only 5 cows (6%) were euthanized or died while 89 and 80% survived for one and four months, respectively. This indicates a high recovery rate from APM. The main reasons for culling reported by the farmers were low milk production or mastitis for which APM may act as a pre-disposing factor [28, 31]. The total proportion of culled cows in the cohort was higher than the national mean reported in the SOMRS (57 vs. 33%).

Although a high recovery rate from APM, only 55% of the cows were inseminated (Table 4) suggesting a decline in fertility or that the farmers' chose not to inseminate these cows again. There was a tendency that fewer *E. coli*- positive than *E. coli*-negative cows were inseminated indicating that especially this species could have a long term negative effect on fertility. However, among the 23 cows diagnosed with *E. coli* that later were inseminated and became pregnant, 17 had been treated with penicillin, which is notably considering the resistance against penicillin. Even though *E. coli* is the most commonly isolated bacterial species it may be more important to treat the other penicillin-susceptible and often tissue-invasive bacteria. New, culture-independent studies report that bacteria other than *E. coli* are the most abundant ones in the uteri of metritic cows one week pp [32], with *Fusobacteriaceae*, *Porphyromonadaceae* and *Streptococcaceae* constituting 59% of the uterine flush sample microbiota and 62% of the uterine biopsy microbiota.

An interesting finding in the present study was that of the six cows not receiving any antimicrobials, three were inseminated and two of these became pregnant (Table 4), suggesting recovery without treatment. The low number of observations and the lack of untreated controls makes it hard to draw conclusions, but our results agree well with self-cure rates in the range of 22 to 87% reported by others [17–19]. It is likely that individual cows would benefit from antimicrobial treatment; the difficulty lies in distinguishing these cows from cases where treatment is unnecessary. A recent review evaluating diagnostic methods for APM indicated that elevated rectal temperature (>39.5 °C) alone is insufficient to diagnose APM since it is also associated with factors such as parity, abnormal calving conditions and hyperketonemia [33]. It was reported that the rectal temperature exceeded 39.5 °C at least once during the first 10 days pp in 66% of healthy cows. In the present study, a tendency was seen for cows with fever ≥40.0 °C not to become pregnant as often as cows with rectal temperatures between 39.5 and 39.9 °C), regardless of antimicrobial treatment and time of the year, which indicates a more severe disease in these animals. Rectal temperature ≥40.0 °C may thus be useful as prognosis for the recovery of individual cases of APM.

In the cows subjected to insemination, the CFI was only increased by 4 days (92 vs. 88 days), and pregnancy rate/AI decreased by 7 percentage units (35 vs. 42%) compared to the national mean, while CLI was even 5 days shorter than the national mean in the cows that eventually got pregnant. This is surprisingly good despite the fact that the majority of cows were *E. coli*-positive and treated with penicillin.

## Conclusion

Although *E. coli* was the most common bacteriological finding in the uterus of cases of APM in the present study, and most cows were treated with only penicillin, acceptable recovery and fertility results were found. This supports the Swedish policy on use of antibiotics in cattle that penicillin is "good enough" as a first line therapy for treatment of bovine APM. This is also concurrent with WHO's and OIE's [34] demand of prudent use of antimicrobial substances in the aim to decelerate emerging antimicrobial resistance.

#### Authors' contributions

RB, HG and HEU designed the study. RB coordinated and supervised the study. AO collected and sorted data and drafted the main manuscript. HEU contributed with competence in bacteriology and antimicrobial susceptibility. AN carried out the statistical analyzes. HG provided data from Swedish official milk and health recording scheme. All authors read and approved the final manuscript.

#### Author details

[1] Department of Clinical Sciences, Swedish University of Agricultural Sciences, SE-750 07 Uppsala, Sweden. [2] Department of Animal Health and Antimicrobial Strategies, National Veterinary Institute, SE-751 89 Uppsala, Sweden. [3] Development and Services for Farmers, Växa Sverige, SE-104 25 Stockholm, Sweden.

#### Acknowledgements

The authors would like to thank the participating practitioners for providing the study with clinical cases and samples. Thanks also to Maria Persson for coordinating the samples and to Kerstin Ekström for performing antimicrobial susceptibility testing at the National Veterinary Institute. The project was funded by the Swedish Farmers' Foundation for Agricultural Research (SLF, V1130023).

#### Competing interests

The authors declare that they have no competing interests.

#### References

1. LeBlanc SJ. Postpartum uterine disease and dairy herd reproductive performance: a review. Vet J. 2008;176:102–14.
2. Löf E, Gustafsson H, Emanuelson U. Factors influencing the chance of cows being pregnant 30 days after the herd voluntary waiting period. J Diary Sci. 2014;97:2071–80.
3. Giuliodori MJ, Magnasco RP, Becu-Villalobos D, Lacau-Mengido IM, Risco CA. Metritis in dairy cows: risk factors and reproductive performance. J Dairy Sci. 2013;96:3621–31.
4. Wittrock JM, Proudfoot KL, Weary DM, von Keyserlingk MA. Short communication: metritis affects milk production and cull rate of Holstein multiparous and primiparous dairy cows differently. J Dairy Sci. 2011;94:2408–12.
5. Fredriksson G, Kindahl H, Sandstedt K, Edqvist LE. Intrauterine bacterial findings and release of PGF2 alpha in the postpartum dairy cow. Zentralbl Veterinarmed A. 1985;32:368–80.
6. Paisley LG, Mickelsen WD, Anderson PB. Mechanisms and therapy for retained fetal membranes and uterine infections of cows: a review. Theriogenology. 1986;25:353–81.
7. Elkjaer K, Ancher ML, Gustafsson H, Friggens NC, Waldman A, Callesen H. Uterine bacterial flora in postpartum Danish Holstein dairy cows determined using DNA based fingerprinting: correlation to uterine condition and calving management. Anim Reprod Sci. 2013;138:39–48.
8. Bekana M. Clinical, ultrasonographic, bacteriological and hormonal studies in post-partum cows with particular emphasis on retained fetal membranes. PhD thesis. Sweden: Swedish university of agricultural sciences, Department of Clinical Science; 1996.
9. LeBlanc SJ, Osawa T, Dubuc J. Reproductive tract defense and disease in postpartum dairy cows. Theriogenology. 2011;76:1610–8.
10. Sheldon IM, Lewis GS, LeBlanc S, Gilbert RO. Defining postpartum uterine disease in cattle. Theriogenology. 2006;65:1516–30.
11. Bondurant RH. Inflammation in the bovine female reproductive tract. J Dairy Sci. 1999;82:101–10.
12. Sheldon IM, Rycroft AN, Zhou C. Association between pyrexia and uterine bacterial infection in dairy cattle. Vet Rec. 2004;154:289–93.
13. Bekana M, Jonsson P, Ekman T, Kindahl H. Intrauterine bacterial findings in postpartum cows with retained fetal membranes. Zentralbl Veterinarmed A. 1994;41:663–70.
14. Kask K, Gustafsson H, Magnusson U, Bertilsson J, Gunnarsson A, Kindahl H. Uterine bacteriology, histology, resumption of ovarian activity and granulocyte function of the postpartum cow in different milking frequencies. Acta Vet Scand. 1999;40:287–97.
15. Königsson K, Gustafsson H, Gunnarsson A, Kindahl H. Clinical and bacteriological aspects on the use of oxytetracycline and flunixin in primiparous cows with induced retained placenta and post-partal endometritis. Reprod Dom Anim. 2001;36:247–56.
16. Smith BI, Donovan GA, Risco C, Littell R, Young C, Stanker LH, et al. Comparison of various antibiotic treatments for cows diagnosed with toxic puerperal metritis. J Dairy Sci. 1998;81:1555–62.
17. Drillich M, Beetz O, Pfützner A, Sabin M, Sabin HJ, Kutzer P, et al. Evaluation of a systemic antibiotic treatment of toxic puerperal metritis in dairy cows. J Dairy Sci. 2001;84:2010–7.
18. Sannmann I, Burfiend O, Voigtsberger R, Heuweiser W. Comparison of two monitoring and treatment strategies for cows with acute puerperal metritis. Theriogenology. 2013;79:961–9.
19. McLaughlin CL, Stanisiewski E, Lucas MJ, Cornell CP, Watkins J, Bryson L, et al. Evaluation of two doses of ceftiofur crystalline free acid sterile suspension for treatment of metritis in lactating dairy cows. J Dairy Sci. 2012;95:4363–71.
20. WHO. Critically important antimicrobials for human medicine. http://apps.who.int/iris/bitstream/10665/77444/1/9789241501439_eng.pdf?ua=1. Accessed 8 Oct 2014.
21. Ozawa T, Kiku Y, Mizuno M, Inumaru S, Kushibiki S, Shingu H, et al. Effect of intramammary infusion of rbGM-CSF on SCC and expression of polymorphonuclear neutrophil adhesion molecules in subclinical mastitis cows. Vet Res Commun. 2012;36:21–7.

22. Chantziaras I, Boyen F, Callens B, Dewulf J. Correlation between veterinary antimicrobial use and antimicrobial resistance in food-producing animals: a report on seven countries. J Antimicrob Chemother. 2014;69:827–34.
23. Swedish Veterinary Association. Guidelines for antimicrobial use in livestock animals. (In Swedish) http://svf.se/Documents/S%C3%A4llskapet/Husdjurssektionen/SVS%20Riktlinjer%20f%C3%B6r%20anv%C3%A4ndning%20av%20antibiotika%20till%20produktionsdjur%202013.pdf. Accessed 3 Sept 2014.
24. Clinical and Laboratory Standards Institute. Performance standards for antimicrobial disc and dilution susceptibility tests for bacteria isolated from animals; approved standard. 3rd ed. Wayne: M31-A3, CLSI; 2008.
25. Växa Sverige-Development and Services for Farmers: animal health 2011/2012. Annual report from the animal health section. (In Swedish) http://vxa.se/Documents/%C3%85rsredog%C3%B6relse%202011_12.pdf Accessed 10 Mar 2014.
26. Dohoo IR, Martin W. Stryhn H. In: McPike SM, editor. Veterinary epidemiologic research. Charlottetown: VER Inc; 2010.
27. Benzaquen ME, Risco CA, Archbald LF, Melendez P, Thatcher MJ, Thatcher WW. Rectal temperature, calving-related factors, and the incidence of puerperal metritis in postpartum dairy cows. J Dairy Sci. 2007;90:2804–14.
28. Ghavi Hossein-Zadeh N, Ardalan M. Cow-specific risk factors for retained placenta, metritis and clinical mastitis in Holstein cows. Vet Res Commun. 2011;35:345–54.
29. Reppert EJ. Evidence for the use of ceftiofur for treatment of metritis in dairy cattle. Vet Clin Food Anim. 2015;31:139–49.
30. Lima FS, Vieira-Neto A, Vasconcellos GS, Mingoti RD, Karakaya E, Solé E, et al. Efficacy of ampicillin trihydrate or ceftiofur hydrochloride for treatment of metritis and subsequent fertility in dairy cows. J Dairy Sci. 2014;97:5401–14.
31. Shwartz G, Hill KL, VanBaale MJ, Baumgard LH. Effects of flunixin meglumine on pyrexia and bioenergetic variables in postparturient dairy cows. J Dairy Sci. 2009;92:1963–70.
32. Knudsen LR, Karstrup CC, Pedersen HG, Angen Ø, Agerholm JS, Rasmussen EL, et al. An investigation of the microbiota in uterine flush samples and endometrial biopsies from dairy cows during the first 7 weeks postpartum. Theriogenology. 2016;86:642–50.
33. Sannmann I, Arlt S, Heuwieser W. A critical evaluation of diagnostic methods used to identify dairy cows with acute post-partum metritis in the current literature. J Dairy Res. 2012;79:436–44.
34. Teale CJ, Moulin G. Prudent use guidelines: a review of existing veterinary guidelines. Rev Sci Tech. 2012;31:343.

# 14

# Weight management in obese pets: the tailoring concept and how it can improve results

Alexander J. German*

*From* Animal Obesity – causes, consequences and comparative aspects
Uppsala, Sweden. 14-16 June 2015

**Abstract**

Obesity is now recognised as the most important medical disease in pets worldwide. All current strategies for weight management involve dietary energy restriction with a purpose-formulated diet. Whilst current weight management regimes can be successful, outcomes are often disappointing with the rate of weight loss progressively slowing down as time goes on. Success is most challenging for the most obese dogs and cats that are more likely to discontinue the programme before reaching target weight. To improve outcomes, clinicians must focus carefully on better tailoring programmes, paying particular to setting an appropriate target weight so as to maximise the benefits for the individual. In this opinionated review, the author will discuss findings from recent clinical research studies examining weight management in obese dogs and cats. A strategy for tailoring weight management targets will then be discussed, illustrated with case examples.

**Keywords:** Overweight, Dog, Cat, Dietary energy restriction, Success, Rebound

## The significance of obesity in pets

In humans, it is now agreed that obesity is a disease [1], which can predispose to the development of various other diseases (e.g. cardiovascular disease, diabetes mellitus, liver disease, respiratory disease, neoplasia, and osteoarthritis) [2–5], and increase mortality risk [6]. Most veterinarians would agree that obesity is also an important medical disease in dogs and cats [7]. Overweight cats are at increased risk of developing diabetes mellitus, neoplasia, skin disease, oral cavity disease and urinary disease [8], whilst overweight dogs can suffer from diabetes mellitus, osteoarthritis, and urinary incontinence [9]. Increased adiposity can also adversely affect respiratory function [10, 11], cause metabolic derangements including insulin resistance [12–15], and also affect renal function and health [16]. Further, dogs that are fed ad libitum are more likely to be overweight, leading to a foreshortened lifespan [17]. Therefore, a wealth of information is now available to demonstrate the adverse health effects that can arise when pet dogs and cats become overweight. However, in light of recent evidence demonstrating that obese dogs have a poorer quality of life [18], the condition also presents a major welfare challenge for veterinary surgeons.

## Overview of obesity management

Successful weight management has two main phases, weight loss and subsequent weight maintenance. During the weight loss phase, it is essential that dietary energy intake is less than energy expenditure. In the last 10 years, two licensed drugs, dirlotapide and mitratapide, were available for the weight loss phase in dogs, both of which primarily acted by reducing appetite and thereby voluntary intake [19, 20]. Despite encouraging results from clinical trials, neither drug received widespread acceptance in clinical practice and, consequently, both have been withdrawn [21, 22]. Therefore, current weight loss strategies involve dietary energy restriction using a

*Correspondence: ajgerman@liverpool.ac.uk; ajgerman@liv.ac.uk
Institute of Ageing and Chronic Disease, University of Liverpool, Leahurst Campus, Chester High Road, Neston, Wirral CH64 7TE, UK

purpose-formulated diet, usually in combination with increasing activity and thereby expenditure [23–27]. Most weight loss diets are less energy dense, with increased amounts of good quality protein and micronutrients so as to reduce the risk of nutrient deficiencies developing and preserving lean tissue mass when food is restricted. For cats, feeding a diet containing 40 % of crude protein (on an as fed basis) during weight loss results in greater loss of fat mass and greater retention of lean body tissue than feeding a diet containing 30 % crude protein [28]. Similar results demonstrating preservation of lean mass during weight loss in obese dogs when comparing high protein (48 % as fed) and moderate protein (24 % as fed) diets [29].

The most effective diets also aim to minimise signs of hunger, in order to reduce begging behaviour and improve compliance, and this is usually achieved by altering macronutrient content [30, 31]. In dogs, supplementing both protein and fibre (e.g. 32 % crude protein and 28 % total dietary fibre, as fed) in a diet is best at reducing voluntary food intake [30], and improving outcomes of weight loss [32]. The protein and fibre content of a feline weight loss diet, must be carefully controlled, so as to inhibit hunger whilst ensuring palatability and, at the same time, preserving lean body mass. Although supplementing dietary fibre decreases voluntary food intake in cats, diets become less palatable if too much fibre diets is added [33]. Further, increasing protein intake generally increases, rather than decreases voluntary food intake [33]. Therefore, diets that minimise signs of hunger, whilst preserving lean tissue and not compromising palatability, have modestly increased dietary fibre (e.g. 23 % total dietary fibre as fed) and protein (e.g. 34 % as fed) [34].

## Success feels good: the benefits of weight loss in obese pets

A mistake many veterinarians make is to focus too heavily on the 'mechanics' of a weight loss programme (i.e. calculating energy intake, diet type, rate of weight loss, estimating target weight), and pay insufficient attention to the overall aim, which is to improve the pet's quality of life, permanently. Thus, rather than worrying if weight loss is too slow, or whether the animal will ever reach its 'perfect weight', the clinician could focus on whether the animal is happier, more active, and less affected by any concurrent disease it may have (e.g. lameness, diabetes mellitus, respiratory diseases etc.). Further, success should be viewed less in terms of reaching a nominal 'perfect weight', than in permanently maintaining any weight lost, so that the health benefits of weight management are maintained. Unless bad owner habits are permanently changed (i.e. avoiding excessive treating, insufficiently exercising their pet), weight management will fail in the long run.

As described above, obesity can affect health in various ways, for instance by decreasing longevity [17], increasing the risk of other diseases developing [8, 9]. Therefore, in theory at least, a range of benefits might be expected for dogs and cats that lose weight successfully, for example longer lifespan, decreased risk of developing new diseases, improved organ function, and improvement in signs of any pre-existing disease. However, as of yet, no published studies have demonstrated that weight loss can either prevent diseases from developing or increase lifespan, possibly because such studies are difficult to perform. That said, there is good evidence that weight loss improves respiratory function [11], insulin sensitivity and other metabolic derangements [12–16], and also improves mobility in obese dogs with concurrent osteoarthritis [35, 36]. Most strikingly, force-plate analysis has demonstrated that mobility benefits begin very quickly during the weight loss process, e.g. once more than 6 % of body weight has been lost [36]. This modest amount of weight loss can readily be achieved in over 80 % of dogs that start a weight loss programme [37].

In addition to health benefits, success of weight loss should also be judged in terms of the impact on wellbeing. Recently, health-related quality of life was assessed in obese dogs before and after weight loss using a validated questionnaire [18]. When the dogs were obese, quality of life was worse than a group of control dogs in optimal body condition. However, quality of life had improved significantly after successful weight loss, with activity-related improvements being most marked. Such improvements were positively correlated with the amount of body fat lost. In summary, although there are many theoretical benefits to weight loss, those that have been clinically proven to date involve benefits in organ function, decreased severity of clinical signs from concurrent diseases, and improvements in quality of life.

## Weight loss is tough: 'real world' outcomes of weight loss in obese pets

Most studies that have assessed weight loss in obese dogs and cats have used colony animals, and protocols are invariably highly successful [19, 23, 27]. Typically, young, healthy dogs and cats are used that are often only modestly (e.g. ≤20 %) overweight. In such a setting, weight loss is predictable, usually progressing at 1–2 %/week, when energy intake is restricted to 50–75 % of maintenance energy requirements [23, 27, 29, 38]. Given such results, the vast majority of weight loss studies in colony was completed in 3–6 months. Whilst there are many advantages to undertaking colony research, the main disadvantage is that the findings cannot easily be generalised to weight loss in obese pets, where weight programmes rely on compliance from owners. It is only by examining the weight loss in clinical studies involving pet animals, that the outcomes of weight loss can be appropriately judged.

In light of this, recent studies have examined a period of weight loss in pet dogs and cats that are overweight. In both species, more marked energy restriction is usually required than in a colony and, despite this, rates of weight loss [0.5–1.0 % of starting bodyweight (SBW) per week in both species] are slower [24–26, 32, 34]. A number of factors account for the differences, such as the fact that most obese pet dogs and cats are neutered, have a variable age range, are more overweight, and commonly have concurrent disease [25]. However, the role of the owner is arguably most critical, most notably through poor compliance with veterinary advice. Indeed, self-reports of both dog and cat owners confirm that feeding extra food (such as table scraps and treats) is common, and the weight management food is not reduced to compensate [25, 26]. This suggests that, in contrast to the findings from colony studies, weight loss in obese pets is extremely challenging, especially for owners.

## Failure of weight loss programmes is common in obese dogs and cats

A number of studies have now assessed weight loss protocols in a clinical setting, but very few have examined success in terms of completion rates. This is because the majority of recent studies are short-term, typically assessing the first 2–3 months of weight loss [24, 27, 34]. Whilst these results are more representative than colony studies, and can demonstrate how successful the early stages of weight loss can be, they do not reflect performance of a complete weight loss cycle, especially in reaching target weight.

One study in dogs examined success of weight loss in terms of completing a programme [24]. Disappointingly, only 32/60 (53 %) completed the 6-month programme, and providing additional education for owners (in terms of classes discussing nutrition-related topics) did not improve compliance. A more recent study has also examined compliance with weight loss protocols in dogs [39]. A total of 143 dogs were studied, all referred to a specialist clinic for weight management, and 87 of these dogs successfully reached their target weight. There were various reasons why the remaining dogs stopped their programme prematurely: 11 (8 %) were euthanased for reasons unrelated to the obesity or stopped because another disease developed (1 dog); in other cases, the owners decided to stop, often because they had second thoughts immediately after enrolment (5 dogs, 3 %), they had struggled to comply with the requirements of the programme (3 dogs, 2 %) or for personal reasons (9, 6 %; including family illness, bereavement, and separation. The reason why the remaining 20 owners (14 %) chose to stop was unclear since they repeatedly refused to respond to any contact from veterinary staff. Multiple regression analysis demonstrated that the main factors that had the greatest effect on success were the rate of weight loss, the degree of obesity, and the type of diet fed. In this respect, rate of weight loss was faster in dogs that completed their programme than in those that stopped. With regard to degree of obesity, the fatter the dog, the less likely it was to complete, with a 15 % increase in the odds of failure for every additional percentage of excess body fat. Finally, a number of weight and dry weight loss diets were used in the study, and owner preferences were taken into account when selecting the particular diet to use. An additional study observation was that, when other factors were taken into account, dogs that had been fed dry food exclusively were significantly more likely to reach their target weight than dogs fed either wet food or a mixture wet and dry food [39].

In addition to the effect of the type of diet used during weight loss, feeding practices before weight loss could also be considered. In another study, possible effects of main meal feeding (type of food, how measured, meal frequency) and the feeding of extras (table scraps or treats) on the success of weight loss programme was assessed [40]. Most feeding practices had no significant effect; however, dietary energy intake during weight loss was less for dogs that were fed purchased snacks before weight loss, most likely because they continued to use these during the weight loss period. A final possible factor in compliance with a weight loss plan could be financial concerns. That said, cost of multiple visits to the veterinarian is unlikely to be a factor because, at least in the UK, these are usually offered free of charge provided that owners pay for the therapeutic weight loss food. Given that such diets are more expensive than standard maintenance diets, cost concerns could be a reason for an owner discontinuing if progress is slow. However, in a recent study, the average daily feeding cost during weight loss in dogs was not significantly different from the daily feeding cost before weight loss [41]. This implies that, for most dogs, the weight management regime is cost-neutral.

In a further recent study, outcomes of weight loss were assessed in cats, which demonstrated similar challenges in this species, with only 28 of 62 cats (45 %) successfully reaching target weight [42]. Again, the degree of obesity was the strongest predictor of failure (fattest cats more likely to fail). Whilst these findings may be disappointing,

85 % of pet dogs and 80 % of pet cats lose more than 6 % weight which, as stated above, would be sufficient to produce measurable health benefits [37, 42].

Therefore, current evidence suggests that approximately half of obese pets that start a weight loss protocol successfully reach their target weight. Perhaps even more disappointing is that fact that many animals subsequently regain weight. For example, in one recent study examining long-term follow up after weight loss protocol in obese dogs, 16 of 42 (48 %) regained some weight [43]. The main risk factor for regain was if the diet was if owners switched back to a standard adult maintenance food during weight loss, rather than continuing with the purpose-formulated weight management diet. In a separate canine study, faster rates weight loss led to more rapid rebound subsequently [38]. Rebound has also been demonstrated in after weight loss in cats, with 12 of 26 cats (46 %) regaining some weight [44]. These studies highlight the fact that weight management is a lifelong process with clinicians needing to continue to monitor body weight after ideal weight has been achieved.

## The law of diminishing returns

As discussed above, weight loss can have many benefits, but the process is challenging, and failure is common. However, a number of studies have suggested that outcomes vary depending upon the stage of the weight management process. Three examples will be discussed, namely changes in body composition, rate and energy intake during weight loss, and overall compliance.

### Changes in body composition during weight loss

Most studies assessing changes in body composition during weight loss in dogs and cats have been undertaken in a colony setting, and often suggest that lean mass is preserved [27, 45]. However, as discussed above, these studies generally examine modest amounts of weight loss (e.g. <20 %), and pets are usually more markedly obese. When a complete weight loss cycle is examined (i.e. restoring ideal weight) in obese pet animals, significant lean tissue loss is seen [25, 26, 32, 39]. The reason such results differ from colony studies is most likely due to the greater degrees of weight loss that are needed. Various factors are associated with lean tissue loss in obese animals during weight management, including rate of weight loss [46], decreased plasma adiponectin [15], and increased plasma clusterin [16]. However, the factor that appears to have greatest influence on how much lean tissue is lost is the overall amount of weight lost [25, 26]. These studies demonstrate that significant lean tissue loss only really occurs when dogs lose more than 20 % of their starting body weight.

### Rate of weight loss and energy intake during a complete weight loss protocol

Recent studies in both dogs and cats have examined rates and energy intake at different stages of a weight loss protocol reported a range of outcomes at key stages during a complete weight loss cycle [35, 39]. In the first 28 days of a weight loss protocol, the median rate of weight loss was 1.2 % body weight per week (BW/wk) in dogs [37] and 0.8 % BW/wk in cats [42]. Thereafter, weight loss rapidly slows in both species such that, after 12 months, median rate is <0.3 %/week in both species [37, 42]. This slowing down of the rate of weight loss occurs despite the energy intake being gradually reduced during the weight programme, by 10–20 % in both species.

### Compliance at different stages of a weight loss protocol

Compliance has also been assessed at different stages of the weight loss cycle in dogs and cats. Early on, compliance is good in both species, with 86 % of dogs and 82 % of cats remaining on the weight loss programme in the first 12 weeks. During this time, dogs and cats will have lost an average of 12 and 8 % of their starting body weight, respectively. Compliance progressively decreases so that, by 48 weeks, only 27 and 32 % of dogs and cats, respectively, are persisting with the programme.

### Summary

Based upon the published research, weight loss in obese pets is a clear example of diminishing returns, whereby the more weight that must be lost, the more difficult it is. Clinicians must accept the fact that failure is common, especially for the most obese animals. Whilst current weight loss strategies are not perfect, there are ways that veterinarians can get the best out of them, and ensure the greatest benefit to quality of life in patients under their care.

## Tailoring weight management protocols: the key to improving success

The research described above has emphasised a number of key aspects of current weight management strategies, which are summarised as follows:

### Successful weight loss has measurable health and welfare benefits when an obese dog loses weight

As described above, clinically proven benefits of successful weight loss include improved respiratory function [11], improved insulin sensitivity [12–15], improved mobility where there is concurrent orthopaedic disease [35, 36], and improved quality of life [18]. Other benefits are possible, including longer lifespan and disease prevention, although these have not yet been proven.

#### Weight management protocols are difficult and many animals fail

In contrast to the results of colony studies, weight loss in obese pets is extremely challenging, requiring marked energy restriction. Rates of weight loss decline steadily over a weight loss cycle, which can be frustrating for the owner and may lead to poor compliance, leading to feeding of extra food or withdrawal.

#### Lean tissue loss is common when obese animals lose significant amounts of weight loss

In the early stages of weight loss, lean tissue mass is preserved. Progressively increased lean tissue loss occurs once dogs and cats have lost more than 20 % of their body weight.

#### Failure is common on current weight loss strategies

Approximately half of obese pet dogs and cats successfully reach their target weight during weight loss, and about half of these subsequently regain some weight. Compliance gradually worsens during a weight loss cycle in both dogs and cats, being good (>80 %) in early stages, but the rate of withdrawal gradually increases thereafter. Not surprisingly, dogs and cats with the most weight to lose are those that are the least likely to succeed.

#### Most dogs lose some weight, even if they do not reach target

Although many dogs and cats are unsuccessful, the majority will lose some weight in the early stages, with at least 80 % losing >6 % weight, the cut-off for improvements in health in one study [36].

Faced with the current reality, clinicians should aim to maximise success by better *tailoring each weight management regime* to the individual animal. Case examples demonstrating how to tailor weight loss are provided in the online supporting information. Attention should be paid to considering what the key priorities for weight management are for the case, such that the most appropriate target weight is set which will maximise the benefit, whilst at the same time minimising the chance of failure. Two opposing strategies for setting target weight will be described, along with benefits and pitfalls. However, in reality, they represent opposite ends of a spectrum for decision making, which are highlighted by the case examples (Additional file 1: S1–S4).

#### Complete weight loss

As the name suggests, the aim *complete weight loss* is to return the animal to its ideal weight, namely a weight whereby body composition is optimal. By reducing adipose tissue mass to this degree, the benefits to health are likely to be maximal. Indeed, the degree of improvement in quality of life is proportional to the amount of body fat lost in obese dogs. Although not yet proven, it might be that complete weight loss will extend lifespan and also prevent other diseases from developing. Such an approach would be most beneficial for young dogs, since their remaining lifespan is likely to be long, effects on organ function will have been short-lived, and associated diseases they are unlikely to have developed yet. Of course, the main disadvantage of attempting complete weight loss is the fact that the overall likelihood of failure is greater, and rebound would be expected.

#### Partial weight loss

The philosophy of *partial weight loss* is for the clinician deliberately to set a target weight, which is above an animal's ideal weight. Thus, rather than striving for the 'perfect weight', the aim is to achieve enough weight loss that quality of life is improved. As mentioned above, even very modest amounts of weight loss (e.g. ≥6 %) are sufficient to alleviate signs of concurrent disease such as osteoarthritis [36]. The main advantage is that such programmes can be relatively quick (2–3 months) and most animals are likely to succeed. The main disadvantages of such a programme is that patients are still likely to be overweight, so there may any benefits on lifespan or disease prevention will be less pronounced. For that reason, this strategy would mainly be used in older animals or for those who already have pre-existing diseases.

A final advantage of partial weight loss is the fact that, if the animals successfully reaches their target, and provided the owner remains committed, a second target weight could then be set. Thus, weight loss could progress in a series of stages, to a point whereby benefits have been maximised but not at the expense of owner compromise.

## Conclusions

Obesity is a major health concern both in pet cats and dogs, and successful weight management brings many benefits. However, the weight loss process is extremely challenging, especially for the most obese animals. Clinicians can get the best out of currently available weight loss strategies by better tailoring the weight loss programme to the individual, most notably by setting a realistic target weight. Returning an obese animal to its ideal weight is not always possible, and may not actually be essential to achieve the desired benefits to health and quality of life.

**Acknowledgements**
The author wishes to thank Shelley Holden for her assistance with the clinical research that underpins this review.

**Competing interests**
The author's academic post at the University of Liverpool is financially supported by Royal Canin. Royal Canin have also supported the author's clinical research into pet obesity. Finally, the author has also received financial remuneration and gifts for providing educational material, speaking at conferences, and consultancy work from various companies including Royal Canin, WALTHAM, Hill's Pet Nutrition, Purina, and Zoetis.

**Declaration**
Publication charges for this article were funded by the research platform Future Animal Health and Welfare at the Swedish University of Agricultural Sciences.

**References**

1. Kopelman PG. Obesity as a medical problem. Nature. 2000;404:635–43.
2. Reisin E, Alpert MA. Definition of the metabolic syndrome: current proposals and controversies. Am J Med Sci. 2005;330:269–72.
3. Shaw DI, Hall WL, Williams CM. Metabolic syndrome: what is it and what are the implications? Proc Nutr Soc. 2005;64:349–57.
4. Marchesini G, Moscatiello S, Di Domizio S, Forlani G. Obesity-associated liver disease. J Clin Endocrinol Metab. 2008;93:s74–8.
5. Calle EE, Thun MJ. Obesity and cancer. Oncogene. 2004;23:6365–78.
6. Adams KF, Arthur Schatzkin A, Harris TB. Overweight, obesity, and mortality in a large prospective cohort of persons 50 to 71 years old. New Engl J Med. 2006;355:763–78.
7. German AJ. The growing problem of obesity in dogs and cats. J Nutr. 2006;136:1940–1946S.
8. Lund EM, Armstrong PJ, Kirk CA, Klausner J. Prevalence and risk factors for obesity in adult cats from private US veterinary practices. Int J Appl Res Vet Med. 2005;3:88–96.
9. Lund EM, Armstrong PJ, Kirk CA, Klausner J. Prevalence and risk factors for obesity in adult dogs from private US veterinary practices. Int J Appl Res Vet Med. 2006;4:177–86.
10. Bach JF, Rozanski EA, Bedenice D, Chan DL, Freeman LM, Lofgren JL, et al. Association of expiratory airway dysfunction with marked obesity in healthy adult dogs. Am J Vet Res. 2007;68:670–5.
11. Mosing M, German AJ, Holden SL, MacFarlane P, Biourge V, Morris PJ, et al. Oxygenation and ventilation characteristics in obese sedated dogs before and after weight loss: a clinical trial. Vet J. 2013;198:367–71.
12. German AJ, Ryan VH, German AC, Wood IS, Trayhurn P. Obesity, its associated disorders and the role of inflammatory adipokines in companion animals. Vet J. 2010;185:4–9.
13. German AJ, Hervera M, Hunter L, Holden SL, Morris PJ, Biourge V, et al. Improvement in insulin resistance and reduction in plasma inflammatory adipokines after weight loss in obese dogs. Domest Anim Endocrinol. 2009;37:214–26.
14. Tvarijonaviciute A, Ceron JJ, Holden SL, Cuthbertson DJ, Biourge V, Morris PJ, et al. Obesity-related metabolic dysfunction in dogs: a comparison with human metabolic syndrome. BMC Vet Res. 2012;8:147. doi:10.1186/1746-6148-8-147.
15. Tvarijonaviciute A, Ceron JJ, Holden SL, et al. Effects of weight loss in obese cats on biochemical analytes related to inflammation and glucose homeostasis. Domest Anim Endocrinol. 2012;42:129–41.
16. Tvarijonaviciute A, Ceron JJ, Holden SL, Morris PJ, Biourge V, German AJ. Effect of weight loss in obese dogs on indicators of renal function or disease. J Vet Intern Med. 2013;27:31–8.
17. Kealy RD, Lawler DF, Ballam JM, Mantz SJ, Biery DN, Greeley EH, et al. Effects of diet restriction on life span and age-related changes in dogs. J Am Vet Med Assoc. 2002;220:1315–20.
18. German AJ, Holden SL, Wiseman-Orr ML, Reid J, Nolan AM, Biourge V, et al. Quality of life is reduced in obese dogs but improves after successful weight loss. Vet J. 2012;192:428–34.
19. Gossellin J, Peachey S, Sherington J, Rowan TJ, Sutherland SJ. Evaluation of dirlotapide for sustained weight loss in overweight Labrador retrievers. J Vet Pharmacol Ther. 2007;30:55–65.
20. Pena C, Suarez L, Bautista-Castano I, Juste MJ, Carreton E, Montoya-Alonso JA. Effects of low-fat high-fibre diet and mitratapide on body weight reduction, blood pressure, and metabolic parameters in obese dogs. J Vet Med Sci. 2014;76:1305–8.
21. European Medicines Agency. Yarvitan; mirtratapide. http://www.ema.europa.eu/ema/index.jsp?curl=pages/medicines/veterinary/medicines/000113/vet_med_000196.jsp&mid=WC0b01ac058008d7a8. Accessed 27 Sep 2015.
22. European Medicines Agency. Slentrol; dirlotapide. http://www.ema.europa.eu/ema/index.jsp?curl=pages/medicines/veterinary/medicines/000116/vet_med_000186.jsp&mid=WC0b01ac058008d7a8. Accessed 27 Sep 2015.
23. Blanchard G, Nguyen P, Gayet C, Leriche I, Siliart B, Paragon BM. Rapid weight loss with a high-protein low energy diet allows the recovery of ideal body composition and insulin sensitivity in obese dogs. J Nutr. 2004;134:2148–2150S.
24. Yaissle JE, Holloway C, Buffington CA. Evaluation of owner education as a component of obesity treatment programs for dogs. J Am Vet Med Assoc. 2004;224:1932–5.
25. German AJ, Holden SL, Bissot T, Hackett RM, Biourge V. Dietary energy restriction and successful weight loss in obese client-owned dogs. J Vet Intern Med. 2007;21:1174–80.
26. German AJ, Holden SL, Bissot T, Morris PJ, Biourge V. Changes in body composition during weight loss in obese client-owned cats: loss of lean tissue mass correlates with overall percentage of weight lost. J Feline Med Surg. 2010;10:452–9.
27. Floerchinger AM, Jackson MI, Jewell DE, MacLeay JM, Pateau-Robinson I, Hahn KA. Effect of feeding a weight loss food beyond a caloric restriction period on body composition and resistance to weight gain in dogs. J Am Vet Med Assoc. 2015;247:375–84.
28. Laflamme DP, Hannah SS. Increased dietary protein promotes fat loss and reduces loss of lean body mass during weight loss in cats. Int J Appl Res Vet Med. 2005;3:62–8.
29. Diez M, Nguyen P, Jeusette I, Devois C, Istasse L, Biourge V. Weight loss in obese dogs: evaluation of a high-protein, low-carbohydrate diet. J Nutr. 2002;132:1685–1687S.
30. Weber M, Bissot T, Servet E, Sergheraert R, Bioruge V, German AJ. A high protein, high fiber diet designed for weight loss improves satiety in dogs. J Vet Intern Med. 2007;21:1203–8.
31. Borne AT, Wolfsheimer KJ, Truett AA, Kiene J, Wojciechowhski T, Davenport DJ, et al. Differential metabolic effects of energy restriction in dogs using diets varying in fat and fiber content. Obes Res. 1996;4:337–45.
32. German AJ, Holden SL, Bissot T, Morris PJ, Biourge V. A high protein high fibre diet improves weight loss in obese dogs. Vet J. 2010;183:294–7.
33. Servet E, Soulard Y, Venet C, Biourge V, German AJ. Ability of diets to generate 'satiety' in cats. J Vet Int Med. 2008;22:1482.
34. Bissot T, Servet E, Vidal S, Deboise M, Sergheraert R, Egron G, et al. Novel dietary strategies can improve the outcome of weight loss programmes in obese client-owned cats. J Feline Med Surg. 2010;12:104–12.
35. Mlacnik E, Bockstahler BA, Müller M, Tetrick MA, Nap RC, Zentek J. Effects of caloric restriction and a moderate or intense physiotherapy program for treatment of lameness in overweight dogs with osteoarthritis. J Am Vet Med Assoc. 2006;229:1756–60.
36. Marshall WG, Hazelwinkel HAW, Mullen D, De Meyer G, Baert K, Carmichael S. The effect of weight loss on lameness in obese dogs with osteoarthritis. Vet Res Commun. 2010;34:241–53.
37. Deagle G, Holden SL, Biourge V, Queau Y, German AJ. The kinetics of weight loss in obese client owned dogs. J Vet Intern Med. 2015;29:443–4.
38. Laflamme DP, Kuhlman G. The effect of weight-loss regimen on subsequent weight maintenance in dogs. Nutr Res. 1995;15:1019–28.
39. German AJ, Titcomb J, Holden SL, Queau Y, Morris PJ, Biourge V, et al. Cohort study of the success of controlled weight loss programs for obese dogs. J Vet Intern Med. 2015;29:1547–55. doi:10.1111/jvim.13629.
40. German AJ, Holden SL, Gernon LJ, Morris PJ, Biourge V, German AJ. Do feeding practices of obese dogs, before weight loss, affect the success of weight management? Br J Nutr. 2011;106:S97–100.
41. German AJ, Luxmore J, Holden SL, Morris PJ, Biourge V. Feeding obese dogs during weight loss is on average cost-neutral. J Small Anim Pract. 2015;56:366–9.

# 15

# Occurrence of cardiorespiratory diseases and impact on lifespan in Swedish Irish Wolfhounds

Lovisa Orleifson[1], Ingrid Ljungvall[1], Katja Höglund[2] and Jens Häggström[1*]

**Abstract**

**Background:** According to Swedish animal insurance data, Irish Wolfhounds (IW) are 29 times more likely to die from cardiac causes than the baseline breed. Dilated cardiomyopathy (DCM) has a high prevalence in the breed and the disease has been shown to be hereditary in IW. Few studies address respiratory diseases in IW, but reports suggest that the incidence of pneumonia is high. Respiratory diseases are reported as a common cause of death in the breed along with cardiac, neoplastic, musculoskeletal and gastrointestinal diseases. The aim of this study was to investigate mortality, morbidity and lifespan in Swedish IW through a questionnaire-based study. Focus was on DCM and pneumonia and potential association between these diseases. Questionnaires were sent to owners of purebred IW registered in the Swedish Kennel Club, born during 2006–2008. Owners were asked for information concerning occurrence of disease, results of clinical examinations, treatments, cause and date of death.

**Results:** Overall response rate was 38% (105 completed questionnaires). Median lifespan was 2720 days (7.5 years). Males had shorter lifespan than females (median 2523 and 2836 days, respectively), $P = 0.02$. The most common causes of death were neoplastic disease (24%), cardiac disease (18%) and respiratory disease (16%). The percentage of dogs with pneumonia on at least one occasion during their lifetime was 37%, with a majority experiencing recurrent episodes (53%). The median lifespan was shorter for dogs affected by pneumonia on at least one occasion (2629 days), compared to dogs without history of pneumonia (2804 days) ($P = 0.04$), whereas the lifespan did not differ between dogs with or without a diagnosis of DCM. No sex predisposition was found regarding DCM or pneumonia.

**Conclusions:** This study showed that DCM and pneumonia are common conditions in IW in Sweden, and that dogs affected by pneumonia have a shorter lifespan than those without history of pneumonia. Considering the results from this study and previous studies regarding these diagnoses in IW; cardiac and respiratory disease should be given further attention in the course of improving the general health of the breed.

**Keywords:** Dilated cardiomyopathy, Irish Wolfhound, Lifespan, Mortality, Pneumonia

## Background

Irish Wolfhounds (IW) have an increased mortality because of neoplastic, musculoskeletal, gastrointestinal, cardiovascular and respiratory disorders [1–3]. Based on Swedish insurance data, the breed had the highest probability of death by 8 and 10 years of age, compared to all other breeds in the insurance database, which included over 350,000 insured Swedish dogs [1]. Indeed, the probability of death by 10 years of age was as high as 91% in IW. The median and mean age at time of death for IW studied in Great Britain and Norway were 6.2 and 7 years, respectively [2, 4].

*Correspondence: jens.haggstrom@slu.se
[1] Department of Clinical Sciences, Faculty of Veterinary Medicine, Swedish University of Agricultural Sciences, Uppsala, Sweden

According to Swedish insurance data, IW were 29 times more likely to die from cardiac disorders, compared to the baseline breeds defined as and including all breeds, except 10 high risk breeds and the 10 most common breeds [1]. Dilated cardiomyopathy (DCM) is a common disease in European IW [5, 6] and is characterized by uni- or bilateral cardiac dilation and reduced systolic function [7]. Generally, DCM in dogs progresses quickly and overall prognosis is poor [8]. However, a difference in progression rate between breeds has been shown [9–11]. Swedish insurance data has shown that median age at death in IW with cardiac disease was 7.5 years [12]. In European studies, the prevalence of DCM among IW has been found to be 24–43% [5, 6, 13], where mean age at diagnosis was 4.2–4.9 years [5, 6, 14]. Genetic factors have been shown to influence the development of DCM in several breeds [10, 15, 16]. Regarding mode of inheritance in IW, a major gene model with a sex-dependent allele effect has been suggested [6], and another study suggested that multiple loci were potentially associated with DCM in this breed [14].

Few reports regarding respiratory diseases in IW are available, but, anecdotally, IW are considered more frequently affected by pneumonias than most other breeds. In a recent study, determining the incidence of pneumonia in dogs admitted to a veterinary hospital, IW had the highest incidence of all breeds [17]. A study describing rhinitis and pneumonia in the breed showed that the majority of affected dogs had clinical signs present since birth [18]. Pedigree analysis revealed that ancestors were shared, which according to the authors, suggested a heritable syndrome. Primary ciliary dyskinesia or primary immunodeficiency were not detected among the affected dogs and signs of cardiac disease were also absent. Rhinitis and pneumonia in IW was early described by Wilkinson [19] who rather suggested the etiology to be a viral infection with secondary bacterial invasion due to the condition being well distributed throughout the breed.

Although insurance data are a valuable source of information to evaluate morbidity and causes of death in specific dog breeds, the resolution of the information is limited and the database does not include old dogs. The aim of this study was, therefore, to investigate mortality, morbidity and lifespan in Swedish IW through a questionnaire-based study, with special focus on DCM and pneumonia and potential associations between the diseases, using the Swedish Kennel Club (SKK) registration database as source of dog and owner related information.

## Methods

### Study design

This retrospective study was performed by distributing a questionnaire (Additional file 1: Questionnaire) to owners of purebred IW born between January 1st 2006 and December 31st 2008 registered in the SKK (460 dogs). The questionnaire was sent by mail to all owners with an address available in the SKK register (n = 280) and since several dogs shared the same owner 280 questionnaires were sent to 232 owners. Recipients that had not responded within the stipulated time received one reminder. Information about the study and reminding notices were published at the webpage and the Facebook page of the Swedish Irish Wolfhound Club. The questionnaire was referred to as a health evaluation of Swedish IW and owners with healthy dogs as well as sick dogs were encouraged to answer.

The questionnaire was divided into three sections, where the first, which was for everyone to answer, covered general information such as sex, identification number, neutering status, weight, coat color, breeding history and the owners contact information. The second section was for dogs that were dead, and the third section for dogs that were still alive. The second section contained questions about cause of death, divided into different main classes, date of death, potential history of DCM or pneumonia, clinical signs observed by the owner and if a post mortem examination had been performed. Questions also concerned medical treatment for DCM and if pneumonias were recurrent. In the third section, there were questions concerning history of DCM or pneumonia, clinical signs observed by the owner and more specific questions whether heart and thorax of the dog had been examined by a veterinarian, and if the dog was subject to ongoing medical treatment as well as if potential pneumonias were recurrent. For all dogs, questions were also asked if known relatives were affected by DCM or pneumonia. In this study, relatives were defined as mother, father, siblings and offspring. The information from the questionnaires was treated confidentially and permission was asked for access to veterinary records if considered required.

### Data management

Complete and correct birth date, as well as sex and coat color, were verified for each dog by use of the SKK register. For owners that had not reported date of death as an exact date, but as a month or a year, date of death was set to the middle of the reported period. Deceased dogs with no information of date of death were excluded from the survival analyses.

Information about clinical signs and results from examinations, that were associated with cardiac disease, were evaluated to determine whether the evidence was sufficiently strong to allow a diagnosis of DCM or not: dogs, for which the owner had reported DCM and/or the diagnosis of DCM had been established by echocardiographic examinations, or a post mortem examination, were classified as DCM. Dogs with other abnormal findings, such as atrial fibrillation, low intensity heart murmur, and/or having developed congestive heart failure (CHF) were classified as "probably" DCM. Dogs diagnosed with CHF at time of euthanasia, but not having undergone more detailed diagnostic procedures, with no prior clinical signs of cardiac disease, were classified as "suspicion of DCM". Dogs with DCM, with suspicion of DCM and those probably affected were all later included when calculating occurrence and lifespan regarding DCM.

### Statistical analyses

The statistical analyses were performed using a commercially available statistical software program (JMP Pro v. 11.2.0, Cary, NC, USA). Level of statistical significance was set at $P < 0.05$. Descriptive statistics were used for dog characteristics, causes of death and occurrence of diagnoses such as DCM and pneumonia. If owners had reported multiple causes of death for one dog, the dog was included in each subgroup in the statistical analysis. Data concerning dogs from the same owner was not clustered in the statistical analysis.

Fisher's exact test was used to test for differences in occurrence of DCM and pneumonia between sexes. Kaplan–Meier curves were generated and the Log Rank test was used to test for difference in lifespan between subgroups in the study population. Lifespan for dogs that were still alive at the time of this study were right censored. Lifespan was reported as median and interquartile range for the whole study population and for subgroups. Multivariable Cox proportional hazard analysis was used to investigate the effect of sex and diagnosis on outcome and for calculating the hazard ratio, variables included in these models were sex and occurrence of pneumonia on at least one occasion, and sex and diagnosis of DCM, respectively.

## Results

Of the 280 distributed questionnaires, 105 were completed and returned by mail to the Swedish University of Agricultural Sciences (SLU). Four letters were undelivered and returned to SLU because of incorrect contact details. This resulted in a total response rate of 38%. In total, 90 owners participated in the study; 80 owners returned one questionnaire, eight owners returned two questionnaires and two owners returned completed questionnaires for three and six dogs each. Not all owners answered all the questions in the questionnaire, resulting in varying response rates for different variables. Case records were retrieved from clinics in eight dogs. The final study population consisted of 52 males and 53 females. Summary statistics for the dogs included in the study are presented in Table 1.

### Causes of death

Of the 105 dogs included in the study, 76 dogs were dead. Two of them had undergone a post mortem examination. Thirteen owners had reported multiple causes of death for their dog, which all were accounted for in the statistical analysis. The most common causes of death were neoplasia, cardiac disease and respiratory disease (Fig. 1). Neoplasia accounted for 24% of the cases of death, where osteosarcoma represented 9% and remaining 15% was neoplasia of unspecified type. Dogs having cardiac disease as cause of death included dogs classified to have DCM (17%) and unspecified cardiac disease (1%). All dogs with respiratory disease as cause of death had pneumonia. Remaining causes of death included a variety of diseases, namely gastric dilation volvulus (6.6%), megaesophagus (3.3%), paresis (3.3%), epilepsy (2.2%), pyometra (2.2%), kidney disease (2.2%), lethargy (2.2%), osteomyelitis or septic arthritis (2.2%) and 1.1% for the following causes; diabetes mellitus, traffic accident, intoxication, behavioral problems, stiffness of the neck, skeletal pain and old age.

Of the deceased dogs, all but five dogs had been euthanized. The remaining five dogs had died suddenly, which result in a sudden death rate of 7%. One of these dogs had undergone a post mortem examination, and was diagnosed with acute circulatory failure with a strong suspicion of DCM. Another dog experiencing sudden death was diagnosed with DCM prior to sudden death, and for

**Table 1 Dog characteristics, number of dogs with dilated cardiomyopathy (DCM) and pneumonia in Irish Wolfhounds born 2006–2008**

| Group | 2006 | 2007 | 2008 |
|---|---|---|---|
| Number of dogs | 45 | 39 | 21 |
| Response rate | 41% | 40% | 30% |
| Alive/dead | 9/36 (45) | 11/28 (39) | 9/12 (21) |
| Sex, male/female | 24/21 (45) | 19/20 (39) | 9/12 (21) |
| Mean weight (kg) | 68 (37) | 67 (36) | 68 (19) |
| Neutered | 4 (39) | 8 (36) | 5 (20) |
| Coat color, B/RB/DB/F/W/Bl | 28/1/0/3/6/7 (45) | 27/2/1/4/3/2 (39) | 16/0/1/1/1/2 (21) |
| Number with offspring | 7 (45) | 6 (38) | 5 (20) |
| DCM | 9 (45) | 7 (39) | 2 (21) |
| Pneumonia | 14 (38) | 14 (36) | 6 (19) |

Total number of values for each specific category is presented in parenthesis. Dogs that had been diagnosed with both DCM and pneumonia appear in both disease groups

Annual response rates; 2006: 45 answers from 109 distributed questionnaires; 2007: 39 answers from 98 distributed questionnaires; 2008: 21 answers from 69 distributed questionnaires

*B* coat color brindle, *RB* red brindle, *DB* dark brindle, *F* fawn, *W* wheaten, *Bl* black

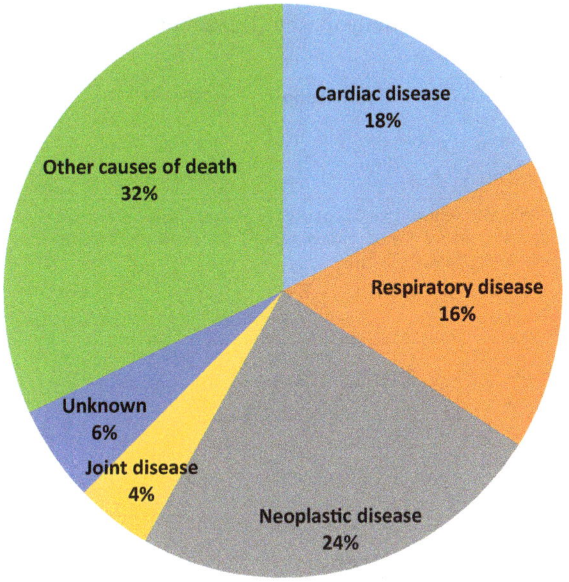


**Fig. 1** Proportional mortality for the 76 dead Irish Wolfhounds

the remaining dogs the owners suspected gastric dilation volvulus in one case, and no specific disease was suspected as cause of death in the remaining two dogs.

### Dilated cardiomyopathy

Overall the owner-reported frequency of DCM in the study was 17% (18 dogs). For a majority of these dogs (n = 14), owners had declared their dog to be diagnosed with DCM, and for two dogs the diagnosis were also confirmed by post mortem examination. The remaining dogs (n = 4) were classified as probably affected by DCM (n = 2), or with a strong suspicion of DCM (n = 2). The proportion of dogs affected by DCM among males was 21% and among females 13%, but no statistical difference between sexes was found (P = 0.31).

### Pneumonia

The proportion of dogs with owners responding that the dog had pneumonia on at least one occasion was 37% (n = 34). The response for this question included 93 answers. The proportion of male and female dogs with at least one episode of pneumonia was 37 and 36%, respectively. There was no significant difference in proportions of dogs with a history of pneumonia between sexes (P = 1.00).

Among dogs with a history of pneumonia, all 34 owners had answered the question regarding recurrence. Eighteen dogs (53%) had recurrent episodes of pneumonia and 11 of them had developed pneumonia three times or more, and two dogs were reported to have developed pneumonia 14 times during their lifetimes.

In the 34 dogs with at least one episode of pneumonia, 15% (n = 5) had also been diagnosed with DCM, and for one of these dogs, the owner had reported the dog to have developed pneumonia 14 times during its lifetime. In three of the 34 dogs, the owners had also reported megaesophagus as a concurrent disease. Two of these dogs had been diagnosed with megaesophagus by radiographic examination, but no information was provided how the diagnosis was established in the third dog. Of the 28 deceased dogs with at least one episode of pneumonia, 50% had pneumonia reported as a cause of death.

### Lifespan

The median lifespan in IW participating in this study is presented in Table 2. Kaplan–Meier survival curves for male and female dogs are presented in Fig. 2, showing that males had a shorter lifespan than females (P = 0.02). Kaplan–Meier survival curves for dogs with and without DCM are shown in Fig. 3, (P = 0.64). The effect of sex on survival was maintained in the multivariable Cox proportional hazard analysis (P = 0.02), which included sex and DCM diagnosis (yes/no). The latter variable remained insignificant on the outcome. Hazard ratios for the variables in the multivariable Cox proportional hazard analysis are presented in Table 3.

The impact of a diagnosis of pneumonia on survival is shown in Fig. 4. Dogs with history of pneumonia on at least one occasion had shorter lifespan compared to those without history of pneumonia (P = 0.04), and this difference remained significant in the multivariable Cox proportional hazard analysis (P = 0.03), which included the variables sex and occurrence of pneumonia in the model. The effect of sex was maintained (P = 0.03) in this model. Hazard ratios for these variables are presented in Table 4.

**Table 2 Median lifespan and interquartile range in days for the entire study population and subgroups**

| Group | Median lifespan | Interquartile range | Number of responses |
|---|---|---|---|
| Deceased dogs | 2477 | 792 | 73 |
| Entire study population[a] | 2720 | 1014 | 101 |
| Males[a] | 2523 | 1238 | 50 |
| Females[a] | 2836 | 890 | 51 |
| DCM[a] | 2699 | 694 | 18 |
| No DCM[a] | 2720 | 1023 | 83 |
| Pneumonia[a] | 2629 | 790 | 34 |
| No pneumonia[a] | 2804 | 985 | 56 |

Dead dogs, in which no date of death was reported; were excluded, as were dogs in the no pneumonia subgroup, if the owner had not provided an answer regarding occurrence of pneumonia

*DCM* dilated cardiomyopathy

[a] Right censored data included

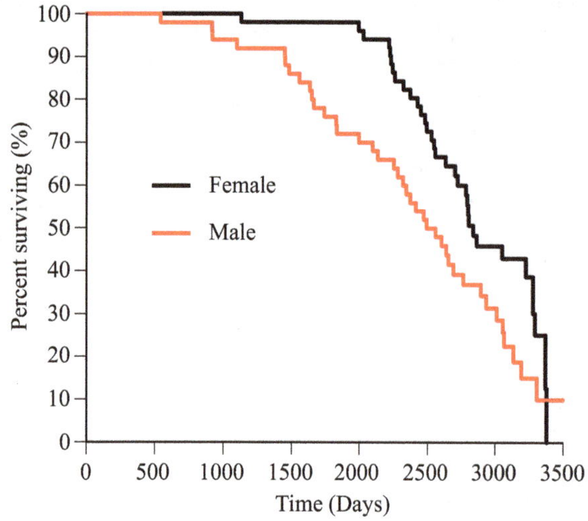


**Fig. 2** Gender-based survival in 101 Irish Wolfhounds. Kaplan–Meier curves for dogs divided into groups based on sex. Males had significantly shorter lifespan than females ($P < 0.05$). Right censored data was included and four dead dogs were excluded because no date of death was reported

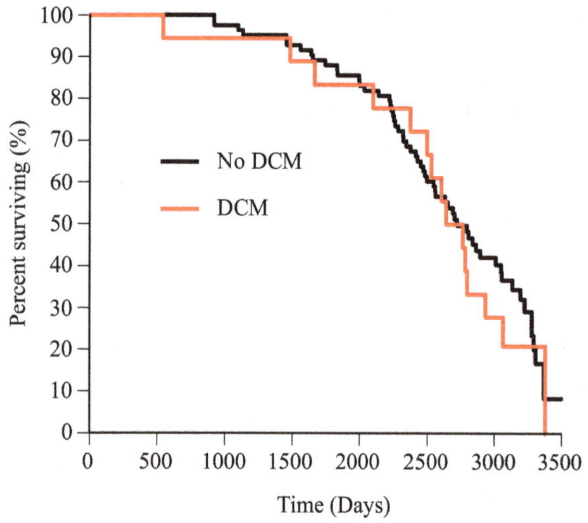


**Fig. 3** Survival in 18 Irish Wolfhounds with dilated cardiomyopathy (DCM) and in dogs without DCM ($n = 83$). Kaplan–Meier curves for dogs divided into subgroups with or without a diagnosis of DCM. The difference in lifespan was not significant. Right censored data was included and four dead dogs were excluded because no date of death was reported

**Table 3 Hazard ratios for the variables sex and a diagnosis of dilated cardiomyopathy (DCM) in the multivariable analysis**

| Variable | Hazard ratio | 95% CI | P value |
|---|---|---|---|
| Male (yes/no) | 1.73 | 1.08–2.77 | 0.02 |
| DCM (yes/no) | 1.17 | 0.64–2.01 | 0.60 |

Result from the multivariable Cox proportional hazard analysis with the variables sex and a diagnosis of dilated cardiomyopathy (DCM), with 95% confidence intervals (95% CI) and P values

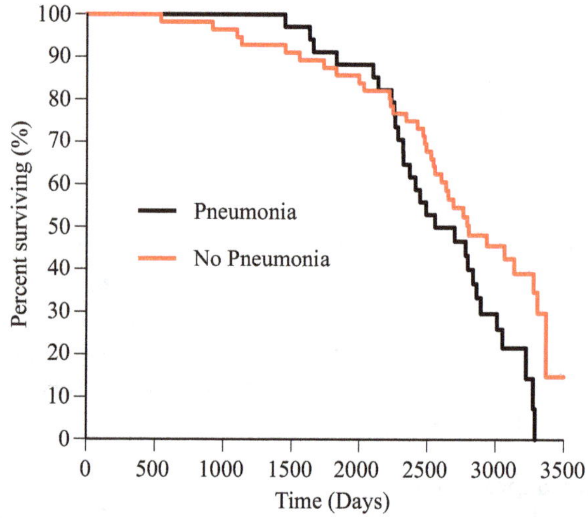


**Fig. 4** Survival in 34 Irish Wolfhounds with history of pneumonia and in dogs ($n = 56$) without a history of pneumonia. Kaplan–Meier curves for dogs divided into subgroups with a history of pneumonia diagnosed at least on one occasion and those without history of pneumonia. The difference in lifespan was statistically significant ($P < 0.05$). Right censored data was included. Four dead dogs were excluded because no date of death was reported and additional 11 dogs were excluded because the owner had not provided an answer regarding occurrence of pneumonia

**Table 4 Hazard ratios for the variables sex and a diagnosis of pneumonia in the multivariable analysis**

| Variable | Hazard ratio | 95% CI | P value |
|---|---|---|---|
| Male (yes/no) | 1.74 | 1.05–2.90 | 0.03 |
| Pneumonia (yes/no) | 1.81 | 1.07–3.03 | 0.03 |

Result from the multivariable Cox proportional hazard analysis with the variables sex and a diagnosis of pneumonia on at least one occasion, with 95% confidence intervals (95% CI) and P values

## Discussion

In this study, we found a high proportion (37%) of pneumonia among the IW and a significant shorter lifespan in dogs affected by pneumonia, the latter has not previously been reported. Most common causes of death among IWs were neoplastic and cardiac diseases along with respiratory disease. The study also showed that females lived longer than males and that the proportion of DCM reported by the owners was high (17%), but the effect of DCM on lifespan was not significant.

**Cause of death**

Results from this study, showing neoplastic and cardiac disease to be the most common causes of death, are supported by previous studies based on Swedish insurance data [1, 20], where the breed was found to have an increased mortality rate for cardiac- and neoplastic disease. In the present study, we found a high proportion of deaths due to pneumonia, which is in agreement with a study by Fleming et al. [3] who reported respiratory disease to be the top four most common causes of death in North American IW.

Neoplastic disease was not the main focus of the present study, but was the most common cause of death and other studies have also reported neoplastic disease to be over-represented as cause of death in the breed [2, 3]. In the present study osteosarcoma accounted for a large portion of all neoplastic diseases, and other studies have also shown bone neoplasia to have an increased incidence rate in the breed [4, 21]. Furthermore, musculoskeletal disorders have previously been reported as a common cause of death in IW [1, 3]. In the study by Egenvall et al. [1], osteosarcoma was not included in musculoskeletal diseases, but in the study by Fleming et al. [3] musculoskeletal diseases included all diseases localized to the specific organ system which allowed neoplasias, such as osteosarcoma, to be included. In the present study, joint disease only accounted for 4% of deaths, which is a low proportion compared to previous studies [3, 20]. However, some owners reported other causes of death, which cannot with certainty be distinguished from musculoskeletal or neurological disorders, such as paresis and stiffness of the neck (accounted for 3% and 1% in the present study, respectively). Previous studies have shown diseases in the gastrointestinal organ system to be a common cause of death [3], and in our study, gastric dilation volvulus accounted for 7% of causes of death.

**Dilated cardiomyopathy**

The owner-reported occurrence of DCM in the studied population was 17%. Among Swedish owners of IW, DCM has gained attention because it is a serious and fatal disease, and because insurance data has identified it as a major cause of death in the breed [1, 12]. This may result in an interest to participate in this study; particularly owners or breeders of dogs having died from DCM, or those highly committed to improve the general health situation of the breed, are likely to respond to surveys like the present. However, a retrospective study like this will only identify dogs diagnosed with DCM, but not dogs with preclinical DCM, unless they had undergone an echocardiographic examination. Brownlie and Cobb [11] reported that 12% of IW without clinical sign of cardiac disease had atrial fibrillation, which they suggested to be a possible indication of preclinical DCM. Therefore, the occurrence of DCM among the IW may be higher than reported in the present study (17%). There is, consequently, a major difference between the present and other studies reporting a higher occurrence of DCM (24–43%), namely that these studies included results from breed screening using echocardiography, and therefore included more cases with preclinical disease [5, 6, 13]. However, four of the dogs classified to have DCM in this study, were classified as probably affected or with suspicion of DCM by the authors based on information from the questionnaire such as presence of atrial fibrillation and/or development of CHF. Dogs with atrial fibrillation were included in the DCM group since reports suggest that atrial fibrillation appears to be associated to DCM in IW [5, 11, 22]. Nevertheless, a few individuals may have been misdiagnosed with DCM.

When comparing the occurrence of DCM by year of birth, the disease seems to be more common among dogs born 2006 and 2007 compared to 2008. This is most probably an effect of a lower response rate for dogs born in 2008, and therefore smaller sample size. Another possibility is that dogs born 2008 were younger (7 years old to current date) and had not yet developed DCM. However, studies have reported the mean age of diagnosis with DCM to be 4–5 years [5, 6, 14]. Most dogs born 2008 would therefore already have developed the disease if they would have had the predisposition. A third possibility is that the disease could be decreasing in incidence in the breed.

In the present study, there was no significant difference in occurrence of DCM between sexes, although the occurrence was 21% among males and 13% among females. A sex predisposition has been shown in a previous study where DCM in IW was more common among males than females [6]. The lack of a significant difference in the present study may be due to the small sample size, with only 18 dogs classified as having DCM.

**Pneumonia**

Our study showed that 37% of the study population had a history of pneumonia and that these dogs had a significantly shorter lifespan than those without history of pneumonia. The occurrence of pneumonia was nearly equally distributed among males and females. Few studies have been published regarding pneumonia in IW. These studies also report that the incidence in the breed is high and respiratory disease is frequently reported as a cause of death [3, 17]. In our study, 53% of the dogs with history of pneumonia had at least one recurrent episode. The comparably high number of dogs where the owner had reported recurrent episodes of pneumonia as well as pneumonia as cause of death, in combination with the documented reduced lifespan and increased hazard ratio, suggest that the pneumonias are severe and that respiratory disease is a serious problem in the breed. Greenwell and Brain [17] found a predisposing cause for aspiration pneumonia in 44% (n = 4) of the IW in their study. In our study, three of the dogs had megaesophagus (two diagnosed by radiology, in the third dog no information was provided on how the diagnosis was established), which may suggest this abnormality as cause for pneumonia in these dogs. Only 15% of the dogs (n = 5) with history of pneumonia had also been diagnosed with DCM. Nevertheless, a possible association between pneumonia and DCM would be of interest to explore further in the future.

### Lifespan

Median lifespan in IW participating in this study were 2720 days (7.5 years), which is longer than previous results in studies from Norway and Great Britain [2, 4]. Dogs with history of pneumonia lived shorter than those without such a history. Our result regarding median lifespan for IW with cardiac disease (7.4 years), is similar to previous studies of Swedish insurance data (7.5 years) [12]. A study concerning age of onset of CHF due to DCM in IW have shown a mean age of 6.4–7.2 years [11], and survival after development of CHF in dogs of different breeds with DCM was only 18% after 1 year [8]. These results are in agreement with ours regarding lifespan in IW with DCM (7.4 years), even though the study by Tidholm et al. [8] included data from dogs of different breeds, and prognostic differences between breeds exist [9, 11]. Moreover, in the present study, data is based on dogs, which likely have been treated with pimobendan, a cardiac drug, which has been shown to significantly increase the lifespan in dogs with DCM [23, 24]. A recent study did show pimobendan to significantly prolong time to CHF or sudden death in IW with preclinical DCM or atrial fibrillation compared to other cardiac drugs [25]. This means that results from the present study, regarding survival among dogs affected by DCM, cannot completely be compared with previous older studies, where dogs were not treated with pimobendan. Moreover, effect of CHF therapy, and course of treatment of pneumonias, have not been evaluated in the present study. They are likely to have affected survival.

### Study limitations

The survey had a response rate of 38% corresponding to 105 dogs, which is a rather small sample size and results in limitations regarding detection of clinically important differences. Furthermore, the small sample size impacts the number of variables that can be included in the statistical models. The response rate in this study is comparable to other similar studies, with small differences in study design, with reported response rates of 21–51% [4, 26–28], and suggests the response rate in this study to be reasonable.

The study population included a cohort of IW born during 2006–2008. During this period 460 dogs were born and registered in the SKK, but for 180 dogs no contact details were available, and these dogs were excluded. Hence, only a minority of the dogs born during these years were included in the study population, and the results may not entirely be representative of the general Swedish IW population. There are, however, no indications that included dogs were biased in either direction with regards to presence and severity of disease. The years were specifically chosen to allow studies of morbidity, mortality and lifespan, because the dogs had reached an age (7–9 years) where many events may have occurred, but not too far back in time for the owner to forget details of their dog's health situation. The latter represents one important limitation with retrospective survey studies, because important details about clinical signs, cause of death and date of death might have been forgotten or mixed up with other dogs in the household. When a retrospective survey, like the present, is performed, information concerning clinical signs and diagnoses are based on the owners' perceptions and knowledge about type of examinations that were performed. Naturally, this is very dependent on how good the communication between owner and veterinarian has been. However, an advantage with a survey compared to clinical case series including dogs visiting veterinary hospitals, is that the results will not be skewed by selection bias. Dogs attending veterinary clinics are more likely to be sick, which would lead to higher prevalence of disease.

Regarding dogs with pneumonia, insufficient information was available to determine how the dogs had been diagnosed and how they had been treated. The results were only based on the information provided by the owner, which, in turn, is dependent on how attentively and vigorously owners monitored health status of their dogs. Questions were asked about course of treatment, time of recurrence and if full recovery was made, but these questions were often answered inadequately, and did not allow any further analysis. The consequence of owner reported diagnoses in this study might have resulted in slightly overrepresented occurrence of pneumonias, depending on the owners' perceptions and interpretation of respiratory clinical signs. However, the presence of DCM was probably more reliable because most of these dogs had undergone diagnostic imaging tests of the heart and thorax.

Regarding cause of death, only two of the deceased dogs had undergone a post mortem examination, which means that causes of death were determined with different degrees of certainty for the dogs.

## Conclusions

The most common causes of death among the IW participating in this study were neoplastic, cardiac and respiratory diseases. The owner-reported occurrence of DCM and pneumonia in the studied population was high. A high proportion of dogs with history of pneumonia had recurrent episodes. Median lifespan was significantly shorter for males than females and for dogs with a history of pneumonia compared to those without history of pneumonia.

Pneumonia, DCM and osteosarcoma are major health problems in IW dogs. The impact of these diseases on the general health in the breed should raise concerns amongst breeders and veterinarians. The results might also provide a basis for clinical decision making and preventive measures aimed at reducing the occurrence of these diseases.

### Abbreviations

CHF: congestive heart failure; DCM: dilated cardiomyopathy; IW: Irish Wolfhound; SKK: Swedish Kennel Club; SLU: Swedish University of Agricultural Sciences.

### Authors' contributions

LO, IL, KH and JH planned the study. LO formed the questionnaire and collected and processed the data. JH performed the statistical analyses. All authors read and approved the final manuscript.

### Author details

[1] Department of Clinical Sciences, Faculty of Veterinary Medicine, Swedish University of Agricultural Sciences, Uppsala, Sweden. [2] Department of Anatomy, Physiology and Biochemistry, Faculty of Veterinary Medicine, Swedish University of Agricultural Sciences, Uppsala, Sweden.

### Acknowledgements

This study was performed with assistance from the Swedish Kennel Club. Many thanks to the Swedish Irish Wolfhound Club and to the owners of Irish Wolfhounds that have participated in this study.

### Competing interests

The authors declare that they have no competing interests.

### Funding

Not applicable.

### References

1. Egenvall A, Bonnett BN, Hedhammar A, Olson P. Mortality in over 350,000 insured Swedish dogs from 1995 to 2000: II. Breed-specific age and survival patterns and relative risk for causes of death. Acta Vet Scand. 2005. doi:10.1186/1751-0147-46-121.
2. Michell AR. Longevity of British breeds of dog and its relationships with sex, size, cardiovascular variables and disease. Vet Rec. 1999;145:625–9.
3. Fleming JM, Creevy KE, Promislow DEL. Mortality in North American dogs from 1984 to 2004: an investigation into age-, size-, and breed-related causes of death. J Vet Intern Med. 2011;25:187–98.
4. Anfinsen KP, Grotmol T, Bruland OS, Jonasdottir TJ. Breed-specific incidence rates of canine primary bone tumors—a population based survey of dogs in Norway. Can J Vet Res. 2011;75:209–15.
5. Vollmar AC. The prevalence of cardiomyopathy in the Irish Wolfhound: a clinical study of 500 dogs. J Am Anim Hosp Assoc. 2000;36:125–32.
6. Distl O, Vollmar AC, Broschk C, Hamann H, Fox PR. Complex segregation analysis of dilated cardiomyopathy (DCM) in Irish Wolfhounds. Heredity. 2007;99:460–5.
7. Richardson P, McKenna W, Bristow M, Maisch B, Mautner B, Oconnell J, et al. Report of the 1995 World Health Organization International Society and Federation of Cardiology Task Force on the definition and classification of cardiomyopathies. Circulation. 1996;93:841–2.
8. Tidholm A, Svensson H, Sylven C. Survival and prognostic factors in 189 dogs with dilated cardiomyopathy. J Am Anim Hosp Assoc. 1997;33:364–8.
9. Calvert CA, Pickus CW, Jacobs GJ, Brown J. Signalment, survival, and prognostic factors in Doberman Pinschers with end-stage cardiomyopathy. J Vet Intern Med. 1997;11:323–6.
10. Dambach DM, Lannon A, Sleeper MM, Buchanan J. Familial dilated cardiomyopathy of young Portuguese water dogs. J Vet Intern Med. 1999;13:65–71.
11. Brownlie SE, Cobb MA. Observations on the development of congestive heart failure in Irish Wolfhounds with dilated cardiomyopathy. J Small Anim Pract. 1999;40:371–7.
12. Egenvall A, Bonnett BN, Haggstrom J. Heart disease as a cause of death in insured Swedish dogs younger than 10 years of age. J Vet Intern Med. 2006;20:894–903.
13. Vollmar AC, Fox PR, Servet E, Biourge V. Determination of the prevalence of whole blood taurine in Irish Wolfhound dogs with and without echocardiographic evidence of dilated cardiomyopathy. J Vet Cardiol. 2013;15:189–96.
14. Philipp U, Vollmar A, Haggstrom J, Thomas A, Distl O. Multiple loci are associated with dilated cardiomyopathy in Irish Wolfhounds. PLoS ONE. 2012. doi:10.1371/journal.pone.0036691.
15. Meurs KM, Fox PR, Norgard M, Spier AW, Lamb A, Koplitz SL, et al. A prospective genetic evaluation of familial dilated cardiomyopathy in the Doberman Pinscher. J Vet Intern Med. 2007;21:1016–20.
16. Stephenson HM, Fonfara S, Lopez-Alvarez J, Cripps P, Dukes-McEwan J. Screening for dilated cardiomyopathy in Great Danes in the United Kingdom. J Vet Intern Med. 2012;26:1140–7.
17. Greenwell CM, Brain PH. Aspiration pneumonia in the Irish Wolfhound: a possible breed predisposition. J Small Anim Pract. 2014;55:515–20.
18. Clercx C, Reichler I, Peeters D, McEntee K, German A, Dubois J, et al. Rhinitis/bronchopneumonia syndrome in Irish Wolfhounds. J Vet Intern Med. 2003;17:843–9.
19. Wilkinson GT. Some observations on the Irish Wolfhound rhinitis syndrome. J Small Anim Pract. 1969;10:5–8.
20. Bonnett BN, Egenvall A, Hedhammar A, Olson P. Mortality in over 350,000 insured Swedish dogs from 1995 to 2000: I. Breed-, gender-, age- and cause-specific rates. Acta Vet Scand. 2005. doi:10.1186/1751-0147-46-105.
21. Egenvall A, Nodtvedt A, von Euler H. Bone tumors in a population of 400 000 insured Swedish dogs up to 10 year of age: incidence and survival. Can J Vet Res. 2007;71:292–9.
22. Vollmar AC, Aupperle H. Cardiac pathology in Irish Wolfhounds with heart disease. J Vet Cardiol. 2016;18:57–70.
23. Fuentes VL, Corcoran B, French A, Schober KE, Kleemann R, Justus C. A double-blind, randomized, placebo-controlled study of pimobendan in dogs with dilated cardiomyopathy. J Vet Intern Med. 2002;16:255–61.
24. O'Grady MR, Minors SL, O'Sullivan ML, Horne R. Effect of pimobendan on case fatality rate in Doberman Pinschers with congestive heart failure caused by dilated cardiomyopathy. J Vet Intern Med. 2008;22:897–904.
25. Vollmar AC, Fox PR. Long-term outcome of Irish Wolfhound dogs with preclinical cardiomyopathy, atrial fibrillation, or both treated with pimobendan, benazepril hydrochloride, or methyldigoxin monotherapy. J Vet Intern Med. 2016;30:553–9.
26. Mandigers PJJ, Senders T, Rothuizen J. Morbidity and mortality in 928 Dobermanns born in the Netherlands between 1993 and 1999. Vet Rec. 2006;158:226–9.

# 16

# A modified oral sugar test for evaluation of insulin and glucose dynamics in horses

Sanna Lindåse*, Katarina Nostell and Johan Bröjer

*From* Animal Obesity – causes, consequences and comparative aspects
Uppsala, Sweden. 14–16 June 2015

**Abstract**

**Background:** An oral sugar test (OST) using Karo® Light Corn Syrup has been developed in the USA as a field test for the assessment of insulin dysregulation in horses but the syrup is not available in Scandinavian grocery stores. The aim of the study was to compare the results of a modified OST between horses with equine metabolic syndrome (EMS) and healthy horses using a Scandinavian commercially available glucose syrup (Dansukker glykossirap). In addition, the effect of breed and the repeatability of the test were evaluated. In the present study, clinically healthy horses (7 Shetland ponies, 8 Icelandic horses, 8 Standardbred horses) and 20 horses of various breeds with EMS underwent the modified OST test. The Icelandic horses and Shetland ponies underwent the OST twice. Insulin and glucose data from the OST were used to calculate peak insulin concentration ($Peak_{INS}$), time to peak insulin concentration ($T\text{-}peak_{INS}$), area under the curve for insulin ($AUC_{INS}$) and glucose ($AUC_{GLU}$) as well as whole body insulin sensitivity index ($ISI_{COMP}$).

**Results:** Compared to the healthy group, the EMS group had 6–7 times higher geometric mean for $Peak_{INS}$ and $AUC_{INS}$ and 8 times lower geometric mean for $ISI_{COMP}$. The EMS group had a delayed $T\text{-}peak_{INS}$ compared to the healthy group. There was no effect of breed in the group of healthy horses on $Peak_{INS}$, $T\text{-}peak_{INS}$, $AUC_{INS}$, $AUC_{GLU}$ and $ISI_{COMP}$. Coefficient of variation for repeated tests was 19.8, 19.0 and 17.6 % for $Peak_{INS}$, $AUC_{INS}$ and $ISI_{COMP}$ respectively.

**Conclusions:** The results of the present study demonstrate that the modified OST appears to be a practical and useful diagnostic tool for assessment of insulin dysregulation in the horse. However, to make it possible to establish the most appropriate sampling interval and to evaluate the accuracy of the modified OST, further studies in horses with a variable degree of insulin resistance are needed, where results from the modified OST are compared with quantitative measurements for IS.

**Keywords:** Horse, Insulin dysregulation, Insulin resistance, Oral sugar test

## Background

Equine metabolic syndrome (EMS) refers to a group of clinical abnormalities including generalized obesity and/or regional adiposity, insulin resistance (IR) and hyperinsulinemia [1]. Postprandial hyperinsulinemia is a risk factor for development of laminitis [2–7], and since EMS is a rising concern in the equine population worldwide, it is important to create appropriate diagnostic tests for abnormalities in insulin regulation. In humans, glucose and insulin data from an oral glucose tolerance test (OGTT) can be used to calculate surrogate estimates for insulin sensitivity (IS) that are well correlated to IS quantified by the euglycemic hyperinsulinemic clamp (EHC) [8–10]. The composite whole-body insulin sensitivity index ($ISI_{COMP}$), also called the Matsuda index, is a commonly used OGTT-derived estimate for IS in humans [10]. The use of $ISI_{COMP}$ as an estimate for IS in the horse has recently been evaluated against quantitative measurements of IS [11]. Despite these relationships OGTT does

*Correspondence: sanna.lindase@slu.se
Department of Clinical Sciences, Swedish University of Agricultural Sciences, Box 7054, 750 07 Uppsala, Sweden

not measure IS per se. Instead, it is a test in which both glucose disposal and insulin secretion are stimulated but the test is influenced by factors such as gastric emptying, degree of hepatic glucose trapping, β-cell responsiveness and incretin effects [12].

Due to the association between hyperinsulinemia and laminitis in the horse [13], identification of individuals with an exaggerated postprandial insulin response using OGTT may enable better management of horses and ponies at risk for pasture-associated laminitis. An alternative to the OGTT, where glucose is used as the only carbohydrate source, is the recently developed oral sugar test (OST) [14]. This test uses a standardized amount of Karo® light corn syrup, which is composed of different unknown carbohydrates. Karo® light corn syrup is, however, not available in Scandinavian grocery stores. The aim of the present study was therefore to compare the results of a modified oral sugar test (OST), using a Scandinavian commercially available glucose syrup (Dansukker glykossirap), in a group of healthy horses and in horses with EMS. In addition, the effect of breed on the test result and the repeatability of the test were studied in clinically healthy horses.

## Methods

### Horses

The study was approved by the Ethical Committee for Animal Experiments, Uppsala, Sweden. Twenty-three clinically healthy horses and 20 horses with EMS were included in the study. The clinically healthy horses were seven Shetland ponies, eight Icelandic horses and eight Standardbred horses. Inclusion criteria for these horses were a body condition score (BCS) of ≤6.5 (scale 1–9) [15], a cresty neck score (CNS) of ≤3.0 (scale 0–5) [16], normal findings on clinical examination, no history of laminitis based on veterinary information and a normal plasma ACTH concentration. The Icelandic horses were used for leisure riding whereas the Standardbred horses and Shetland ponies were sedentary horses. The horses with EMS were two Fjord horses, one Swedish warmblood, ten Icelandic horses, two Shetland ponies, one Welsh Cob, one Highland pony, one Swedish riding pony, one crossbreed horse and one crossbreed pony. The horses with EMS were recruited from a group of horses referred for an extended evaluation of EMS at the University Animal hospital, Swedish University of Agricultural Sciences. Criteria for inclusion were IR, defined as a M/I ratio of ≤3.5 calculated from an EHC, and a normal plasma ACTH. In addition, horses had to have either ≥1 previous episode of laminitis not associated with other predisposing conditions or a CNS >3 [16]. Also, horses eligible to participate had no significant findings on clinical examination, were fed a roughage based diet without grain supplementation and had no ongoing episode of laminitis. Physical characteristics for the two groups of horses are reported in Table 1. All horses were privately owned except for the clinically healthy Standardbred horses, which belonged to the Swedish University of Agricultural Sciences research herd. All horses in the study were fed a hay or haylage diet supplemented with minerals and six of the Icelandic horses were feed 50–100 g of grain 3–5 times/week as a treat. Horses were housed in individual box stalls and allowed daily turnout in a dirt or a sand paddock. None of the horses had been at grass pasture for at least 2 month prior to testing.

### Experimental design

The healthy horses were examined in their home environment whereas the horses diagnosed with EMS were examined at the large animal clinic at the Swedish University of Agricultural Sciences after an acclimatization period of 2 days. All horses in the study were examined once with the modified OST. The Icelandic horses and Shetland ponies in the healthy group were examined twice with 8 days in between, to assess the repeatability of the OST. Horses in the EMS group were tested with an EHC 24 h after the OST. Both the OST and the EHC commenced after 12 h of feed withdrawal overnight but with free access to water.

**Table 1 Baseline physical characteristics of horses in healthy (n = 23) and equine metabolic syndrome (EMS) (n = 20) groups**

| Group | Age (years) | Body weight (kg) | Body condition score (1–9) | Cresty neck score (0–5) |
|---|---|---|---|---|
| EMS (n = 20) | 13.9 ± 4.6 (5–22)$^{a}$ | 395 ± 117 (124–558)$^{a}$ | 6.9 ± 1.1 (5.5–9.0)$^{a}$ | 3.7 ± 0.6 (2.5–5.0)$^{a}$ |
| Healthy (n = 23) | | | | |
| Shetland pony (n = 7) | 3.9 ± 2.7 (1–9)$^{c}$ | 152 ± 29 (115–194)$^{b}$ | 5.6 ± 0.6 (5.0–6.5)$^{b}$ | 2.6 ± 0.4 (2.0–3.0)$^{b}$ |
| Icelandic horse (n = 8) | 7.0 ± 2.0 (5–10)$^{bc}$ | 342 ± 21 (298–360)$^{ac}$ | 6.0 ± 0.4 (5.5–6.5)$^{ab}$ | 2.6 ± 0.2 (2.5–3.0)$^{b}$ |
| Standardbred horses (n = 8) | 10.5 ± 4.7 (5–20)$^{ab}$ | 507 ± 56 (441–595)$^{d}$ | 5.0 ± 0.5 (4.5–5.5)$^{b}$ | 2.0 ± 0.5 (1.5–2.5)$^{b}$ |

Data are presented as mean ± standard deviation (SD) (range)

Means with different superscript letters within column differ at P < 0.02

#### OST—oral sugar test

The day before the OST an intravenous catheter (Intranule, 2.0 × 105 mm. Vygon, Ecouen, France) was inserted aseptically into one of the jugular veins under local anesthesia (EMLA, AstraZenica AB, Södertälje, Sweden). On the morning of the OST, Dan Sukker Glykossirap (Nordic Sugar A/S, Copenhagen, Denmark) was syringed per os at a dosage of 0.2 ml/kg body weight, providing 216 mg/kg BW of saccharides (Table 2). Blood samples were collected from the jugular catheter into evacuated tubes (Vacuette 9 ml, Greiner Bio-One GmbH, Kremsmünster, Austria) containing lithium heparin, immediately before (−5 min), and at 30, 60, 90, 120, 150 and 180 min after the oral administration of syrup. After collection of each blood sample the catheter line was immediately flushed with 10 ml 0.9 % sterile saline solution. Sample tubes were centrifuged for 10 min at 2700×*g* and plasma was subsequently harvested and stored at −80 °C until analysis of plasma glucose and plasma insulin.

Insulin and glucose data from the OST were used to calculate the following variables: Peak insulin concentration ($Peak_{INS}$), time to peak insulin concentration ($T\text{-}peak_{INS}$), area under the curve for insulin ($AUC_{INS}$), area under the curve for glucose ($AUC_{GLU}$) and composite whole-body insulin sensitivity index ($ISI_{COMP}$) [10]. $AUC_{INS}$ and $AUC_{GLU}$ were calculated by use of the trapezoid method (GraphPad Prism, version 6.0 for windows; GraphPad Software Inc, San Diego, CA). $ISI_{COMP}$ was calculated by the following formula: $1000/\sqrt{(G \cdot I) \cdot (MG \cdot MI)}$, where G = baseline glucose concentration, I = baseline insulin concentration, MG = mean glucose concentration during the OST and MI = mean insulin concentration during the OST. A numerator of 1000 was used in the formula, to transform the data into manageable values.

#### EHC—euglycemic hyperinsulinemic clamp

For horses in the EMS group, a second intravenous catheter (Intranule, 2.0 × 105 mm. Vygon, Ecouen, France) was inserted into the contralateral jugular vein after the OST examination. On the morning of the following day blood samples for the determination of baseline concentrations of plasma glucose and plasma insulin were drawn from one of the intravenous catheters immediately before (−10, −5, and −1 min) the start of the EHC.

**Table 2 Chemical composition of the Dan Sukker Glykossirap**

| Dry matter (%) | Glucose (%) | Maltose (%) | Maltotriose (%) | Other sugars (%) | Density (20 °C) |
|---|---|---|---|---|---|
| 77 | 12 | 11 | 10 | 44 | 1.40 kg/L |

Product specification | PS 236654-1.3EN. Nordic Sugar A/S, Copenhagen, Denmark

The EHC technique has previously been described for use in horses [17, 18]. Briefly, a continuous rate infusion of glucose (Glucose Fresenius Kabi 500 mg/ml, Fresenius Kabi AB, Uppsala, Sweden) and recombinant human insulin (Humulin Regular, Eli Lilly Sweden AB, Solna, Sweden) was initiated through one of the jugular catheters, using a multi-channel volumetric infusion pump (Colleague, Volumetric infusion pump, Baxter Healthcare SA, Zurich, Switzerland). The infusion rate for insulin was constant at 3 mU/kg/min and a variable rate of glucose was infused to maintain blood glucose concentration at euglycemia (5 mmol/L) during the 3 h long infusion. The glucose infusion rate was adjusted if the concentration deviated by more than 0.2 mmol/L from euglycemia. Blood samples were obtained every 5 min for analysis of blood glucose using a handheld glucometer (Accu-Check Aviva, Roche Diagnostics Scandinavia AB, Bromma, Sweden) and every 10 min throughout the EHC for subsequent determination of plasma glucose (10 min intervals) and plasma insulin (20 min intervals). After collection of each blood sample, the catheter line was immediately flushed with 10 ml 0.9 % sterile saline solution.

The first 120 min of the EHC were considered an equilibration period. Glucose and insulin data from the final 60 min (steady-state) were used for calculation of insulin sensitivity (M/I ratio). The M/I ratio was calculated for each 20-min interval where M is the mean glucose infusion rate and I is the plasma insulin concentration for the interval. The $M/I_{60}$ is the mean of the three M/I ratios during steady state [17].

#### Analysis of blood samples

Plasma glucose concentrations were measured enzymatically with an automated clinical chemistry analyzer (YSI 2300 Stat Plus Analyzer, YSI Incorporated, Yellow Spring, Ohio). Endogenous equine plasma insulin concentrations from the OST were determined using a commercial equine-optimized ELISA (Mercodia Equine Insulin ELISA, Mercodia AB, Uppsala, Sweden) evaluated for use in horses [19] and insulin levels were controlled with a commercial kit (Mercodia Animal Insulin Control (Low, Medium, High), Mercodia AB, Uppsala, Sweden). Plasma insulin concentrations from the continuous rate infusion of recombinant human insulin during the EHC procedures were determined using a commercial human ELISA (Mercodia Insulin ELISA, Mercodia AB, Uppsala, Sweden) and a commercial kit (Mercodia Diabetes Antigen Control (Low, High)/Human, Mercodia AB, Uppsala, Sweden) was used as a control. All analyses of plasma glucose and insulin were performed in duplicate. The mean intra-assay CVs for glucose, equine insulin (equine-optimized ELISA) and human insulin (human ELISA) were 0.4, 2.7 and 2.7 % respectively, as determined from duplicate analyses.

### Statistical analysis

All data were analyzed in JMP® Pro 11.0.0. (SAS Institute Inc., Cary, North Carolina, USA). Differences in plasma glucose and insulin concentrations for the healthy and the EMS groups were compared at different time points during the OST, by use of a 2-way ANOVA for repeated measures. Differences in physical characteristics (age, BCS, CNS and body weight) and OST derived calculated variables ($AUC_{GLU}$, $AUC_{INS}$, $ISI_{COMP}$, $Peak_{INS}$ and $T\text{-}peak_{INS}$) were compared between breeds and between the healthy and EMS groups by use of an independent t test or a 1-way ANOVA as appropriate. Differences in calculated variables for repeated OST tests were compared by use of a paired t test. The repeatability of the OST was determined by the mean coefficient of variation (mean CV), the intraclass correlation coefficient (ICC) and the repeatability coefficient (RC). The ICC was calculated according to the formula $1-S_W^2/(s_b^2 + S_w^2)$ and the RC was calculated as $2.77S_w$, where $S_w^2$ is the within subject variance and $s_b^2$ is the between subject variance calculated from the analysis of variance table of a 1-way ANOVA [20]. Values of $P < 0.05$ were considered as significant for all analyses. If residuals were not normally distributed data were logarithmically transformed. Logarithmically transformed data were then expressed as the geometric mean ± 95 % CI on the original scale after back transformation. All other results were expressed as mean ± SD, whereas data for age, body weight, BCS and CNS were additionally presented with the range.

## Results

All horses included in the study fulfilled the inclusion criteria for the separate groups. All horses tolerated the administration of syrup well. The loss of syrup was negligible comprising the small amount that got stuck to the outside of the syringe during administration.

### Comparison of EMS and healthy groups

All horse in the EMS group were defined as insulin resistant by a $M/I_{60}$ of <3.5 (μg/kg/min)/(mU/L). Fourteen of 20 included horses with EMS had a severe IR i.e. $M/I_{60} < 2.0$ (μg/kg/min)/(mU/L). Sixteen of the 20 horses included in the EMS group had previous episodes of laminitis. The EMS group had a higher mean CNS compared to the breeds included in the healthy group ($P < 0.0004$). Mean BCS was higher in the EMS group compared to the Standardbred horses and Shetland ponies of the healthy group ($P < 0.010$), but no difference was found between the EMS group and the healthy Icelandic horses ($P = 0.074$) (Table 1).

There was an overall effect of time between the group of healthy horses and EMS horses during the OST for insulin ($P < 0.0001$) but not for glucose ($P = 0.178$). An overall interaction between group of horses (clinically healthy vs EMS) and time was identified for both insulin ($P < 0.0001$) and glucose ($P = 0.003$) (Fig. 1).

Compared to the healthy group, the EMS group had 6–7 times higher geometric mean for $Peak_{INS}$ ($P < 0.0001$) and $AUC_{INS}$ ($P < 0.0001$) and 8 times lower geometric mean for $ISI_{COMP}$ ($P < 0.0001$) (Fig. 2). Horses in the healthy group reached the maximum insulin concentration ($T\text{-}peak_{INS}$) on average 69 ± 25 min from the start of the OST. Horses in the EMS group had delayed insulin peak compared to the healthy group ($P = 0.007$) with an average of 92 ± 27 min from the start of OST. In the healthy group geometric means (95 % CI) for insulin were 222 (172–288) ng/L and 206 (159–267) ng/L at the 60 and 90 min sampling respectively. For the EMS group the geometric means (95 % CI) for insulin for the corresponding time points were 1329 (1006–1756) ng/L and 1452 (1099–1919) ng/L, respectively.

### Breed comparison

There was no effect of breed on $AUC_{GLU}$, $AUC_{INS}$, $Peak_{INS}$, $ISI_{COMP}$ and $T\text{-}peak_{INS}$ in the group of healthy horses (Table 3).

### Repeatability testing

The $AUC_{GLU}$, $AUC_{INS}$, $Peak_{INS}$, $ISI_{COMP}$ and $T\text{-}peak_{INS}$ did not significantly differ between repeated tests performed in the group of healthy horses (Table 4). Among the variables derived from the OST, the $AUC_{GLU}$ had the best combination of repeatability measures i.e., a low mean CV, a high ICC and a relatively small RC. In contrast, $Peak_{INS}$ and $T\text{-}peak_{INS}$ had higher mean CVs as well as larger RC in relation to each of the means. Further, the $Peak_{INS}$ had a similar ICC as $AUC_{GLU}$, whilst $T\text{-}peak_{INS}$ had the lowest ICC of all calculated variables.

## Discussion

A modified OST test was developed and evaluated using a Scandinavian commercially available glucose syrup (Dan Sukker Glykossirap). Higher OST glucose and insulin plasma concentrations and accordingly lower $ISI_{COMP}$ as well as higher $AUC_{GLU}$, $AUC_{INS}$ and $Peak_{INS}$ were found in the EMS group compared to the healthy group. Moreover, the calculated parameters from the OST had moderate to high repeatability and there was no effect of breed on the test results. These results show that the modified OST appears to be a practical and useful diagnostic tool for assessment of dysinsulinemia in the horse.

It has been suggested that the OGTT and OST more closely mimic the glucose and insulin dynamics during

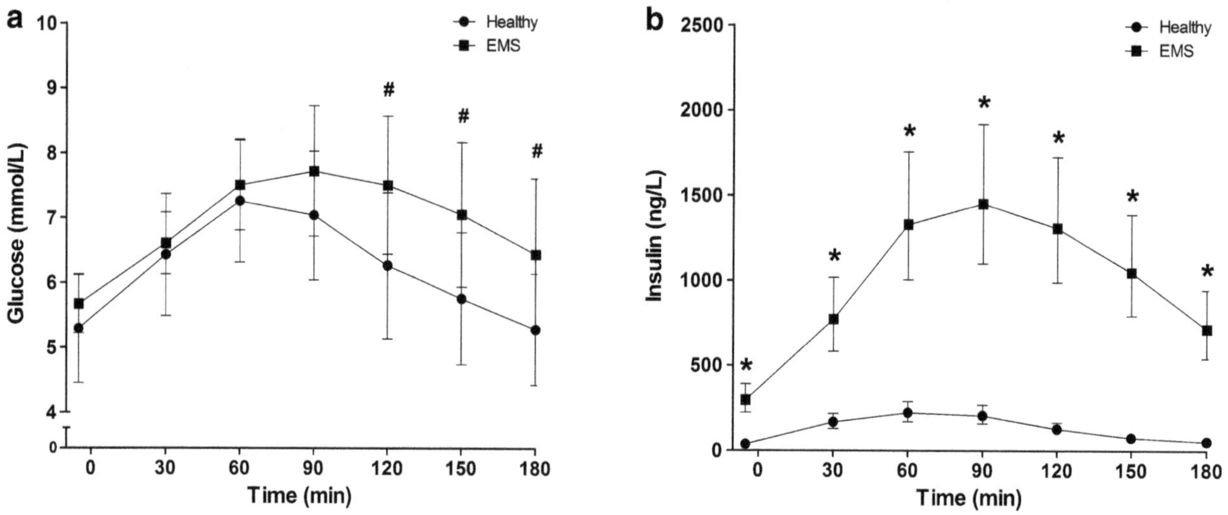


**Fig. 1** Plasma glucose (**a**) and plasma insulin (**b**) concentrations measured during the OST in healthy (n = 23) and EMS (n = 20) groups. Data are presented as mean ± SD for plasma glucose and as geometric mean, 95 % confidence interval for plasma insulin. *Groups differ at $P < 0.0001$. #Groups differ at $P < 0.0036$. *OST* oral sugar test; *EMS* equine metabolic syndrome; *SD* standard deviation

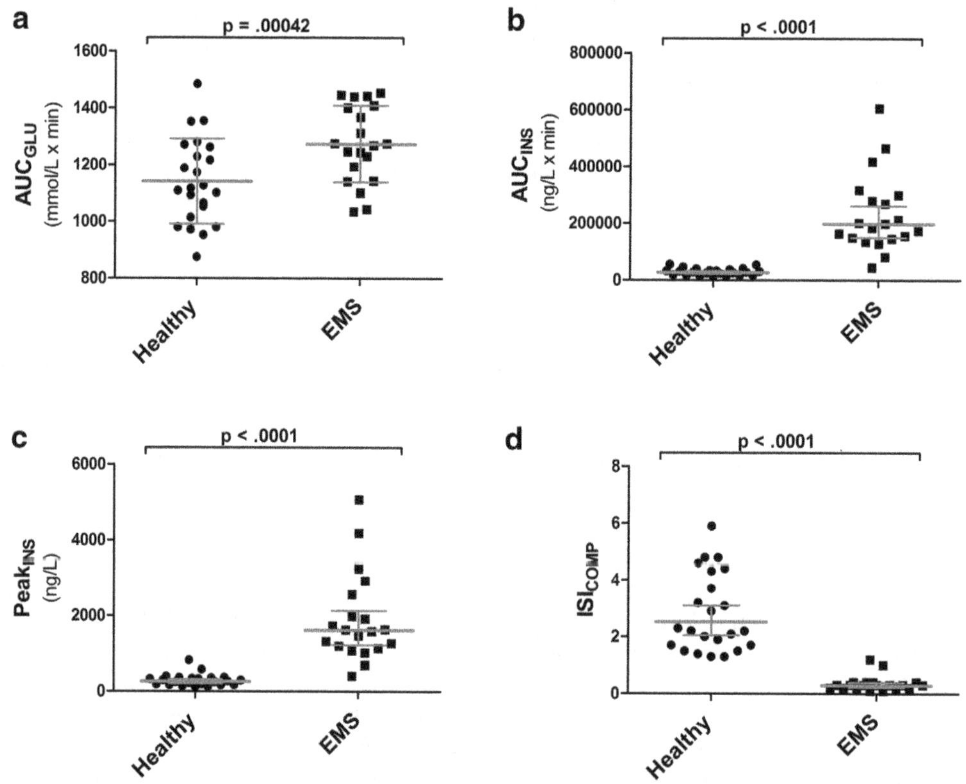


**Fig. 2** $AUC_{GLU}$ (**a**), $AUC_{INS}$ (**b**), $Peak_{INS}$ (**c**) and $ISI_{COMP}$ (**d**) values for OST performed in healthy (n = 23) and EMS (n = 20) groups. Horizontal lines present mean, SD for $AUC_{GLU}$; and geometric mean, 95 % confidence interval for $AUC_{INS}$, $Peak_{INS}$ and $ISI_{COMP}$. $P < 0.05$ represents statistical differences. *OST* oral sugar test; $AUC_{GLU}$ area under the curve for glucose; $AUC_{INS}$ area under the curve for insulin; $Peak_{INS}$ peak concentration for insulin; $ISI_{COMP}$ composite whole-body insulin sensitivity index; EMS, equine metabolic syndrome; *SD* standard deviation

**Table 3 Calculated variables and measures for the oral sugar test (OST) in healthy Shetland ponies (n = 7), Icelandic horses (n = 8) and Standardbred horses (n = 8)**

| | Shetland ponies | Icelandic horses | Standardbred horses | P value |
|---|---|---|---|---|
| $AUC_{GLU}$ (mmol/L × min) | 1071 ± 136 | 1239 ± 167 | 1100 ± 96 | 0.055 |
| $AUC_{INS}$ (ng/L × min) | 32,235 ± 14,797 | 29,130 ± 14,655 | 26,967 ± 7600 | 0.728 |
| $ISI_{COMP}$ | 2.2 (1.5–3.2) | 2.6 (1.8–3.7) | 2.8 (1.9–4.0) | 0.608 |
| $Peak_{INS}$ (ng/L) | 301 (203–446) | 237 (164–342) | 259 (179–374) | 0.652 |
| $T\text{-}peak_{INS}$ (min) | 56 ± 27 | 75 ± 23 | 75 ± 23 | 0.234 |

Data are presented as mean ± SD for $AUC_{GLU}$ and $AUC_{INS}$; and as geometric mean (95 % confidence interval) for $Peak_{INS}$ and $ISI_{COMP}$

*$AUC_{GLU}$* area under the curve for glucose; *$AUC_{INS}$* area under the curve for insulin; *$ISI_{COMP}$* composite whole-body insulin sensitivity index; *$Peak_{INS}$* peak concentration for insulin; *$T\text{-}peak_{INS}$* time to peak concentration for insulin; *SD* standard deviation

**Table 4 Calculated variables and measures of repeatability for the oral sugar test (OST) in 15 healthy horses (7 Shetland ponies, 8 Icelandic horses)**

| | Test 1 | Test 2 | P value | Mean CV (%) | ICC | RC |
|---|---|---|---|---|---|---|
| $AUC_{GLU}$ (mmol/L × min) | 1161 ± 171 | 1153 ± 116 | 0.823 | 6.7 | 0.79 | 237.7 |
| $AUC_{INS}$ (ng/L × min) | 30,579 ± 14,276 | 31,706 ± 15,526 | 0.623 | 16.9 | 0.91 | 16,556.4 |
| $ISI_{COMP}$ | 2.7 ± 1.5 | 2.8 ± 1.6 | 0.912 | 17.3 | 0.85 | 2.1 |
| $Peak_{INS}$ (ng/L) | 309 ± 190 | 308 ± 153 | 0.976 | 18.3 | 0.83 | 255.5 |
| $T\text{-}peak_{INS}$ (min) | 66 ± 26 | 74 ± 34 | 0.334 | 18.5 | 0.64 | 60.7 |

Data are presented as mean ± standard deviation (SD)

*$AUC_{GLU}$* area under the curve for glucose; *$AUC_{INS}$* area under the curve for insulin; *$ISI_{COMP}$* composite whole-body insulin sensitivity index; *$Peak_{INS}$* peak concentration for insulin; *$T\text{-}peak_{INS}$* time to peak concentration for insulin; *mean CV* mean coefficient of variation; *ICC* intraclass correlation coefficient; *RC* repeatability coefficient

physiological conditions than the EHC and the frequently sampled IV glucose tolerance test (FSIGTT). However, it is important to recognize that glucose and insulin responses after oral glucose delivery are not equivalent to insulin sensitivity. The glucose and insulin response after oral administration of glucose are dependent on factors such as gastric emptying, absorption, glucose uptake in the liver, incretin effects, insulin secretion and clearance as well as insulin sensitivity [12]. Thus, the OGTT and OST provide information about the efficiency of the homeostatic mechanisms including insulin-dependent mechanisms to restore blood glucose concentration to basal levels but not IS/IR per se. Nevertheless, several studies in humans, but also in the horse, have used different surrogate indices based on dynamic data from OGTT in order to estimate IS [8–11]. The most commonly used index in humans, $ISI_{COMP}$, reflects a composite estimate of both hepatic and peripheral insulin sensitivity based on fasting glucose and insulin data as well as the mean of glucose and insulin values obtained during the OGTT. The square-root conversion in the formula is used to correct for non-linear distribution of data in relation to the IS determined by the EHC [10]. Studies in humans and horses have shown that $ISI_{COMP}$ has a relatively good linear correlation to quantitative measurements of IS obtained by the EHC and the surrogate index therefore provides a reasonable estimate of IS [10, 11].

Compensatory hyperinsulinemia can develop in horses with IR [21, 22] by two mechanisms: increased insulin secretion from the ß-cells in the pancreas and reduced insulin clearance by the liver [21, 23–26]. This hyperinsulinemia is more pronounced and thereby easier to detect after feed intake compared to pre-prandial conditions [27, 28]. The OST is a dynamic test that mimics a feeding situation and makes it possible to study postprandial hyperinsulinemia under controlled conditions. In the present study horses in the EMS group had higher plasma insulin concentrations at all time points during the OST compared to the healthy group. The higher insulin response in the EMS group resulted in higher $AUC_{INS}$, $Peak_{INS}$ and lower $ISI_{COMP}$ compared to the healthy group. In contrast, plasma glucose concentrations only differed between the healthy and the EMS group at 120, 150 and 180 min. Repeated blood sampling is necessary for calculation of $AUC_{INS}$, $AUC_{GLU}$ and $ISI_{COMP}$, making these parameters less useful during field conditions. Instead, $Peak_{INS}$ requires only a single sample, which reduces the costs for laboratory analyses as well as the time spent on sampling in the field during the test.

For the USA-developed OST [14] researchers found that peak concentrations for insulin was recorded at blood sampling at 60 or 90 min after syrup administration. Hence, the time interval between 60 and 90 min after sugar administration is recommended for single blood sampling for measurements of peak insulin concentrations. In the present study, there was a longer mean time to peak insulin in the EMS group (92 ± 27 min) compared to the healthy group (69 ± 25 min). Nevertheless, plasma insulin concentration differed between the healthy and the EMS group at all time points during the OST and there was no overlap of confidence intervals. This suggests that the time frame for single blood sampling could be extended, making the test protocol more time flexible. The largest difference in plasma insulin concentrations between the two groups of horses occurred at sampling times between 60 and 150 min. However, the majority of horses included in the EMS group of the present study had a severe IR, as determined by the EHC. Severe IR is associated with a pronounced compensatory β-cell response as well as decrease in insulin clearance [22, 25], leading to a prolonged insulin response during the OST. On the other hand, a horse in an early stage of disease with a mild to moderate degree of IR, is likely to have a shorter and less prominent insulin response. Thus, if a blood sample is taken later during the OST in these horses (for example at 150 min) the insulin concentration may then have decreased to a level seen in a normal horse. The most optimal time point for sampling in order to distinguish normal horses from those with insulin dysregulation, can therefore not be concluded from the present study since it would have required a larger number of horses with a wider range of IR and β-cell responses.

The Karo® Light Corn Syrup is not available in Scandinavian grocery stores wherefore the agreement between the USA-developed OST and the modified OST could not be assessed. For the modified OST a dose of 0.2 ml/kg syrup is used, providing 216 mg saccharides/kg of body weight compared to 0.15 ml/kg of syrup for the USA developed OST that is estimated to provide the horse with 150 mg/kg of body weight of dextrose-derived digestible sugars. The total dose of sugar is thereby 44 % higher for the modified test. The glucose and insulin response after administration of syrup is not only influenced by the total amount of sugar but also the relative composition of the different sugar types. Information about the composition of the Karo® Light Corn Syrup is withheld by the manufacturer, which therefore makes it difficult to design an identical test for the Scandinavian market. Another aspect that further complicates comparisons between the two tests is that different assays have been used for measurement of plasma insulin (Coat-A-Count Insulin RIA vs Mercodia Equine Insulin ELISA). Earlier performed work [19] showed that results were in good agreement between these two assays for samples with equine insulin concentrations <150 μU/ml, but for samples with higher insulin concentrations the agreement between assays was poor [29]. The calculated conversion factor for equine insulin from mU/L, determined with the radioimmunoassay (RIA) method, to the quantitative unit ng/L, determined with the equine specific ELISA is 10 [19]. The cutoff for dysinsulinemia for the USA developed OST is >60 mU/L (measured by the RIA) at sampling at 60–90 min [30, 31], corresponding to >600 ng/L for insulin concentrations measured by the equine ELISA. In the present study, 21 of the 23 horses in the healthy group had plasma insulin concentrations <400 ng/L at the 60 min sampling and at the 90 min sampling all healthy horses had plasma insulin concentrations <400 ng/L. In the EMS group 19 of 20 horses had plasma insulin concentrations >600 ng/L at 60 and 90 min. If the same sampling interval is used for the modified OST as for the USA developed OST (i.e. 60–90 min) it seems reasonable to use the same cut off values for the two tests.

No differences were found between breeds for any of the OST calculated variables ($AUC_{GLU}$, $AUC_{INS}$, $ISI_{COMP}$, $Peak_{INS}$ and $T\text{-}peak_{INS}$). Previous studies have shown differences in IS between healthy horses of different breeds using other diagnostic tests such as the CGIT [32] or the FSIGTT [28]. A small sample in combination with a relatively large within breed variation could possibly explain why no effect of breed was found in the present study. Another aspect is that only the Icelandic horses were exercised and used for leisure riding whereas the remainder (Shetland ponies and Standardbred horses) were sedentary horses. Since exercise can affect the degree of IS [33, 34], it is possible that the outcome would have been different if the degree of activity had been similar between breeds. Another explanation might be that the test is not sensitive enough to detect small differences in IS between different breed populations.

One limitation of the present study is that one group of horses (the EMS group) was tested during hospitalization whereas all other horses were tested in their home environment. In a previous study [35] no effect of housing and diet on results from the OST were found. The EMS horses in our study were acclimatized 48 h prior to testing at the large animal clinic and horses were only fed their own hay or haylage in order to minimize the possible effect of housing and feeding. Another limitation is that normal IS evaluated by EHC was not used as inclusion criteria for the healthy group. Whereas the IS of the Standardbred horses is known to be normal based on information from previous research projects where the horses' IS have been quantified (data not shown), the IS of the privately owned control horses is unknown. However, all control horses had normal fasting plasma insulin and glucose concentrations suggesting normal IS.

The definition of general obesity has varied among studies, e.g., BCS > 6 [5], BCS ≥ 7 [23, 36], BCS ≥ 8 [16]. Another study suggested BCS 7–7.5 as overweight but not obese [16]. The Henneke score [15] is originally adapted for use in Quarter Horses but there are no studies evaluating how well this scoring system agrees between different breeds. In addition, there seems to be breed variations as well as seasonal variations in CNS [37]. There is thus no consensus on how overweight or abnormal local adiposity should be defined for different breeds of horses. It is possible that the inclusion criteria for BCS and CNS among the normal horses in the present study should have used a narrower range. To test the hypothesis that BCS or CNS among the normal horses were associated with fasting insulin concentrations, $Peak_{INS}$ or $ISI_{COMP}$ linear regressions were performed. These regression models showed no significant correlations ($P > 0.160$, data not shown) suggesting no effect of BCS or CNS on the insulin response or estimates for IS in the normal horses.

The CV values for repeated tests in the present study varied between 6.7 and 18.5 % for calculated variables, where $AUC_{GLU}$ showed the lowest variation between tests. Higher intra-assay variability was found for analysis of insulin than for glucose in the present study, possibly affecting the CV values for the calculated parameters. In comparison, a previous study [14] using the USA developed OST, reported a similar CV for $AUC_{GLU}$ (6.4 %) but a higher CV for the $AUC_{INS}$ (45.1 %). One reason for the discrepancy of results is that fewer horses were used for repeatability testing in the aforementioned study. The insulin derived variables from the modified OST were generally considered to have a moderate to high repeatability based on CV, ICC and RC. Thus, repeatability of the OST appears to be comparable to the calculated variables from the insulin curve of another non-quantitative dynamic tests, the CGIT [32].

## Conclusions

The results of the present study demonstrate that the modified OST appears to be a practical and useful diagnostic tool for assessment of dysinsulinemia in the horse. However, to make it possible to establish the most appropriate sampling interval and to evaluate the accuracy of the modified OST, further studies in horses with a variable degree of insulin resistance are needed, where results from the modified OST are compared with quantitative measurements for IS.

### Abbreviations

$AUC_{INS}$: area under the curve for insulin during OST; $AUC_{GLU}$: area under the curve for glucose during OST; BCS: body condition score; CNS: cresty neck score; CV: coefficient of variation; EHC: euglycemic hyperinsulinemic clamp; EMS: equine metabolic syndrome; FSIGTT: frequently sampled IV glucose tolerance test; ICC: intraclass correlation coefficient; IS: insulin sensitivity; $ISI_{COMP}$: composite whole-body insulin sensitivity index; IR: insulin resistance; $M/I_{60}$: mean rate of glucose disposal per unit of insulin during the last 60 min of the; OGTT: oral glucose tolerance test; OST: oral sugar test; $Peak_{INS}$: peak concentration of insulin during OST; RC: repeatability coefficient; SD: standard deviation; T-$peak_{INS}$: time (min) to peak concentration for insulin during OST.

### Authors' contributions

All authors participated in the design of the study and in the collection of the data. SL interpreted the data and performed the statistical analysis in cooperation with JB. SL drafted the manuscript, but all authors have contributed substantially to the final manuscript. All authors read and approved the final manuscript.

### Acknowledgements

A special thanks to all of the horse owners and to Dr. Ida Askerfelt.

### Competing interests

None of the authors of this paper has a financial or personal relationship with other people or organizations that could inappropriately influence or bias the content of the article.

### About this supplement

This article has been published as part of *Acta Veterinaria Scandinavica* Volume 58 Supplement 1, 2016: Animal Obesity—causes, consequences and comparative aspects: current research. The full contents of the supplement are available online at http://www.actavetscand.biomedcentral.com/articles/supplements/volume-58-supplement-1.

### Funding

Publication charges for this article were funded by the research platform Future Animal Health and Welfare at the Swedish University of Agricultural Sciences.

### References

1. Frank N, Geor R, Bailey S, Durham A, Johnson P. Equine metabolic syndrome. J Vet Intern Med. 2010;24:467–75.
2. Bailey SR, Habershon-Butcher JL, Ransom KJ, Elliott J, Menzies-Gow NJ. Hypertension and insulin resistance in a mixed-breed population of ponies predisposed to laminitis. Am J Vet Res. 2008;69:122–9.
3. Geor RJ. Metabolic predispositions to laminitis in horses and ponies: obesity, insulin resistance and metabolic syndromes. J Equine Vet Sci. 2008;28:753–9.
4. Carter RA, Treiber K, Geor R, Douglass L, Harris PA. Prediction of incipient pasture-associated laminitis from hyperinsulinaemia, hyperleptinaemia and generalised and localised obesity in a cohort of ponies. Equine Vet J. 2009;41:171–8.
5. Treiber KH, Kronfeld DS, Hess TM, Byrd BM, Splan RK, Staniar WB. Evaluation of genetic and metabolic predispositions and nutritional risk factors for pasture-associated laminitis in ponies. J Am Vet Med Assoc. 2006;228:1538–45.

6. Treiber KH, Kronfeld DS, Geor RJ. Insulin resistance in equids: possible role in laminitis. J Nutr. 2006;136:2094S–8S.
7. Geor RJ. Current concepts on the pathophysiology of pasture-associated laminitis. Vet Clin North Am Equine Pract. 2010;26:265–76.
8. Stumvoll M, Mitrakou A, Pimenta W, Jenssen T, Yki-Jarvinen H, Van Haeften T, et al. Use of the oral glucose tolerance test to assess insulin release and insulin sensitivity. Diab Care. 2000;23:295–301.
9. Gutt M, Davis CL, Spitzer SB, Llabre MM, Kumar M, Czarnecki EM, et al. Validation of the insulin sensitivity index (ISI0,120): comparison with other measures. Diab Res Clin Pract. 2000;47:177–84.
10. Matsuda M, DeFronzo RA. Insulin sensitivity indices obtained from oral glucose tolerance testing: comparison with the euglycemic insulin clamp. Diab Care. 1999;22:1462–70.
11. Pratt-Phillips SE, Geor RJ, McCutcheon LJ. Comparison among the euglycemic-hyperinsulinemic clamp, insulin-modified frequently sampled intravenous glucose tolerance test, and oral glucose tolerance test for assessment of insulin sensitivity in healthy Standardbreds. Am J Vet Res. 2015;76:84–91.
12. Kronfeld DS, Treiber KH, Geor RJ. Comparison of nonspecific indications and quantitative methods for the assessment of insulin resistance in horses and ponies. J Am Vet Med Assoc. 2005;226:712–9.
13. Asplin KE, Sillence MN, Pollitt CC, McGowan CM. Induction of laminitis by prolonged hyperinsulinaemia in clinically normal ponies. Vet J. 2007;174:530–5.
14. Schuver A, Frank N, Chameroy KA, Elliott SB. Assessment of insulin and glucose dynamics by using an oral sugar test in horses. J Equine Vet Sci. 2013;34:465–70.
15. Henneke D, Potter G, Kreider J, Yeates B. Relationship between condition score, physical measurements and body fat percentage in mares. Equine Vet J. 1983;15:371–2.
16. Carter RA, Geor RJ, Burton Staniar W, Cubitt TA, Harris PA. Apparent adiposity assessed by standardised scoring systems and morphometric measurements in horses and ponies. Vet J. 2009;179:204–10.
17. Lindåse SS, Nostell KE, Müller CE, Jensen-Waern M, Bröjer JT. Effects of diet-induced weight gain and pasture turnout on insulin sensitivity in moderately insulin resistant horses. Am J Vet Res. 2016;77:300–9.
18. Firshman AM, Valberg SJ, Baird JD, Hunt L, DiMauro S. Insulin sensitivity in Belgian horses with polysaccharide storage myopathy. Am J Vet Res. 2008;69:818–23.
19. Öberg J, Bröjer J, Wattle O, Lilliehöök I. Evaluation of an equine-optimized enzyme-linked immunosorbent assay for serum insulin measurement and stability study of equine serum insulin. Comp Clin Pathol. 2012;21:1291–300.
20. Bland M. An introduction to medical statistics. 3rd ed. New York: Oxford University Press; 2000. p. 269–72.
21. Carter RA, McCutcheon LJ, George LA, Smith TL, Frank N, Geor RJ. Effects of diet-induced weight gain on insulin sensitivity and plasma hormone and lipid concentrations in horses. Am J Vet Res. 2009;70:1250–8.
22. Toth F, Frank N, Martin-Jimenez T, Elliott SB, Geor RJ, Boston RC. Measurement of C-peptide concentrations and responses to somatostatin, glucose infusion, and insulin resistance in horses. Equineet Vet J. 2010;42:149–55.
23. Hoffman R, Boston R, Stefanovski D, Kronfeld D, Harris P. Obesity and diet affect glucose dynamics and insulin sensitivity in Thoroughbred geldings. J Anim Sci. 2003;81:2333–42.
24. Erdmann J, Kallabis B, Oppel U, Sypchenko O, Wagenpfeil S, Schusdziarra V. Development of hyperinsulinemia and insulin resistance during the early stage of weight gain. Am J Physiol Endocrinol Metab. 2008;294:E568–75.
25. Mittelman SD, Van Citters GW, Kim SP, Davis DA, Dea MK, Hamilton-Wessler M, et al. Longitudinal compensation for fat-induced insulin resistance includes reduced insulin clearance and enhanced beta-cell response. Diabetes. 2000;49:2116–25.
26. Ader M, Stefanovski D, Kim SP, Richey JM, Ionut V, Catalano KJ, et al. Hepatic insulin clearance is the primary determinant of insulin sensitivity in the normal dog. Obesity (Silver Spring). 2014;22:1238–45.
27. Borgia L, Valberg S, McCue M, Watts K, Pagan J. Glycaemic and insulinaemic responses to feeding hay with different non-structural carbohydrate content in control and polysaccharide storage myopathy-affected horses. J Anim Physiol Anim Nutr (Berl). 2011;95:798–807.
28. Bamford NJ, Potter SJ, Harris PA, Bailey SR. Breed differences in insulin sensitivity and insulinemic responses to oral glucose in horses and ponies of moderate body condition score. Domest Anim Endocrinol. 2014;47:101–7.
29. Borer-Weir KE, Bailey SR, Menzies-Gow NJ, Harris PA, Elliott J. Evaluation of a commercially available radioimmunoassay and species-specific ELISAs for measurement of high concentrations of insulin in equine serum. Am J Vet Res. 2012;73:1596–602.
30. Tadros EM, Frank N. Endocrine disorders and laminitis. Equine Vet Educ. 2013;25:152–62.
31. Frank N. Equine metabolic syndrome. Vet Clin North Am Equine Prac. 2011;27:73–92.
32. Brojer J, Lindase S, Hedenskog J, Alvarsson K, Nostell K. Repeatability of the combined glucose-insulin tolerance test and the effect of a stressor before testing in horses of 2 breeds. J Vet Intern Med. 2013;27:1543–50.
33. Pratt S, Geor R, McCutcheon L. Effects of dietary energy source and physical conditioning on insulin sensitivity and glucose tolerance in Standardbred horses. Equine Vet J. 2006;38:579–84.
34. Steward-Hunt L, Geor R, McCutcheon L. Effects of short-term training on insulin sensitivity and skeletal muscle glucose metabolism in Standardbred horses. Equine Vet J. 2006;38:226–32.
35. Banse HE, McFarlane D. Comparison of three methods for evaluation of equine insulin regulation in horses of varied body condition score. J Equine Vet Sci. 2014;34:742–8.
36. Frank N, Elliott SB, Brandt LE, Keisler DH. Physical characteristics, blood hormone concentrations, and plasma lipid concentrations in obese horses with insulin resistance. J Am Vet Med Assoc. 2006;228:1383–90.
37. Giles SL, Nicol CJ, Rands SA, Harris PA. Assessing the seasonal prevalence and risk factors for nuchal crest adiposity in domestic horses and ponies using the cresty neck score. BMC Vet Res. 2015;11:13.

# 17

# Comparative review of human and canine osteosarcoma: morphology, epidemiology, prognosis, treatment and genetics

Siobhan Simpson[1], Mark David Dunning[1], Simone de Brot[1], Llorenç Grau-Roma[1], Nigel Patrick Mongan[1,2*] and Catrin Sian Rutland[1]

**Abstract**

Osteosarcoma (OSA) is a rare cancer in people. However OSA incidence rates in dogs are 27 times higher than in people. Prognosis in both species is relatively poor, with 5 year OSA survival rates in people not having improved in decades. For dogs, 1 year survival rates are only around ~ 45%. Improved and novel treatment regimens are urgently required to improve survival in both humans and dogs with OSA. Utilising information from genetic studies could assist in this in both species, with the higher incidence rates in dogs contributing to the dog population being a good model of human disease. This review compares the clinical characteristics, gross morphology and histopathology, aetiology, epidemiology, and genetics of canine and human OSA. Finally, the current position of canine OSA genetic research is discussed and areas for additional work within the canine population are identified.

**Keywords:** Bone cancer, Canine, Genetics, Human, Molecular diagnostics, Osteosarcoma, Treatment

## Background

Cancer is a leading cause of non-communicable morbidity and mortality throughout the world, second only to cardiovascular disease in the number of deaths of adults between the ages of 30 and 70 years old [1, 2]. For dogs, the most frequent causes of mortality in order are (i) cancer, (ii) trauma, (iii) locomotor (skeletal, muscles and joints), (iv) cardiac disease, and (v) neurological disease [3]. The development of new and superior cancer treatments has long been a priority in medicine, more recently there has been a drive to develop new approaches to treat and manage cancer in companion animals. Indeed, cancer in dogs is increasingly a concern for pet owners, in particular as some types of cancer occur at much higher rates in certain dogs breeds [4–7]. These cases of cancer in dogs themselves require treatment, in addition these spontaneous cancers in dogs represent effective models for the human disease equivalent [8]. Although developing new treatments in companion animals with naturally occurring disease is less contentious than inducing disease in experimental animals, ethical concerns with regards to the treatment of individuals enrolled on studies and gaining informed consent from owners remain [9].

Cancer is more common in adults than children, adolescents, and young adults (< 30 years old) [10, 11]. Despite this, bone cancer is most common in the young (< 20 years old) and elderly (over 60 years old) than individuals of intermediary age (20–60 years old) [10–12]. For many cancer types 5 year survival rates are improving, reflecting the development of earlier diagnostic techniques and improved treatments [1, 13]. In contrast to many other cancers OSA, the most common bone cancer, has not shown comparable improvements in mortality

*Correspondence: Nigel.mongan@nottingham.ac.uk
[1] Faculty of Medicine and Health Sciences, School of Veterinary Medicine and Science, The University of Nottingham, Sutton Bonington Campus, Loughborough LE12 5RD, UK

rates [13–15]. There is thus an urgent need to develop improved treatments for OSA.

In both human and canine patients the predominant bone cancer diagnosis is OSA [15, 16]. OSA is still considered rare in humans. For example, there were 217,440 estimated breast cancer cases in the NIH–NCI surveillance, epidemiology, evidence and end results (SEER) database in 2004 alone, compared to 3482 cases of OSA in the same database between 1973 and 2004 [15, 17]. Although OSA is also not very common in dogs, it is much more common than in people. Norwegian owner questionnaire data from four breeds (Labrador retriever, Newfoundland, Leonberger and Irish wolfhound) showed OSA incidences of between 0.2 and 8.9% depending on the breed [18]. The percentage of dogs positively identified with OSA in two Polish clinics was estimated to be between 2.7 and 10.7%, again depending on breed [19]. Between 1995 and 2002 of 394,061 insured Swedish dogs, 764 (0.19%) developed a bone cancer [16]. This is an incidence rate of 27.2 dogs per 100,000 included in the dataset each year. While the canine data only includes insured dogs, it is a large dataset so is likely to be representative of the dog population of the country as whole. In the comparable Swedish population, 234 men and 164 women had bone cancer between 1998 and 2002, which is roughly 0.89 cases of bone cancer per 100,000 people each year [11]. The human data records all bone cancer cases in the country and the average population size between 1998 and 2002 was calculated from government census data. In addition all other countries in the "Cancer Incidence in Five Continents" registry report human incidence rates similar to Sweden [11, 12]. Thus, the incidence of canine bone cancer is 27 times higher than in humans. The higher incidence rate of canine OSA makes the pet dog population a good model for human disease. While there is potential for any dog to develop OSA, a subset of larger dog breeds are at increased risk of developing OSA [16].

The purpose of this review is to give an insight into the morphology, epidemiology, prognosis, treatment and genetics of osteosarcoma and to compare these aspects, in light of the published literature, between humans and dogs. Such knowledge is required to translate advances made in the clinical management of OSA in people to dogs; and to advance our understanding of where disease processes are similar across species.

## Search strategy

This review is based on a search in PubMed (http://www.ncbi.nlm.nih.gov/pubmed) using the terms "canine, dog, human, osteosarcoma, cancer, tumour, oncology". Each title and abstract of the obtained hits were evaluated and articles referring to genetics, epidemiology, treatment, histology and prognosis were assessed in detail (full text). Searches were carried out from 06/2016 to 02/2017 an additionally 08/2017. All titles, abstracts and full texts were read and obtained by all authors. Searches included web of science and PubMed. All papers published prior to, and including 08/2017 were included. Our personal photograph archives were used to illustrate OSA (with appropriate ethical permissions) and our experience within the field was used to evaluate the literature.

## Gross and histological similarities and differences between canine and human OSA

A sarcoma is a malignant tumour originating in tissues derived from the mesoderm; affecting bone, cartilage and other connective tissues [20]. OSA is a sarcoma which produces bone or osteoid [21]. In both people and dogs, the gross appearance of the OSA is markedly variable, some being predominantly lytic (soft, fleshy and with areas of haemorrhage and necrosis), productive (hard consistency and variably grey in colour), or being a mix of both. It frequently transgresses the cortex at the same time that it grows within the medulla, rarely penetrating the joint (Fig. 1) [22]. World Health Organisation (WHO) defines OSA as a primary malignant bone tumour in which the neoplastic cells produce osteoid [22]. In both people and dogs, OSA is characterized by a highly pleomorphic and heterogeneous microscopic appearance, and it is divided into several histologic subtypes similar in both species (Table 1) [22, 23]. Commonly, these subtypes are typically mixed in the same tumour, which questions the significance of histologic tumour classification for prognostic purposes. Indeed, histologic subtype could not be demonstrated to influence biological

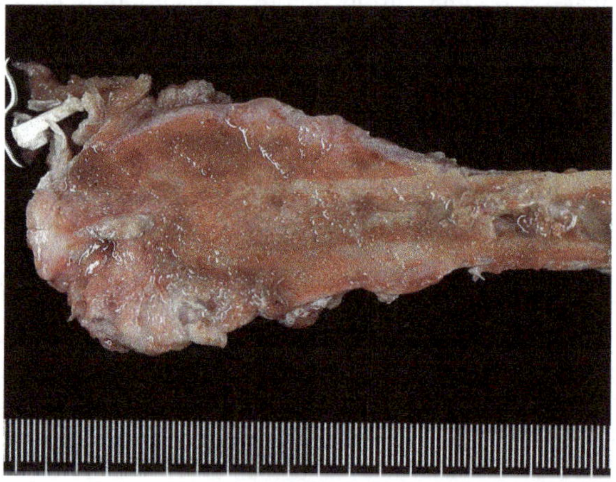

**Fig. 1** Femoral osteosarcoma. Greyhound, 7 years and 7 months old. Dense sclerotic neoplastic proliferation with hard consistency at the level of the proximal metaphysis. The tumour infiltrates the medullary cavity and transgresses the cortical bone

**Table 1 Histologic subtypes of human and canine osteosarcoma**

| Species | Canine[a] | Human[b] |
|---|---|---|
| Subtypes | A. Central | Osteosarcoma |
| | Osteosarcoma | Low-grade central osteosarcoma |
| | a. Poorly differentiated | Conventional |
| | b. Osteoblastic | Chondroblastic |
| | Nonproductive | Fibroblastic |
| | Productive | Osteoblastic |
| | c. Chondroblastic | Secondary |
| | d. Fibroblastic | Telangiectatic |
| | e. Telangiectatic | Small cell |
| | f. Giant cell type | Parosteal |
| | B. Peripheral | Periosteal |
| | 1. Periosteal osteosarcoma | High grade surface |
| | 2. Parosteal osteosarcoma | |

[a] Based on World Health Organization (WHO) International Histological Classification of Tumors of Domestic Animals [23]

[b] Based on WHO Classification of Tumours of Bone [22]

tumour behavior in dogs [24] and is controversially discussed in human literature. The most common subtype is the osteoblastic form in both people and dogs (Fig. 2) [21, 25, 26]. Furthermore, OSAs are classified on tumour grade, which is based on microscopic features such as cellular pleomorphism, mitotic index, tumour matrix and degree of necrosis [25–27]. The vast majority of canine and human OSAs are high grade tumours [21, 26, 28]. Regarding the prognostic effect of OSA grading, the veterinary literature remains divided [26, 29, 30], whereas it is considered important and relevant for prognosis in human medicine [27].

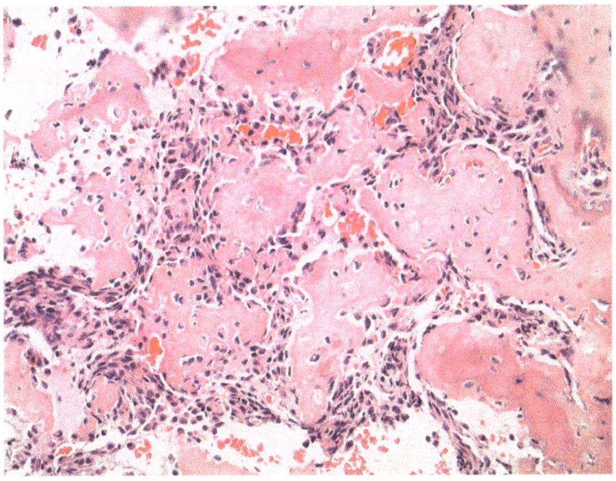

**Fig. 2** Microphotograph of a productive osteoblastic osteosarcoma. Abundant accumulation of extracellular lakes of osteoid between malignant osteoblasts. Haematoxylin and eosin stain. Obj. 20x

The vast majority of OSAs in both dogs and humans arise from within bones, particularly in the metaphyseal regions of long bones [22, 23] but can also originate on the surface of the bone or be extra-osseous [21]. In both humans and large dogs, OSA has a clear preference for the appendicular skeleton (up to 80% in dogs and 90% in humans) over the axial skeleton, with different bone percentages of involvement associated to the main weight bearing regions in each species. In people, ~ 50% of cases occur in the region of the knee (distal femur > proximal tibia followed by proximal humerus in approximately 25% of cases), in dogs the forelimbs are affected twice as often as the hind limbs (mainly distal radius and proximal humerus followed by distal and proximal femur and distal tibia) [31].

## Treatment of osteosarcoma in humans and dogs

In both humans and dogs, treatment for OSA involves surgery to remove primary tumours and on occasion distant metastasis, combined with neoadjuvant and/or adjuvant chemotherapy [32, 33]. Surgery involves either amputation of the limb or limb salvage/sparing procedures [34, 35]. Limb salvage is most frequently performed on patients with lower grade tumours and has been associated with similar outcomes to conventional approaches using amputation [35]. The proposed advantage of limb salvage surgery over amputation is that these patients have a better return-to-function and consequently quality-of-life than those undergoing amputation [36]. A recent meta-analysis supported this benefit in addition to a lower incidence of metastasis with limb salvage [37]. Similar advantages have yet to be reported in dogs undergoing limb salvage, perhaps suggesting poor cross-species efficacy. Canine reports suggest a similar metastatic frequency and survival time with limb salvage compared with the more conventional approach of amputation and adjuvant chemotherapy [38]. The failure to identify a significant difference in the outcomes in dogs compared with humans may be related to fewer numbers of dogs undergoing limb salvage procedures and therefore a more limited experience with the procedure. It is also possible that differences in case selection between humans and dogs impacts on outcome, in dogs clearly this may be the result of both patient factors and owner factors. Until a greater number of cases appear in the canine literature, the reason for the differences in outcomes remains unclear. Of note however from the canine literature on limb salvage, is that post-operative infections are associated with increased survival times [39–42]. The mechanism responsible for this prolonged survival and disease-free interval has yet to be elucidated, but is hypothesised to be due to up-regulation of antitumor immunity [39]. This is phenomenon is not unique to the dog and has also been reported in humans, with a similarly unclear aetiology [43, 44].

In human OSA, surgery with adjuvant chemotherapy remains the treatment of choice [45, 46]. The standard adjuvant chemotherapeutic approach uses a combination of methotrexate, doxorubicin and cisplatin using either a high, moderate, or standard dose protocols [47–50]. This approach has remained relatively unaltered for many years. The inclusion of additional chemotherapeutics including ifosfamide has met with mixed results and meta-analyses have provided conflicting evidence as to whether this provides a clear benefit in all cases [51, 52]. Whilst a large number of protocol modifications and experimental therapies have been reported, these at present do not offer credible therapeutic alternatives to improve outcome in affected individuals [49]. However there is evidence suggesting six doses of carboplatin may be superior to alternating doxorubicin and carboplatin regimens [53]. In canine OSA adjuvant chemotherapy with either doxorubicin or the platinum-based compounds including cisplatin and carboplatin have been associated with increased survival times over amputation alone [54–57]. The relative merits of the individual chemotherapy drugs have been evaluated. Reports indicate no significant difference in disease free interval or survival times in those dogs receiving either post-operative doxorubicin or carboplatin or combinations thereof for OSA [32]. However, those dogs receiving carboplatin experienced fewer side-effects improving the quality of life during therapy, an important consideration for most owners. Combination protocols with doxorubicin and carboplatin have also been evaluated for their potential benefit in improving disease free interval and survival times [58]. This combination protocol has been associated with a greater degree of chemotherapy induced toxicity [59]. A recent prospective study comparing carboplatin with an alternating carboplatin-doxorubicin protocol showed no benefit of the combination in improving survival over carboplatin alone [53]. Other (retrospective) publications using this combination have failed to demonstrate a clear benefit over single-agent carboplatin [58, 59]. Limited publications exist evaluating the benefits of additional chemotherapeutic agents for canine OSA e.g. gemcitabine; none provide a clear improvement in outcome above the use of carboplatin [60].

The use of bisphosphonate therapy as an adjunct to standard approaches for treating OSA has received reasonable coverage in the literature. A wide variety of experimental data exists on their efficacy in vitro and in models of OSA [61–65]. There has however been equivocal clinical benefit from their use in both in vivo models and in naturally occurring disease [66–68]. Whilst their value in management of the primary disease is unclear, perhaps more compelling evidence exists for their role in managing metastatic disease [63, 69–71]. This is a very important feature in managing OSA, given the importance of metastatic disease in overall mortality.

More recent reports on the use of immunotherapy based on an attenuated recombinant *Listeria monocytogenes* expressing a chimeric HERS/neu fusion protein have shown some encouraging results [72]. Dogs having undergone surgery (with amputation or limb salvage) with post-operative chemotherapy with four doses of carboplatin were enrolled in this study. In these dogs, 3 weeks after completion of their chemotherapy protocol they received the immunotherapy agent. There was an overall increase in survival time and reduction in the incidence of metastasis compared with historic controls. Newer therapeutic treatments including immunotherapies are also being investigated and developed in people given the failure to improve the outcome of human patients significantly in the past 30 years [73–75].

Given the failure to significantly improve the treatment approach and therefore outcome of OSA in humans over the past 3 decades [76, 77] and in dogs over the same period [78–80], novel approaches are clearly required. One particular area of medicine that may provide improved treatment approaches for OSA focuses on the field of pharmacogenomics. Here specific pharmacogenetic biomarkers and targets can provide a personalised approach to therapy for OSA [81, 82]. This approach whilst desirable remains in its infancy but clearly provides exciting potential for future management of OSA in both humans and dogs.

## Prognostic factors for osteosarcoma in humans and dogs

Key factors affecting treatment outcome are diagnostic and prognostic tools. Typical OSA disease progression consists of a primary tumour, usually originating within the medullary cavity, which grows, proliferates, and invades, and left unchecked frequently metastasises to the lungs [83]. Prognosis for individuals with metastatic tumours is much poorer than for individuals with only primary tumours. The 5-year-event-free-survival for humans with metastatic tumours at diagnosis reported to be 27.4%, while individuals with no metastases at diagnosis the 5-year-event-free-survival is ~ 70% [15, 83]. The prognosis for canine OSA is poor with 1 year survival rates following diagnosis and treatment typically less than 45% [84–86]. Of those dogs surviving beyond 1 year, ~ 54% will develop metastatic disease with a median survival time of 243 days [40]. In dogs with evidence for metastatic disease at the time of diagnosis, the median survival time is 76 days [23]. There is gathering evidence in some cases (although limited by study numbers) that in addition to the understanding that certain breeds are predisposed to developing OSA, there are also specific genetic differences within the tumours encountered in certain breeds which may have prognostic significance [87, 88].

A number of factors have been suggested to have prognostic significance in canine OSA. Bodyweight and tumour location have been suggested to be of particular importance and are readily available parameters for all patients. Dogs with lower body weight have a longer survival time [39, 89, 90] and dogs with proximal humeral tumours experience a shorter survival time [91]. Serum biomarkers have also been evaluated, such markers are clearly desirable particularly if routinely measured as this helps clinicians to begin discussions around prognosis with clients without recourse to advanced diagnostics. Increased serum alkaline phosphatase activity in dogs has been associated with a shorter disease free interval and survival time [92]. Histological grading is relevant for prognosis in human medicine [27], but remains controversial in dogs [26, 29, 30]. A recent meta-analysis in dogs has suggested that ALP and a proximal humeral location are significant negative prognostic factors. The importance of other factors was difficult to determine in this meta-analysis due to limited numbers of dogs and studies in which these had been reviewed [91]. In humans, the extent of any histological response to pre-operative chemotherapy has significant predictive value for both local and distant disease control [48, 77]. A similar effect has not been reported in dogs, this may be due to pre-operative chemotherapy not being part of routine treatment for canine OSA. In both humans and dogs molecular and genetic factors have also been identified as having potential prognostic significance. Many of these have been identified in OSA cell lines and therefore their clinical significance needs clarifying, however a number of cell lines have shown similarities between human and canine OSA, these therefore represent a very valuable evaluation tool [93]. Some of the factors observed in cell lines include HER-2 and PTEN, which have also been identified in some tissue samples [31]. The expression of matrix metalloproteases have also been demonstrated in some tissue samples (MMPs 2 and 9), however the clinical and prognostic significance of these is unclear. In humans, the literature often has conflicting data on the significance of particular markers. For example, the human epidermal growth factor 2 oncogene (HER-2) has been suggested in some reports to have prognostic significance, though further study is required to definitively confirm this [94–96]. Epidermal growth factor has been evaluated in dogs, whilst expressed in primary and metastatic tumour cells, it has not been shown to be an effective prognostic marker clinically [97]. Vascular endothelial growth factor A (VEGFA) has also been implicated in prognosis and over-expression has been associated with shorter survival times in humans [98]. However, at present the actual value of VEGFA in prognostication remains to be clarified [98, 99]. In humans p53 has been shown to be an effective prognostic marker and upregulated p53 is associated with a shorter survival time [100]. This has also been associated with prognosis canine OSA [101]. Strong expression of CXCL-12 is also associated with a more favourable outcome in humans with OSA [96]. The significance of CXCL-12 expression has yet to be investigated in dogs. MicroRNA transcripts have also been investigated for their prognostic significance. It would seem that down-regulation of 14q32 miRNA expression is a conserved mechanism in both human and canine OSA samples and influences tumour behaviour [102]. One particularly promising molecule however is ezrin, a membrane cytoskeleton linking molecule. This has been associated with a shorted survival time in both humans and dogs with OSA [103–106]. In addition to overall prognosis, a number of factors have been implicated in the development of metastatic disease. Given that local disease control is not the major life-limiting aspect to both canine and human OSA, identifying factors affecting metastasis are crucial. A number of markers have been identified in humans including Hes4 [107] and in canine OSA the proto-oncogene c-Met has been implicated in lymphatic spread [108].

## Epidemiology and genetics of osteosarcoma in humans

Some cases of human OSA are associated with heritable cancer syndromes, and the genetic bases of these have been established [109–111]. Most instances of OSA, however are not associated with heritable cancer syndromes and there have only been two heritable genetic loci identified, but there are some risk factors associated with OSA development including growth, puberty, sex, and race [15, 112, 113]. Evidence that growth plays a part in the development of OSA comes from the age of onset frequently coinciding with rapid bone growth during puberty, tumour sites most frequently at the end of bones where active growth occurs, and people affected by OSA are on average taller than the unaffected population [15, 112]. There is a difference between sexes in the development of OSA with males more commonly affected than females, and there is some evidence of variation in the incidence rate between races in the USA [15, 112]. Although OSA itself does not appear to be directly heritable in most instances, there are heritable components to the risk factors [114].

There have been somatic mutations in tumour suppressor genes identified in individuals with heritable cancer syndromes, and there have been mutations identified in OSA tumours compared to non-tumours [109, 115–117]. There have, however, only been two somatic genetic mutations associated with OSA specifically [113]. This lack of identified somatic genetic associations is not surprising based on the lack of heritability observed in human OSA. Despite the lack of heritability and somatic genetic mutations identified there have been over 900 genes associated with human OSA [118]. These genes have been associated with OSA due to either differences in expression between tumour and non-tumour tissue, or due to mutations that have arisen in the tumour tissue compared to the non-tumour tissue [119–121]. Mutations in OSA tumour tissue, but not non-tumour tissue, and differences in gene expression between tumour and non-tumour tissue could be either the cause of the tumour or a result of the tumour. A possible cause of both differences in expression between tumour and non-tumour tissue, and mutations in tumour but not non-tumour tissue, is genomic and chromosomal instability [122, 123]. Genomic and chromosomal instability is a reported factor in many types of cancer progression [122, 123]. OSA has been shown to display chromosomal instability associated with mutations in the *TP53* gene [124]. A consequence of this chromosomal instability is aneuploidy, which can lead to the overexpression of some genes within malignant cells, disrupting normal cell processes [125]. Although mutations in *TP53* appear to be associated with chromosomal instability, the gene itself does not seem to be subsequently over expressed following aneuploidy [124, 125].

## Epidemiology and genetics of osteosarcoma in dogs

As outlined above, canine OSA is more common than human OSA [11, 12, 16]. Despite this there are similar risk factors associated with the development of OSA in dogs as in people, including growth and sex [16, 126]. In addition, OSA in dogs is also influenced by breed and neutering status [16, 126]. Large dogs constitute the majority of OSA cases [16, 94]. Similarly, people with OSA are commonly taller than average [112]. In the canine population, as with the human population, there also appears to be a sex disparity, with males more likely to develop OSA than females [12, 16]. Neutering status, although not relevant in the human context, appears to contribute to OSA risk where neutered dogs are more likely to develop OSA than non-neutered dogs [126]. This, combined with the association with puberty, suggests a complex role for sex hormone signalling in OSA risk. In contrast to human OSA, canine OSA appears to be heritable, with some breeds appearing to be predisposed to developing OSA compared to others [16, 127]. Interestingly of the 15 breeds with the highest reported incidence of OSA 12 are within a clear clade on the canine phylogeny [16, 128]. This relationship between affected breeds could indicate a potential common genetic origin of canine OSA across breeds, however the clade is large and contains many breeds that are not highly affected by OSA, thus this seems less likely [128].

Four breeds of dog that have a high incidence of OSA are the Rottweiler, Greyhound, Deerhound and Irish Wolfhound. The Irish Wolfhound, the largest breed, has the highest prevalence of OSA within the insured Swedish dog population once numbers within the population are taken into account [16]. It also has one of the lower median ages of onset at 6.6 years, only the greyhound has a lower median age of onset at 6.2 years [16]. Greyhounds are recognised to frequently develop OSA—accounting for around 25% of mortality in some cohorts [129, 130]. Although The Irish Wolfhound history includes a period when they were close to extinction [131]. In the process of conserving the breed the few remaining Irish Wolfhounds were crossed with Great Danes, Deerhounds, Borzois, and Mastiffs [131, 132]. This out-crossing will have introduced some genetic diversity, but to retain the Irish Wolfhound phenotype a large amount of inbreeding will have been required, therefore as with most modern breeds, genetic diversity is low within the breed [133]. Importantly for the Irish Wolfhound breed both Great Danes and Deerhounds have a high prevalence of OSA, and these were two breeds used to help rescue Irish Wolfhounds from extinction [16, 127, 131]. Combined with inbreeding, the use of two breeds predisposed to developing OSA could have led to Irish Wolfhounds acquiring OSA predisposition genes from both breeds. The Deerhound, a hunting dog, with references as far back as the third century; was split into various strains in the early nineteenth century, which is likely to have had an effect on genetic diversity. The Rottweiler is also a large breed of dog and within the insured Swedish dog population they have the 5th highest incidence ranking (after correction for actual numbers of dogs) for OSA with a median age of onset of 7.9 years [16]. The Rottweiler originated in Germany being used for guarding, droving, and as a draught dog [134]. Following the creation of breed standards in the 1930s, when the breed was registered with the UK and American Kennel Clubs it is likely that Rottweilers have exclusively been mated with other Rottweilers leading to a closed gene pool within the pedigree Rottweiler population [134, 135].

There have been 34 genetic loci associated with canine OSA across four breeds [136, 137]. One study identified 33 loci as associated with canine OSA across three breeds [136] and another identified a single locus associated with OSA in Deerhounds [137]. None of the loci were consistently associated across breeds, further suggesting that there may be a difference between breeds in the genetic predisposition to developing canine OSA [136, 137]. There have been 4 loci associated with the development of OSA in Irish Wolfhounds [136]. In Rottweilers 15 loci were associated with the development of OSA [136]. Deerhounds also have a high prevalence of OSA with an incidence rate of 15% and a heritability value of 0.69 [126, 127]. Those Deerhounds carrying putative high-risk dominant allele are considered to have a > 75% risk of developing OSA compared with those not carrying the allele. This has been mapped to CFA34 [137]. Unusually, in this breed, females appear to have an increased risk of developing OSA; this is not influenced by the neuter status [127]. Genetic analysis of Greyhounds has shown 14 inherited risk loci, the strongest in this breed was located 150 kb upstream of the tumour suppressor genes CDKN2A/B [136]. Interestingly the risk of developing OSA seems not to be a general feature of derivative breeds such as Whippets. Despite close clustering of molecular microsatellite markers, Whippets rarely suffer from OSA [138]. This raises the question of whether genetic factors alone account for the incidence of OSA in this breed. The influence of IGF-1 on size variation in dogs may have an influence in this regard, given the possible association with the development of canine OSA [139].

Currently none of the genetic variants identified as associated with canine OSA have been mechanistically verified. Verification of the mode of action could lead to the identification of novel therapeutic targets, and if these loci can be shown to consistently predict an increased risk of OSA, the number of affected individuals could be reduced. Breeders could genotype prospective sires and dams prior to mating and choose parents to reduce the risk of offspring having multiple deleterious OSA alleles in conjunction with minimising the epidemiological factors. In addition to the 34 genetic loci identified as associated with canine OSA, there have been genes identified as differentially expressed in canine OSA compared to non-tumour tissue that have implications for growth and metastasis, and are potential drug targets [140–143]. These genes have been identified utilising canine OSA tumour tissue, and canine OSA cell lines. There has also been variation in the expression of genes within tumours associated with survival time in canine OSA [97, 144–146].

## Conclusions

There are several dog breeds that appear to have a genetic predisposition to OSA for which no OSA associated loci have been identified, these breeds could benefit from the identification of OSA predisposition loci. Additional work is required to confirm the effect of the genetic loci identified as associated with canine OSA, and account for the variation observed in the development of disease. This is also the case with humans, therefore comparing the two species may provide valuable insights into disease origins and progression, given the many similarities between the tumour in both species. Further work is also required to establish improved treatment regimens for individuals that develop disease, the identification of particular genetic pathways that are altered in OSA tumour tissue compared to non-tumour tissue could facilitate this. Any genetic loci identified as associated with canine OSA have the potential to be examined for an association with human OSA, and any treatments shown to be effective in either species could be applied to the other.

### Abbreviations

HER-2: human epidermal growth factor 2 oncogene; OSA: osteosarcoma; SEER: surveillance, epidemiology, evidence and end results; VEGFA: vascular endothelial growth factor A; WHO: World Health Organisation.

### Authors' contributions

All authors contributed towards the writing. CSR and NPM fostered the idea of the review and coordinated the writing process. CSR, SS and NPM drafted the background, and sections on epidemiology and genetics, MD and SS drafted the section on clinical treatment and prognostics, SDB and LGR drafted the section on histology. All authors read and approved the final manuscript.

### Authors' information

SS (BSc, MSc, PhD) under took her PhD in osteosarcoma genomics and epidemiology, under the supervision of CSR and NPM. MD is a Clinical Associate Professor in Small Animal Internal Medicine (MA, VetMB, PhD, CertSAM, DipECVIM-CA, MRCVS), European Veterinary Specialist in Small Animal Internal Medicine and RCVS Recognised Specialist in Small Animal Internal Medicine. SdB is a Clinical Assistant Professor in Veterinary Pathology (DVM, Dr.med. vet., ECVP Diplomate) who has been active in comparative (primarily canine and human) cancer research since 2004. LGR is a Clinical Assistant Professor in Veterinary Pathology (BSc, DVM, PhD, ECVP Diplomate). NPM is an Associate Professor of Cancer Biology [BSc (Hons) PhD]. He is a Fellow of the Royal College of Pathology with more than 15 years' experience in translational cancer research and genomics. CSR is an Assistant Professor in Anatomy and Developmental Genetics [BSc (Hons), MSc, MMedSci, PhD, FAS], Fellow of the Anatomical Society and the Galton Institute with over 15 years research experience in histology and genomics.

### Author details

[1] Faculty of Medicine and Health Sciences, School of Veterinary Medicine and Science, The University of Nottingham, Sutton Bonington Campus, Loughborough LE12 5RD, UK. [2] Department of Pharmacology, Weill Cornell Medicine, 1300 York Avenue, New York, NY 10065, USA.

### Acknowledgements

We would like to thank Professor Malcolm Cobb, School of Veterinary Medicine and Science, University of Nottingham for his insight and expertise.

### Competing interests

The authors declare that they have no competing interests.

**Funding**

The authors declare that they have no competing interests. This work was supported by the Biotechnology and Biological Sciences Research Council (Grant Number BB/J014508/1), by generous funding to Nigel P. Mongan and Catrin S. Rutland from the BBSRC University of Nottingham Doctoral Training Programme. The funders did not participate in any aspect of the manuscript.

**References**

1. Siegel RL, Miller KD, Jemal A. Cancer statistics, 2015. CA Cancer J Clin. 2015;65:5–29.
2. World Health Organisation. Noncommunicable diseases country profiles 2014. http://apps.who.int/iris/bitstream/10665/128038/1/9789241507509_eng.pdf (2014). Accessed 28 May 2017.
3. Bonnett B, Egenvall A, Hedhammar A, Olson P. Mortality in over 350,000 insured Swedish dogs from 1995–2000: I. Breed-, gender-, age- and cause-specific rates. Acta Vet Scand. 2005;46:105–20.
4. DeVita VT, Chu E. A history of cancer chemotherapy. Cancer Res. 2008;68:8643–53.
5. Grüntzig K, Graf R, Hässig M, Welle M, Meier D, Lott G, Erni D, Schenker NS, Guscetti F, Boo G, et al. The swiss canine cancer registry: a retrospective study on the occurrence of tumours in dogs in Switzerland from 1955 to 2008. J Comp Pathol. 2015;152:161–71.
6. Ranieri G, Gadaleta CD, Patruno R, Zizzo N, Daidone MG, Hansson MG, Paradiso A, Ribatti D. A model of study for human cancer: spontaneous occurring tumors in dogs. Biological features and translation for new anticancer therapies. Crit Rev Oncol Hematol. 2013;88:187–97.
7. Schneider R. Comparison of age, sex, and incidence rates in human and canine breast cancer. Cancer. 1970;26:419–26.
8. Pinho SS, Carvalho S, Cabral J, Reis CA, Gärtner F. Canine tumors: a spontaneous animal model of human carcinogenesis. Transl Res. 2012;159:165–72.
9. Page R, Baneux P, Vail D, Duda L, Olson P, Anestidou L, Dybdal N, Golab G, Shelton W, Salgaller M, Hardy C. Conduct, oversight, and ethical considerations of clinical trials in companion animals with cancer: report of a workshop on best practice recommendations. J Vet Intern Med. 2016;30:527–35.
10. Forman D, Bray F, Brewster DH, Gombe Mbalawa C, Kohler B, Piñeros MSF, Swaminathan R, Ferlay J. Cancer incidence in five continents, vol. X. IARC Scientific Publication No. 164. Lyon: International Agency for Research on Cancer; 2014.
11. Parkin DM, Ferlay J, Curado M-P, Bray F, Edwards B, Shin H-R, Forman D. Fifty years of cancer incidence: CI5 I-IX. Int J Cancer. 2010;127:2918–27.
12. Mirabello L, Troisi RJ, Savage SA. International osteosarcoma incidence patterns in children and adolescents, middle ages and elderly persons. Int J Cancer. 2009;125:229–34.
13. Siegel R, Naishadham D, Jemal A. Cancer statistics, 2013. CA Cancer J Clin. 2013;63:11–30.
14. Dorfman HD, Czerniak B. Bone cancers. Cancer. 1995;75:203–10.
15. Mirabello L, Troisi RJ, Savage SA. Osteosarcoma incidence and survival rates from 1973 to 2004: data from the surveillance, epidemiology, and end results program. Cancer. 2009;115:1531–43.
16. Egenvall A, Nødtvedt A, von Euler H. Bone tumors in a population of 400 000 insured Swedish dogs up to 10 y of age: incidence and survival. Can J Vet Res. 2007;71:292–9.
17. Jemal A, Tiwari RC, Murray T, Ghafoor A, Samuels A, Ward E, Feuer EJ, Thun MJ. Cancer statistics, 2004. CA Cancer J Clin. 2004;54:8–29.
18. Anfinsen KP, Grotmol T, Bruland OS, Jonasdottir TJ. Breed-specific incidence rates of canine primary bone tumors—a population based survey of dogs in norway. Can J Vet Res. 2011;75:209–15.
19. Sapierzynski R, Czopowicz M. The animal-dependent risk factors in canine osteosarcomas. Pol J Vet Sci. 2017;20:293–8.
20. Souhami R, Tobias J, editors. Bone and soft-tissue sarcomas. In: Cancer and its management. Chichester: Blackwell Publishing Ltd; 2005. p. 386–404.
21. Klein MJ, Siegal GP. Osteosarcoma: anatomic and histologic variants. Am J Clin Pathol. 2006;125:555–81.
22. Fletcher CDM, Bridge JA, Hogendoorn PCW, Mertens F. Who classification of tumours of soft tissue and bone. 4th ed. Geneva: WHO Press; 2013.
23. Slayter MV, Boosinger TR, Pool RR, Dammrich K, Misdrop W, Larsen S, World Health Organization. International histologic classification of tumors of domestic animals, histological classification of bone and joint tumors of domestic animals. Washington, DC: Armed Forces Institute of Pathology American Registry of Pathology; 1994.
24. Nagamine E, Hirayama K, Matsuda K, Okamoto M, Ohmachi T, Kadosawa T, Taniyama H. Diversity of histologic patterns and expression of cytoskeletal proteins in canine skeletal osteosarcoma. Vet Pathol. 2015;52:977–84.
25. Fenger JM, London CA, Kisseberth WC. Canine osteosarcoma: a naturally occurring disease to inform pediatric oncology. ILAR J. 2014;55:69–85.
26. Loukopoulos P, Robinson WF. Clinicopathological relevance of tumour grading in canine osteosarcoma. J Comp Pathol. 2007;136:65–73.
27. Righi A, Paioli A, Dei Tos AP, Gambarotti M, Palmerini E, Cesari M, Marchesi E, Donati DM, Picci P, Ferrari S. High-grade focal areas in low-grade central osteosarcoma: high-grade or still low-grade osteosarcoma? Clin Sarcoma Res. 2015;5:23.
28. Withrow SJ, Wilkins RM. Cross talk from pets to people: translational osteosarcoma treatments. ILAR J. 2010;51:208–13.
29. Kirpensteijn J, Kik M, Rutteman GR, Teske E. Prognostic significance of a new histologic grading system for canine osteosarcoma. Vet Pathol. 2002;39:240–6.
30. Kruse MA, Holmes ES, Balko JA, Fernandez S, Brown DC, Goldschmidt MH. Evaluation of clinical and histopathologic prognostic factors for survival in canine osteosarcoma of the extracranial flat and irregular bones. Vet Pathol. 2013;50:704–8.
31. Morello E, Martano M, Buracco P. Biology, diagnosis and treatment of canine appendicular osteosarcoma: similarities and differences with human osteosarcoma. Vet J. 2011;189:268–77.
32. Selmic LE, Burton JH, Thamm DH, Withrow SJ, Lana SE. Comparison of carboplatin and doxorubicin-based chemotherapy protocols in 470 dogs after amputation for treatment of appendicular osteosarcoma. J Vet Intern Med. 2014;28:554–63.
33. Ta HT, Dass CR, Choong PFM, Dunstan DE. Osteosarcoma treatment: state of the art. Cancer Metastasis Rev. 2009;28:247–63.
34. Liptak JM, Dernell WS, Ehrhart N, Lafferty MH, Monteith GJ, Withrow SJ. Cortical allograft and endoprosthesis for limb-sparing surgery in dogs with distal radial osteosarcoma: a prospective clinical comparison of two different limb-sparing techniques. Vet Surg. 2006;35:518–33.
35. Reddy KIA, Wafa H, Gaston CL, Grimer RJ, Abudu AT, Jeys LM, Carter SR, Tillman RM. Does amputation offer any survival benefit over limb salvage in osteosarcoma patients with poor chemonecrosis and close margins? Bone Joint J. 2015;97(B):115–20.
36. Mavrogenis A, Abati C, Romagnoli C, Ruggieri P. Similar survival but better function for patients after limb salvage versus amputation for distal tibia osteosarcoma. Clin Orthop Relat Res. 2012;470:1735–48.
37. Li X, Zhang Y, Wan S, Li H, Li D, Xia J, Yuan Z, Ren M, Yu S, Li S, et al. A comparative study between limb-salvage and amputation for treating osteosarcoma. J Bone Oncol. 2016;5:15–21.
38. Mitchell KE, Boston SE, Kung M, Dry S, Straw RC, Ehrhart NP, Ryan SD. Outcomes of limb-sparing surgery using two generations of metal endoprosthesis in 45 dogs with distal radial osteosarcoma. A veterinary society of surgical oncology retrospective study. Vet Surg. 2016;45:36–43.
39. Lascelles BD, Dernell WS, Correa MT, Lafferty M, Devitt CM, Kuntz CA, Straw RC, Withrow SJ. Improved survival associated with postoperative wound infection in dogs treated with limb-salvage surgery for osteosarcoma. Ann Surg Oncol. 2005;12:1073–83.
40. Culp WT, Olea-Popelka F, Sefton J, Aldridge CF, Withrow SJ, Lafferty MH, Rebhun RB, Kent MS, Ehrhart N. Evaluation of outcome and prognostic factors for dogs living greater than one year after diagnosis of osteosarcoma: 90 cases (1997–2008). J Am Vet Med Assoc. 2014;245:1141–6.
41. Sottnik JL, U'Ren LW, Thamm DH, Withrow SJ, Dow SW. Chronic bacterial osteomyelitis suppression of tumor growth requires innate immune responses. Cancer Immunol Immunother. 2010;59:367–78.

42. Seo K, Holt R, Jung YS, Rodriguez CO Jr, Chen X, Rebhun RB. Fluoroquinolone-mediated inhibition of cell growth, S-G2/M cell cycle arrest, and apoptosis in canine osteosarcoma cell lines. PLoS ONE. 2012;7:e42960.
43. Jeys LM, Grimer RJ, Carter SR, Tillman RM, Abudu A. Post operative infection and increased survival in osteosarcoma patients: are they associated? Ann Surg Oncol. 2007;14:2887–95.
44. Chen YU, Xu SF, Xu M, Yu XC. Postoperative infection and survival in osteosarcoma patients: reconsideration of immunotherapy for osteosarcoma. Mol Clin Oncol. 2015;3:495–500.
45. Anderson ME. Update on survival in osteosarcoma. Orthop Clin North Am. 2016;47:283–92.
46. Luetke A, Meyers PA, Lewis I, Juergens H. Osteosarcoma treatment—where do we stand? A state of the art review. Cancer Treat Rev. 2014;40:523–32.
47. Winkler K, Bielack SS, Delling G, Jurgens H, Kotz R, Salzer-Kuntschik M. Treatment of osteosarcoma: experience of the cooperative osteosarcoma study group (COSS). Cancer Treat Res. 1993;62:269–77.
48. Zhang FY, Tang W, Zhang ZZ, Huang JC, Zhang SX, Zhao XC. Systematic review of high-dose and standard-dose chemotherapies in the treatment of primary well-differentiated osteosarcoma. Tumour Biol. 2014;35:10419–27.
49. Ferrari S, Serra M. An update on chemotherapy for osteosarcoma. Expert Opin Pharmacother. 2015;16:2727–36.
50. Wang WG, Wan C, Liao GJ. The efficacy of high-dose versus moderate-dose chemotherapy in treating osteosarcoma: a systematic review and meta-analysis. Int J Clin Exp Med. 2015;8:15967–74.
51. Fan XL, Cai GP, Zhu LL, Ding GM. Efficacy and safety of ifosfamide-based chemotherapy for osteosarcoma: a meta-analysis. Drug Des Dev Ther. 2015;9:5925–32.
52. Su W, Lai Z, Wu F, Lin Y, Mo Y, Yang Z, Wu J. Clinical efficacy of preoperative chemotherapy with or without ifosfamide in patients with osteosarcoma of the extremity: meta-analysis of randomized controlled trials. Med Oncol. 2015;32:481.
53. Skorupski KA, Uhl JM, Szivek A, Allstadt Frazier SD, Rebhun RB, Rodriguez CO Jr. Carboplatin versus alternating carboplatin and doxorubicin for the adjuvant treatment of canine appendicular osteosarcoma: a randomized, phase iii trial. Vet Comp Oncol. 2016;14:81–7.
54. Berg J. Canine osteosarcoma: amputation and chemotherapy. Vet Clin North Am Small Anim Pract. 1996;26:111–21.
55. Phillips B, Powers BE, Dernell WS, Straw RC, Khanna C, Hogge GS, Vail DM. Use of single-agent carboplatin as adjuvant or neoadjuvant therapy in conjunction with amputation for appendicular osteosarcoma in dogs. J Am Anim Hosp Assoc. 2009;45:33–8.
56. Saam DE, Liptak JM, Stalker MJ, Chun R. Predictors of outcome in dogs treated with adjuvant carboplatin for appendicular osteosarcoma: 65 cases (1996–2006). J Am Vet Med Assoc. 2011;238:195–206.
57. Alvarez FJ, Kisseberth W, Hosoya K, Lara-Garcia A, Kosarek C, Murahari S, Au JL, Wientjes MG, Couto J, Couto G. Postoperative adjuvant combination therapy with doxorubicin and noncytotoxic suramin in dogs with appendicular osteosarcoma. J Am Anim Hosp Assoc. 2014;50:12–8.
58. Kent MS, Strom A, London CA, Seguin B. Alternating carboplatin and doxorubicin as adjunctive chemotherapy to amputation or limb-sparing surgery in the treatment of appendicular osteosarcoma in dogs. J Vet Intern Med. 2004;18:540–4.
59. Bacon NJ, Ehrhart NP, Dernell WS, Lafferty M, Withrow SJ. Use of alternating administration of carboplatin and doxorubicin in dogs with microscopic metastases after amputation for appendicular osteosarcoma: 50 cases (1999–2006). J Am Vet Med Assoc. 2008;232:1504–10.
60. McMahon M, Mathie T, Stingle N, Romansik E, Vail D, London C. Adjuvant carboplatin and gemcitabine combination chemotherapy postamputation in canine appendicular osteosarcoma. J Vet Intern Med. 2011;25:511–7.
61. Evdokiou A, Labrinidis A, Bouralexis S, Hay S, Findlay DM. Induction of cell death of human osteogenic sarcoma cells by zoledronic acid resembles anoikis. Bone. 2003;33:216–28.
62. Horie N, Murata H, Kimura S, Takeshita H, Sakabe T, Matsui T, Maekawa T, Kubo T, Fushiki S. Combined effects of a third-generation bisphosphonate, zoledronic acid with other anticancer agents against murine osteosarcoma. Br J Cancer. 2007;96:255–61.
63. Zekri J, Mansour M, Karim SM. The anti-tumour effects of zoledronic acid. J Bone Oncol. 2014;3:25–35.
64. Ohba T, Cates JM, Cole HA, Slosky DA, Haro H, Ichikawa J, Ando T, Schwartz HS, Schoenecker JG. Pleiotropic effects of bisphosphonates on osteosarcoma. Bone. 2014;63:110–20.
65. Wu CC, Huang YF, Hsieh CP, Chueh PJ, Chen YL. Combined use of zoledronic acid augments ursolic acid-induced apoptosis in human osteosarcoma cells through enhanced oxidative stress and autophagy. Molecules. 2016;21(12):1640.
66. Endo-Munoz L, Cumming A, Rickwood D, Wilson D, Cueva C, Ng C, Strutton G, Cassady AI, Evdokiou A, Sommerville S, et al. Loss of osteoclasts contributes to development of osteosarcoma pulmonary metastases. Cancer Res. 2010;70:7063–72.
67. Wolfe TD, Pillai SPS, Hildreth BE, Lanigan LG, Martin CK, Werbeck JL, Rosol TJ. Effect of zoledronic acid and amputation on bone invasion and lung metastasis of canine osteosarcoma in nude mice. Clin Exp Metastasis. 2011;28:377–89.
68. Piperno-Neumann S, Le Deley MC, Redini F, Pacquement H, Marec-Berard P, Petit P, Brisse H, Lervat C, Gentet JC, Entz-Werle N, et al. Zoledronate in combination with chemotherapy and surgery to treat osteosarcoma (os2006): a randomised, multicentre, open-label, phase 3 trial. Lancet Oncol. 2016;17:1070–80.
69. Koto K, Horie N, Kimura S, Murata H, Sakabe T, Matsui T, Watanabe M, Adachi S, Maekawa T, Fushiki S, Kubo T. Clinically relevant dose of zoledronic acid inhibits spontaneous lung metastasis in a murine osteosarcoma model. Cancer Lett. 2009;274:271–8.
70. Conry RM, Rodriguez MG, Pressey JG. Zoledronic acid in metastatic osteosarcoma: encouraging progression free survival in four consecutive patients. Clin Sarcoma Res. 2016;6:6.
71. Byrum ML, Pondenis HC, Fredrickson RL, Wycislo KL, Fan TM. Downregulation of CXCR4 expression and functionality after zoledronate exposure in canine osteosarcoma. J Vet Intern Med. 2016;30:1187–96.
72. Mason NJ, Gnanandarajah JS, Engiles JB, Gray F, Laughlin D, Gaurnier-Hausser A, Wallecha A, Huebner M, Paterson Y. Immunotherapy with a HER2-targeting listeria induces HER2-specific immunity and demonstrates potential therapeutic effects in a phase i trial in canine osteosarcoma. Clin Cancer Res. 2016;22:4380–90.
73. Bishop MW, Janeway KA, Gorlick R. Future directions in the treatment of osteosarcoma. Curr Opin Pediatr. 2016;28:26–33.
74. Wan J, Zhang X, Liu T. Strategies and developments of immunotherapies in osteosarcoma. Oncol Lett. 2016;11:511–20.
75. Botter SM, Neri D, Fuchs B. Recent advances in osteosarcoma. Curr Opin Pharmacol. 2014;16:15–23.
76. Murakami T, Igarashi K, Kawaguchi K, Kiyuna T, Zhang Y, Zhao M, Hiroshima Y, Nelson SD, Dry SM, Li Y, et al. Tumor-targeting salmonella typhimurium A1-R regresses an osteosarcoma in a patient-derived xenograft model resistant to a molecular-targeting drug. Oncotarget. 2017;8:8035–42.
77. Bielack SS, Hecker-Nolting S, Blattmann C, Kager L. Advances in the management of osteosarcoma. F1000Research. 2016;5:2767.
78. Shapiro W, Fossum TW, Kitchell BE, Couto CG, Theilen GH. Use of cisplatin for treatment of appendicular osteo-sarcoma in dogs. J Am Vet Med Assoc. 1988;192:507–11.
79. Thompson JP, Fugent MJ. Evaluation of survival times after limb amputation, with and without subsequent administration of cisplatin, for treatment of appendicular osteosarcoma in dogs—30 cases (1979–1990). J Am Vet Med Assoc. 1992;200:531–3.
80. MacEwen EG, Kurzman ID. Canine osteosarcoma: amputation and chemoimmunotherapy. Vet Clin North Am Small Anim Pract. 1996;26:123–33.
81. Serra M, Hattinger CM. The pharmacogenomics of osteosarcoma. Pharmacogenomics J. 2017;17:11–20.
82. Vos HI, Coenen MJ, Guchelaar HJ, Te Loo DM. The role of pharmacogenetics in the treatment of osteosarcoma. Drug Discov Today. 2016;21:1775–86.
83. Bacci G, Rocca M, Salone M, Balladelli A, Ferrari S, Palmerini E, Forni C, Briccoli A. High grade osteosarcoma of the extremities with lung metastases at presentation: treatment with neoadjuvant chemotherapy and simultaneous resection of primary and metastatic lesions. J Surg Oncol. 2008;98:415–20.
84. Frimberger AE, Chan CM, Moore AS. Canine osteosarcoma treated by post-amputation sequential accelerated doxorubicin and carboplatin chemotherapy: 38 cases. J Am Anim Hosp Assoc. 2016;52:149–56.

85. Moore AS, Dernell WS, Ogilvie GK, Kristal O, Elmslie R, Kitchell B, Susaneck S, Rosenthal R, Klein MK, Obradovoich J, et al. Doxorubicin and bay 12–9566 for the treatment of osteosarcoma in dogs: a randomized, double-blind, placebo-controlled study. J Vet Intern Med. 2007;21:783–90.
86. Straw RC, Withrow SJ, Richter SL, Powers BE, Klein MK, Postorino NC, LaRue SM, Ogilvie GK, Vail DM, Morrison WB, et al. Amputation and cisplatin for treatment of canine osteosarcoma. J Vet Intern Med. 1991;5:205–10.
87. Thomas R, Wang HJ, Tsai PC, Langford CF, Fosmire SP, Jubala CM, Getzy DM, Cutter GR, Modiano JF, Breen M. Influence of genetic background on tumor karyotypes: evidence for breed-associated cytogenetic aberrations in canine appendicular osteosarcoma. Chromosome Res. 2009;17:365–77.
88. Angstadt AY, Motsinger-Reif A, Thomas R, Kisseberth WC, Guillermo Couto C, Duval DL, Nielsen DM, Modiano JF, Breen M. Characterization of canine osteosarcoma by array comparative genomic hybridization and Rt-qPCR: signatures of genomic imbalance in canine osteosarcoma parallel the human counterpart. Gene Chromosome Cancer. 2011;50:859–74.
89. Bergman PJ, MacEwen EG, Kurzman ID, Henry CJ, Hammer AS, Knapp DW, Hale A, Kruth SA, Klein MK, Klausner J, et al. Amputation and carboplatin for treatment of dogs with osteosarcoma: 48 cases (1991 to 1993). J Vet Intern Med. 1996;10:76–81.
90. Amsellem PM, Selmic LE, Wypij JM, Bacon NJ, Culp WT, Ehrhart NP, Powers BE, Stryhn H, Farese JP. Appendicular osteosarcoma in small-breed dogs: 51 cases (1986–2011). J Am Vet Med Assoc. 2014;245:203–10.
91. Boerman I, Selvarajah GT, Nielen M, Kirpensteijn J. Prognostic factors in canine appendicular osteosarcoma—a meta-analysis. BMC Vet Res. 2012;8:56.
92. Garzotto CK, Berg J, Hoffmann WE, Rand WM. Prognostic significance of serum alkaline phosphatase activity in canine appendicular osteosarcoma. J Vet Intern Med. 2000;14:587–92.
93. Wilson H, Huelsmeyer M, Chun R, Young KM, Friedrichs K, Argyle DJ. Isolation and characterisation of cancer stem cells from canine osteosarcoma. Vet J. 2008;175:69–75.
94. Zhang Q, Liu F, Wang B, Li Z, Zhou D, Yang Q, Dong J, Li J. HER-2 expression in biopsy and surgical specimen on prognosis of osteosarcoma: a systematic review and meta-analysis of 16 studies. Medicine (Baltimore). 2016;95:e3661.
95. Gill J, Geller D, Gorlick R. HER-2 involvement in osteosarcoma. Adv Exp Med Biol. 2014;804:161–77.
96. Baumhoer D, Smida J, Specht K, Bink K, Quintanilla-Martinez L, Rosemann M, Siggelkow H, Nathrath WB, Atkinson MJ, Bielack S, et al. Aberrant expression of the human epidermal growth factor receptor 2 oncogene is not a common feature in osteosarcoma. Hum Pathol. 2011;42:859–66.
97. Selvarajah GT, Verheije MH, Kik M, Slob A, Rottier PJM, Mol JA, Kirpensteijn J. Expression of epidermal growth factor receptor in canine osteosarcoma: association with clinicopathological parameters and prognosis. Vet J. 2012;193:412–9.
98. Yu XW, Wu TY, Yi X, Ren WP, Zhou ZB, Sun YQ, Zhang CQ. Prognostic significance of VEGF expression in osteosarcoma: a meta-analysis. Tumour Biol. 2014;35:155–60.
99. Qu JT, Wang M, He HL, Tang Y, Ye XJ. The prognostic value of elevated vascular endothelial growth factor in patients with osteosarcoma: a meta-analysis and systemic review. J Cancer Res Clin Oncol. 2012;138:819–25.
100. Fu HL, Shao L, Wang Q, Jia T, Li M, Yang DP. A systematic review of p53 as a biomarker of survival in patients with osteosarcoma. Tumour Biol. 2013;34:3817–21.
101. Kirpensteijn J, Kik M, Teske E, Rutteman GR. TP53 gene mutations in canine osteosarcoma. Vet Surg. 2008;37:454–60.
102. Sarver AL, Thayanithy V, Scott MC, Cleton-Jansen AM, Hogendoorn PC, Modiano JF, Subramanian S. Micrornas at the human 14q32 locus have prognostic significance in osteosarcoma. Orphanet J Rare Dis. 2013;8:7.
103. Jaroensong T, Endo Y, Lee SJ, Kamida A, Mochizuki M, Nishimura R, Sasaki N, Nakagawa T. Effects of transplantation sites on tumour growth, pulmonary metastasis and ezrin expression of canine osteosarcoma cell lines in nude mice. Vet Comp Oncol. 2012;10:274–82.
104. Ren L, Hong SH, Chen QR, Briggs J, Cassavaugh J, Srinivasan S, Lizardo MM, Mendoza A, Xia AY, Avadhani N, et al. Dysregulation of ezrin phosphorylation prevents metastasis and alters cellular metabolism in osteosarcoma. Cancer Res. 2012;72:1001–12.
105. Khanna C, Wan X, Bose S, Cassaday R, Olomu O, Mendoza A, Yeung C, Gorlick R, Hewitt SM, Helman LJ. The membrane-cytoskeleton linker ezrin is necessary for osteosarcoma metastasis. Nat Med. 2004;10:182–6.
106. Xu-Dong S, Zan S, Shui-er Z, Li-na T, Wen-xi Y, Feng L, Yang Y. Expression of ezrin correlates with lung metastasis in Chinese patients with osteosarcoma. Clin Invest Med. 2009;32:E180–8.
107. McManus M, Kleinerman E, Yang Y, Livingston JA, Mortus J, Rivera R, Zweidler-McKay P, Schadler K. Hes4: A potential prognostic biomarker for newly diagnosed patients with high-grade osteosarcoma. Pediatr Blood Cancer. 2016. doi:10.1002/pbc.26318.
108. Fieten H, Spee B, Ijzer J, Kik MJ, Penning LC, Kirpensteijn J. Expression of hepatocyte growth factor and the proto-oncogenic receptor c-Met in canine osteosarcoma. Vet Pathol. 2009;46:869–77.
109. Ognjanovic S, Olivier M, Bergemann TL, Hainaut P. Sarcomas in tp53 germline mutation carriers. Cancer. 2012;118:1387–96.
110. Stinco G, Governatori G, Mattighello P, Patrone P. Multiple cutaneous neoplasms in a patient with Rothmund–Thomson syndrome: case report and published work review. J Dermatol. 2008;35:154–61.
111. Thomas DM, Ballinger ML. Etiologic, environmental and inherited risk factors in sarcomas. J Surg Oncol. 2015;111:490–5.
112. Mirabello L, Pfeiffer R, Murphy G, Daw NC, Patiño-Garcia A, Troisi RJ, Hoover RN, Douglass C, Schüz J, Craft AW, Savage SA. Height at diagnosis and birth-weight as risk factors for osteosarcoma. Cancer Causes Control. 2011;22:899–908.
113. Savage SA, Mirabello L, Wang Z, Gastier-Foster JM, Gorlick R, Khanna C, Flanagan AM, Tirabosco R, Andrulis IL, Wunder JS, et al. Genome-wide association study identifies two susceptibility loci for osteosarcoma. Nature Genet. 2013;45:799–803.
114. Yang J, Benyamin B, McEvoy BP, Gordon S, Henders AK, Nyholt DR, Madden PA, Heath AC, Martin NG, Montgomery GW, et al. Common SNPs explain a large proportion of the heritability for human height. Nature Genet. 2010;42:565–9.
115. Chen X, Bahrami A, Pappo A, Easton J, Dalton J, Hedlund E, Ellison D, Shurtleff S, Wu G, Wei L, et al. Recurrent somatic structural variations contribute to tumorigenesis in pediatric osteosarcoma. Cell Rep. 2014;7:104–12.
116. Srivastava S, Zou Z, Pirollo K, Blattner W, Chang EH. Germ-line transmission of a mutated p53 gene in a cancer-prone family with Li-fraumeni syndrome. Nature. 1990;348:747–9.
117. Zhang J, Walsh MF, Wu G, Edmonson MN, Gruber TA, Easton J, Hedges D, Ma X, Zhou X, Yergeau DA, et al. Germline mutations in predisposition genes in pediatric cancer. N Engl J Med. 2015;373:2336–46.
118. Poos K, Smida J, Nathrath M, Maugg D, Baumhoer D, Neumann A, Korsching E. Structuring osteosarcoma knowledge: An osteosarcoma-gene association database based on literature mining and manual annotation. Database. 2014. doi:10.1093/database/bau042.
119. Man T-K, Lu X-Y, Jaeweon K, Perlaky L, Harris CP, Shah S, Ladanyi M, Gorlick R, Lau CC, Rao PH. Genome-wide array comparative genomic hybridization analysis reveals distinct amplifications in osteosarcoma. BMC Cancer. 2004;4:45.
120. Xiao X, Wang W, Zhang H, Gao P, Fan B, Huang C, Fu J, Chen G, Shi L, Zhu H, et al. Individualized chemotherapy for osteosarcoma and identification of gene mutations in osteosarcoma. Tumour Biol. 2015;36:2427–35.
121. Yuan D, Liu B, Liu K, Zhu G, Dai Z, Xie Y. Overexpression of fibroblast activation protein and its clinical implications in patients with osteosarcoma. J Surg Oncol. 2013;108:157–62.
122. de Bruin EC, McGranahan N, Mitter R, Salm M, Wedge DC, Yates L, Jamal-Hanjani M, Shafi S, Murugaesu N, Rowan AJ, et al. Spatial and temporal diversity in genomic instability processes defines lung cancer evolution. Science. 2014;346:251–6.
123. Galanos P, Vougas K, Walter D, Polyzos A, Maya-Mendoza A, Haagensen EJ, Kokkalis A, Roumelioti F-M, Gagos S, Tzetis M, et al. Chronic p53-independent p21 expression causes genomic instability by deregulating replication licensing. Nat Cell Biol. 2016;18:777–89.
124. Al-Romaih K, Bayani J, Vorobyova J, Karaskova J, Park PC, Zielenska M, Squire JA. Chromosomal instability in osteosarcoma and its

association with centrosome abnormalities. Cancer Genet Cytogenet. 2003;144:91–9.

125. Carter SL, Eklund AC, Kohane IS, Harris LN, Szallasi Z. A signature of chromosomal instability inferred from gene expression profiles predicts clinical outcome in multiple human cancers. Nature Genet. 2006;38:1043–8.

126. Ru G, Terracini B, Glickman LT. Host related risk factors for canine osteosarcoma. Vet J. 1998;156:31–9.

127. Phillips JC, Stephenson B, Hauck M, Dillberger J. Heritability and segregation analysis of osteosarcoma in the Scottish deerhound. Genomics. 2007;90:354–63.

128. von Holdt BM, Pollinger JP, Lohmueller KE, Han E, Parker HG, Quignon P, Degenhardt JD, Boyko AR, Earl DA, Auton A, et al. Genome-wide SNP and haplotype analyses reveal a rich history underlying dog domestication. Nature. 2010;464:898–902.

129. Caro JT, Marin LM, Iazbik MC, Zaldivar-Lopez S, Borghese H, Couto CG. Markers of iron metabolism in retired racing greyhounds with and without osteosarcoma. Vet Clin Pathol. 2013;42:360–3.

130. Lord LK, Yaissle JE, Marin L, Couto CG. Results of a web-based health survey of retired racing greyhounds. J Vet Intern Med. 2007;21:1243–50.

131. Samaha J. The new complete Irish wolfhound. Howell Book House; 1991.

132. Philipp U, Vollmar A, Häggström J, Thomas A, Distl O. Multiple loci are associated with dilated cardiomyopathy in Irish wolfhounds. PLoS ONE. 2012;7:e36691.

133. Jansson M, Laikre L. Recent breeding history of dog breeds in Sweden: modest rates of inbreeding, extensive loss of genetic diversity and lack of correlation between inbreeding and health. J Anim Breed Genet. 2014;131:153–62.

134. The Kennel Club UK. Breed information centre—rottweiler. 2016. http://www.thekennelclub.org.uk/services/public/breed/display.aspx?id=5137. Accessed 29 Aug 2017.

135. American Kennel Club. Rottweiler. 2017. http://www.akc.org/dog-breeds/rottweiler/. Accessed 28 Aug 2017.

136. Karlsson EK, Sigurdsson S, Ivansson E, Thomas R, Elvers I, Wright J, Howald C, Tonomura N, Perloski M, Swofford R, et al. Genome-wide analyses implicate 33 loci in heritable dog osteosarcoma, including regulatory variants near CDKN2A/B. Genome Biol. 2013;14:R132.

137. Phillips JC, Lembcke L, Chamberlin T. A novel locus for canine osteosarcoma (OSA1) maps to CFA34, the canine orthologue of human 3q26. Genomics. 2010;96:220–7.

138. Dobson JM. Breed-predispositions to cancer in pedigree dogs. ISRN Vet Sci. 2013;2013:941275.

139. MacEwen EG, Pastor J, Kutzke J, Tsan R, Kurzman ID, Thamm DH, Wilson M, Radinsky R. IGF-1 receptor contributes to the malignant phenotype in human and canine osteosarcoma. J Cell Biochem. 2004;92:77–91.

140. McCleese JK, Bear MD, Kulp SK, Mazcko C, Khanna C, London CA. Met interacts with EGFR and Ron in canine osteosarcoma. Vet Comp Oncol. 2013;11:124–39.

141. Millanta F, Asproni P, Cancedda S, Vignoli M, Bacci B, Poli A. Immunohistochemical expression of COX-2, mPGES and EP2 receptor in normal and reactive canine bone and in canine osteosarcoma. J Comp Pathol. 2012;147:153–60.

142. Pang LY, Argyle SA, Kamida A, Morrison K, Argyle DJ. The long-acting COX-2 inhibitor mavacoxib (Trocoxil™) has anti-proliferative and pro-apoptotic effects on canine cancer cell lines and cancer stem cells. BMC Vet Res. 2014;10:184.

143. Shahi MH, York D, Gandour-Edwards R, Withers SS, Holt R, Rebhun RB. BMI1 is expressed in canine osteosarcoma and contributes to cell growth and chemotherapy resistance. PLoS ONE. 2015;10:e0131006.

144. Maniscalco L, Iussich S, Morello E, Martano M, Gattino F, Miretti S, Biolatti B, Accornero P, Martignani E, Sánchez-Céspedes R, et al. Increased expression of insulin-like growth factor-1 receptor is correlated with worse survival in canine appendicular osteosarcoma. Vet J. 2015;205:272–80.

145. Selvarajah GT, Kirpensteijn J, van Wolferen ME, Rao NAS, Fieten H, Mol JA. Gene expression profiling of canine osteosarcoma reveals genes associated with short and long survival times. Mol Cancer. 2009;8:72.

146. Selvarajah GT, Bonestroo FAS, Kirpensteijn J, Kik MJL, van der Zee R, van Eden W, Timmermans-Sprang EPM, Slob A, Mol JA. Heat shock protein expression analysis in canine osteosarcoma reveals HSP60 as a potentially relevant therapeutic target. Cell Stress Chaperon. 2013;18:607–22.

# 18

# Adoptive cell transfer: new perspective treatment in veterinary oncology

Joanna Katarzyna Bujak[1], Rafał Pingwara[1], Michelle Hase Nelson[2] and Kinga Majchrzak[1*]

**Abstract**

Cancer immunotherapy is recently considered the most promising treatment for human patients with advanced tumors and could be effectively combined with conventional therapies such as chemotherapy or radiotherapy. Patients with hematological malignancies and melanoma have benefited greatly from immunotherapies such as, adoptive cell transfer therapy, experiencing durable remissions and prolonged survival. In the face of increasing enthusiasm for immunotherapy, particularly for the administration of tumor-specific T lymphocytes, the question arises whether this method could be employed to improve treatment outcomes for canine patients. It is warranted to determine whether veterinary clinical trials could support comparative oncology research and thus facilitate the development of new cell-based therapies for humans. Herein, we discuss adoptive transfer of T lymphocytes and lymphokine-activated cells for application in veterinary oncology, in the context of human medicine achievements. Furthermore, we discuss potential benefits of using domestic dog as a model for immunotherapy and its advantages for translational medicine. We also focus on an emerging genome-editing technology as a useful tool to improve a T cells' phenotype.

**Keywords:** Adoptive cell transfer, Canine oncology, Gene editing, Immunotherapy, T lymphocytes

## Background

Cancer is a complex disease caused by the impairment in a cells' physiology leading to uncontrolled proliferation and inhibition of apoptosis [1]. Disease progression results from a complicated interplay between genetic alterations of transformed cells and cancer immunoediting by the hosts immune defense mechanisms [2]. It has been indicated in multiple human and canine studies that the dysfunction of immune system, enabling tumor growth and metastasis, is associated with tumor immune escape. This process is mainly manifested by downregulated expression of major histocompatibility complex (MHC) class I and tumor specific antigens, as well as, by production of anti-inflammatory cytokines such as IL-10 and TGF-β by malignant cells [3, 4]. Local immunosuppression is further supported by active recruitment of myeloid-derived suppressor cells (MDSC) into tumor microenvironment and activation of suppressive T regulatory cells (Tregs). This unfavorable niche alters the fate of immune cells and contributes to the functional inhibition of effector T and NK cells (Natural Killer cells), resulting in immunologic tolerance [5]. Unresponsiveness of T cells is caused by chronic stimulation and the expression of co-inhibitory receptors such as Programmed cell death protein 1 (PD-1) and cytotoxic T cell antigen 4 (CTLA-4), which leads to T cell exhaustion [6]. Moreover, cancer cells can induce deactivation of circulating monocytes and polarization of macrophages to M2-like phenotype, which not only foster existing tumor but also facilitate spread of transformed cells [7, 8]. Promotion of cancer progression is also linked with production of pro-angiogenic and pro-metastatic factors by tumor-associated macrophages (TAMs) and MDSCs [8–10]. Given the complex and dynamic crosstalk within the tumor microenvironment, the development of an effective anticancer immunotherapy has been a challenging endeavor.

*Correspondence: kinga_majchrzak@sggw.pl

[1] Department of Physiological Sciences, Faculty of Veterinary Medicine, Warsaw University of Life Sciences, ul. Nowoursynowska 159, 02-776 Warsaw, Poland

The first report of ACT therapy date back to mid-1960's, when allogeneic T lymphocytes have been transferred into rats to treat primary fibrosarcoma [11]. The goal of the study was to harness cytotoxic $CD8^+$ T cells (CTLs), capable of mediating direct target cell lysis, to fight against cancer. These landmark experiments paved the way for the development of cellular immunotherapy. Further advances have resulted in the discovery of cancer-associated antigens and the improvement of genetic engineering.

Currently, ACT therapy has demonstrated great promise in eliciting curative responses against hematological malignancies and melanoma in human patients. Veterinary oncology is highly translatable for human medicine and results obtained in the canine patients can facilitate the design of the next-generation clinical trials to treat advanced solid tumors in humans.

## Search strategy

This review is based on a search in PubMed (http://www.ncbi.nlm.nih.gov/pubmed) using the terms "adoptive cell transfer" OR "adoptive cell transfer in dogs" AND "tumor infiltrating lymphocytes" OR "TILs" AND "TCR engineered T cells" AND "CAR T cells" OR "canine CAR T cells" AND "canine T-LAK" AND "genome editing" OR "genome editing therapy". Only papers written in English were included in the review. The vast majority of the literature cited, is less than 15 years old. Exceptions are the papers that describe for the first time the crucial method or discovered phenomenon in the field of immunotherapy (i.e. first studies that paved the way for immunotherapy as a historical link).

All original research related to the canine immunotherapy (more specifically canine adoptive cell transfer and T-LAK therapy) were incorporated. Studies related to adoptive cell immunotherapy and genome editing, were evaluated and the most relevant to the review were selected. Our systematic review comprises the current knowledge on adoptive cell transfer therapy in canine oncology, in the context of human medicine achievements.

## Advantages of using a dog model for comparative oncology

The domestic dog (*Canis lupus familiaris*) is an attractive and useful model for comparative medicine for the evaluation and development of novel therapeutic strategies and ensuing immunological assessments [12–16]. Unlike transplantable xenograft rodent models, canine tumors share with human tumors similar epidemiology, genetic, biology, treatment responses, prognosis factors and clinical outcomes. Cancer occurs in dogs naturally and spontaneously and the progression of disease (e.g. metastatic cascade) is similar to humans. Finally, dogs share the same life environment and thus cancerogenic and risk factors with people [17]. Similar to people, the incidence of cancer in dogs increases with age, with a frequency of 45% in animals older than 10 years [18]. Therefore, the domestic dog is a recommended model for multiple human diseases including cancers such as non-Hodgkin lymphoma, osteosarcoma, leukemia, melanoma and lung, head and neck, prostate, mammary, and bladder carcinomas [12, 19, 20].

Cancer research has been revolutionized through the advances in genome sequencing and assembly. Knowledge about the genetic basis and molecular mechanisms of cancer progression greatly accelerated the development of novel therapies. In 2005, the canine genome was sequenced, leading to more advanced studies in the field of veterinary sciences [21]. It was an important step for comparative studies that improved the understanding of mammalian evolution as well as enhanced our knowledge of tumorigenesis, cancer growth and metastasis, and tumor immunology in animals.

The innate and adaptive immune system in dogs is comparable to humans. Additionally, the main immune cells subsets identified in dogs, as well as their surface markers, exhibit similarities to human [16]. Although many similarities have been found our understanding of canine immune system functioning is still highly affected by lack of specific reagent to fully define all immune subsets. Furthermore, factors regulating immune response and subsequent signaling pathways responsible for induction of anticancer immunity are yet to be determined. Nevertheless, domestic dog model offer possibilities of clinical studies that will benefit and inform design of human clinical trials. Advantages of using canine animal models are summarized in Fig. 1.

## Adoptive T cell transfer therapy

Among the four different categories of immunotherapies including: checkpoint inhibitors, monoclonal antibodies, therapeutic vaccines and cellular therapies, it is adoptive T cells transfer (ACT) therapy that has recently shown clinical outcomes of record efficiency in human hematological malignances and melanoma [22, 23].

ACT treatment involves the infusion of tumor-specific T lymphocytes into the circulatory system of cancer patients. The immune cells can be derived from one of two sources: (1) natural host T cells identified in the tumor mass—the autologous tumor infiltrating lymphocytes (TILs), (2) autologous T cells from patients' peripheral blood that have been genetically engineered ex vivo to express specific antitumor T cell receptors (TCRs) or chimeric antigen receptors (CARs) [24, 25]. The cells obtained from patients are activated and extensively

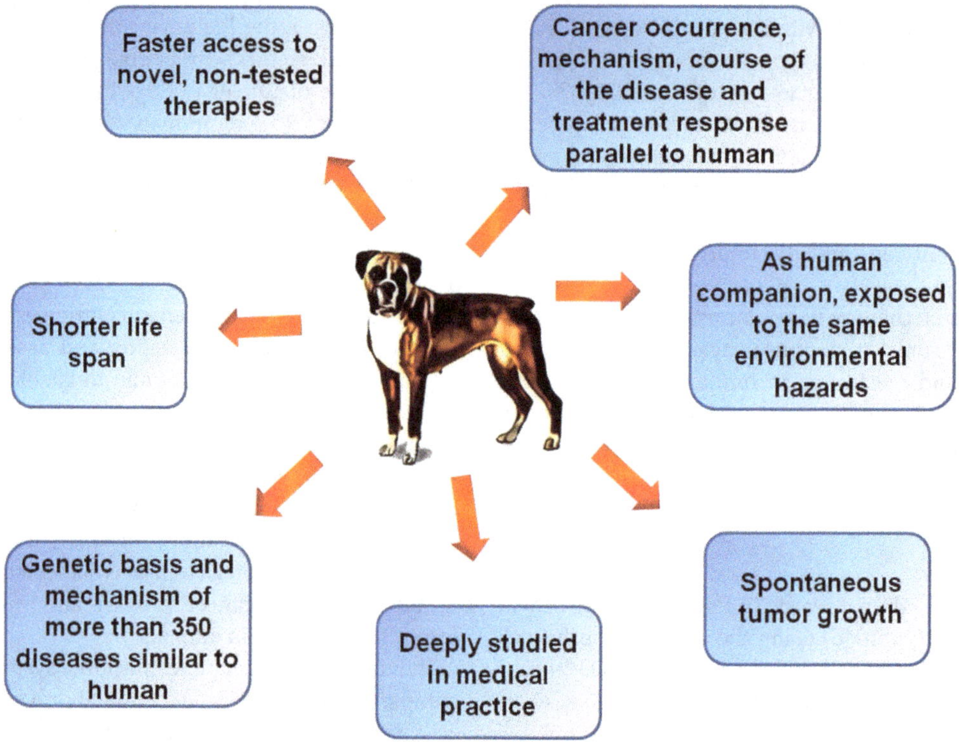


**Fig. 1** The domestic dog can serve as an attractive model in comparative oncology. Dogs and humans share the same environment and possess multiple similarities in genetics, physiology as well as tumorigenesis and cancer progression. For this reason, canine models are of great importance to cancer and immunological studies and can contribute to improvement of human immunotherapy

expanded to large numbers ($1 \times 10^{11}$) ex vivo in the presence of high dose IL-2 (a T cell growth factor) before re-infusion. Recently, additional genome editing has been proposed to enhance the function of engineered T lymphocytes.

In veterinary medicine, due to the similarities between canine and human antitumor immunity, a parallel approach can be applied (Fig. 2). Herein, we will compare ACT therapy in human versus veterinary settings.

## Tumor infiltrating T lymphocytes

The tumor microenvironment consists of transformed cancer cells and non-transformed stromal and inflammatory cells including fibroblasts, endothelial cells, T lymphocytes, dendritic cells, MDSCs and macrophages. Dynamic crosstalk between all of them via released cytokines and growth factors, and direct cell–cell interactions is responsible for either promotion or inhibition of tumor growth and metastasis (Fig. 3).

Among the immune cells that penetrate a tumor, the tumor infiltrating lymphocytes (TILs), are capable of mediating cancer cells eradication. Increased T cell infiltration is a good prognostic marker for multiple solid tumors including, breast cancer (reviewed: [26, 27]) head and neck squamous cell carcinoma [28], melanoma [29, 30], muscle-invasive bladder cancer [31], seminoma [32], pancreatic adenocarcinoma [33], cervical [34], ovarian [35], gastric [36] and colorectal [37] tumors.

Most of the TILs in the tumor environment, due to the immunoediting process, experience chronic activation and exhaustion leading to the attenuation of proliferation and effector functions via activation of checkpoint co-inhibitory receptors such as PD-1 or CTLA-4 [6]. In some solid tumors, TILs are present in too low frequency to mediate a potent immune response [38]. Thus, TILs are retrieving from tumor mass, expanded ex vivo and re-infused back to the cancer patients. Tumor-specificity of TILs is selected based on IFN-γ production while co-cultured with cancer cells. Rosenberg et al. [39] were the first to demonstrate the regression of metastatic melanoma in patients that received autologous TILs along with high doses of IL-2 treatment.

However, after initial success with TIL therapy, further investigation revealed that transferred T cells do not persist long-term. In fact, infused T cells diminished over time and were undetectable in the blood of some cancer patients 2 weeks post-transfer, which resulted in a lack of objective responses [40]. The cytotoxic T cells

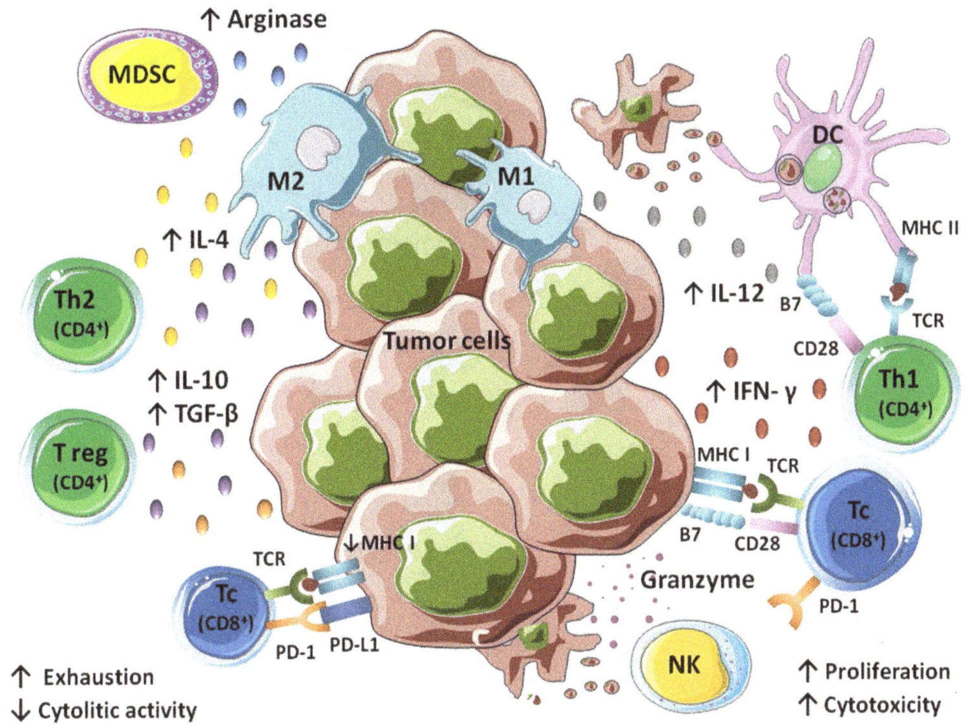


**Fig. 2** Tumor microenvironment consists of malignant cells, stroma and different populations of immune cells. Complex crosstalk between them shapes the final outcome of neoplastic disease. Anticancer response is driven mainly by cytotoxic CD8$^+$ T cells and NK cells, which release IFN-γ and granzymes, thus are involved in direct lysis of the tumor cells. Th1 subpopulation of CD4$^+$ T cells, M1 macrophages and activated dendritic cells (DCs) support anticancer immunity by antigen presentation and cytokine production (IL-12, IFN-γ). CD8$^+$ and CD4$^+$ T cells recognize tumor antigens in the context of MHC class I and II respectively, followed by costimulatory signaling via CD28 molecule, necessary for their full activation, proliferation and function. Tumor progression, in turn, is associated with the presence of the Th2 and T regulatory CD4$^+$ lymphocytes, M2 macrophages and MDSC. These cells secrete immunosuppressive factors such as IL-4, IL-10, or TGF-β and exhibit high activity of arginase, respectively. Unresponsiveness of cytotoxic CD8$^+$ T cells is caused by decreased expression of MHC I on the cancer cells surface and activation of coinhibitory receptors such as PD-1. Adapted from Servier Medical Art

used for transfer were comprised of terminally differentiated effector cells, without self-renewal capacity. Moreover, for CTLs to induce a potent antitumor response they depend on the activity of effector CD4$^+$ T cells and the availability of homeostatic cytokines [41–43]. Thus, upon transfer into an immunocompetent recipient, CTLs were not able to survive and mount an effective response.

Preconditioning of cancer patients significantly improves the therapeutic efficiency of TIL therapy. This involves the systemic destruction of the recipient immune system (lymphodepletion) before ACT-based treatment. It was shown that chemotherapy consisting of high-dose of cyclophosphamide and fludarabine or total body irradiation of non-myeloablative (2 Gy) dose caused lymphodepletion, which significantly enhanced ACT efficiency [44, 45]. Such a regimen, prior to infusion, is necessary to destroy host immune cells and create 'space' for expansion of adoptively transferred T lymphocytes. The mechanism relies also on the elimination of immunosuppressive Tregs and MDSCs and by augmenting the innate immune system. Lymphodepletion excludes immune cells termed "cytokine sinks" that compete with infused T cells for homeostatic cytokines, thereby increasing access to those cytokines, particularly IL-15 and IL-7, which promote T lymphocyte proliferation in vivo [46].

Autologous TIL treatment was currently demonstrated to induce durable, complete, and in some cases curative metastatic melanoma regression with objective tumor response observed in around 50% of patients [47, 48]. Nevertheless, adaptation of this therapy for other types of solid tumor is limited due to low availability of TILs from tumor mass [49, 50]. To date, melanoma remains most immunogenic type of tumor and even patients in advanced stage IV of melanoma can benefit from autologous TIL transfer. However, still short-term persistence of infused T cells that are fully differentiated and exhausted constitutes an obstacle [51, 52]. Thus, extensive studies are ongoing to improve the protocols of ex vivo expansion and preparation of TILs (i.e. using pharmacological modifications). As of September 2018

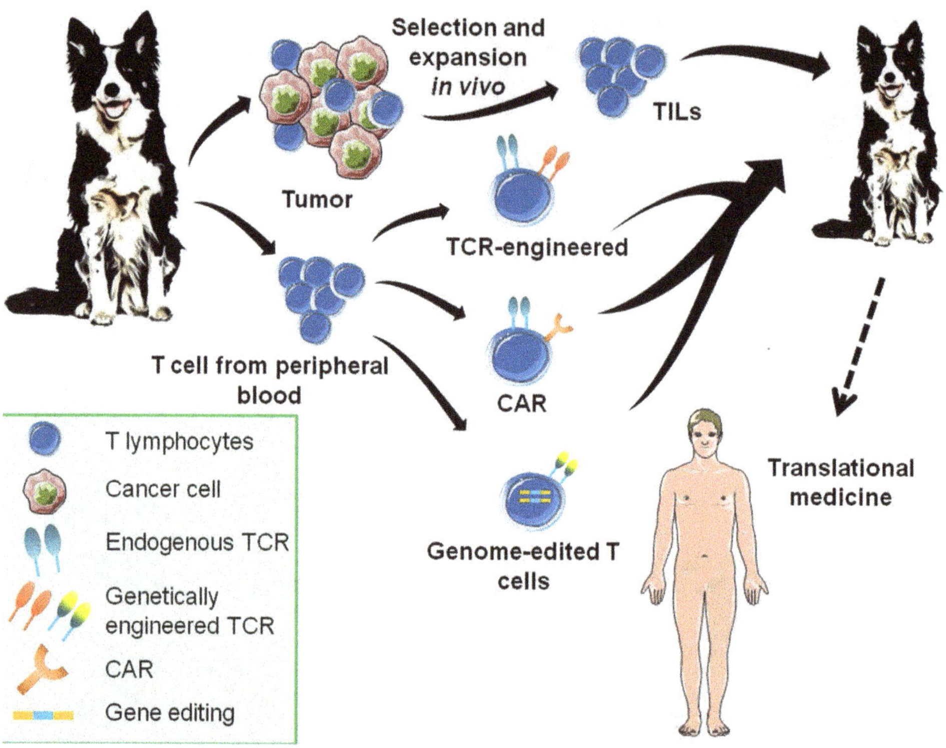


**Fig. 3** Adoptive cell immunotherapy possibilities for cancer in dogs include transfer of TILs, TRC-modified and CAR-engineered T lymphocytes. Tumor reactive T cells can be derived from tumor mass or peripheral blood lymphocytes can be genetically engineered to recognize tumor-specific antigens. Obtained T cells are expanded ex vivo and then administrated back to the tumor-bearing patient. Recently, genome editing technologies are using to confer additional modifications to T cells such as disruption of endogenous TCR and MHC. Introduction of ACT treatment into veterinary medicine can greatly facilitate the design of the new clinical trials for humans. Adapted from Servier Medical Art

there are 158 open clinical studies regarding administration of TILs to human cancer patients (http://www.clinicaltrials.gov). Advantages and disadvantages of using TILs are summarized in Table 1.

## TILs in veterinary oncology

Tumor infiltrating lymphocytes in canine cancers are not well characterized, therefore there is still much to be gleaned. An increase in T lymphocyte infiltration was correlated with spontaneous, rapid regression of transmissible venereal sarcoma [53], oral papilloma [54] and cutaneous histiocytoma [55].

Lymphocyte infiltration has been studied in canine mammary gland tumors as it is an attractive biological model for the investigation of human breast cancer immunology [56]. Initial studies showed an increase in infiltrating T cells in the tumors that gave metastasis, suggesting that TILs, especially $CD4^+$ T cells promote tumor expansion [57, 58]. In contrast, the lab of Carvalho [59] demonstrated that malignant mammary tumors had a reduced number of intratumoral T cells compared to benign tumors. However, the proportion was reversed when $CD3^+$ T cells were counted in the peripheral parts of the tumor or in the adjacent non-malignant mammary gland, indicating that T cells from that region might be engaged in tumor progression. In addition, an increase of TILs was associated with increased canine mammary tumor malignancy [60]. Unfortunately, the published data lacks in-depth T cell subset analysis, specifically the identification of Tregs, which are known to exhibit immunosuppressive properties thereby supporting cancer development [60].

Recent data confirms that a high frequency of T cells found within malignant tumors is due to a high percentage of Tregs [61]. Similarly, Mucha et al. [62] demonstrate an increased population of $FoxP3^+$ (regulatory T cell-associated transcription factor) cells in canine malignant and metastatic mammary cancers compared to benign tumors. Likewise, Tominaga et al. [63] found, high Treg frequency in the peripheral blood and even higher in the tumor mass of dogs with oral melanoma.

Although, no studies have utilized TILs for ACT therapy in dogs with solid tumor, there is ongoing research which exploits T cells from canine patients with lymphoma [64]. In this case, however, the use of the term "TILs" can be speculative since in the hematological

**Table 1 The major advantages and disadvantages of various methods of generating T cells for the purpose of adoptive transfer**

| Therapy type | Advantages | Disadvantages |
|---|---|---|
| Tumor-infiltrating lymphocytes (TILs) | Recognize tumor-specific antigens | Isolation difficulties—not applicable for all of the cancer types |
| | High objective response against cancer reaching even up to 70% | Labor and time consuming |
| | Sustained remission | Not applicable for larger group of patients |
| | Low recurrence rate | Not all of the TILs are reactive to tumor antigens |
| | | Presence of tumor-reactive T cells is indispensable |
| TCR-engineered lymphocytes | Does not require presence of tumor antigen-specific T cells | Competition between transgenic TCR and endogenous TCR |
| | Lymphocytes can be obtained from blood not from tumor tissue | Heterodimer formation and possibility of gaining unknown antigen-specificity |
| | | Expression of two distinct TCR was associated with autoimmunity |
| Chimeric antigen receptor (CAR)—engineered T lymphocytes | Specific for broad-range of antigens including non-proteinaceous Ag | Fusion of various signaling domains may alter proper signaling cascade |
| | MHC-independent antigen recognition | CAR expression may not be stable |
| | Suitable for a relatively wide range of patients—not HLA-restricted | Uncertainties regarding the type of signaling domains and their order for proper T cell function |
| | Production of large quantities in relatively short time | Antigen specificity must be selected with caution |
| | Putative improvement of T cell properties such as proliferation, activation or cytokine secretion by insertion of specially designed CAR | May cause toxicity (on target/off tumor effect) |
| | | CAR biology and interaction with different cancer types and TME not well defined yet |
| | | Identification of optimal CAR still based on experimental procedures |
| Genome editing technologies (ZFN, TALENS, CRISPR/Cas) | Enhancement of T cells biology (e.g. resistance to TMI, cytokine secretion) | Possible off-target effect |
| | Applicable for wide-range of dysfunctions | Technical problems with delivery and efficiency |
| | Allow to overcome limitations of TCR-engineered and CAR T cells (elimination of endogenous TCR expression) | May induce immune response against bacterial components of GE technology |
| | Applicable for greater number of patients | Controversial, ethical issues |

malignancies T cells do not truly infiltrate the tumor. T cells used in the following study were memory T cells which exhibit anticancer activity. These studies revealed that the transfer of autologous T lymphocytes from dogs with non-Hodgkin lymphoma, previously treated with chemotherapy, improved clinical outcomes. T cells isolated from the blood of lymphoma-bearing dogs were co-cultured with γ-irradiated K562 cells genetically modified to function as artificial antigen presenting cells (aAPC), in the presence of rhIL-21 and rhIL-2. Recently, this approach was also used to expand canine CAR T cells [65]. For the purpose of ACT, the majority of the cells were $CD3^+/CD8^+$ (88%). Importantly, 70% of the cells were memory T cells ($CD3^+$, $CCR7^+$) characterized by high production of IFN-γ. Dogs treated with chemotherapy and ACT therapy achieved complete remission lasting at least 338 days post T cell transfer. Overall percentage of $CD8^+$ T cells was higher in the blood for up to 42 days of canine patients that received ACT therapy compared to their non-treated counterparts. The increase of $CD8^+$ T cells was correlated with increased expression of thymidine kinase, enhanced granzyme B production and decreased neutrophil to lymphocyte ratio. The study demonstrated the successful application and clinical outcomes of tumor immunotherapy for canine patients. Of note, this was the first study to show the power of this effective therapy in in vivo study providing a solid foundation for further studies in the field of veterinary oncology.

## Utilizing T cell receptor transduction for ACT therapy

Antitumor activity of T cells is based on the ability of a T cells to recognize antigen via its endogenous T cell receptor (TCR). TCR is a transmembrane protein complex, consisting of α- and β-chains (more rarely δ- and γ-chains). Although, it was demonstrated that tumor-specific T cells can be successfully isolated from both tumor microenvironment and the blood for the purpose of ACT [66, 67], the limitations of this approach still hinder its wide application in medicine. The major drawback is related to accessibility of TILs in certain tumor types [50]. To overcome this limitation, the use of TCR-engineered T cells has been extensively studied.

The first studies, performed with mouse models, demonstrated that transfer of TCR α and β genes, targeted to tumor antigens, into T cells confers tumor antigen-specificity [68, 69]. These pioneering studies led to significant progress in the field of TCR-engineering for T cell therapy. To date, TCR-engineered T cells have been used against renal cell carcinoma antigen (RCC) [70], Wilms tumor antigen-1 (WT1) for leukemia cells [71], melanoma antigen recognized by T cells 1 (MART1) for patients suffering from melanoma [72] or cancer–testis antigen (NY-ESO-1) to treat myeloma [73]. Each of the studies showed the benefit with objective responses and potent antitumor activity.

The advantage of TCR-engineered T cells is that lymphocytes can be easily obtained from the peripheral blood and then transformed into tumor-reactive cells. Nevertheless, the major limitation of this method arises from off-target TCR heterodimer formation (Table 1). With the addition of a second α and β TCR chain, it is probable for the expression of four different TCR receptors due to interactions of endogenous and introduced α and β TCR chains [74]. Studies by Sommermeyer laboratory [75] have indicated that TCR with strong antigen affinity may replace TCR with weak antigen affinity, resulting in T cells with altered or novel antigen specificity. Furthermore, simultaneous expression of two distinct TCR was associated with an induction of autoimmunity [76–78].

Numerous clinical trials reveal potential toxicity of TCR-redirected T cell therapy, arising from on-target but off-tumor effects that in extreme cases lead to lethal outcomes [79]. For this reason, the crucial step in development of effective and safe treatment is selection of tumor-specific TCR.

TCR-engineered T cells have not been used in veterinary oncology primarily due to the fact that antigen recognition is based on MHC-restricted epitopes. Recently, however, Barth et al. [80] successfully identified a binding motif of canine MHC I allele DLA-88*50101. Interestingly, this binding motif exhibited high similarity to human leukocyte antigen HLA-A*02:01. Therefore, the authors stressed that canine models would be suitable for testing TCR-transduced T cell-based immunotherapies. Importantly, the canine genome has been sequenced which will help in the development of novel targets that can be implemented in both human and veterinary medicine.

## Chimeric antigen receptor (CAR) engineered T cells

The main restriction in using TCR-engineered T cells results from heterodimer formation resulting in undefined antigen specificity. Importantly, T cells can recognize antigen via its TCR only when it is processed into a peptide and presented in the context of an MHC molecule. However, malignant cells often downregulate expression of MHC molecules in order to avoid immune response [81]. Due to these limitations, researchers have developed a novel solution. The chimeric antigen receptor (CAR) fuses a single chain variable fragment (scFv) of an antibody that recognizes antigen with the intracellular signaling domains of the CD3ζ. The initial studies, conducted by Gross et al. [82], proved that T cells can successfully express chimeric receptors that recognize specific antigens and trigger T cell response. To date, three generations of CARs can be distinguished, based on the signaling endodomains [83]. First generation CARs consist solely of an antigen binding domain and the CD3ζ signaling domain necessary for T cell activation, while the 2nd generation incorporated a co-stimulatory signaling such as CD28 or inducible T cell costimulator (ICOS) [84]. Third generation of CARs combine additional co-stimulatory molecules to enhance the potency [85]. It was demonstrated that each generation of CARs exhibited distinctive properties with regard to the T cells' antitumor activity, proliferation, cytotoxic properties, and persistence [86]. Studies by Hombach and Abken [87] have revealed significant differences, mainly related to proliferation and cytokine secretion, between lymphocytes expressing CARs recognizing the same epitope but with various costimulatory endodomains. Also, Bridgeman et al. [88] pointed out that results may differ significantly from each other even if the same chimeric receptors were used. Consequently, the design of artificial chimeric receptors requires further refinements and definition of the most optimal CAR structure.

There is great potential for adoptive therapy with CAR-engineered T cells as a treatment for some types of the cancer such as neuroblastoma and leukemia [89, 90], yet in other cancer types (e.g. ovarian cancer and metastatic renal cell carcinoma) the therapy have demonstrated poor responses [91, 92]. Additionally, these studies have documented on-target/off-tumor toxicities after CAR-T cell treatments. Nonetheless, it was proposed that on-target toxic effects of CAR-T cell therapy can be abolished by administration of agents that block specific epitopes, such as monoclonal antibodies [93].

Many aspects of CAR-T cell therapy require further investigation however, the therapy induce a powerful antitumor response. The latest trends in CAR-T cell research are designing the next-generation CAR-T cells that will be engineered with suicide genes or dual-antigen receptors. It is believed that it will be easier to control the function of the next generation CAR-T cells and thereby minimizing their side effects [94].

## CAR-T cells in veterinary oncology

ACT therapy in dogs is not as advanced as in humans and therefore the literature on the subject is still limited. To date, just two groups have attempted to use CAR technology to treat canine osteosarcoma (OS) and B cell lymphoma. These tumors are considered as valuable model of human cancers as they share similar tumor-associated antigens such as HER2 (osteosarcoma associated antigen) and CD20 (marker of transformed B cells).

The ACT study to treat osteosarcoma was performed with T cells obtained from peripheral blood of healthy dogs [65]. The T lymphocytes were activated using irradiated K562 aAPCs, genetically modified to express human CD80, CD83, CD86, 41BBL. Additionally, cells were stimulated with phytohemagglutinin (PHA) and rhIL-21. Interestingly, other methods of activation, such as administration of Concanavalin A (ConA) or anti-human CD3 (OKT-3 clone) antibodies coated-plates were insufficient to effectively stimulate canine T cell proliferation for ACT therapy purpose [65, 95]. Activated T cells were subsequently transfected with a 2nd generation α-canine HER2 CAR (containing CD3ζ and CD28 domains). The authors demonstrated that HER2-CAR-T cells in co-culture with several HER2 positive canine OS cell lines secreted more IFN-γ and exhibited superior ability to eliminate $HER2^+$ OS cells in vitro. The results were not observed in $HER2^-$ OS-phenotype cell lines or non-transfected T cells. Despite these promising results, this approach has not yet been evaluated in vivo.

Building on these encouraging in vitro data, Panjwani et al. [95] performed in vivo studies on dogs suffering from B cell lymphoma. Autologous canine T cells were transiently transfected with α-canine CD20 CAR using electroporation. In the presence of canine lymphoma cells the CD20-CAR-T cells secreted significantly more of IFN-γ, than non-modified T cells or CD19-CAR-T cells (used as non-specific CAR transfection control). Additionally, antigen-specific CAR-T cells actively lysed the target cancer cells. Dogs with B cell lymphoma that relapsed after chemotherapy (L-asparaginase, vincristine, cyclophosphamide, doxorubicin or prednisone) were given three doses of 700,000 CD20-CAR-T cells per kg. Serious adverse side effects were not observed. Each injection resulted in an enlargement of the target lymph node, decreased frequency of cancer $CD79a^+$/$CD20^+$ cells and increase of non-transformed $CD5^+$ B lymphocytes in the lymph nodes. In addition, increased serum levels of IL-6 and IFN-γ were measured after the first dose of CD20-CAR-T cells [95]. Unfortunately, due to the transient transfection of these CAR-T cells, durable remission was not attained.

## Lymphokine-activated killer (LAK) cells for adoptive cell therapy

In contrast to adoptive T cell transfer therapy which exploits tumor-specific T cells, passive immunotherapy involves administration of autologous lymphocytes, without cancer specificity. In human medicine, this type of immunotherapy is referred to as lymphokine-activated killer (LAK) cell therapy and was among one of the first cell transfers [96] discarded in a favor of newer technologies (ACT therapy using TCR- or CAR-engineered T cells). However, LAK cells transfer was preferentially investigated in veterinary medicine, due to the low cost of cell generation. LAK cells are derived from PBMC stimulated with α-CD3 antibody-coated plates and soluble hrIL-2. Initially, LAK cell therapy was tested in healthy beagles [97]. Sequential administration of LAK cells increased host immune cell proliferation and IFN-γ levels in the serum without inducing severe side effects. These results suggested that LAK cell therapy is safe and could promote an immune response. Several papers described LAK cells' generation and anticancer activity against canine thyroid carcinoma and melanoma cell lines in vitro [97–99]. Recently, LAK cell therapy, in combination with surgery, was evaluated in vivo in 15 tumor-bearing dogs [100]. Patients received five rounds of LAK cell transfer with 2–4 weeks intervals. Single transfer resulted in an increase of $CD8^+$ T cells' frequency and a decreased ratio of $CD4^+$ to $CD8^+$ T cells. Although the immunoenhancing effect of LAK cell transfer was confirmed, this type of immunotherapy alone has not mediated potent anticancer immune response or complete tumor eradication. Therefore, LAK cell transfer is not suitable as a monotherapy, but its application is promising as an adjuvant treatment.

A summary of different immunotherapeutic approaches in veterinary medicine have been compiled in Table 2.

**Table 2 Adoptive cell transfer immunotherapies in veterinary medicine**

| Therapy type | Attempts to use in veterinary oncology | |
|---|---|---|
| TIL therapy | Non-Hodgkin's lymphoma | In vivo [64] |
| CAR-T cell transfer | Osteosarcoma | In vitro [65] |
| | B-cell lymphoma | In vitro and in vivo [95] |
| T-LAK cell transfer | Thyroid cancer | In vitro and in vivo [98, 100] |
| | Melanoma | In vitro and in vivo [98, 100] |
| | Hepatocarcinoma | In vivo [100] |
| | Fibrosarcoma | In vivo [100] |

## Exploiting genome-editing technology to improve T cell phenotype

Genetic engineering technology is used for modifying of both TCR- and CAR-engineered T cells. Novel approaches focused on modulation of chemokine receptor expression and cytokine secretion of T lymphocytes or resistance to immunosuppressive tumor microenvironment by effector cells.

To date, three methods of genome editing have been implemented in the clinic: (1) zinc finger nucleases (ZFN), (2) transcription activator-like effector nuclease (TALEN) and the most recent (3) clustered regularly interspaced short palindromic repeats (CRISPR) associated protein system (CRISPR/Cas9) (Fig. 4) [101]. ZFN and TALEN are chimeric nucleases that contain a DNA-binding domain (engineered to recognize specific sequences) and a DNA cleavage enzyme (usually FokI) [102–104]. CRISPR/Cas9 system is based on RNA-guided DNA sequence recognition followed by cleavage by Cas9 endonuclease [105]. Each of these methods introduces nuclease-induced DNA double strand breaks into the sequence of interest. Importantly, these technologies not only improve gene silencing, but also allows for other genetic manipulations such as gene correction, deletion or insertion (Fig. 4) [106]. Thus, they appear to be a promising and useful tool for biomedical research.

The first in vivo success of this technology was achieved using ZFN to treat haemophilia in a murine model-correcting this genetic disorder and restorating normal blood coagulation [107]. Genome-editing technologies were also employed for treating of hereditary tyrosinemia

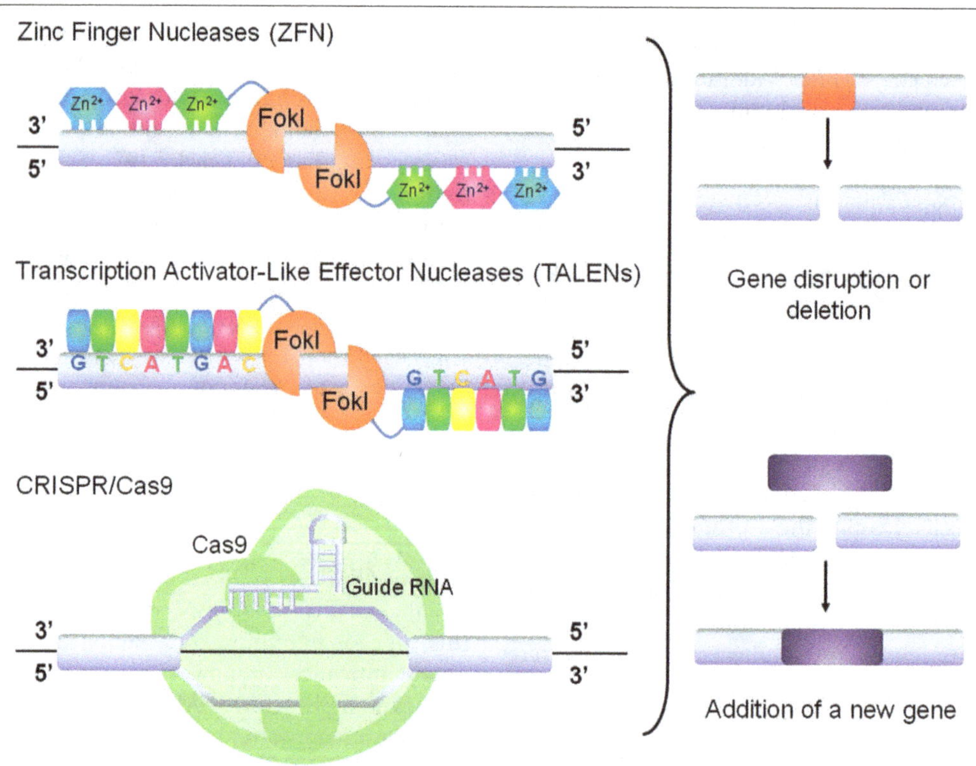


**Fig. 4** Genome editing systems are used to introduce double-strand breaks into DNA, which allow for gene correction, deletion or addition ZFNs, TALENs and CRISPR/Cas9 are versatile nuclease-based platforms of genome editing technology. ZFNs and TALENs consist of DNA-binding domain, which is engineered to recognize specific sequences and nuclease domain—FokI—responsible for DNA cleavage. CRISPR/Cas9 is based on RNA-guided DNA recognition complex which interacts with Cas9 nuclease catalyzing site-specific breaks in DNA. Genome editing technologies can be used for the immunotherapy purposes to enhance T cells properties

(HTI), Duchenne muscular dystrophy (DMD) and hepatitis B virus (HBV) infection [108–110].

Recently, T cells modified using TALEN-based technology were transferred to leukemia patients [111]. Allogeneic healthy donor T cells were genetically engineered to prevent graft-versus-host disease (GVHD) upon adoptive cell transfer. Infused T cells did not cause an immune response in the recipient. This technique has been used just to prolong a patients' survival time until suitable donor is found. In followup studies, CD19 CAR-T cells with disrupted TCR and CD52 coding genes were used to effectively treat B cell malignancies in infant [112]. Authors speculated that due to the lack of TCR expression, heterologous CAR-T cells can potentially be utilized for every patient with B cell leukemia [112, 113]. These study confirmed that gene editing technology may help to solve problems associated with engineering T cells. Similarly, ZFN-mediated disruption of the endogenous TCR genes in WT1 antigen-specific T cells prevented GVHD upon transfer into mice. This procedure prevents TCR heterodimmer formation, which is one of the major drawbacks of TCR-engineered T cell transfer therapy [114]. Recent advances in genetic manipulations can allowed to reduce adverse effects of ACT therapy and make it more widely applicable for the treatment for a range of malignancies. However, there are still several limitations of using genome editing technologies, which comprise: low efficiency of the method in some cell types, construct delivery problems, single-instead of double-stranded breaks, and off-target effects of nucleases and genetically modified cells (Table 1) [106, 115].

Genome editing has not been fully exploited in canine patients. Nevertheless, CRISPR/Cas9 method has been used to generate beagles with a myostatin gene knockout [116]. The study proved the feasibility of canine genome editing technique and has paved the way to generate other knockout dogs, potentially serving as models of multiple disease in the biomedical sciences.

## Conclusion

In the past few years, we have witnessed amazing successes in harnessing immune system to fight against cancer. The American Society of Clinical Oncology selected cancer immunotherapy as the 2016 "Advance of the Year" for its unprecedented effectiveness in eradicating various types of tumors. In the future, more efforts should be made to utilize translational veterinary medicine to benefit human health. The domestic dog model offer multiple advantages to move cancer immunotherapies forward. Most importantly, these treatments may be also the silver lining in veterinary oncology giving hope for canine patients.

### Abbreviations

aAPC: artificial antigen presenting cells; ACT: adoptive cell transfer; ADCC: antibody-dependent cellular cytotoxicity; CAR: chimeric antigen receptor; CCL-20: chemokine (C-C motif) ligand 20; CCR5: chemokine receptor 5; CCR7: C-C chemokine receptor type 7; CD: cluster of differentiation; ConA: concanavalin A; CRISPR/Cas9: clustered regularly interspaced short palindromic repeats (CRISPR) associated protein system with Cas9 endonuclease; CTLA-4: cytotoxic T cell antigen 4; CTLs: cytotoxic T lymphocytes, $CD8^+$ positive cells; DC: dendritic cells; DLA: dog leukocyte antigen; DMD: Duchenne muscular dystrophy; GVHD: graft-versus-host disease; HBV: hepatitis B virus; HER2: human epidermal growth factor receptor 2; HLA: human leukocyte antigen; HTI: hereditary tyrosinemia I; ICOS: inducible T cell costimulator; IFN-γ: interferon-γ; IL: interleukin; LAK: lymphokine-activated killer cells; MART1: melanoma antigen recognized by T cells 1; MDSC: myeloid-derived suppressor cells; MHC: major histocompatibility complex; NK cells: natural killer cells; NKT cells: natural killer T cells; NY-ESO-1: cancer–testis antigen; OS: canine osteosarcoma; PD-1: programmed cell death protein 1; PHA: phytohemagglutinin; RCC: renal cell carcinoma antigen; rhIL: recombinant human interleukin; ROR: retinoic acid-related orphan receptor; scFv: single chain variable fragment; TALEN: transcription activator-like effector nuclease; TAMs: tumor-associated macrophages; TCR: T cell receptor; TGF-β: tumor growth factor β; Th cells: helper $CD4^+$ T cells; TILs: tumor infiltrating lymphocytes; TNF-α: tumor necrosis factor α; Tregs: T regulatory cells; WT1: Wilms tumor antigen-1; ZFN: zinc finger nucleases.

### Authors' contributions

JKB provided the design of the paper, reviewed the literature and wrote the major part of the manuscript, prepared figures and tables. RP reviewed the literature, wrote the TILs and Lymphokine-activated killer cells paragraphs, formatted references list, and completed the tables, significantly contributed to the final outcome of the draft. MHN provided the human immunotherapy expertise, critically reviewed and contributed to the final draft of the manuscript. KM helped in conception and design of the paper, critically reviewed the manuscript, provided veterinary oncology expertise, and significantly contributes to the final draft of the manuscript. All authors read and approved the final manuscript.


### Author details

[1] Department of Physiological Sciences, Faculty of Veterinary Medicine, Warsaw University of Life Sciences, ul. Nowoursynowska 159, 02-776 Warsaw, Poland. [2] Department of Microbiology and Immunology, Medical University of South Carolina, 86 Jonathan Lucas Street HCC-612, Charleston, SC 29425, USA.


### Competing interests

The authors declare that they have no competing interests.


### Funding

This work was supported, in part, by NCN UMO-2016/21/N/NZ6/02137 grant (to JKB) and programme First TEAM/2017-3/25 of Foundation for Polish Science co-financed by the European Union under the European Regional Development Fund (to KM).


### References


1. Hanahan D, Weinberg RA. The hallmarks of cancer. Cell. 2000;100:57–70.
2. Mittal D, Gubin MM, Schreiber RD, Smyth MJ. New insights into cancer immunoediting and its three component phases–elimination, equilibrium and escape. Curr Opin Immunol. 2014;27:16–25.
3. Kim R, Emi M, Tanabe K. Cancer immunoediting from immune surveillance to immune escape. Immunology. 2007;121:1–14.

4. Grivennikov SI, Greten FR, Karin M. Immunity, inflammation, and cancer. Cell. 2010;140:883–99.
5. Horna P, Sotomayor EM. Cellular and molecular mechanisms of tumor-induced T-cell tolerance. Curr Cancer Drug Targets. 2007;7:41–53.
6. Intlekofer AM, Thompson CB. At the bench: preclinical rationale for CTLA-4 and PD-1 blockade as cancer immunotherapy. J Leukoc Biol. 2013;94:25–39.
7. Mytar B, Wołoszyn M, Szatanek R, Baj-Krzyworzeka M, Siedlar M, Ruggiero I, et al. Tumor cell-induced deactivation of human monocytes. J Leukoc Biol. 2003;74:1094–101.
8. Chanmee T, Ontong P, Konno K, Itano N. Tumor-associated macrophages as major players in the tumor microenvironment. Cancers. 2014;6:1670–90.
9. Król M, Pawłowski KM, Majchrzak K, Dolka I, Abramowicz A, Szyszko K, et al. Density of tumor-associated macrophages (TAMs) and expression of their growth factor receptor MCSF-R and CD14 in canine mammary adenocarcinomas of various grade of malignancy and metastasis. Pol J Vet Sci. 2011;14:3–10.
10. Mucha J, Majchrzak K, Taciak B, Hellmén E, Król M. MDSCs mediate angiogenesis and predispose canine mammary tumor cells for metastasis via IL-28/IL-28RA (IFN-λ) signaling. PLoS ONE. 2014;9:e103249.
11. Delorme E. Treatment of primary fibrosarcoma in the rat with immune lymphocytes. Lancet. 1964;284:117–20.
12. Paoloni M, Khanna C. Translation of new cancer treatments from pet dogs to humans. Nat Rev Cancer. 2008;8:147–56.
13. Schiffman JD, Breen M. Comparative oncology: what dogs and other species can teach us about humans with cancer. Philos Trans R Soc B Biol Sci. 2015;370:20140231.
14. Mata M, Gottschalk S. Man's best friend: utilizing naturally occurring tumors in dogs to improve chimeric antigen receptor T-cell therapy for human cancers. Mol Ther. 2016;24:1511–2.
15. Stroud C, Dmitriev I, Kashentseva E, Bryan JN, Curiel DT, Rindt H, et al. A one health overview, facilitating advances in comparative medicine and translational research. Clin Transl Med. 2016;5. http://clintransmed.springeropen.com/articles/10.1186/s40169-016-0107-4. Accessed 30 Jun 2017.
16. Park JS, Withers SS, Modiano JF, Kent MS, Chen M, Luna JI, et al. Canine cancer immunotherapy studies: linking mouse and human. J Immunother Cancer. 2016; 4. http://jitc.biomedcentral.com/articles/10.1186/s40425-016-0200-7. Accessed 29 Jun 2017.
17. Khanna C, Lindblad-Toh K, Vail D, London C, Bergman P, Barber L, et al. The dog as a cancer model. Nat Biotechnol. 2006;24:1065–6.
18. Bronson RT. Variation in age at death of dogs of different sexes and breeds. Am J Vet Res. 1982;43:2057–9.
19. Anderson KL, Modiano JF. Progress in adaptive immunotherapy for cancer in companion animals: success on the path to a cure. Vet Sci. 2015;2:363–87.
20. Nishiya A, Massoco C, Felizzola C, Perlmann E, Batschinski K, Tedardi M, et al. Comparative aspects of canine melanoma. Vet Sci. 2016;3:7.
21. Lindblad-Toh K, Wade CM, Mikkelsen TS, Karlsson EK, Jaffe DB, Kamal M, et al. Genome sequence, comparative analysis and haplotype structure of the domestic dog. Nature. 2005;438:803–19.
22. Muranski P, Restifo NP. Adoptive immunotherapy of cancer using CD4(+) T cells. Curr Opin Immunol. 2009;21:200–8.
23. Rosenberg SA, Restifo NP. Adoptive cell transfer as personalized immunotherapy for human cancer. Science. 2015;348:62–8.
24. Rosenberg SA, Restifo NP, Yang JC, Morgan RA, Dudley ME. Adoptive cell transfer: a clinical path to effective cancer immunotherapy. Nat Rev Cancer. 2008;8:299–308.
25. Raval RR, Sharabi AB, Walker AJ, Drake CG, Sharma P. Tumor immunology and cancer immunotherapy: summary of the 2013 SITC primer. J Immunother Cancer. 2014;2:14.
26. Mahmoud SMA, Paish EC, Powe DG, Macmillan RD, Grainge MJ, Lee AHS, et al. Tumor-infiltrating CD8+ lymphocytes predict clinical outcome in breast cancer. J Clin Oncol Off J Am Soc Clin Oncol. 2011;29:1949–55.
27. Wang K, Xu J, Zhang T, Xue D. Tumor-infiltrating lymphocytes in breast cancer predict the response to chemotherapy and survival outcome: a meta-analysis. Oncotarget. 2014. http://www.oncotarget.com/abstract/9988. Accessed 29 Jun 2017.
28. Nguyen N, Bellile E, Thomas D, McHugh J, Rozek L, Virani S, et al. Tumor infiltrating lymphocytes and survival in patients with head and neck squamous cell carcinoma: tumor infiltrating lymphocytes. Head Neck. 2016;38:1074–84.
29. Piras F, Colombari R, Minerba L, Murtas D, Floris C, Maxia C, et al. The predictive value of CD8, CD4, CD68, and human leukocyte antigen-D-related cells in the prognosis of cutaneous malignant melanoma with vertical growth phase. Cancer. 2005;104:1246–54.
30. van Houdt IS, Sluijter BJR, Moesbergen LM, Vos WM, de Gruijl TD, Molenkamp BG, et al. Favorable outcome in clinically stage II melanoma patients is associated with the presence of activated tumor infiltrating T-lymphocytes and preserved MHC class I antigen expression. Int J Cancer. 2008;123:609–15.
31. Sjödahl G, Lövgren K, Lauss M, Chebil G, Patschan O, Gudjonsson S, et al. Infiltration of CD3$^+$ and CD68$^+$ cells in bladder cancer is subtype specific and affects the outcome of patients with muscle-invasive tumors. Urol Oncol. 2014;32:791–7.
32. Hadrup SR, Braendstrup O, Jacobsen GK, Mortensen S, Pedersen LØ, Seremet T, et al. Tumor infiltrating lymphocytes in seminoma lesions comprise clonally expanded cytotoxic T cells. Int J Cancer. 2006;119:831–8.
33. Fukunaga A, Miyamoto M, Cho Y, Murakami S, Kawarada Y, Oshikiri T, et al. CD8+ tumor-infiltrating lymphocytes together with CD4+ tumor-infiltrating lymphocytes and dendritic cells improve the prognosis of patients with pancreatic adenocarcinoma. Pancreas. 2004;28:e26–31.
34. Piersma SJ, Jordanova ES, van Poelgeest MIE, Kwappenberg KMC, van der Hulst JM, Drijfhout JW, et al. High number of intraepithelial CD8+ tumor-infiltrating lymphocytes is associated with the absence of lymph node metastases in patients with large early-stage cervical cancer. Cancer Res. 2007;67:354–61.
35. Li J, Wang J, Chen R, Bai Y, Lu X. The prognostic value of tumor-infiltrating T lymphocytes in ovarian cancer. Oncotarget. 2017. http://www.oncotarget.com/abstract/14919. Accessed 29 Jun 2017.
36. Lee HE, Chae SW, Lee YJ, Kim MA, Lee HS, Lee BL, et al. Prognostic implications of type and density of tumour-infiltrating lymphocytes in gastric cancer. Br J Cancer. 2008;99:1704–11.
37. Mei Z, Liu Y, Liu C, Cui A, Liang Z, Wang G, et al. Tumour-infiltrating inflammation and prognosis in colorectal cancer: systematic review and meta-analysis. Br J Cancer. 2014;110:1595–605.
38. Hershkovitz L, Schachter J, Treves AJ, Besser MJ. Focus on adoptive T cell transfer trials in melanoma. Clin Dev Immunol. 2010;2010:1–11.
39. Rosenberg SA, Packard BS, Aebersold PM, Solomon D, Topalian SL, Toy ST, et al. Use of tumor-infiltrating lymphocytes and interleukin-2 in the immunotherapy of patients with metastatic melanoma. N Engl J Med. 1988;319:1676–80.
40. Dudley ME, Wunderlich J, Nishimura MI, Yu D, Yang JC, Topalian SL, et al. Adoptive transfer of cloned melanoma-reactive T lymphocytes for the treatment of patients with metastatic melanoma. J Immunother. 2001;24:363–73.
41. Dudley ME. Cancer regression and autoimmunity in patients after clonal repopulation with antitumor lymphocytes. Science. 2002;298:850–4.
42. Walter EA, Greenberg PD, Gilbert MJ, Finch RJ, Watanabe KS, Thomas ED, et al. Reconstitution of cellular immunity against cytomegalovirus in recipients of allogeneic bone marrow by transfer of T-cell clones from the donor. N Engl J Med. 1995;333:1038–44.
43. Matloubian M, Concepcion RJ, Ahmed R. CD4+ T cells are required to sustain CD8+ cytotoxic T-cell responses during chronic viral infection. J Virol. 1994;68:8056–63.
44. Dudley ME, Wunderlich JR, Yang JC, Sherry RM, Topalian SL, Restifo NP, et al. adoptive cell transfer therapy following non-myeloablative but lymphodepleting chemotherapy for the treatment of patients with refractory metastatic melanoma. J Clin Oncol. 2005;23:2346–57.
45. Dudley ME, Yang JC, Sherry R, Hughes MS, Royal R, Kammula U, et al. Adoptive cell therapy for patients with metastatic melanoma: evaluation of intensive myeloablative chemoradiation preparative regimens. J Clin Oncol. 2008;26:5233–9.
46. Gattinoni L, Finkelstein SE, Klebanoff CA, Antony PA, Palmer DC, Spiess PJ, et al. Removal of homeostatic cytokine sinks by lymphodepletion

enhances the efficacy of adoptively transferred tumor-specific CD8+ T cells. J Exp Med. 2005;202:907–12.
47. Besser MJ, Shapira-Frommer R, Treves AJ, Zippel D, Itzhaki O, Hershkovitz L, et al. Clinical responses in a phase II study using adoptive transfer of short-term cultured tumor infiltration lymphocytes in metastatic melanoma patients. Clin Cancer Res Off J Am Assoc Cancer Res. 2010;16:2646–55.
48. Pilon-Thomas S, Kuhn L, Ellwanger S, Janssen W, Royster E, Marzban S, et al. Efficacy of adoptive cell transfer of tumor-infiltrating lymphocytes after lymphopenia induction for metastatic melanoma. J Immunother. 2012;35:615–20.
49. Clay TM, Custer MC, Sachs J, Hwu P, Rosenberg SA, Nishimura MI. Efficient transfer of a tumor antigen-reactive TCR to human peripheral blood lymphocytes confers anti-tumor reactivity. J Immunol. 1999;163:507–13.
50. Kunert A, Straetemans T, Govers C, Lamers C, Mathijssen R, Sleijfer S, et al. TCR-engineered T cells meet new challenges to treat solid tumors: choice of antigen, T cell fitness, and sensitization of tumor milieu. Front Immunol. 2013;4:363.
51. Robbins PF, Dudley ME, Wunderlich J, El-Gamil M, Li YF, Zhou J, et al. Cutting edge: persistence of transferred lymphocyte clonotypes correlates with cancer regression in patients receiving cell transfer therapy. J Immunol. 2004;173:7125–30.
52. Zhou J, Shen X, Huang J, Hodes RJ, Rosenberg SA, Robbins PF. Telomere length of transferred lymphocytes correlates with in vivo persistence and tumor regression in melanoma patients receiving cell transfer therapy. J Immunol. 2005;175:7046–52.
53. Knowles G, O'Neil BW, Campo MS. Phenotypical characterization of lymphocytes infiltrating regressing papillomas. J Virol. 1996;70:8451–8.
54. Nicholls PK, Moore PF, Anderson DM, Moore RA, Parry NR, Gough GW, et al. Regression of canine oral papillomas is associated with infiltration of CD4+ and CD8+ lymphocytes. Virology. 2001;283:31–9.
55. Pires I, Queiroga FL, Alves A, Silva F, Lopes C. Decrease of E-cadherin expression in canine cutaneous histiocytoma appears to be related to its spontaneous regression. Anticancer Res. 2009;29:2713–7.
56. Carvalho MI, Pires I, Prada J, Queiroga FL. A role for T-lymphocytes in human breast cancer and in canine mammary tumors. Biomed Res Int. 2014;2014:130894.
57. Kim J-H, Yu C-H, Yhee J-Y, Im K-S, Sur J-H. Lymphocyte infiltration, expression of interleukin (IL)-1, IL-6 and expression of mutated breast cancer susceptibility gene-1 correlate with malignancy of canine mammary tumours. J Comp Pathol. 2010;142:177–86.
58. Estrela-Lima A, Araujo MS, Costa-Neto JM, Teixeira-Carvalho A, Barrouin-Melo SM, Cardoso SV, et al. Immunophenotypic features of tumor infiltrating lymphocytes from mammary carcinomas in female dogs associated with prognostic factors and survival rates. BMC Cancer. 2010;10. http://bmccancer.biomedcentral.com/articles/10.1186/1471-2407-10-256. Accessed 29 Jun 2017.
59. Carvalho MI, Pires I, Prada J, Queiroga FL. T-lymphocytic infiltrate in canine mammary tumours: clinic and prognostic implications. Vivo Athens Greece. 2011;25:963–9.
60. Saeki K, Endo Y, Uchida K, Nishimura R, Sasaki N, Nakagawa T. Significance of tumor-infiltrating immune cells in spontaneous canine mammary gland tumor: 140 cases. J Vet Med Sci. 2012;74:227–30.
61. Kim ST, Jeong H, Woo OH, Seo JH, Kim A, Lee ES, et al. Tumor-infiltrating lymphocytes, tumor characteristics, and recurrence in patients with early breast cancer. Am J Clin Oncol. 2013;36:224–31.
62. Mucha J, Rybicka A, Dolka I, Szymańska J, Manuali E, Parzeniecka-Jaworska M, et al. Immunosuppression in dogs during mammary cancer development. Vet Pathol. 2016;53:1147–53.
63. Tominaga M, Horiuchi Y, Ichikawa M, Yamashita M, Okano K, Jikumaru Y, et al. Flow cytometric analysis of peripheral blood and tumor-infiltrating regulatory T cells in dogs with oral malignant melanoma. J Vet Diagn Investig. 2010;22:438–41.
64. O'Connor CM, Sheppard S, Hartline CA, Huls H, Johnson M, Palla SL, et al. Adoptive T-cell therapy improves treatment of canine non-Hodgkin lymphoma post chemotherapy. Sci Rep. 2012;2:249.
65. Mata M, Vera JF, Gerken C, Rooney CM, Miller T, Pfent C, et al. Toward immunotherapy with redirected T cells in a large animal model: ex vivo activation, expansion, and genetic modification of canine T cells. J Immunother. 2014;37:407–15.
66. Yee C, Thompson JA, Byrd D, Riddell SR, Roche P, Celis E, et al. Adoptive T cell therapy using antigen-specific CD8+ T cell clones for the treatment of patients with metastatic melanoma: in vivo persistence, migration, and antitumor effect of transferred T cells. Proc Natl Acad Sci USA. 2002;99:16168–73.
67. Butler MO, Friedlander P, Milstein MI, Mooney MM, Metzler G, Murray AP, et al. Establishment of antitumor memory in humans using in vitro-educated CD8+ T cells. Sci Transl Med. 2011;3:80ra34.
68. Gabert J, Langlet C, Zamoyska R, Parnes JR, Schmitt-Verhulst AM, Malissen B. Reconstitution of MHC class I specificity by transfer of the T cell receptor and Lyt-2 genes. Cell. 1987;50:545–54.
69. DembiĆ Z, Haas W, Weiss S, McCubrey J, Kiefer H, von Boehmer H, et al. Transfer of specificity by murine α and β T-cell receptor genes. Nature. 1986;320:232–8.
70. Engels B, Noessner E, Frankenberger B, Blankenstein T, Schendel DJ, Uckert W. Redirecting human T lymphocytes toward renal cell carcinoma specificity by retroviral transfer of T cell receptor genes. Hum Gene Ther. 2005;16:799–810.
71. Xue S-A, Gao L, Hart D, Gillmore R, Qasim W, Thrasher A, et al. Elimination of human leukemia cells in NOD/SCID mice by WT1-TCR gene-transduced human T cells. Blood. 2005;106:3062–7.
72. Morgan RA, Dudley ME, Wunderlich JR, Hughes MS, Yang JC, Sherry RM, et al. Cancer regression in patients after transfer of genetically engineered lymphocytes. Science. 2006;314:126–9.
73. Rapoport AP, Stadtmauer EA, Binder-Scholl GK, Goloubeva O, Vogl DT, Lacey SF, et al. NY-ESO-1-specific TCR-engineered T cells mediate sustained antigen-specific antitumor effects in myeloma. Nat Med. 2015;21:914–21.
74. Thomas S, Stauss HJ, Morris EC. Molecular immunology lessons from therapeutic T-cell receptor gene transfer. Immunology. 2010;129:170–7.
75. Sommermeyer D, Neudorfer J, Weinhold M, Leisegang M, Engels B, Noessner E, et al. Designer T cells by T cell receptor replacement. Eur J Immunol. 2006;36:3052–9.
76. Sarukhan A, Garcia C, Lanoue A, von Boehmer H. Allelic inclusion of T cell receptor alpha genes poses an autoimmune hazard due to low-level expression of autospecific receptors. Immunity. 1998;8:563–70.
77. Gladow M, Uckert W, Blankenstein T. Dual T cell receptor T cells with two defined specificities mediate tumor suppression via both receptors. Eur J Immunol. 2004;34:1882–91.
78. Bendle GM, Linnemann C, Hooijkaas AI, Bies L, de Witte MA, Jorritsma A, et al. Lethal graft-versus-host disease in mouse models of T cell receptor gene therapy. Nat Med. 2010;16:565–70 **(1p following 570)**.
79. Linette GP, Stadtmauer EA, Maus MV, Rapoport AP, Levine BL, Emery L, et al. Cardiovascular toxicity and titin cross-reactivity of affinity-enhanced T cells in myeloma and melanoma. Blood. 2013;122:863–71.
80. Barth SM, Schreitmüller CM, Proehl F, Oehl K, Lumpp LM, Kowalewski DJ, et al. Characterization of the Canine MHC Class I DLA-88*50101 Peptide binding motif as a prerequisite for canine T cell immunotherapy. PLoS ONE. 2016;11:e0167017.
81. Garrido F, Ruiz-Cabello F, Cabrera T, Pérez-Villar JJ, López-Botet M, Duggan-Keen M, et al. Implications for immunosurveillance of altered HLA class I phenotypes in human tumours. Immunol Today. 1997;18:89–95.
82. Gross G, Waks T, Eshhar Z. Expression of immunoglobulin-T-cell receptor chimeric molecules as functional receptors with antibody-type specificity. Proc Natl Acad Sci USA. 1989;86:10024–8.
83. Jena B, Dotti G, Cooper LJN. Redirecting T-cell specificity by introducing a tumor-specific chimeric antigen receptor. Blood. 2010;116:1035–44.
84. Gilham DE, Debets R, Pule M, Hawkins RE, Abken H. CAR–T cells and solid tumors: tuning T cells to challenge an inveterate foe. Trends Mol Med. 2012;18:377–84.
85. Berry LJ, Moeller M, Darcy PK. Adoptive immunotherapy for cancer: the next generation of gene-engineered immune cells. Tissue Antigens. 2009;74:277–89.
86. Dai H, Wang Y, Lu X, Han W. Chimeric antigen receptors modified t-cells for cancer therapy. J Natl Cancer Inst. 2016. https://doi.org/10.1093/jnci/djv439.
87. Hombach AA, Abken H. Costimulation by chimeric antigen receptors revisited the T cell antitumor response benefits from combined CD28-OX40 signalling. Int J Cancer. 2011;129:2935–44.

88. Bridgeman JS, Hawkins RE, Hombach AA, Abken H, Gilham DE. Building better chimeric antigen receptors for adoptive T cell therapy. Curr Gene Ther. 2010;10:77–90.
89. Grupp SA, Kalos M, Barrett D, Aplenc R, Porter DL, Rheingold SR, et al. Chimeric antigen receptor-modified T cells for acute lymphoid leukemia. N Engl J Med. 2013;368:1509–18.
90. Louis CU, Savoldo B, Dotti G, Pule M, Yvon E, Myers GD, et al. Antitumor activity and long-term fate of chimeric antigen receptor-positive T cells in patients with neuroblastoma. Blood. 2011;118:6050–6.
91. Kershaw MH, Westwood JA, Parker LL, Wang G, Eshhar Z, Mavroukakis SA, et al. A phase I study on adoptive immunotherapy using gene-modified T cells for ovarian cancer. Clin Cancer Res. 2006;12:6106–15.
92. Lamers CHJ, Sleijfer S, Vulto AG, Kruit WHJ, Kliffen M, Debets R, et al. Treatment of metastatic renal cell carcinoma with autologous T-lymphocytes genetically retargeted against carbonic anhydrase IX: first clinical experience. J Clin Oncol. 2006;24:e20–2.
93. Lamers CH, Sleijfer S, van Steenbergen S, van Elzakker P, van Krimpen B, Groot C, et al. Treatment of metastatic renal cell carcinoma with CAIX CAR-engineered T cells: clinical evaluation and management of on-target toxicity. Mol Ther J Am Soc Gene Ther. 2013;21:904–12.
94. Zhang E, Xu H. A new insight in chimeric antigen receptor-engineered T cells for cancer immunotherapy. J Hematol Oncol. 2017;10:1.
95. Panjwani MK, Smith JB, Schutsky K, Gnanandarajah J, O'Connor CM, Powell DJ, et al. Feasibility and Safety of RNA-transfected CD20-specific chimeric antigen receptor T cells in dogs with spontaneous B cell lymphoma. Mol Ther. 2016;24:1602–14.
96. Rosenberg SA, Lotze MT. Cancer immunotherapy using interleukin-2 and interleukin-2-activated lymphocytes. Annu Rev Immunol. 1986;4:681–709.
97. Hoshino Y, Takagi S, Osaki T, Okumura M, Fujinaga T. Phenotypic analysis and effects of sequential administration of activated canine lymphocytes on healthy beagles. J Vet Med Sci. 2008;70:581–8.
98. Helfand SC, Soergel SA, Modiano JF, Hank JA, Sondel PM. Induction of lymphokine-activated killer (LAK) activity in canine lymphocytes with low dose human recombinant interleukin-2 in vitro. Cancer Biother. 1994;9:237–44.
99. Itoh H, Kakuta T, Kudo T, Sakonju I, Hohdatsu T, Ebina T, et al. Bulk cultures of canine peripheral blood lymphocytes with solid phase anti-CD3 antibody and recombinant interleukin-2 for use in immunotherapy. J Vet Med Sci. 2003;65:329–33.
100. Mie K, Shimada T, Akiyoshi H, Hayashi A, Ohashi F. Change in peripheral blood lymphocyte count in dogs following adoptive immunotherapy using lymphokine-activated T killer cells combined with palliative tumor resection. Vet Immunol Immunopathol. 2016;177:58–63.
101. Cox DBT, Platt RJ, Zhang F. Therapeutic genome editing: prospects and challenges. Nat Med. 2015;21:121–31.
102. Urnov FD, Rebar EJ, Holmes MC, Zhang HS, Gregory PD. Genome editing with engineered zinc finger nucleases. Nat Rev Genet. 2010;11:636–46.
103. Nemudryi AA, Valetdinova KR, Medvedev SP, Zakian SM. TALEN and CRISPR/Cas genome editing systems: tools of discovery. Acta Nat. 2014;6:19–40.
104. Joung JK, Sander JD. TALENs: a widely applicable technology for targeted genome editing. Nat Rev Mol Cell Biol. 2013;14:49–55.
105. Hsu PD, Lander ES, Zhang F. Development and applications of CRISPR-Cas9 for genome engineering. Cell. 2014;157:1262–78.
106. Gaj T, Gersbach CA, Barbas CF. ZFN, TALEN, and CRISPR/Cas-based methods for genome engineering. Trends Biotechnol. 2013;31:397–405.
107. Li H, Haurigot V, Doyon Y, Li T, Wong SY, Bhagwat AS, et al. In vivo genome editing restores haemostasis in a mouse model of haemophilia. Nature. 2011;475:217–21.
108. Yin H, Xue W, Chen S, Bogorad RL, Benedetti E, Grompe M, et al. Genome editing with Cas9 in adult mice corrects a disease mutation and phenotype. Nat Biotechnol. 2014;32:551–3.
109. Lin S-R, Yang H-C, Kuo Y-T, Liu C-J, Yang T-Y, Sung K-C, et al. The CRISPR/Cas9 system facilitates clearance of the intrahepatic HBV templates in vivo. Mol Ther Nucleic Acids. 2014;3:e186.
110. Ousterout DG, Perez-Pinera P, Thakore PI, Kabadi AM, Brown MT, Qin X, et al. Reading frame correction by targeted genome editing restores dystrophin expression in cells from duchenne muscular dystrophy patients. Mol Ther. 2013;21:1718–26.
111. Reardon S. Leukaemia success heralds wave of gene-editing therapies. Nature. 2015;527:146–7.
112. Qasim W, Zhan H, Samarasinghe S, Adams S, Amrolia P, Stafford S, et al. Molecular remission of infant B-ALL after infusion of universal TALEN gene-edited CAR T cells. Sci Transl Med. 2017;9:eaaj2013.
113. Torikai H, Reik A, Liu P-Q, Zhou Y, Zhang L, Maiti S, et al. A foundation for universal T-cell based immunotherapy: T cells engineered to express a CD19-specific chimeric-antigen-receptor and eliminate expression of endogenous TCR. Blood. 2012;119:5697–705.
114. Provasi E, Genovese P, Lombardo A, Magnani Z, Liu P-Q, Reik A, et al. Editing T cell specificity towards leukemia by zinc finger nucleases and lentiviral gene transfer. Nat Med. 2012;18:807–15.
115. Peng R, Lin G, Li J. Potential pitfalls of CRISPR/Cas9-mediated genome editing. FEBS J. 2016;283:1218–31.
116. Zou Q, Wang X, Liu Y, Ouyang Z, Long H, Wei S, et al. Generation of gene-target dogs using CRISPR/Cas9 system. J Mol Cell Biol. 2015;7:580–3.

# Farm characteristics and management routines related to cow longevity: a survey among Swedish dairy farmers

Karin Alvåsen[1*], Ian Dohoo[2], Anki Roth[3] and Ulf Emanuelson[1]

**Abstract**

**Background:** Longevity is an important trait for increasing the profitability of dairy production. Long cow longevity is also essential to reduce the environmental impact of milk production, and to maintain positive consumer attitude. Genetic selection for increased longevity has been effective, but the phenotypic trend of longevity in Swedish dairy cows has not been improved. The objective of this study was to identify herd characteristics and management routines that are associated with the average cow longevity in a herd. To obtain this information, a questionnaire was developed and sent out to 661 Swedish dairy farmers.

**Results:** The response rate was 35%. Seventeen of the 62 characteristics investigated had either a univariable association with the outcome (days from birth to culling) at $P < 0.15$, or were identified as confounders in the causal diagram and were therefore considered as candidates for the multivariable analysis. Multiple imputation was used to fill in the missing data from the questionnaires, and this increased the number of usable observations in the multivariable modeling from 156 to 228. Only a few of the investigated herd characteristics and management routines were associated with average cow longevity. The results demonstrated that using herd health advisory services shortened the average longevity, while using breeding advisory services prolonged the average longevity in the herd. Furthermore, having a greater interest in animal breeding (i.e. genetic selection) decreased the longevity, and calling the veterinarian when discovering an unhealthy cow increased the average longevity. Higher age of the farmer was also associated with longer average herd longevity.

**Conclusions:** The herd average cow longevity was only associated with some of the farm characteristics and management routines studied. The results demonstrate that the use of advisory services and farmers' attitudes could be targeted for increasing the herd longevity. Further, the results indicate that other e.g. qualitative factors influencing farmers' decisions play an important role.

**Keywords:** Dairy cattle, Life expectancy, Lifespan, Longevity, Management, Multiple imputation

*Correspondence: karin.alvasen@slu.se
[1] Department of Clinical Sciences, Swedish University of Agricultural Sciences, P.O. Box 7054, 75007 Uppsala, Sweden
Full list of author information is available at the end of the article

## Background

Cow longevity refers to how long the cow stays in the herd. The modern dairy cow has a short longevity, far below their biological potential. In Sweden, between 35 and 40% of the cows are culled from the herd each year, and this is done at an average age of 60.5 months [1]. Longevity is an important economic trait in dairy production [2, 3]. Increasing the productive lifetime of dairy cows would improve the efficiency of dairy production as cows must typically reach the second lactation to produce sufficient milk to break even on rearing costs [4, 5]. Herd replacement is the second highest variable cost in a dairy enterprise [6], and with increased longevity fewer replacement heifers would be required to achieve the same herd output, which would reduce replacement costs [3, 7, 8]. Surplus heifers could instead be sold or a larger proportion of the cows could be inseminated with beef semen [9]. Furthermore, with increased longevity the mean production of the herd could be higher because a large proportion of the culling decisions are based on production, and also because the proportion of mature cows, which generally produce more milk than young cows, would be increased [2, 3, 7, 10]. In addition, the carbon footprint per kilogram of product is reduced with increased lifetime productivity [11]. High culling rates and, in particular, high on-farm mortality, are indicators of poor welfare status and are not compatible with sustainable dairy production [12–14].

Longevity has been included in genetic selection in Sweden and in many other countries for many years, and a positive genetic trend has been observed (Jan-Åke Eriksson, personal communication). However, the phenotypic trend in Swedish cows has shown no improvement, and the average age at culling was still approximately 60 months in 1990 [1]. The longevity of a dairy cow is determined mainly by the culling decision made by the farmer, and such decisions are the result of intrinsic cow factors such as health, milk production, and reproductive status and extrinsic factors such as the availability of replacement heifers, the number of cow-places, the capacity of the milking system, and milk prices [15–18]. Studies have shown that pregnancy, higher milk production, younger age, and the absence of health issues such as metabolic problems, lameness, or mastitis are intrinsic cow factors that reduce the risk of culling [12, 19, 20]. On the herd level, Strandberg and Emanuelson [21] used data retrieved from the Swedish official milk recording scheme (SOMRS) and found that an expanding herd size and a high proportion of culling in early lactation were associated with both a short total lifespan and a short productive life (from first calving to culling). Management at the time around calving was suggested as a key area to improve cow longevity.

Although many intrinsic and extrinsic factors affecting longevity have been identified, very little is known about the actual herd management practices that affect these factors and thus have an impact on cow longevity. Information about such associations would be useful so that advisory activities can be more targeted. The objective of this study was therefore to identify herd management practices that are associated with average cow longevity under Swedish production conditions.

## Methods

### Study design and study population

The target population in this study was dairy farms with short or long average herd longevity (described below) and a herd size of at least 35 cows enrolled in the SOMRS. The SOMRS is a voluntary service that in 2012/2013 included 84% of the Swedish dairy cows [1]. Herds in the SOMRS are categorized into long or short longevity based on the average longevity of all cows in the herd. To avoid including herds with either temporary short or long longevity, data from three consecutive years were used. The herds were categorized into short longevity or long longevity herds based on their average longevity during 2008/2009, 2009/2010, and 2010/2011 (the SOMRS uses fiscal years running from September 1 to August 31, and this classification of year is used in the present study, with years referred to as 2009/2010, etc.). Long longevity herds had an average longevity, based on total lifespan (from birth to culling) in the fourth quartile of all SOMRS herds during 2009/2010 and 2010/2011 (1742 and 1748 days, respectively) and above the median during 2008/2009 (1579 days). Short longevity herds had an average longevity in the first quartile during 2009/2010 and 2010/2011 (1429 and 1437 days, respectively), and below the median during 2008/2009. The median was used as the threshold during 2008/2009 to increase the number of eligible herds. Out of 3698 herds with > 35 cows registered in the SOMRS, 350 and 311 herds met the criteria for short and long longevity, respectively.

### Data collection

A questionnaire was developed to acquire information on management routines that we hypothesized to be related to cow longevity in Swedish dairy herds. The questionnaire was also used in another study about on-farm cow mortality, and a more detailed description of the development of the questionnaire can therefore be found in Alvåsen et al. [14]. The questionnaire consisted of 49 questions in Swedish of which 32 were of multiple choice type, 10 were open-ended and 7 were answered on a visual analog scale. An English version of the questionnaire can be found in Additional file 1.

Questionnaires were distributed by mail in October 2012 to all farmers whose herds met the inclusion criteria. In total, 1000 questionnaires were sent, of which 661 went to the long and short longevity herds described above and 339 went to herds that were targeted for the on-farm cow mortality study. The respondents were informed that all information they provided would be treated as confidential, but they were not made aware of the study design or purpose. After 7 weeks, a reminder in the form of a postcard was sent to the non-responders. In total, 353 questionnaires were returned, of which 233 were from the 661 long and short longevity herds.

Data on average herd longevity for 2011/2012 was retrieved from the SOMRS. This average herd longevity data corresponded to the period that was covered by the questionnaire. We also retrieved data from the SOMRS on some common herd characteristics (e.g. housing and milking systems, geographic location and herd size) and average herd production parameters (e.g. milk yield and quality, reproductive performance and age at first calving) for all targeted herds. These latter data were used to compare certain parameters among respondents and non-respondents using *t* test for continuous variables and the $\chi^2$ test for categorical variables.

### Causal diagram

Analyses were guided by the causal diagram shown in Fig. 1. The causal diagram was created by the authors using DAGitty [22]. Predictor variables were categorized as farmer characteristics, herd characteristics, farmer attitudes, or management practices. Variables in the latter two groups were the main exposures of interest while those in the first two groups were potential confounders. One farmer characteristic (age) and two herd characteristics (region and number of milking cows) were considered confounders in all analyses and were forced to remain in all models. Management factors were considered to be intervening variables for the evaluation of the effects of farmer attitudes and consequently were not included in these regression models.

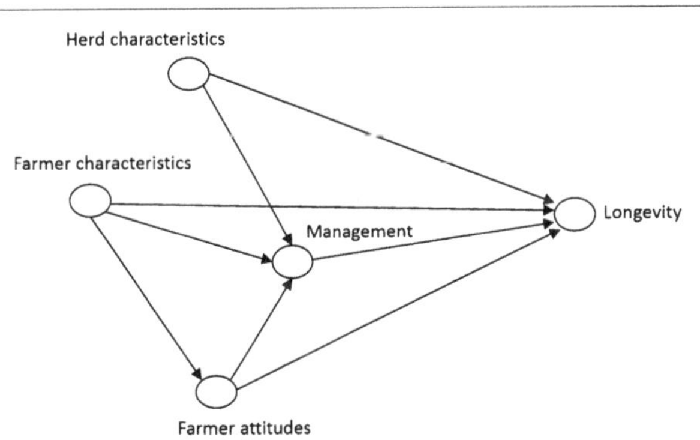


**Fig. 1** Causal diagram for analysis of the effects of farmer attitudes and management practices on longevity in dairy cows

### Outcome variable

The outcome variable of interest was the average longevity (days from birth to culling) of milking cows in the herd for the period 2011/2012. Culling was defined as the departure of cows from the herd because of sale, slaughter, salvage, or death. It was first ascertained that this variable had no missing values. Although many of the study herds had been selected based on historically long or short longevity, the variable was approximately normally distributed, although the tails of the distribution were slightly longer than expected under the assumption of normality. No transformation was employed, but the assumption of normality of residuals was checked after model building.

### Predictors

All possible predictors for which data were collected in the questionnaire were reviewed, and obvious errors were corrected. Some variables were dropped (n = 8) because there was an obvious misunderstanding of the question by some respondents (i.e., they gave completely illogical answers). Categorical variables were recoded as needed to eliminate categories with very small numbers of observations. All of the continuous variables related to farmer attitude and management factors (Table 1) were answered on a visual analogue scale where a higher number refers to "very likely" for all variables except for "Interest in animal breeding" where a high value refers to "high interest". Visual analogue scale variables related to the diagnosis of lameness or unhealth were combined using Cronbach's alpha into a single scale variable (an average score of standardized values). The number of valid observations for each variable was determined. A complete listing of all categorical and continuous predictors considered in the analyses (including the number of valid observations) can be found in Additional files 2, 3.

### Unconditional associations

Associations between predictors of interest and longevity were evaluated one at a time in linear regression models in which region, herd size, and age of farmer were forced in as confounders. P-values for the associations are shown in Additional file 2. Variables with $P < 0.15$ were retained for use in multivariable modeling (Table 1). Following this evaluation, housing was also identified as a potentially important confounding variable and was forced into all subsequent multivariable models.

**Table 1 Predictors selected as candidates for multivariable modeling**

| Variable | n | Continuous mean, SD (min, max) | Categorical | | Overall |
|---|---|---|---|---|---|
| | | | Categories | n (%) | P-value[a] |
| Farmer characteristics | | | | | |
| Age of farmer (year) | 225 | 48.7, 11.3 (20, 79) | | | < 0.001 |
| Herd characteristics | | | | | |
| Herd size (no. of cows) | 213 | 87.6, 84.6 (26, 1000) | | | 0.192 |
| Housing type | 227 | | Tie stall | 100 (56) | 0.017 |
| | | | Free stall | 127 (44) | |
| Region | 228 | | South Sweden | 32 (14) | 0.089 |
| | | | East Sweden | 62 (27) | |
| | | | West Sweden | 74 (32) | |
| | | | Middle Sweden | 20 (9) | |
| | | | North Sweden | 40 (18) | |
| Farmer attitudes | | | | | |
| Expected future herd size | 224 | | Same or fewer | 163 (73) | 0.046 |
| | | | Expand | 61 (27) | |
| Expectation that the farm will still be operating in 5 year | 227 | 7.6, 2.7 (1, 10) | | | 0.144 |
| Interest in animal breeding (genetic selection) | 223 | 7.9, 2.0 (0.5, 10) | | | 0.145 |
| Management factors | | | | | |
| Composition of workforce | 222 | | Only family members | 94 (42) | 0.141 |
| | | | Employee(s) | 128 (58) | |
| Used herd health advice during the last year | 182 | | No | 82 (45) | 0.029 |
| | | | Yes | 100 (55) | |
| Used breeding advice during the last year | 204 | | No | 55 (27) | 0.123 |
| | | | Yes | 149 (73) | |
| Calving occurs in individual calving pens | 227 | | Yes | 78 (34) | 0.017 |
| | | | No | 149 (66) | |
| Time required for drying off (d) | 214 | 7.8, 4.3 (0, 21) | | | 0.019 |
| Call veterinarian for lame cows | 210 | 4.4, 3.1 (0, 10) | | | 0.003 |
| Move lame cows to isolation pen | 202 | 5.3, 3.2 (0, 10) | | | 0.029 |
| Call veterinarian for unhealthy cows | 219 | 7.5, 2.4 (0.1, 10) | | | 0.011 |
| Move unhealthy cows to isolation pen | 213 | 6.1, 3.2 (0, 10) | | | 0.121 |
| Initiate treatment of unhealthy cows on my own | 215 | 5.0, 3.4 (0, 10) | | | 0.148 |

Predictors selected as candidates for multivariable modeling of associations with average herd longevity according to the categories identified in the causal diagram

[a] Univariable P-values for the confounders (age, herd size, region), but multivariable P-values for the predictors

### Complete case analyses

Several multivariable linear regression models were fitted, in which region, herd size, age of farmer, and housing were forced in as confounders. Attitude variables were included in the model as potential confounders but were not forced to remain in the model if not significant. A manual backwards elimination procedure was used in which the variables with the largest P-values were sequentially removed while watching for changes in the coefficients of the retained variables. Ultimately, only management factors with $P < 0.05$ were retained. For the final model, graphical evaluations were used to assess the normality of residuals and to check for evidence of heteroscedasticity. The model was refitted without observations that had standardized residuals $> |2.5|$ in order to evaluate the impact of the outliers.

The process was repeated for the evaluation of attitude variables except that management variables were excluded from the model because they were intervening variables (Fig. 1). Any attitude variables with $P < 0.05$ were retained in the final model.

### Multiple imputation

Multiple imputation is a flexible, simulation-based statistical technique for handling missing data [23, 24]. It has been shown that multiple imputation analyses generally produce less biased results than complete case analyses [24]. Multiple imputation of missing predictor values was carried out using the outcome variable and all predictors for which data were missing. Chained equations were used and categorical predictors were imputed using a multinomial logit function, while ordinal, dichotomous, and continuous predictors were imputed using predictive mean matching. Problems with convergence were observed for a few categorical variables, so these were converted to a set of dichotomous predictors (1 for each category). Twenty imputed data sets were generated, and diagnostic plots comparing the distribution of the observed values with the imputed values were examined for the selected predictor variables.

### Analyses of multiply imputed data

A model-building procedure (manual backwards elimination) similar to that employed in the complete case analysis was applied to the multiply imputed data. Again, separate models were built to evaluate the effects of management factors and farmers' attitudes. A comparison of the coefficient estimates and their statistical significance was carried out for the management practice models.

All statistical analyses were performed in Stata version 14 (StataCorp LP, College Station, TX).

## Results

Of the 233 returned questionnaires, 3 herds had ceased milk production and 2 herds had sent in blank questionnaires. The number of usable questionnaires was thus 228 for a response rate of 34%. The distribution of herd characteristics was similar in the respondent and non-respondent groups (Table 2). The median of the average herd longevity of the 228 herds was 1554 days (Q1 = 1404 days, Q3 = 1752 days).

### Variables and missing data

Only four predictors had complete data for all 228 herds, and 20% of the herds had complete data for all of the variables that were evaluated. The number of observations with valid data for each variable is shown in Additional file 2, 3. In general, the number of missing values for each variable was small, with a maximum of 57 missing. The variables with unconditional associations $P < 0.15$, as well as the confounders, are presented in Table 1 according to the groups identified in the causal diagram (Fig. 1).

### Multivariable models

Results from the final multivariable models, including the complete case and the models using imputed data, can be found in Tables 3, 4, respectively. In both models, four variables (Age, Herd size, Region, and Housing) were included as confounders. The final model with imputed data (Table 4) demonstrated that farmers that used herd health advisory services during the last year had shorter average herd longevity (− 124 days), while farmers that used breeding advisory services had a longer average longevity (117 days). Farmers that were more likely to contact the veterinarian when detecting an unhealthy cow and farmers that did not consider themselves as interested in genetic selection had longer average longevity (23 and 21 days, respectively). The four confounders forced into the model were all non-significant except for

**Table 2 Distribution of herd characteristics among respondents and non-respondents**

| Variable | Category | Respondents (n = 228) | Non-respondents (n = 443) | P-value[1] |
|---|---|---|---|---|
| Age at 1st calving (days) | | 866 (99.1)[2] | 898 (115.3) | < 0.01 |
| BMSCC (1000 cells/ml) | | 254 (85) | 256 (88) | 0.37 |
| Breed[3] | SR | 18.5 | 18.0 | 0.19 |
| | SH | 20.3 | 26.6 | |
| | Mixed | 61.2 | 55.4 | |
| Calving interval (mo) | | 13.4 (1.1) | 13.8 (1.3) | < 0.01 |
| Herd size (cow-year) | | 94 (107) | 88 (73) | 0.79 |
| Milk yield (kg ECM/cow-year) | | 9264 (1457) | 9191 (1656) | 0.71 |
| Region | North | 20.2 | 22.4 | 0.60 |
| | Middle | 57.0 | 52.9 | |
| | South | 22.8 | 24.7 | |

Distribution of herd characteristics (percentage of observations for categorical variables and means with standard deviations for continuous variables) among respondents and non-respondents to the questionnaire

*BMSCC* bulk milk somatic cell count

[1] Significance level (*t*-test for continuous variables and $\chi^2$ test for categorical variables)

[2] Mean (standard deviation)

[3] SR = > 80% Swedish Red; SH = > 80% Swedish Holstein; Mixed = all other herds

**Table 3 Final complete case model of associations between management practices and average herd longevity**

| Variable | Coefficient | SE | P>t | 95% CI |
|---|---|---|---|---|
| Age of farmer[a] (year) | 7.15 | 1.65 | 0.000 | 3.89; 10.40 |
| Herd size[a] | −0.03 | 0.22 | 0.887 | −0.47; 0.41 |
| Housing[a] | | | | |
| Tie stall | Reference | | | |
| Free stall | 73.65 | 42.96 | 0.089 | −11.27; 158.56 |
| Region[a,b] | | | | |
| South Sweden | Reference | | | |
| East Sweden | 10.02 | 61.68 | 0.871 | −111.89; 131.93 |
| West Sweden | −53.10 | 59.35 | 0.372 | −170.41; 64.21 |
| Middle Sweden | −119.62 | 93.33 | 0.202 | −304.09; 64.85 |
| North Sweden | −70.88 | 66.68 | 0.290 | −202.67; 60.90 |
| Initiate treatment on my own when recognizing unhealthy cows | −16.14 | 5.80 | 0.006 | −27.61; −4.68 |
| Use of breeding advisory services | | | | |
| No | Reference | | | |
| Yes | 108.87 | 44.38 | 0.015 | 21.15; 196.59 |
| Use of preventive herd health advisory services | | | | |
| No | Reference | | | |
| Yes | −121.41 | 43.32 | 0.006 | −207.03; −35.78 |
| Intercept | 1317.05 | 103.75 | | |

Final model of associations between management practices and average herd longevity (days) from the complete case analysis based on data from 156 herds

[a] Confounders forced into the model

[b] Region: overall P-value = 0.38 (Wald test)

age, where higher age of the farmer was associated with an increased herd longevity (5 days per year of age).

## Model evaluation

Coefficients from the complete case and the multiple imputation models are shown in Table 5. The complete case analysis had reasonable normality and showed no evidence of heteroscedasticity. There were six observations with standardized residuals > |2.5|. Removal of these observations reduced the coefficient and significance of the variable "Use of preventive herd health advisory services". None of the attitude variables were significant after controlling for the four confounders (data not shown).

All missing values were successfully imputed, and comparison of the distribution of imputed and original values showed good imputation. We used the coefficient of determination ($R^2$) statistic to compare the predictive abilities of the complete case and the multiple imputation procedures. The two procedures produced different final models, but regardless of whether the comparison was based on applying each procedure to the complete observations (n = 156) or to a larger subset where the variables in the two models had complete information (n = 182), the model derived from the imputation procedure had better predictive ability ($R^2 = 26.2\%$ vs. 24.2% if n = 156, $R^2_{\text{(average d over 20 imputations)}} = 21.4\%$ vs 18.1% if n = 182).

## Discussion

This study aimed to identify herd management practices and characteristics associated with average cow longevity in the herd. We found surprisingly few predictors that had a significant impact on cow longevity. Herds that are using herd health advisory services were associated with shorter cow longevity, but this does not necessarily imply that dairy farms should not use herd health advisory services. Instead, these services might be used to a higher degree by farms with herd health problems and thus possibly also shorter longevity. In any cross-sectional study (such as this) it is difficult to sort out the time sequence between predictors and the outcome of interest. In some situations, it is necessary to use strategies that involve higher culling rates, e.g., when combating aggressive pathogens in a herd [25, 26]. This approach can result in improved herd health in the future, but will result in a higher culling rate and hence reduce the average longevity of the herd in the short term. Also, preventive herd health services offered by veterinarians or other advisors in Sweden are not fully recognized among the dairy farmers. In a qualitative study about preventive

**Table 4 Final model multiple imputation model of associations between management practices and average herd longevity**

| Variable | Coefficient | SE | P>t | 95% CI |
|---|---|---|---|---|
| Age of farmer[a] (year) | 5.45 | 1.65 | 0.001 | 2.21; 8.70 |
| Herd size[a] | 0.01 | 0.23 | 0.977 | − 0.44; 0.46 |
| Housing[a] | | | | |
| Tie stall | Reference | | | |
| Free stall | 30.55 | 40.91 | 0.456 | − 50.10; 111.19 |
| Region[ab] | | | | |
| South Sweden | Reference | | | |
| East Sweden | − 49.54 | 59.77 | 0.408 | − 167.37; 68.29 |
| West Sweden | − 104.32 | 57.31 | 0.070 | − 217.30; 8.65 |
| Middle Sweden | − 143.15 | 78.27 | 0.069 | − 297.45; 11.15 |
| North Sweden | − 140.06 | 64.89 | 0.032 | − 267.98; − 12.14 |
| Call the veterinarian when recognizing unhealthy cows | 22.59 | 8.26 | 0.007 | 6.28; 38.91 |
| Interest in animal breeding (genetic selection) | − 21.09 | 9.87 | 0.034 | − 40.56; − 1.62 |
| Used breeding advisory services during the last year | | | | |
| No | Reference | | | |
| Yes | 116.88 | 48.34 | 0.017 | 21.19; 212.58 |
| Used preventive herd health advisory services during the last year | | | | |
| No | Reference | | | |
| Yes | − 124.26 | 43.15 | 0.005 | − 209.48; − 39.04 |
| Intercept | 1366.83 | 144.22 | | |

Final model of associations between management practices and average herd longevity (days) following multiple imputation of missing data. The analysis is based on data from 228 herds

[a] Confounders forced into the model

[b] Region: overall P-value = 0.13 (Wald test)

herd health management, Swedish dairy farmers had difficulties in defining the concept of preventive herd health and in telling what roles the veterinarian could fill in this regard [27]. One key barrier for using veterinarians more proactively in herd health management that has been mentioned by farmers is that veterinarians are associated only with their curative role in acute illness [28, 29]. Thus there is a great need for veterinarians to communicate and improve the herd health services being offered—both in Sweden and in some other countries—in order to change the current stereotype of being seen as “fire fighters” who are only treating unhealthy cows [29, 30]. These difficulties for farmers in defining the concept of preventive herd health management, along with the limited experience of this type of advisory service, could have introduced observational bias in our data.

Using breeding advisory services was, however, beneficial for the average cow longevity even though being interested in animal breeding reduced the average longevity. This suggests that farmers with low interest in animal breeding might be the ones using breeding advisory services, which might result in having a more structured breeding plan and thus more robust cows. Farmers interested in animal breeding might also have a more “active” culling strategy and hence end up with a shorter average lifespan in the herd. In face-to-face interviews with Swedish dairy farmers, Bergeå et al. [31] discovered a management-related phenomenon where farmers interested in genetic selection and breeding improvements are more likely to accept that heifers “push out” older cows. This was mainly a consequence of farmers breeding too many heifers combined with a greater interest in genetic improvements. The difference in genetic potential has been shown in Swedish dairy herds; for example, herds with the lowest average estimated breeding value in milk were four times more likely to have a long average productive life and total life span than average herds [21]. One way to extend the average cow longevity is to bring fewer heifers into the herd and therefore to cull fewer cows [8, 15]. One management option would be the use of sexed semen with genetically superior cows and inseminating a proportion of the remaining cows with beef semen—which will also improve the farm economy [9]. It is likely that farms taking breeding advice receive support in these kinds of breeding strategies as genetic improvement is important but does not warrant short cow longevity [32].

Moreover, the results of the present study indicate that farmers that are more likely to contact the veterinarian as a first step when recognizing an unhealthy cow were associated with longer average cow longevity. Prompt and adequate treatment is in most situations crucial to solving health issues and thus reducing the need for premature culling. Also, achieving greater longevity through improved cow health will improve cow welfare [32].

The only confounder in the model that was statistically significant was the age of the farmer, and older farmers generally had a longer average longevity in their herds. The age of the farmer and the farmer's experience were highly correlated, and having greater experience in running a dairy enterprise appears to improve longevity. An older and more experienced farmer might be better at keeping the animals healthy, which will reduce the number of forced culls. Another suggestion is that an older farmer might approach dairying as a lifestyle rather than a business, and therefore have a different view on ownership of their cows that transcends economic decision-making and rationale culling. Younger farmers could be more economically driven and therefore have a higher interest in genetic and herd heath improvement which could result in a shorter average cow longevity.

**Table 5 Comparison of complete case and multiple imputation models**

| Variable | Models with all 17 selected predictors[a] | | Final models[b] | |
|---|---|---|---|---|
| | Complete case analysis (n = 131) | Multiple imputation (n = 228) | Complete case analysis (n = 156) | Multiple imputation (n = 228) |
| Confounders forced into model | | | | |
| Age of farmer | 4.71** | 5.06*** | 7.15*** | 5.45*** |
| Herd size | 0.13 | 0.1 | − 0.03 | 0.01 |
| Housing | | | | |
| Tie stall | Reference | | | |
| Free stall | 95.80* | − 18.21 | 73.65* | 30.55 |
| Region | | | | |
| South Sweden | Reference | | | |
| East Sweden | 13.21 | − 67.1 | 10.02 | − 49.54 |
| West Sweden | − 43.05 | − 103.93* | − 53.1 | − 104.32* |
| Middle Sweden | − 117.93 | − 171.90** | − 119.62 | − 143.15* |
| North Sweden | − 49.84 | − 130.49* | − 70.88 | − 140.06** |
| Predictors available for selection | | | | |
| Expected future herd size | | | | |
| Same or fewer | Reference | | | |
| Expand | − 48.23 | − 77.56* | | |
| Probability that the farm will still be operating in 5 year | − 7.8 | − 0.94 | | |
| Interest in animal breeding (genetic selection) | − 0.6 | − 16.11 | | − 21.09** |
| Composition of workforce | | | | |
| Only family members | Reference | | | |
| Employee(s) | − 37.05 | − 50.03 | | |
| Used preventive herd health advisory services during the last year | | | | |
| No | Reference | | | |
| Yes | − 43.1 | − 107.33** | − 121.41*** | − 124.26*** |
| Used breeding advisory services during the last year | | | | |
| No | Reference | | | |
| Yes | 86.87* | 113.21** | 108.87** | 116.88** |
| Calving occurs in individual calving pens | | | | |
| No | Reference | | | |
| Only individual calving pens | − 24.02 | − 60.42 | | |
| Average time for dry-off (d) | − 1.11 | 1.69 | | |
| Call veterinarian when recognizing a lame cow | 8.62 | 6.04 | | |
| Move to isolation pen when recognizing a lame cow | − 7.14 | − 9.89 | | |
| Call veterinarian when recognizing an unhealthy cow | 15.08 | 16.70* | | 22.59*** |
| Move to isolation pen when recognizing an unhealthy cow | 9.39 | 5.12 | | |
| Initiate treatment on my own when recognizing unhealthy cows | − 8.79 | − 4.69 | − 16.14*** | |
| Intercept | 1295.35*** | 1483.90*** | 1317.05*** | 1366.83*** |

Comparison of full and final models from both the complete case and the multiple imputation models of associations between management practices and average herd longevity (*P < 0.1, **P < 0.05, ***P < 0.001)

In this study we used two different models: one complete case analysis and one analysis of the data material that had undergone multiple imputation. The complete case analysis had somewhat different variables in the final model. The use of breeding and herd health advice services was similar to the multiple imputation model, and the directions of the effects were the same. However, instead of calling the veterinarian when discovering a sick cow, this data set showed a negative association between the average longevity of the herd and farmers that most likely "Initiated treatment on one's own" when discovering an unhealthy cow. As multiple imputation analyses generally produce less biased results than complete case analyses [24], more weight is put on the results from the multiple imputation model. It is generally recommended to use a large number of predictors in the imputation process, and in this case we used all available data from the questionnaires. When comparing $R^2$ on the same number of observations for the two models, the gain in explanation was rather small, but an important benefit with the imputation is that it increased the number of usable observations from 156 to 228. Being able to use the data from these observations most likely contributed to less biased results in this study.

The questionnaires were sent to herds in the lowest and highest quartiles of average longevity. Our initial intention was to use these classifications for the analyses, but instead we retrieved additional data from the SOMRS on average longevity for the responding herds. In this way we were able to analyze the actual average herd longevity for the same period in which the farmers filled out the questionnaire. Even though the selection criteria were based on three consecutive years, there were some herds that had changed group, and basing the analysis on the currently used farm characteristics was therefore considered to give more valid results regarding management routines and average longevity of the herd.

Because not all of the farmers responded to the questionnaire, selection bias might have been present. However, when comparing some of the herd characteristics, only two characteristics differed between respondents and non-respondents. Respondents had herds with significantly lower age at first calving and shorter calving intervals, which could reflect the level of management. Most herd characteristics showed no differences between respondents and non-respondents, and we therefore believe that the study population was reasonably similar to the target population and thus had an acceptable level of external validity.

We did not find many management-related associations, which was contrary to our expectation. Either we did not have the correct questions in our questionnaire, or a questionnaire is not the best way to capture the type of factors that we were interested in, or other unknown factors are more important, or there simply are not many management-related associations. Fetrow et al. [33] point out that a short lifespan of a dairy cow is primarily the result of an economic decision on the part of the dairy farmer and making a decision to replace one cow with another could sometimes be a strategic economic option. Different herd conditions will most likely play a significant role in culling decisions, and characteristics such as the availability of heifers, cultural influences, farmer's attitude, and prices on the milk and beef market are some of the possible factors that have an impact on the decisions taken by the farmer [34]. Furthermore, using averages on herd level for a trait like longevity could cause bias because the same averages may come from herds with vastly different age patterns.

Longevity has been ranked as the most important trait by both organic and conventional Swedish dairy producers [35]. The longevity-related decisions taken by dairy farmers are however complex to understand, and longevity is not usually visible in farm-management data. Even though the average herd longevity is highly dependent on the decisions taken by the individual farmer, farmers themselves have expressed a low level of consciousness of the power they have to influence the longevity in their herd [31]. These kinds of qualitative factors are difficult to capture in a questionnaire of the type used in this study, but they might have a significant influence on the longevity of dairy herds.

## Conclusions

The present questionnaire study identified only a few predictors that were associated with average longevity in Swedish dairy herds. This indicates that there might be other important factors that influence herd longevity and that more effort is needed to identify which herd-specific actions need to be taken by Swedish farmers to increase the productive life of dairy cows.

#### Authors' contributions

KA, AR and UE participated in the study and questionnaire design. AR and KA coordinated the distribution of questionnaires. IRD, UE and KA participated in the statistical analyses. All authors contributed to writing the manuscript. All authors read and approved the final manuscript.

#### Author details

[1] Department of Clinical Sciences, Swedish University of Agricultural Sciences, P.O. Box 7054, 75007 Uppsala, Sweden. [2] Department of Health Management, Atlantic Veterinary College, University of Prince Edward Island, Charlottetown, PEI C1A 4P3, Canada. [3] Växa Sverige, P.O. Box 1146, 63220 Eskilstuna, Sweden.

#### Acknowledgements

The authors acknowledge all farmers for their participation. The authors would also like to thank Hanna Bergeå, Sigrid Agenäs, Kjell Holtenius, and Nils Fall (Swedish University of Agricultural Sciences), Johan Waldner (Swedish Board of Agriculture), and Thure Bjerketorp and Anna-Lena Hegrestad (Växa Sverige) for valuable input and interesting discussions.

#### Competing interests

The authors declare that they have no competing interests.

**Funding**
This study was funded by the Swedish Farmers' Foundation for Agricultural Research.

**References**

1. Växa Sverige. Cattle statistics. 2017. http://www.vxa.se/fakta/styrning-och-rutiner/mer-om-mjolk. Accessed 28 Aug 2017.
2. Allaire FR, Gibson JP. Genetic value of herd life adjusted for milk production. J Dairy Sci. 1992. https://doi.org/10.3168/jds.S0022-0302(92)77886-2.
3. Pritchard T, Coffey M, Mrode R, Wall E. Understanding the genetics of survival in dairy cows. J Dairy Sci. 2013. https://doi.org/10.3168/jds.2012-6219.
4. Archer SC, Mc Coy F, Wapenaar W, Green MJ. Association between somatic cell count early in first lactation and the longevity of Irish dairy cows. J Dairy Sci. 2013. https://doi.org/10.3168/jds.2012-6115.
5. Boulton AC, Rushton J, Wathes DC. An empirical analysis of the cost of rearing dairy heifers from birth to first calving and the time taken to repay these costs. Animal. 2017. https://doi.org/10.1017/S1751731117000064.
6. Chamberlain T. Understanding the economics of dairy farming Part 1: income, costs and profit. Livestock. 2012. https://doi.org/10.111 1/j.2044-3870.2012.00137.x.
7. Brickell JS, Wathes DC. A descriptive study of the survival of Holstein-Friesian heifers through to third calving on English dairy farms. J Dairy Sci. 2011. https://doi.org/10.3168/jds.2010-3710.
8. Kelleher MM, Amer PR, Shalloo L, Evans RD, Byrne TJ, Buckley F, Berry DP. Development of an index to rank dairy females on expected lifetime profit. J Dairy Sci. 2015. https://doi.org/10.3168/jds.2014-9073.
9. Ettema J, Thomasen J, Hjorto L, Kargo M, Ostergaard S, Sorensen A. Economic opportunities for using sexed semen and semen of beef bulls in dairy herds. J Dairy Sci. 2017. https://doi.org/10.3168/jds.2016-11333.
10. VanRaden PM, Wiggans GR. Productive life evaluations: calculation, accuracy, and economic value. J Dairy Sci. 1995. https://doi.org/10.3168/jds.S0022-0302(95)76674-7.
11. Knapp JR, Laur GL, Vadas PA, Weiss WP, Tricarico JM. Invited review: enteric methane in dairy cattle production: quantifying the opportunities and impact of reducing emissions. J Dairy Sci. 2014. https://doi.org/10.3168/jds.2013-7234.
12. Weigel KA, Palmer RW, Caraviello DZ. Investigation of factors affecting voluntary and involuntary culling in expanding dairy herds in Wisconsin using survival analysis. J Dairy Sci. 2003. https://doi.org/10.3168/jds.S0022-0302(03)73733-3.
13. de Vries M, Bookers EAM, Dijkstra T, van Schaik G, de Boer IJM. Invited review: associations between variables of routine herd data and dairy cattle welfare indicators. J Dairy Sci. 2011. https://doi.org/10.3168/jds.2011-4169.
14. Alvåsen K, Roth A, Jansson Mörk M, Hallén Sandgren C, Thomsen PT, Emanuelson U. Farm characteristics related to on-farm cow mortality in dairy herds: a questionnaire study. Animal. 2014. https://doi.org/10.1017/S1751731114001633.
15. De Vries A. Cow longevity economics: The cost benefit of keeping the cow in the herd. In: Proc. of the cow longevity conference. 2013. http://www.milkproduction.com/Library/Editorial-articles/Cow-Longevity-Conference-2013—proceedings. Accessed 15 June 2016.
16. Rajala-Schultz PJ, Gröhn YT. Culling of dairy cows. Part II. Effects of diseases and reproductive performance on culling in Finnish Ayrshire cows. Prev Vet Med. 1999. https://doi.org/10.1016/S0167-5877(99)00045-8.
17. Rajala-Schultz PJ, Gröhn YT. Culling of dairy cows. Part III. Effects of diseases, pregnancy status and milk yield on culling in Finnish Ayrshire cows. Prev Vet Med. 1999. https://doi.org/10.1016/s0167-5877(99)00047-1.
18. Schneider MDP, Strandberg E, Emanuelson U, Grandinson K, Roth A. The effect of veterinary-treated clinical mastitis and pregnancy status on culling in Swedish dairy cows. Prev Vet Med. 2007. https://doi.org/10.1016/prevetmed.2007.02.006.
19. Pinedo PJ, De Vries A, Webb DW. Dynamics of culling risk with disposal codes reported by dairy herd improvement dairy herds. J Dairy Sci. 2010. https://doi.org/10.3168/jds.2009-2572.
20. Rajala-Schultz PJ, Gröhn YT. Culling of dairy cows. Part I. Effects of diseases on culling in Finnish Ayrshire cows. Prev Vet Med. 1999. https://doi.org/10.1016/S0167-5877(99)00046-X.
21. Strandberg E, Emanuelson U. Herd-level factors associated with longevity in Swedish dairy cattle. Acta Agric Scand. 2016. https://doi.org/10.1080/09064702.2016.1221986.
22. Textor J, Hardt J, Knüppel S. DAGitty: a graphical tool for analyzing causal diagrams. Epidemiology. 2011. https://doi.org/10.1097/EDE.0b013e318225c2be.
23. Rubin DB. Multiple imputation for nonresponse in surveys. Jersey: Wiley; 1987.
24. Dohoo IR, Nielsen CR, Emanuelson U. Multiple imputation in veterinary epidemiological studies: a case study and simulation. Prev Vet Med. 2016. https://doi.org/10.1016/j.prevetmed.2016.04.003.
25. Kudahl AB, Nielsen SS, Østergaard S. Strategies for time of culling in control of paratuberculosis in dairy herds. J Dairy Sci. 2011. https://doi.org/10.3168/jds.2010-3933.
26. Nicholas RAJ, Fox LK, Lysnyansky I. Mycoplasma mastitis in cattle: To cull or not to cull. Vet J. 2016. https://doi.org/10.1016/j.tvjl.2016.08.001.
27. Svensson C, Alvåsen K, Eldh AC, Frössling J, Lomander H. Veterinary herd health management—experience among farmers and farm managers in Swedish dairy production. Prev Vet Med. 2018. https://doi.org/10.1016/j.prevetmed.2018.04.012.
28. Kaler J, Green LE. Sheep farmer opinions on the current and future role of veterinarians in flock health management on sheep farms: a qualitative study. Prev Vet Med. 2013. https://doi.org/10.1016/j.prevetmed.2013.09.009.
29. Duval JE, Bareille N, Fourichon C, Madouasse A, Vaarst M. Perceptions of French private veterinary practitioners' on their role in organic dairy farms and opportunities to improve their advisory services for organic dairy farmers. Prev Vet Med. 2016. https://doi.org/10.1016/j.prevetmed.2016.09.008.
30. Ruston A, Shortall O, Green M, Brennan M, Wapenaar W, Kaler J. Challenges facing the farm animal veterinary profession in England: a qualitative study of veterinarians' perceptions and responses. Prev Vet Med. 2016. https://doi.org/10.1016/j.prevetmed.2016.03.008.
31. Bergeå H, Roth A, Emanuelson U, Agenäs S. Farmer awareness of cow longevity and implications for decision-making at farm level. Acta Agric Scand. 2016. https://doi.org/10.1080/09064702.2016.1196726.
32. De Vries A. Economic trade-offs between genetic improvement and longevity in dairy cattle. J Dairy Sci. 2017. https://doi.org/10.3168/jds.2016-11847.
33. Fetrow J, Nordlund KV, Norman HD. Invited review: culling: nomenclature, definitions, and recommendations. J Dairy Sci. 2006. https://doi.org/10.3168/jds.S0022-0302(06)72257-3.
34. Beaudeau F, Seegers H, Ducrocq V, Fourichon C, Bareille N. Effect of health disorders on culling in dairy cows: a review and a critical discussion. Ann Zootech. 2000. https://doi.org/10.1051/animres:2000102.
35. Ahlman T, Ljung M, Rydhmer L, Röcklinsberg H, Strandberg E, Wallenbeck A. Differences in preferences for breeding traits between organic and conventional dairy producers in Sweden. Livest Sci. 2014. https://doi.org/10.1016/j.livsci.2013.12.014.

# 20

# Sperm quality in frozen beef and dairy bull semen

Jane Margaret Morrell[1*], Andra Sabina Valeanu[1,2], Nils Lundeheim[3] and Anders Johannisson[1]

**Abstract**

**Background:** There is speculation that beef bull semen quality is inferior to that of dairy bulls although few scientific studies are available in the literature. The aim of this study was to evaluate sperm quality in beef bull semen and to determine which parameters could be indicative of fertility after insemination. Sperm quality, assessed by computer assisted sperm motility analysis and flow cytometric evaluation of membrane integrity, levels of reactive oxygen species, mitochondrial membrane potential, acrosome status and DNA fragmentation index, was evaluated in beef and dairy bull semen.

**Results:** For beef bulls, normal morphology ($r = 0.62$, $P < 0.05$) and WOBBLE ($r = 0.57$, $P < 0.05$) were significantly correlated with 56-day non-return rate, whereas sperm quality was not significantly correlated with the fertility index score for dairy bulls. Membrane integrity ($46 \pm 8.0\%$ versus $40 \pm 11\%$, $P < 0.05$), normal morphology ($87 \pm 6\%$ versus $76 \pm 8\%$; $P < 0.05$), and high respiratory activity ($52 \pm 13$ versus $12 \pm 4\%$; $P < 0.001$) were higher for dairy bulls than for beef bulls. The DNA fragmentation index was lower for dairy bull spermatozoa than beef ($3.8 \pm 1.1\%$ versus $6.1 \pm 2.9\%$; $P < 0.01$), whereas some sperm kinematics were higher. Multivariate analysis indicated that type of bull (beef versus dairy) had an impact on sperm quality.

**Conclusions:** Different assays of sperm quality may be needed for appropriate analysis of beef and dairy bull semen. These finding could be important for cattle breeding stations when evaluating semen quality.

**Keywords:** Chromatin integrity, Membrane integrity, Mitochondrial membrane potential, Motility, Reactive oxygen species

## Background

Artificial insemination (AI) is one of the most effective tools available to dairy cattle producers to improve herd productivity and profitability [1]. Whereas more than 80% of dairy cows are artificially inseminated in e.g. North America or Europe, less than 5% of beef cows are bred by this method [1, 2]. The main reasons for this difference are that beef cows are managed under more extensive husbandry conditions than dairy cows, which makes oestrus detection problematic, and they may not be accustomed to being handled. Seasonal differences in fertility may occur and oestrus signs may not be as obvious as in dairy breeds; some of these issues may be overcome by hormonal manipulation of ovulation [3]. However, there is also speculation that beef bull semen quality is inferior to that of dairy bulls [4], although few scientific studies have been reported in the literature. Fertility is believed to vary up to 20% among bulls classified as having a satisfactory breeding soundness evaluation [5].

Although the market for beef bull semen for inseminating beef cows is generally stable, it is increasing in countries such as Brazil, where sales of beef semen have risen from approximately 3 million to nearly 12 million in less than 20 years [6]. Therefore, there is considerable potential to increase the use of AI in beef breeds in other countries. There is also a market for inseminating dairy heifers with beef bull semen to produce a crossbred calf with better beef-producing qualities than a purebred dairy calf, and an increasing interest in using sexed semen in

*Correspondence: jane.morrell@slu.se
[1] Division of Reproduction, Department of Clinical Sciences, Faculty of Veterinary Medicine and Animal Science, Swedish University of Agricultural Sciences (SLU), 75007 Uppsala, Sweden

beef cattle [7]. Thus, quality evaluation of beef bull semen is important. The aim of the present study was to make a retrospective analysis of sperm quality in commercial doses of frozen beef bull semen and to identify some parameters of sperm quality that could be used as indicators of potential fertility. A further aim was to identify where potential differences in sperm quality occur between beef and dairy bull semen.

## Methods

### Semen

Commercial straws of frozen semen from 14 beef bulls (6 Limousin, 3 Charolais, 2 Simmental, 2 Hereford, 1 Angus) frozen in Triladyl extender (Minitüb, Tiefenbach, Germany) were available from the Estonian Animal Breeders Association, Rapla, Estonia. Semen from 19 dairy bulls (10 Swedish Red and 9 Holstein) and 4 beef bulls (2 Limousin, 1 Charolais and 1 Blonde D'Aquitaine) frozen in Andromed (Minitüb) was supplied by Viking-Genetics, Skara, Sweden. The straws were thawed in a water bath at 37 °C for 12 s.

### Sperm concentration

A Nucleocounter SP-100 (Chemometec) was used to measure sperm concentration. Aliquots (50 μL) of frozen-thawed semen were diluted with 5 mL S100 reagent to permeabilise the sperm membranes and a cassette containing propidium iodide (PI) was loaded with the mixture. The cassette was inserted into the fluorescence reader, which displayed the sperm concentration after approximately 30 s.

### Sperm morphology assessment

Wet smears were air dried and stained with carbolfuchsin-eosin, [8] for evaluation of five hundred spermatozoa at 1000× magnification under oil immersion. Additionally, sperm head morphology of 200 spermatozoa was assessed at 1000× magnification using aliquots of semen fixed in formol-saline. The sperm morphology assessment was carried out by skilled personnel at the Swedish Sperm Reference Laboratory, Swedish University of Agricultural Sciences (SLU). The proportions of morphological abnormalities such as proximal cytoplasmic droplets, acrosome defects, detached heads, nuclear pouches and tail defects were calculated. Normal morphology was calculated as 100 − % spermatozoa with abnormal morphology.

### Computer assisted semen analysis (CASA)

Sperm kinematics were assessed objectively using a CASA system, consisting of a phase-contrast Olympus BX 51 microscope (Olympus, Japan) connected to the SpermVision™ (Minitüb, Tiefenbach, Germany). An aliquot (5 μL) of semen was deposited on a warmed microscope slide at 38 °C and covered with a coverslip (18 × 18 mm). Sperm images in 8 fields were digitized for analysis of the kinematic patterns using the SpermVision™ software. The mean values were calculated for each of the following parameters based on approximately 1000 spermatozoa [9]: total motility (TM%), progressive motility (PM %), VCL (velocity curved line, μm/s), VSL (velocity straight line, μm/s), VAP (velocity average path, μm/s), ALH (amplitude of lateral head displacement, μm), BCF (beat cross frequency, Hz) and the ratios STR (straightness, VSL/VAP), LIN (linearity, VSL/VCL), and WOB (wobble, VAP/VCL).

### Plasma membrane integrity

Membrane integrity was analysed by flow cytometry after SYBR14-PI staining [10]. Aliquots of thawed semen were extended to a concentration of approximately $2 \times 10^6$ spermatozoa/mL for staining with the Live-Dead Sperm Viability KIT L-7011 (Invitrogen). An aliquot (300 μL) of the sperm suspension was stained with 0.6 μL SYBR14 (final stain concentration 0.02 μM) and 3 μL PI (final stain concentration 12 μM), and incubated for 10 min at 38 °C. The stained samples were evaluated using a BD LSR flow cytometer (Beckon Dickinson, San José, CA, USA), the excitation being induced by an argon-ion laser (488 nm). Green fluorescence was detected with a FL 1 band-pass filter (530/30 nm) while red fluorescence was measured using a FL 3 long-pass filter (> 670 nm). A total of 50,000 sperm-specific events was evaluated and classified as membrane intact (SYBR14 positive; live), membrane damaged (dying: SYBR14 positive, PI positive; dead: SYBR14 negative, PI positive).

### Reactive oxygen species (ROS)

Reactive oxygen species were determined using a modification of the protocol described by Guthrie and Welch [11], in which the spermatozoa were stained with hydroethidine (HE; Molecular Probes, Inc.), 2′,7′-dichlorodihydrofluorescein diacetate (DCFDA; Molecular Probes, Inc.) and Hoechst 33258 (HO). The ROS superoxide (SO·) and hydrogen peroxide ($H_2O_2$) were determined using HE and DCFDA, respectively, while HO was added to enable live and dead cells to be differentiated.

After adjusting the sperm concentration to approximately $2 \times 10^6$ spermatozoa/mL, the spermatozoa were stained as follows: two aliquots (300 μL) of each sample were stained with 9 μL of HO (40 μM), 9 μL HE (40 μM) and 9 μL DCFDA, (2 mM). In addition, 3 μL Menadione (MEN, 20 mM) were added to one of the aliquots to stimulate ROS production. After mixing gently, the samples were incubated at 38 °C for 30 min.

The analysis was carried out using the BD LSR flow cytometer (Beckon Dickinson, San José, CA, USA). Excitation was achieved with an argon-ion laser (488 nm) and a HeCd laser (325 nm); green fluorescence was detected with a FL1 band pass filter (530/30 nm), red fluorescence with a FL3 long pass filter (>670 nm) and blue fluorescence with a FL4 band pass filter (510/20 nm). In total, 30,000 sperm-specific events were evaluated and classified as the proportions of: Live, Superoxide negative; Live, Superoxide positive; Dead superoxide positive; Live, $H_2O_2$ negative; Live, $H_2O_2$ positive; Dead, $H_2O_2$ negative; Dead, $H_2O_2$ positive (%).

### Mitochondrial membrane status

Aliquots of semen (300 μL) at a sperm concentration of approximately $2.5 \times 10^6$/mL, were mixed with 1.2 μL 5,5′,6,6′-tetrachloro-1,1′,3,3′-tetraethylbenzimidazolylcarbocyanineiodide (JC-1) (stock 3 mM) and incubated for 40 min at 38 °C as described by Garner and Thomas [12]. The JC-1 fluorescence was measured in the FL1 (530/30 nm) and FL2 (585 nm) channels of the flow cytometer. In total, 10,000 cells were evaluated and classified in two categories: high respiratory activity (orange fluorescence) and low respiratory activity (green fluorescence).

### Sperm chromatin structure assay

Chromatin integrity was evaluated using the metachromatic dye acridine orange (AO). The DNA fragmentation index (%DFI) was expressed as the proportion of cells with denatured, single stranded DNA (red fluorescence) out of the total population (stable, double stranded DNA [green fluorescence] + single stranded DNA). An aliquot (20 μL) of thawed semen was mixed 1:1 (v/v) with TNE buffer, snap-frozen in liquid nitrogen and stored at −80 °C. For analysis, samples were thawed on ice, and an aliquot (10 μL) was mixed with 90 μL of TNE followed by 200 μL of acid-detergent solution. After 30 s, AO (600 μL) was added and the sample was analyzed within 3–5 min using a FACStar Plus Flow cytometer with settings and software as described previously by Morrell et al. [13].

### Acrosome status

Sperm acrosome status and cell viability were assessed using fluorescein isothiocyanate-PNA (FITC-PNA) labeling and PI, respectively. An aliquot (300 μL) of semen, previously diluted to a sperm concentration of $2 \times 10^6$/mL, was mixed with 3 μL of FITC-PNA (previously diluted tenfold with buffer enriched with 10 mM Calcium and Magnesium) and 3 μL of PI, and was incubated at 38 °C for 10 min [14, 15]. The fluorescence from 50,000 sperm-events was recorded after gating out the non-sperm events. PI was detected using the FL 3 long-pass filter (>670 nm), while FITC-PNA fluorescence was detected at 515–545 nm in the FL1. The sperm subpopulations were categorized as live acrosome reacted, dead acrosome damaged, live non-reacted acrosome and dead non-reacted acrosome (%).

### Fertility

The 56-day non-return rate after first insemination in 130 to > 1000 cows was available for the beef bulls. For the 19 dairy bulls, a fertility index score was provided for inseminations in > 1000 cows, which had been calculated by adjusting the non-return rate to account for factors such as the age and parity of the female, farm location, inseminator etc.

### Statistical analysis

The statistical analyses were performed using the SAS software (ver. 9.3; SAS Inst.). To evaluate the difference between the two groups of bulls, analysis of variance (PROC GLM) was applied, using a statistical model including the effect of breed. The relationships between sperm quality and fertility (either the 56-day non-return rate or the fertility index score) were analysed within bull type (beef or dairy) using Spearman rank correlation. Only bulls with more than 130 cows were included in the correlation analysis. In all cases, $P < 0.05$ was considered to be significant.

To investigate the interaction of extender and type of semen i.e. beef or dairy bull semen, multivariate analysis was performed with Partial Least Squares Regression (PLS) using Simca software (version 14; MKS Data Analytics Solutions, Umeå, Sweden), as described on the website http://onlinelibrary.wiley.com/doi/10.1002/cem.1006/full.

## Results

### Sperm concentration

The mean concentration (±SD) was $88 \pm 20 \times 10^6$/mL and $55 \pm 19 \times 10^6$/mL for beef and dairy bull semen, respectively ($P < 0.001$).

### Sperm morphology

Normal morphology for beef and dairy bulls was 76 ± 8% and 87 ± 6%, respectively ($P < 0.05$).

### CASA kinematics

Except for total motility, progressive motility and BCF, the sperm kinematics were significantly different for the two types of semen (Table 1). Most kinematics were higher for dairy bull spermatozoa than for beef bull

**Table 1 Sperm motility parameters (mean ± SD) measured by computer assisted sperm analysis in semen from beef to dairy bulls (n = 37)**

| Parameters | Beef (n = 17) | Dairy (n = 20) | Significance |
|---|---|---|---|
| Motility (%) | 64 ± 14 | 59 ± 14 | NS |
| Progressive motility (%) | 58 ± 13 | 55.6 ± 14 | NS |
| Hyperactivity (%) | 6 ± 3 | 11 ± 5 | P < 0.01 |
| VAP (μm/s) | 52 ± 4 | 65 ± 8 | P < 0.001 |
| VCL (μm/s) | 87 ± 8 | 128 ± 18 | P < 0.001 |
| VSL (μm/s) | 39 ± 3 | 45 ± 7 | P < 0.01 |
| STR | 0.75 ± 0.03 | 0.70 ± 0.05 | P < 0.001 |
| LIN | 0.44 ± 0.02 | 0.35 ± 0.04 | P < 0.001 |
| WOB | 0.59 ± 0.01 | 0.50 ± 0.03 | P < 0.001 |
| ALH (μm) | 4.1 ± 0.6 | 4.98 ± 0.5 | P < 0.001 |
| BCF (Hz) | 23 ± 1.4 | 22 ± 2.5 | NS |

*NS* not significant (P > 0.05)

spermatozoa, with the exception of STR, LIN and WOB which were higher for beef than for dairy.

### Membrane integrity

Beef bull semen contained a lower proportion of membrane intact spermatozoa (Table 2) than dairy bull semen (40 ± 11% versus 46 ± 8%, respectively; P = 0.053).

### Oxidative stress

In both control samples and samples stimulated with menadione (Table 3), there was a significant difference (P < 0.001) between dairy and beef bulls in live superoxide negative and live superoxide positive spermatozoa (P < 0.001). Additionally, in the samples not stimulated with menadione, there was a trend towards significance (P < 0.08) for dead $H_2O_2$ negative sperm cells between the two types of bulls, although no significant differences were observed for the other categories of ROS. In samples stimulated with menadione, trends towards significance were seen for live $H_2O_2$ positive spermatozoa (P < 0.055) and dead, $H_2O_2$ negative spermatozoa (P < 0.066) between the two types of bulls.

**Table 2 Living, dying, dead sperm cells, %DFI, acrosome status, and mitochondrial membrane potential in frozen-thawed AI doses (mean ± SD) from beef to dairy bulls (n = 37)**

| Parameter | Beef (n = 17) | Dairy (n = 20) | Significance |
|---|---|---|---|
| Living (%) | 40 ± 11 | 46 ± 8 | Trend P = 0.053 |
| Dying (%) | 6 ± 3 | 5 ± 3 | NS |
| Dead (%) | 55 ± 14 | 49 ± 8 | NS |
| % DFI | 6 ± 3 | 4 ± 1 | P < 0.01 |
| Live not acrosome reacted (%) | 59 ± 12 | 52 ± 8 | P < 0.05 |
| Dead not acrosome reacted (%) | 18 ± 12 | 32 ± 8 | P < 0.001 |
| Live acrosome reacted (%) | 0.3 ± 0.3 | 0.3 ± 0.2 | NS |
| Dead damaged (%) | 21 ± 11 | 17 ± 10 | P < 0.001 |
| High respiratory activity (%) | 36 ± 10 | 58 ± 12 | P < 0.001 |
| Low respiratory activity (%) | 64 ± 10 | 42 ± 12 | P < 0.001 |

*NS* not significant (P > 0.05)

**Table 3 ROS-production (mean ± SD) in beef and dairy bull semen (n = 17 and 20 respectively)**

| ROS category | Beef | Dairy | Beef + MEN | Dairy + MEN |
|---|---|---|---|---|
| Live superoxide negative (%) | 57 ± 18$^a$ | 35 ± 14$^a$ | 62 ± 23$^b$ | 37 ± 12$^b$ |
| Live superoxide positive (%) | 8 ± 3$^a$ | 25 ± 7$^a$ | 6 ± 6$^b$ | 24 ± 10$^b$ |
| Dead superoxide positive (%) | 36 ± 17 | 40 ± 11 | 32 ± 20 | 39 ± 9 |
| Live hydrogen peroxide negative (%) | 61 ± 23 | 61 ± 11 | 68 ± 20 | 62 ± 9 |
| Live hydrogen peroxide positive (%) | 4 ± 14 | 0.2 ± 0.3 | 0.6 ± 1.2* | 0.1 ± 0.1* |
| Dead hydrogen peroxide negative (%) | 31 ± 16* | 39 ± 11* | 30 ± 19* | 39 ± 9* |
| Dead hydrogen peroxide positive (%) | 4 ± 11 | 0.08 ± 0.2 | 1.2 ± 2.9 | 0.05 ± 0.08 |

Same superscripts within a row indicate significant difference (P < 0.001)

*MEN* menadione

* Denotes trend towards significance: for live hydrogen peroxide positive with menadione P < 0.055; for dead hydrogen peroxide negative P < 0.08; for dead hydrogen peroxide negative with menadione P < 0.066

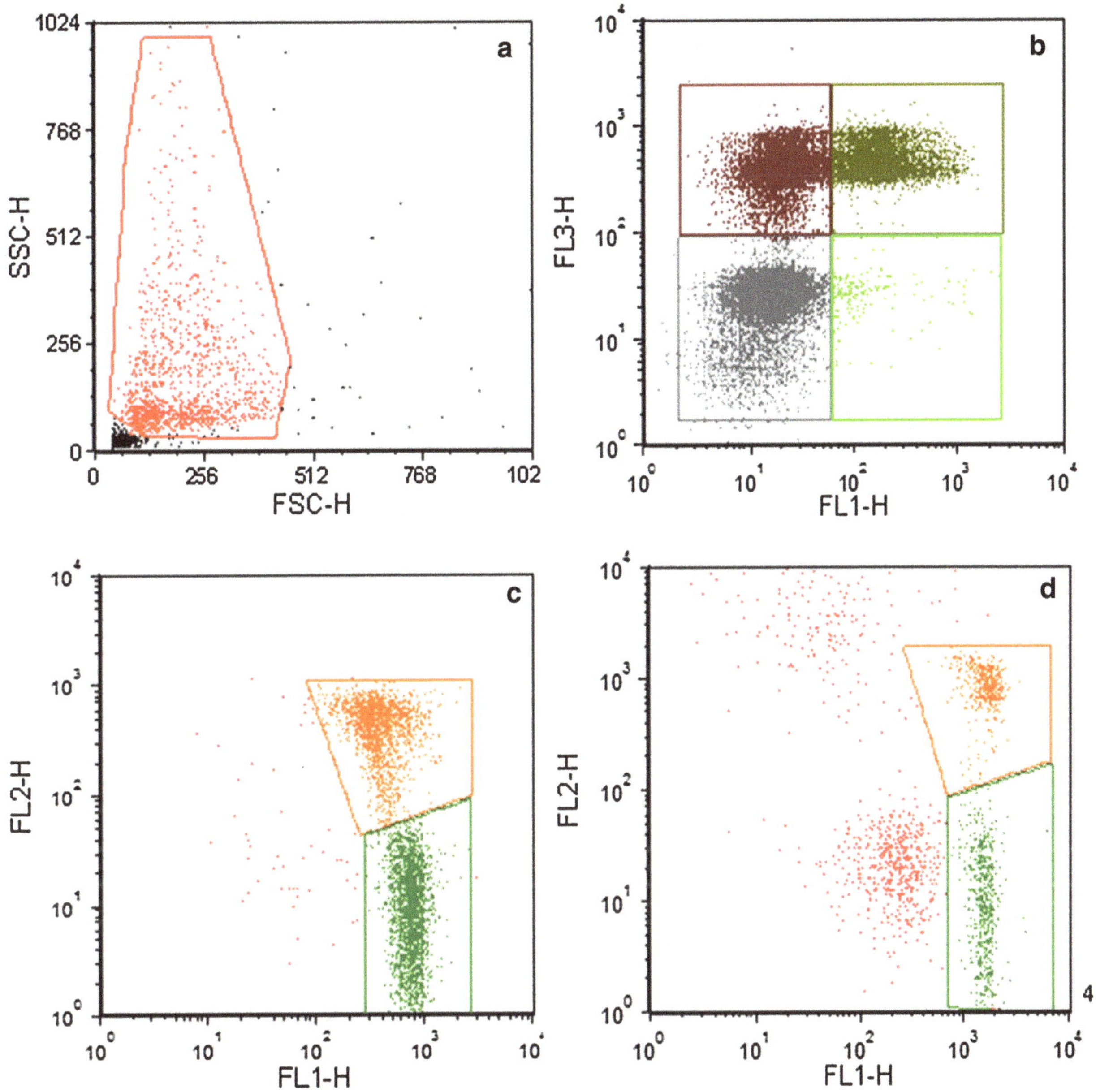


**Fig. 1** Flow cytometry data: **a** FSC-SSC pattern obtained as well as the gate used to select spermatozoa for further analysis steps; **b** shows the regions of analysis used in the acrosome status assay. Lower right: live, reacted, green; Upper right: dead damaged, olive; Lower left: live, non-reacted, grey; Upper left: dead, non-reacted, dark red; **c**, **d** results from analysis of mitochondrial membrane status of spermatozoa from a dairy bull and a beef bull, respectively. Indicated are the regions of analysis for spermatozoa with high MMP (orange) and low MMP (green). Events inside the gate for spermatozoa, but outside the regions of analysis, are shown in red

### Acrosome integrity

The FSC-SSC pattern obtained and the regions of analysis used in the assay for acrosome status are shown in Fig. 1a, b, respectively. There were significant differences (Table 2) in the proportions of live acrosome intact ($59 \pm 12$ versus $52 \pm 8$; $P < 0.05$), dead acrosome intact ($18 \pm 12$ versus $32 \pm 8$; $P < 0.001$), and dead acrosome damaged sperm cells between beef and dairy semen ($21 \pm 11$ versus $17 \pm 10\%$; $P < 0.001$).

### Mitochondrial potential

Figure 1c, d show the FSC-SSC pattern obtained with JC-1 staining of dairy and beef bulls, respectively, as well as the gate used to select spermatozoa for further analysis steps. For beef bulls, the proportion of sperm with high respiratory activity (Table 2) was 36 ± 10%, significantly lower ($P < 0.001$) than for dairy bulls (52 ± 12%). The proportion of sperm with low respiratory activity was higher for beef bulls than dairy bulls (64 ± 10% versus 42 ± 12%; $P < 0.001$).

### Sperm chromatin structure assay

The %DFI was significantly higher ($P < 0.01$) for beef bulls (6.1 ± 2.9) than for dairy bulls (3.8 ± 1.1).

### Correlations of sperm quality with fertility

For beef bulls, the kinematic WOBBLE (Fig. 2a) was significantly correlated with 56-day non-return rate ($r = 0.59$, $P < 0.05$), as was normal morphology (Fig. 2b; $r = 0.517$, $P = 0.059$). In addition, there were negative relationships between live superoxide-negative spermatozoa and 56-day non-return rate ($r = -0.63$, $P < 0.05$, Fig. 2c), and between live hydrogen peroxide-negative spermatozoa and 56-day non-return rate ($r = -0.62$, $P < 0.05$; Fig. 2d). In contrast, for dairy bulls there were no significant relationships between fertility index and sperm quality.

### Multivariate analysis

The PLS scatter plot showing the distribution of the individual bulls according to type (beef or dairy) and extender is shown in Fig. 3. The values for beef bulls clustered on the right side of the scatter plot, irrespective of extender, whereas those for dairy bulls clustered on the left. The PLS loading plot of the variables obtained by analysing type of bull (beef versus dairy) against all other variables (Fig. 4) showed that normal morphology, mitochondrial membrane potential, live reacted acrosomes, and the kinematics VCL, VSL, VAP and ALH clustered together with dairy bull semen and Andromed extender. In contrast, %DFI, categories of hydrogen peroxide producing spermatozoa, Linearity and Wobble, and dead reacted

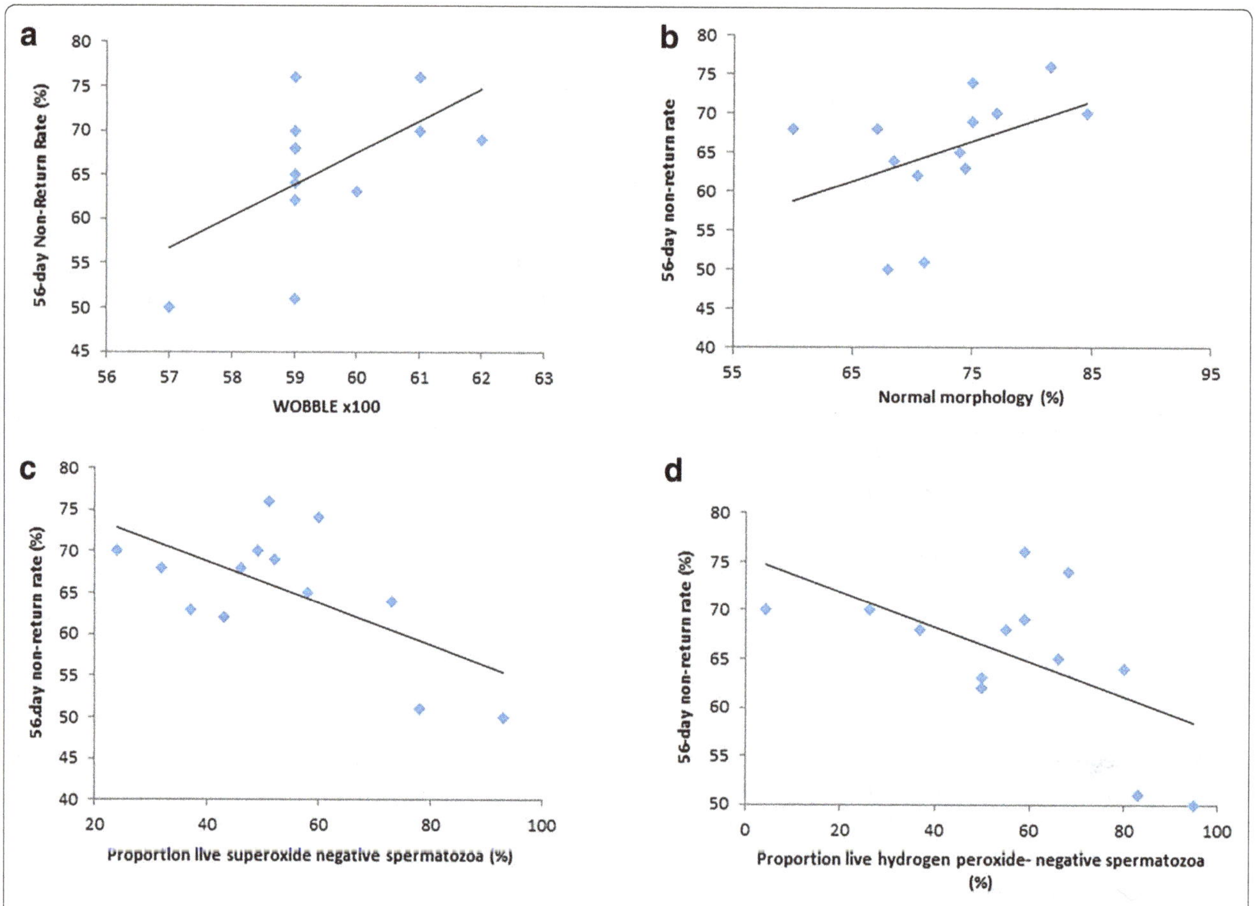


**Fig. 2** Relationship between various sperm characteristics and 56-day non-return rate for beef bulls (n = 13). **a** WOBBLE; **b** normal morphology; **c** live superoxide negative; **d** live hydrogen peroxide negative

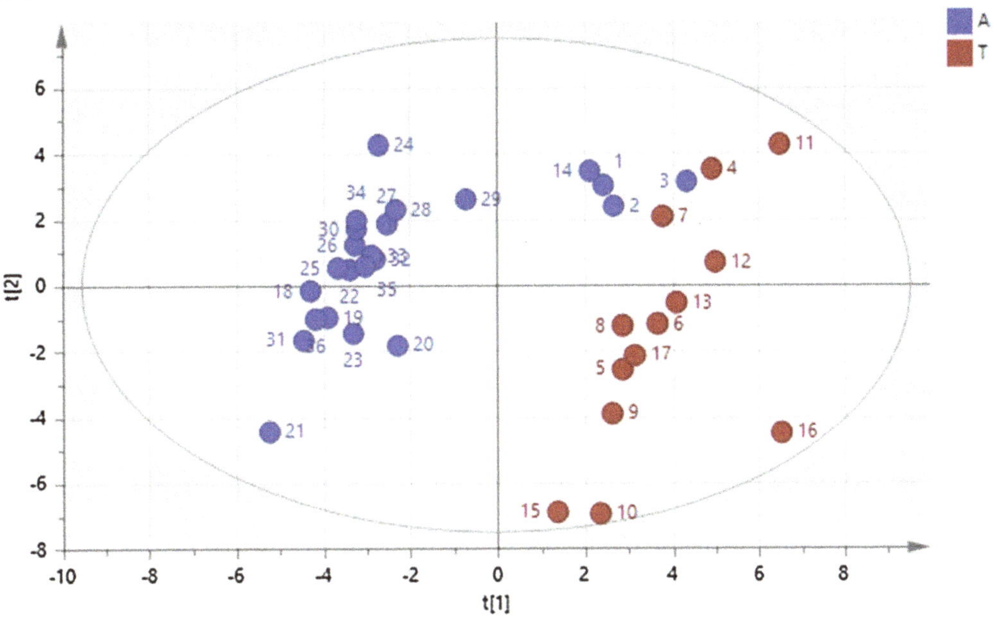


**Fig. 3** Scatter plot of beef and dairy bulls according to sperm quality (n = 37)

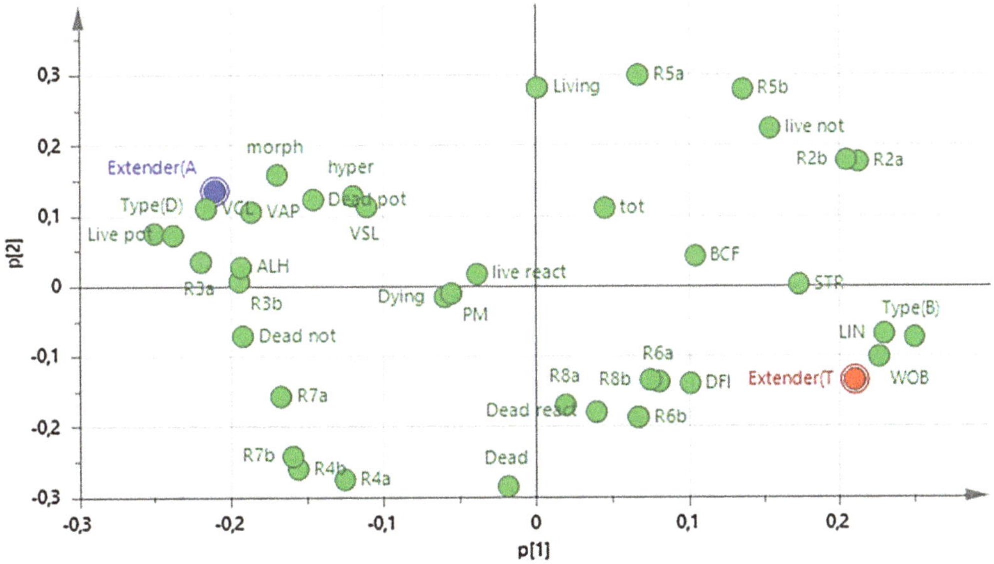


**Fig. 4** Partial Least Squares loading plot showing the relationship of breed to the various parameters of sperm quality. Type B and D refer to beef and dairy bulls respectively, Extender A and T refer to Andromed and Triladyl, respectively; *morph* morphology, *living, dead and dying* refer to membrane integrity, *hyper* hypermotility, *VCL* curvilinear velocity, *VSL* straight line velocity, *VAP* velocity of the average path, *STR* straightness, *LIN* linearity, *WOB* wobble, *ALH* amplitude of lateral head deviation, *BCF* beat cross frequency; high and low potential: high and low mitochondrial membrane potential; *live react, dead react, live not and dead not* acrosome status (acrosome reacted or not reacted) in relation to viability, *R2* live superoxide negative, *R3* live superoxide positive, *R4* dead superoxide positive, *R5* live hydrogen peroxide negative, *R6* live hydrogen peroxide positive, *R7* dead hydrogen peroxide negative, *R8* dead hydrogen peroxide positive; a or b in connection with R2-R8 refer to non-stimulated and stimulated with menadione, respectively

acrosomes clustered together with beef bull semen and Triladyl. The clusters appeared in opposite quadrants on the plot (top left for variables associated with dairy bulls and bottom right for those associated with beef bulls), indicating that they are different.

## Discussion

In this study, some interesting relationships between sperm quality and pregnancy rates were observed, not the least the fact that sperm motility (the most widely-used assessment of sperm quality) was not significantly related to pregnancy rate for these bulls. Significant differences in sperm quality between the two types of bulls were seen, as were correlations between sperm quality and pregnancy rate for beef bulls (namely WOBBLE and normal morphology), whereas there were no links between sperm quality parameters and fertility for the dairy bulls. There were significant differences between sperm motility patterns in semen from beef and dairy bulls; however, the semen was frozen in different extenders on the two commercial cattle stations, which could have affected the assessment of kinematics. Multivariate analysis showed that the sperm quality of beef bull semen frozen in Andromed was more similar to that of beef bull semen frozen in Triladyl than to sperm quality of dairy bull semen frozen in Andromed. Therefore, we deduce that type of bull semen (beef versus dairy) has more effect on sperm quality than the extender itself (or differences in the semen handling and freezing protocols on the two commercial semen stations), and therefore it is justifiable to combine the data for all of the beef bulls in this study, regardless of extender.

The sperm concentration in the straws was different for beef and dairy semen. However, this should not have affected the motility analysis since the sperm concentration was not too high to be analysed by the CASA instrument. Sperm concentration was adjusted to the same levels in all samples for staining in the flow cytometric analyses. However, sperm concentration could be important depending on the type of abnormality that is present. So-called compensable abnormalities are ones that impede the ability of the spermatozoa to reach the oviducts or to interact with the oocyte [16]; increasing the sperm concentration improves the chances of conception by increasing the number of normal spermatozoa that are present until the required threshold for conception is reached. Although originally described for some morphological defects [17], the idea of other sperm characteristics being compensable has gained ground e.g. membrane integrity, mitochondrial membrane potential, whereas sperm chromatin damage, protamine status etc. are considered to be non-compensable [16], because increasing the number of spermatozoa inseminated does not increase the chances of pregnancy.

According to a study in fresh bull semen [18], high sperm concentration may cause an increase in oxidative stress, with negative effects on cell viability. Superoxide production was significantly less in the semen from beef bulls than from dairy bulls but the extenders used may contain differing amounts of antioxidants, which would remove these ROS. It was proposed that ROS damage sperm DNA, at least in human patients with oligoasthenozoospermia [19], but this may not be the case in semen from normal bulls, especially where extenders containing antioxidants are used. In the beef bulls in the present study, there was a negative relationship between live spermatozoa with no superoxide or hydrogen peroxide production and fertility. These results indicate that lack of ROS-production could indicate low metabolic activity in these thawed spermatozoa, and that sperm cells with low metabolism did not result in pregnancies.

Reactive oxygen species are believed to cause decreased motility, decreased viability, and a number of morphological defects, particularly in the mid-piece. Although viability was superior in the dairy bulls in the present study, no significant differences were observed in total and progressive motility between breed types. These results are in contrast to those obtained by Fiaz et al. [20], who observed significantly higher total mobility ($P < 0.05$) in dairy bulls compared with beef ones. There were significant differences in all velocity kinematics in our study, being higher in spermatozoa from dairy bulls although they showed lower linearity ($P < 0.001$) than spermatozoa from beef bulls. In contrast, beef bull spermatozoa showed a higher beat cross-frequency and lower amplitude of lateral head displacement than dairy bull spermatozoa. Our results are in contrast to those of Hoflack et al. [21], who reported that Holstein bull spermatozoa showed superior total motility, progressive motility and linearity than spermatozoa from Belgian Blue bulls. However, as previously stated, the extenders used for dairy and beef bull semen were different (Andromed and Triladyl, respectively), which may have had an impact on sperm motility assessment. Zhang et al. [22] suggested that an improvement of boar sperm motility in extender containing soybean milk could be due to the lower viscosity and less debris compared to egg yolk.

A comparative study on AndroMed®, Bioxcell® and Triladyl® extender for cryopreservation of bull semen [23] showed that total and progressive motility were better in the ejaculates processed with Andromed, compared to those processed with Triladyl or Bioxcell. For sperm viability, however, significantly better results were obtained using Triladyl compared to Andromed and Bioxcell. In contrast, mitochondrial membrane potential and the DNA fragmentation index are improved in the soy-based extender compared to the milk-based extender during liquid storage [24]. According to the study that we conducted, both DNA fragmentation and low mitochondrial membrane potential were significantly higher for beef bull spermatozoa (extended with Triladyl) than for dairy bull spermatozoa (in Andromed).

The effect of bull type on other sperm quality parameters such as sperm morphology, may be explained by breed differences in adaptability to environmental conditions [25] and scrotal circumference. Studies showed a significant positive correlation ($P < 0.05$) between primary morphological defects and sperm DNA fragmentation in Holstein-Frisian bulls [26], although such a relationship was not seen in our study (data not shown). However, in the present study, dairy bull spermatozoa showed fewer primary morphological defects than beef bulls, and a statistically significant difference ($P < 0.01$) was observed between breeds for the proportion of sperm cells with fragmented DNA. These results correspond with other studies where lower sperm DNA fragmentation was found in dairy breeds than beef breeds [27]. Damage to sperm DNA does not impede oocyte fertilization or completion of early stages of cleavage but may block blastocyst formation by inducing an apoptosis-like phenomenon [28]. Sperm DNA lesions have been correlated with deficiencies in embryonic development [29, 30]. The significant differences between dairy and beef bulls for plasma membrane integrity, acrosomal integrity and mitochondrial function could indicate potentially higher fertility for the dairy semen since these parameters were found to be related to pregnancy rate in Nellore cows [31], although they were not correlated with higher fertility index score in our study.

Interestingly, multivariate analysis indicated that the type of bull (beef or dairy) had more of an effect on sperm quality than the extender. Since different extenders were used on the two commercial semen stations, the variable "extender" could also reflect differences in sperm handling procedures or freezing protocols. However, regardless of such potential sources of variation, beef bulls clustered together rather than clustering according to extender.

The observed differences in sperm quality between beef and dairy breeds may be due in part to intensive selection among dairy sires both in terms of production traits in their offspring and in sperm quality. The relationships between sperm quality and pregnancy rate for the beef bulls are interesting and warrant further study with a larger number of bulls. It would also be interesting to study possible breed differences among beef breeds, especially since a breed effect has been observed in dairy bulls [32]. The lack of significant correlations between sperm quality parameters and the dairy bull fertility index may be due to the use of an adjusted score instead of the unadjusted 56-day non-return rate, or to the relatively similar values in fertility index score for these bulls. It would be interesting to include bulls with higher and lower fertility scores than the ones used here. Unfortunately, it was only possible to use retrospective non-return data to look for associations with various parameters of sperm quality; thus, no account is taken of differences in female factors or herd management [33], which are likely to be different between dairy and beef cows. Nevertheless, the findings presented here are of interest in the context of the questions posed, namely whether some parameters of sperm quality could be identified that might be useful as indicators of fertility for beef bulls, and whether different parameters are needed for beef bull semen than for dairy bull semen.

## Conclusions

Significant relationships were seen between normal morphology and the 56-day non-return rate for beef bulls, and also for WOBBLE and the 56-day non-return rate, although no correlations were found between sperm quality and the fertility index score for dairy bulls. There were some differences in sperm quality between dairy and beef bulls. Multivariate analysis indicated that type of bull (beef versus dairy) had more effect on sperm quality than the extender used. Thus, different parameters of sperm quality may be needed as indicators of fertility for the two types of bull. These finding could be important for cattle breeding stations when evaluating semen quality.

#### Authors' contributions

JMM organized the collection of material, data analysis, and critically revised the manuscript; SV helped with the laboratory analysis and wrote the first draft of the manuscript; AJ ran the flow cytometric analyses; NL did the statistical analysis; all authors approved the submission of the manuscript. All authors read and approved the final manuscript.


#### Author details

[1] Division of Reproduction, Department of Clinical Sciences, Faculty of Veterinary Medicine and Animal Science, Swedish University of Agricultural Sciences (SLU), 75007 Uppsala, Sweden. [2] University of Agricultural Sciences and Veterinary Medicine Iaşi, 3, Mihail Sadoveanu Alley, 700490 Iaşi, Romania. [3] Department of Animal Breeding and Genetics, Faculty of Veterinary Medicine and Animal Science, Swedish University of Agricultural Sciences, 75007 Uppsala, Sweden.



#### Acknowledgements

We thank the staff of Viking Genetics and Estonian Cattle Breeders Association for the semen, especially Anders Edman and Peter Padrik for sending us the samples, and Dr. Triin Hallap for organizing the contact with the latter. We are very grateful to Karin Selin-Wretling and Annika Rikberg for the morphology evaluation.


#### Competing interests

The authors declare that they have no competing interests.


#### Funding

The study was financed by the Swedish Farmers' Association (Stiftelsen Lantbruksforskning, Stockholm, Sweden) awarded to Profs. Morrell and

Johannisson. In addition, ASV received a scholarship from USAMV IASI, Romania, POSDRU PROJECT—CPP107-DMI1/5/S/77222, for a Ph.D. internship in Uppsala, Sweden. The sponsors played no part in collection, analysis and interpretation of data, the writing of the report or the decision to submit the article for publication.

## References


1. Vishwanath R. Artificial insemination: the state of the art. Theriogenology. 2003;59:571–84.
2. Colazo MG, Mapletoft RJ. A review of current timed-AI (TAI) programs for beef and dairy cattle. Can Vet J. 2015;55:772–80.
3. Pfeifer LFM, Castro NA, Meloc VTO, Nevesc PMA, Cestaroc JP, Schneider A. Timed artificial insemination in blocks: a new alternative to improve fertility in lactating beef cows. Anim Reprod Sci. 2015;16:89–96.
4. Borges-Silva JC, Silva MR, Marinho DB, Nogueira E, Sampaio DC, Oliveira LOF, et al. Cooled semen for fixed-time artificial insemination in beef cattle. Reprod Fertil Dev. 2016;28:1004–8.
5. Thundathil JC, Dance AL, Kastelic JP. Fertility management of bulls to improve beef cattle productivity. Theriogenology. 2016;86:397–405.
6. Dahlen C, Larson J, Lamb GC. Impacts of reproductive technologies on beef production in the United States. Adv Exp Med Biol. 2014;752:97–114.
7. Sales JN, Neves KAL, Souza AH, Crepaldi GA, Sala RV, Fosado M, et al. Timing of insemination and fertility in dairy and beef cattle receiving timed artificial insemination using sex-sorted sperm. Theriogenology. 2011;76:427–35.
8. Kavak A, Lundeheim N, Aidnik M, Einarsson S. Sperm morphology in Estonian and Tori breed stallions. Acta Vet Scand. 2004;45:11–8.
9. Farrell P, Trouern-Trend V, Foote RH, Douglas-Hamilton D. Repeatability of measurements on human, rabbit, and bull sperm by computer assisted sperm analysis when comparing individual fields and means of 12 fields. Fertil Steril. 1995;64:208–10.
10. Januskauskas A, Johannisson A, Rodriguez-Martinez H. Subtle membrane changes in cryopreserved bull semen in relation with sperm viability, chromatin structure, and field fertility. Theriogenology. 2003;60:743–58.
11. Guthrie HD, Welch GR. Determination of intracellular reactive oxygen species and high mitochondrial membrane potential in Percoll-treated viable boar sperm using fluorescence-activated flow cytometry. J Anim Sci. 2006;84:2089–100.
12. Garner DL, Thomas CA. Organelle-specific probe JC-1 identifies membrane potential differences in the mitochondrial function of bovine sperm. Mol Reprod Dev. 1999;53:222–9.
13. Morrell JM, Johannisson A, Dalin A-M, Hammar L, Sandebert T, Rodriguez-Martinez H. Sperm morphology and chromatin integrity in Swedish warmblood stallions and their relationship to pregnancy rates. Acta Vet Scand. 2008;50:2–8.
14. Januskauskas A, Johannisson A, Soderquist LK, Rodríguez-Martínez H. Assessment of sperm characteristics post-thaw and response to calcium ionophore in relation to fertility in Swedish dairy AI bulls. Theriogenology. 2000;53:859–75.
15. Nagy S, Jansen J, Topper E, Gadella B. A triple-stain flow cytometric method to assess plasma- and acrosome-membrane integrity of cryopreserved bovine sperm immediately after thawing in presence of egg-yolk particles. Biol Reprod. 2003;68:1828–35.
16. Kastelic JP. Male involvement in fertility and factors affecting semen quality in bulls. Anim Front. 2013;3:20–5.
17. Saacke RG. Sperm morphology: its relevance to compensable and uncompensable traits in semen. Theriogenology. 2008;70:473–8.
18. Murphy C, Fahey AG, Shafat A, Fair S. Reducing sperm concentration is critical to limiting the oxidative stress challenge in liquid bull semen. J Dairy Sci. 2013;96:1–8.
19. Aitken RJ, Harkiss D, Buckingham DW. Analysis of lipid peroxidation mechanisms in human spermatozoa. Mol Reprod Dev. 1993;35:302–15.
20. Fiaz M, Usmani RH, Abdullah M, Ahmad T. Evaluation of semen quality of Holstein Friesian and Jersey bulls maintained under subtropical environment. Pak Vet J. 2010;30:75–8.
21. Hoflack G, Opsomer G, Rijsselaere T, Van Soom A, Maes D, de Kruif A, et al. Comparison of computer-assisted sperm motility analysis parameters in semen from Belgian Blue and Holstein Friesian bulls. Reprod Domest Anim. 2007;42:153–61.
22. Zhang SS, Hu JH, Li QW, Jiang ZL, Xiaoying Z. The cryoprotective effects of soybean lecithin on boar spermatozoa quality. Afr J Biotechnol. 2009;8:6476–80.
23. Janett F, Keo S, Bollwein H, Hässig M, Thun R. Comparison of AndroMed, Bioxcell and Triladyl extender for cryopreservation of bull semen. Schweiz Arch Tierheilk. 2005;147:62.
24. Kasimanickam R, Kasimanickam V, Tibracy A, Pelzer K. Effect of semen extenders on sperm parameters of ram semen during liquid storage at 4 °C. Small Rumin Res. 2011;99:208–13.
25. Bonsma JC. Livestock production: a global approach. Cape Town: Tafelberg Publishers; 1980.
26. Enciso M, Cisale H, Johnston SD, Sarasa J, Fernández JL, Gosálvez J. Major morphological sperm abnormalities in the bull are related to sperm DNA damage. Theriogenology. 2011;76:23–32.
27. Bocknek M, Smorag Z. The level of sperm DNA fragmentation in bulls of different breeds. Ann Anim Sci. 2010;10:379–84.
28. Fatehi AH, Bevers MM, Schoevers E, Roelen BA, Colenbrander B, Gadella BM. DNA damage in bovine sperm does not block fertilization and early embryonic development but induces apoptosis after the first cleavages. J Androl. 2006;27:76–88.
29. Hargreave T. Genetically determined male infertility and assisted reproduction techniques. J Endocrinol Invest. 2000;23:697–710.
30. Shi Q, Martin RH. Aneuploidy in human sperm: a review of the frequency and the distribution of aneuploidy, effects of donor age and lifestyle factors. Cytogenet Cell Genet. 2000;90:219–26.
31. Oliveira BM, Arruda RP, Thorné HE, Filho MM, Oliveira G, Guimarães C, et al. Fertility and uterine hemodynamic in cows after artificial insemination with semen assessed by fluorescent probes. Theriogenology. 2014;82:767–72.
32. Morrell JM, Nongbua T, Valeanu S, Lundstedt-Enkel K, Edman A, Johannisson A. Sperm quality variables as indicators of fertility may be breed dependent. Anim Reprod Sci. 2017;185:42–52.
33. Amann RP. Weaknesses in reports of "fertility" for horses and other species. Theriogenology. 2005;63:698–715.

# 21

# Treatment of 503 cattle with traumatic reticuloperitonitis

Ueli Braun[1*], Sonja Warislohner[1], Christian Gerspach[1], Stefanie Ohlerth[2] and Karl Nuss[1]

**Abstract**

**Background:** The treatment of traumatic reticuloperitonitis (TRP) in cattle has a long and impressive history that goes back more than 100 years. This study describes treatment for TRP in 503 cattle. Initial treatment was based on radiographic findings; cattle with a foreign body attached to a magnet were treated conservatively using antibiotics, anti-inflammatory drugs and intravenous fluids. Cattle with a foreign body lying on the ventral aspect of the reticulum or penetrating or perforating the reticulum received a magnet in addition to medical treatment. Cattle were radiographed again the next day. When the foreign body was completely attached to the magnet, medical treatment was continued. When the foreign body was not attached or still penetrated/perforated the reticulum, a rumenotomy was carried out.

**Results:** Of the 503 cattle, 232 were treated conservatively, 206 underwent surgery, 61 were slaughtered or euthanased and four were treated after discharge at home with a magnet and antibiotics. Surgical treatment was significantly more successful than conservative treatment; 90% of 206 operated and 82% of 232 medically-treated cattle were discharged.

**Conclusions:** For practical purposes, cattle suspected of having traumatic reticuloperitonitis should initially be treated with a magnet and antibiotics and re-evaluated, ideally radiographically, when response to treatment does not occur within 3 or 4 days. Surgery is limited to cases in which the foreign body fails to completely attach to the magnet.

**Keywords:** Cattle, Traumatic reticuloperitonitis, Treatment, Rumenotomy

## Background

The treatment of traumatic reticuloperitonitis (TRP) in cattle has a long and impressive history that goes back more than 100 years and has been documented in detail [1]. In the pre-antibiotic era, cows suspected of having TRP were fasted 2 or 3 days and positioned on an incline to elevate the front end for 1–2 weeks [2]. In addition, cows were treated with antibacterial drugs and laxatives. The first account of removal of a foreign body by means of rumenotomy was in the nineteenth century. Attempts were made to remove metallic foreign bodies using a magnetic probe that was introduced orally [3–5]. Even though this method was sometimes successful in removing superficial and non-perforating foreign bodies, penetrating or perforating foreign bodies that caused disease were rarely retrieved [6]. Currently, treatment of TRP may be conservative or surgical [2, 7, 8]. Conservative treatment consists of oral administration of a regular magnet or a magnet with a plastic cage combined with the administration of antibiotics. The success of treatment with a magnet is well documented [9–12] and in one study could be confirmed radiographically [13]. However, not all magnets fall directly into the reticulum; some fall into the anterior blind sac or possibly elsewhere in the rumen. Attempts to guide a magnet into the reticulum on a piece of string were unsuccessful in one study [14] as were attempts to direct the course of an orally-administered magnet using a second magnet externally. Another study showed that fasting the cow for 1 day, or lowering the position of the forelimbs during application increases the likelihood of a magnet

*Correspondence: ubraun@vetclinics.uzh.ch
[1] Department of Farm Animals, Vetsuisse Faculty, University of Zurich, Zurich, Switzerland

falling into the reticulum [15]. Subcutaneous administration of 40–60 mg atropine 10 min before administration of a magnet was yet another attempt to guide it directly into the reticulum [12, 14]. A compass was used to monitor the final position of the magnet. Follow-up studies showed that the administration of atropine does not affect the placement of a magnet [16–19] even though atropine delays the passage of the magnet through the oesophagus and causes reticular atony [20]. Likewise, lowering the position of the forefeet and pre-treatment with scopolamine or xylazine had no effect [18, 19]. According to current opinion, it is not possible to influence reticular placement of a magnet by means of external manipulations or drugs. Acute and uncomplicated TRP is treated with a magnet combined with antibiotics for several days [2] using penicillin or broad-spectrum antibiotics including tetracyclines or trimethoprim sulfonamide combinations [8]. However, the choice of antibiotics is arbitrary and not based on scientific studies. If no improvement occurs within 2–4 days, surgical treatment to remove the foreign body or euthanasia should be considered [2]. There are two main surgical techniques for rumenotomy [2]; the first involves permanently suturing the rumen to the peritoneum and transverse fascia, which allows extraperitoneal access to the rumen as well as extraperitoneal healing of the rumenotomy incision, and the second is the Weingarth's ring rumenotomy, in which the rumen is closed after exploration and returned to its normal abdominal position [2]. There have been other studies of laparorumenotomy techniques [21–23], one of which determined that skin suture fixation was superior to the Weingarth's ring technique [22]. Of 38 cattle that underwent rumenotomy, 34% were still in the herd, 37% had been removed from the herd and 29% had died or been euthanased at follow-up 5 months to 5 years after surgery [24]. The goal of the present study was to describe the treatment and course of the disease in 503 cattle diagnosed with TRP based on the results of clinical, ultrasonographic and radiographic findings.

## Methods

### Animals

A total of 503 cattle treated for TRP at the Department of Farm Animals of the Vetsuisse Faculty, University of Zurich, between January 1, 2001 and December 31, 2014 were analysed [25]. Radiography was used to diagnose TRP in 484 cattle, and laparoruminotomy (206) and postmortem examination (61) were additional diagnostic aids. There were 496 females and 7 males, which ranged in age from 1.0 to 14.9 years (median, 4.1 years) with 97% of the cattle being more than 2 years of age. Breeds included Swiss Braunvieh (208), Holstein–Friesian (155), Simmental (124), Jersey (3), Eringer (1), Hinterwälder (1) and crossbred cattle (11). The month when the animal became ill and the history were recorded in all cattle. The clinical, laboratory, ultrasonographic and radiographic findings obtained on admission to the clinic were published separately [26, 27]. Based on the ultrasonographic findings, 33 cattle with severe and extensive or generalised peritonitis were euthanased.

### Overview of the treatment of TRP

Initial treatment was selected on the basis of radiographic findings at the time of admission (Fig. 1). Cattle with a foreign body attached to a magnet were treated conservatively, and cattle with radiographic evidence of a foreign body (non-penetrating, penetrating or perforating) were treated with antibiotics and a magnet with a plastic cage (Bovivet Magnet, Kruuse, Denmark). The magnet was administered using an appropriate balling gun without premedication of the animal. Radiographic examination was repeated on the following day [28–30] and the results were used to guide subsequent treatment. Conservative treatment was continued when the foreign body was completely attached to the magnet and another radiograph was made. In cases where the foreign body was not in contact with the magnet or was still penetrating or perforating the reticulum, surgery was carried out.

### Conservative treatment

Conservative treatment included amoxicillin (7 mg/kg body weight, Clamoxyl®, Zoetis Switzerland) or penicillin G procaine (12,000 IU/kg body weight, Procacillin®, MSD Animal Health) given intramuscularly for 1–13 days, in most cases for 7 (n = 42) to 8 (n = 30) days (median 6 days). Seventy-nine cattle received a daily injection of a non-steroidal anti-inflammatory drug (flunixin meglumine, 1 mg/kg, Flunixine®, Biokema, Crissier, or ketoprofen, 3 mg/kg, Rifen®, Streuli Pharma) or a pyrazolone preparation (metamizole, 35 mg/kg, Vetalgin®, MSD Animal Health). All cattle received 10 l of a solution containing 50 g glucose and 9 g sodium chloride per litre daily for 3 days administered as a slow intravenous drip via an indwelling jugular vein catheter (Abbocath-T 14 g, length 14 cm, Abbott AG, Baar). Cows with hypocalcaemia (calcium < 2.0 mmol/L), hypophosphataemia (inorganic phosphorus < 1.0 mmol/L) or hypomagnesaemia (magnesium < 0.7 mmol/L) were treated orally with monocalcium phosphate, sodium dihydrogen phosphate and/or magnesium oxide. Clinical examinations were carried out daily.

### Surgical treatment

Cattle were fasted for 24 h before surgery to reduce rumen fill. After paravertebral anaesthesia of the last thoracic and the first two lumbar nerves on the left, a

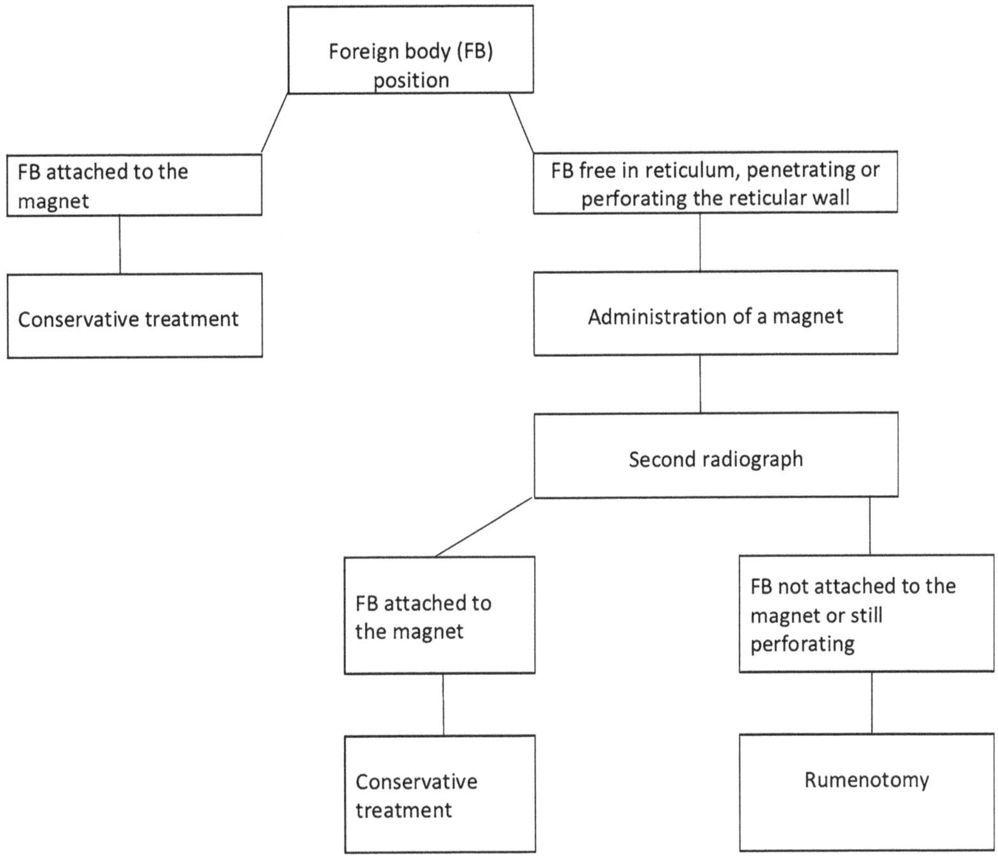


**Fig. 1** Treatment flowchart. Treatment flowchart for 503 cattle with traumatic reticuloperitonitis

25–30 cm incision was made in the abdominal wall parallel to the contour of the last rib. A perforating foreign body was removed from the reticulum during exploration of the abdomen in three cows. In all other cases, foreign bodies were removed via rumenotomy. Adhesive drapes and surgical drapes moistened with sterile saline solution were used to prevent contamination of the surgical field and abdominal cavity. Twenty-one cattle had perireticular abscesses adherent to the reticulum, which were drained after aspiration of the contents and ultrasound-guided incision from within the reticulum. A new cage magnet was placed into the reticulum, and 4–5 L of rumen liquor from a healthy donor cow supplemented with hay chaff was added to the rumen contents before the rumen was closed using a two-layer Cushing suture pattern (PDS 2®, Ethicon; since 2011 MonoPlus®, B. Braun). The suture line was lavaged with sterile saline-iodine solution, and the abdominal wall was closed routinely in four layers. The cattle were fasted for 24 h after surgery and treated with antibiotics for 1–19 days (median, 8 days), and 201 cattle received flunixin meglumine daily for 3 days, both at the doses outlined for conservative treatment. Two animals were euthanased during surgery because of severe inflammatory changes. Intravenous treatment with glucose and electrolytes was the same as that used for conservative treatment.

### Statistical analysis

The program IBM SPSS Statistics 22.0 was used for analysis. Means ± standard deviations were calculated for normal data and medians were calculated for non-normal data. For normal data, differences between two groups were analysed using a t-test. The Mann–Whitney U-test was used to analyse differences of non-normal data between two groups, and the Chi square test was used to analyse differences of nominal data between two groups. Differences were considered significant at $P < 0.05$.

## Results

Of the 503 cattle, 232 received conservative treatment, 206 were operated, 61 were slaughtered or euthanased and four were discharged and treated conservatively at home at the request of the owner (Fig. 2). Treatment at home consisted of administration of a magnet as well as antibiotics, such as amoxicillin or penicillin, for several days.

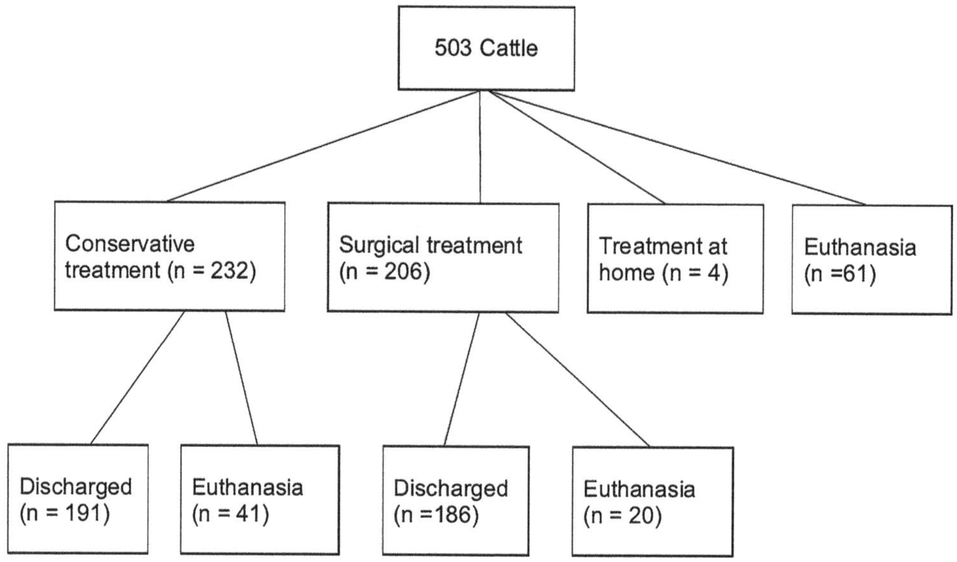


**Fig. 2** Treatment choices in 503 cattle. Treatment choices in 503 cattle with traumatic reticuloperitonitis

**Table 1 Position and efficacy of a magnet administered orally in 177 cattle with traumatic reticuloperitonitis**

| Variable | Outcome | n | % |
|---|---|---|---|
| Position of magnet (n = 177) | Reticulum | 146 | 82.5 |
| | Anterior blind sac of rumen | 16 | 9.0 |
| | Not visible | 15 | 8.5 |
| Efficacy of magnet in reticulum (n = 177) | Magnet not in reticulum | 31 | 17.5 |
| | Entire foreign body attached to magnet | 94 | 53.0 |
| | Parts of foreign body protruding from magnet | 10 | 6.0 |
| | No contact between magnet and foreign body | 35 | 20.0 |
| | Not all foreign bodies attached to magnet | 6 | 3.0 |
| | Foreign body not seen on first radiograph | 1 | 0.5 |

**Table 2 Efficacy of a magnet in the reticulum dependent on the position of the foreign body in 146 cattle with traumatic reticuloperitonitis**

| Position of foreign body | Efficacy of magnet | |
|---|---|---|
| | n | % |
| Upright on ventral aspect of reticulum at an angle of > 30 degrees (n = 32) | 24 | 75 |
| Flat on ventral aspect of reticulum (n = 56) | 32 | 57 |
| No contact with ventral aspect of reticulum (n = 36) | 16 | 44 |
| Perforating reticular wall (n = 22) | 7 | 32 |

$\chi^2 = 11.6$
$P < 0.01$

## Supplemental radiographs

A second radiograph was taken in 177 cattle one the day after the administration of a magnet. A third radiograph was taken in 37 cattle 2 days, and a fourth in eight cattle 3 days after the administration of a magnet. Radiographs taken in 177 cattle after administration of a magnet showed the magnet in the reticulum in 146 (82.5%) and in the anterior blind sac of the rumen in 16 (9%). A magnet was not seen on 15 (8.5%) radiographs, most likely because it was in the rumen (Table 1).

In 94 (53%) cattle with a magnet in the reticulum, the foreign body was attached to the magnet in its entirety and treatment was considered successful. In 10 (6%) cattle, a part of the foreign body was attached to the magnet but one end was protruding and possibly still penetrating the reticulum, and in 35 (20%) cases, the foreign body had maintained its position and had no contact with the magnet. In 6 (3%) cattle with multiple foreign bodies, at least one had remained penetrating or perforating and was not in contact with the magnet. In one (0.5%) animal, the second radiograph showed a foreign body that was missed on the initial radiograph.

The efficacy of treatment with a magnet was significantly associated with the position of the foreign body ($P < 0.01$, $\chi^2 = 11.6$). The best efficacy was achieved when the foreign body had an upright position on the ventral aspect of the reticulum; this occurred in 32 cattle and treatment was successful in 24 (75%) (Table 2). Of 56 foreign bodies lying on the ventral aspect of the reticulum,

32 (57%) were attached to the magnet. Of 36 foreign bodies that did not contact the ventral aspect of the reticulum, 16 (44%) were attached to the magnet. Perforation of the reticulum by a foreign body was confirmed radiographically in 22 cattle and in 32% of these, the foreign body was attached to the magnet and completely removed from the reticular wall.

In 37 cattle in which a penetrating foreign body was seen on the second radiograph, a third radiograph showed the foreign body completely attached to the magnet in 24 cattle and without attachment in 13. Five of the latter underwent rumenotomy and eight underwent radiography for the fourth time. In four cattle, the foreign body was attached to the magnet and in four it was not; the latter underwent rumenotomy.

### Efficacy of conservative treatment

Of 232 cattle, 191 (82%) were treated successfully and discharged (Fig. 2) and 41 did not respond to treatment and were euthanased. Nonresponse to treatment was defined as complete or partial anorexia, absent or reduced rumination or pyrexia for several days after the start of treatment. The general health condition and the appetite normalised after 2–14 days (median 2 days) in all but 5 of the cattle that were discharged. The rectal temperature decreased from 39.0 ± 0.61 °C on admission to 38.7 ± 0.35 °C 8 days after the start of treatment, and successfully treated cattle were discharged after 2–18 days (median 8 days).

### Efficacy of surgical treatment

Of 206 cattle that had surgical treatment, 195 underwent standing laparoruminotomy using the Weingarth's ring, 1 had a laparotomy in dorsal recumbency under general anaesthesia and 10 underwent draining of a reticular abscess through a transcutaneous incision without laparotomy. Surgical treatment was successful in 186 (90%) of 206 cases (Fig. 2), and a foreign body was removed in 184. A return to satisfactory general health and appetite occurred one to 20 days (median 3 days) after surgery. The rectal temperature decreased from 39.0 ± 0.61 °C on admission to 38.8 ± 0.43 °C 8 days after surgery, and successfully treated cattle were discharged after 5–39 days (median 11 days). Twenty animals did not respond to treatment and were euthanased.

### Comparison of conservative and surgical treatment

The efficacy of surgical treatment was significantly greater than that of conservative treatment (90 vs. 82%, $P < 0.05$), but recovery with regard to general health, appetite and rectal temperature after the start of treatment did not differ between the two groups. Hospitalisation was significantly shorter in conservatively treated cattle (8 vs. 11 days, $P < 0.01$).

### Type of foreign bodies

The type of 299 foreign bodies retrieved from 271 cattle was documented. There were 141 pieces of fencing wire, 121 nails, 13 screws, 8 flat pieces of metal, 5 pieces of barbed wire, 4 arms from eye glasses, 2 staples, 1 hair clip, 1 piece of aluminium, 1 fence insulator, 1 buckle and 1 set of nail clippers. The foreign bodies were from 1.5 to 18 cm in length (median 6 cm), and 273 were ferromagnetic.

## Discussion

Traumatic reticuloperitonitis may be treated conservatively or surgically [2, 7, 8]. In the present study, the choice of treatment was based on the radiographic findings of the reticulum: cattle with a foreign body attached to a magnet were treated conservatively, and cattle without a magnet were given one orally and radiographed again the next day. Thirty-seven cattle were radiographed a third time and eight cattle a fourth time because the efficacy of the magnet was poor and the owners declined rumenotomy. From a clinical standpoint, it was important to learn that attachment of the foreign body to the magnet was not seen radiographically until the third radiograph in 24 of 37 cattle and the fourth radiograph in four of eight cattle. Thus, the clinical recommendation to wait several days after magnet administration before opting for surgical treatment or euthanasia is reasonable because attachment of a foreign body to a magnet may require a few days. Eating and rumination variables of cows with TRP were shown to normalise rapidly within 3–4 days after successful treatment with a magnet [31]. On the other hand, unnecessary delay of surgery in cattle with a perforating foreign body carries the risk of complications such as traumatic pericarditis or abscess of the liver or spleen.

The efficacy of the magnet in the present study was similar to that of a previous study of 100 cows with TRP [18, 30], in which 85% of magnets were in the reticulum (compared with in 82.5% in the present study), 9% were in the anterior blind sac of the rumen (same as present study) and 6% were not seen on radiographs (compared with 8.5%), most likely because they were in the rumen. Thus, 15–20% of magnets administered orally are likely to end up in the anterior blind sac or other parts of the rumen rather than in the reticulum. This is irrelevant when a magnet is administered prophylactically because most magnets that fall into the rumen are moved into the reticulum within one to 3 days by reticulo-ruminal contractions [2]. However, this process may be delayed or does not occur in sick cows with reduced ruminal contractility, and in some cows, severe pathological changes that affect reticular structure and function preclude placement of a magnet into the reticulum altogether.

It was surprising that only 53% of the foreign bodies were attached to the magnet at the time of the second radiograph even though this rate was similar to 54% obtained in an earlier study of 100 cows with TRP [18, 30]. Other authors reported much higher efficacy rates of magnets of up to 97% [9, 10, 14]. A possible explanation for this difference is that field studies involve primarily acute and often uncomplicated cases, whereas the present study involved cases that did not respond to treatment by the referring veterinarian. Furthermore, unless radiography was part of the diagnostic procedure, it can be assumed that not all cattle treated successfully with a magnet indeed had TRP and that part of the high efficacy rates may be based on misdiagnosis [30]. The efficacy of a magnet depends greatly on the position of the foreign body within the reticulum; foreign bodies lying on the ventral aspect of the reticulum or in an upright position are more likely to become attached to a magnet than foreign bodies that have no contact with the ventral aspect of the reticulum or have perforated the reticulum. In a previous study [30] magnets were most effective (92%) when foreign bodies were lying flat on the ventral aspect of the reticulum, whereas in the present study magnets were most efficacious with foreign bodies in an upright position on the ventral aspect of the reticulum (75%). The efficacy of a magnet administered orally in cattle with foreign bodies that had no contact with the ventral aspect of the reticulum (54 vs. 44%) or that had perforated the reticulum (30 vs. 32%) was similar in the present and the former study. Even though a perforating foreign body is less likely to become attached to a magnet than a non-perforating foreign body, our findings show that radiographs cannot be used to determine whether administration of a magnet will be successful. Furthermore, there was no association between the severity of perforation or the length and shape of the foreign body and the efficacy of treatment. This supports our earlier recommendation that the first line of treatment in cows with TRP is administration of a magnet [30] except when a large part or the entire foreign body is situated outside of the reticulum. The response to treatment is considered positive when the rectal temperature normalises and eating and rumination improve [31] but can also be confirmed radiographically. Ultrasonography is not a suitable tool for determining the short-term response to treatment because attachment of a foreign body to a magnet cannot be visualised and it takes several months for inflammatory lesions to heal [32].

Surgical removal of foreign bodies situated on the ventral aspect of the reticulum or perforating the reticulum was generally straightforward, and the outcome of surgery was often successful even though most cases were chronic and had severe adhesions. This indicates that delaying the surgical removal of a foreign body after a period of conservative treatment is not necessarily a disadvantage. This is also supported by the observation that most fibrinous changes involving the reticulum can regress within 6 months [32]. Foreign bodies that were entirely outside of the reticulum (n = 9) could not always be found. Before a reticular abscess is incised and drained from within the reticulum, the surgeon must confirm that the abscess is closely adhered to the reticulum.

The success rates of conservative and surgical treatment were 82 and 90%, respectively, which was similar to previously reported rates of 84 [33] and 89% [34] for conservative treatment and 90–95% [2] for surgical treatment of acute cases.

Of 299 foreign bodies retrieved surgically, 141 (47.2%) were pieces of fence wire and 121 (40.5%) were nails, confirming observations of other authors that these types of foreign bodies are most common [35–37]. Aluminium foreign bodies were rare, which was in agreement with another study [38], and wires from cut tires used to weigh down tarps covering silage were not identified [38–40], because silage in Switzerland is usually stored in upright silos rather than in bunker silos that are covered with a tarp and tyres. Non-magnetic foreign bodies have been reported to be rare [36] and we encountered only 6%. These foreign bodies are difficult to treat medically and may be diagnosed when a magnet and a foreign body are seen together in the reticulum, but there is no contact between them [41]. There also have been two reports of an increased incidence of TRP in the vicinity of small airports where adjacent hay fields were contaminated with worn wire bristles from brushes used to clean the runways [42, 43].

## Conclusions

Initial treatment for TRP should include a magnet administered orally and antibiotics. When there is no response to conservative treatment within 3–4 days, the cow is re-assessed, ideally using radiography, and the treatment options are re-evaluated. Surgery is indicated only when a foreign body that has penetrated or perforated the reticulum fails to fully attach to the magnet.

**Authors' contributions**

UB initiated and planned the study and he prepared the manuscript together with KN. SW analysed the medical histories of the cows as part of her dissertation. CG made substantial contributions to acquisition and interpretation of data and he was involved in revising the manuscript. Radiography was performed by the technicians of the Clinic of Diagnostic Imaging under the supervision of SO, who also analysed the radiographs. Surgical treatment was performed by KN and his assistants. All authors read and approved the final manuscript.

**Author details**
[1] Department of Farm Animals, Vetsuisse Faculty, University of Zurich, Zurich, Switzerland. [2] Clinic of Diagnostic Imaging, Vetsuisse Faculty, University of Zurich, Zurich, Switzerland.

**Acknowledgements**
The authors thank the agricultural assistants for their help with the clinical examinations and the veterinary students for monitoring the cows during the night. Thanks also go out to the many veterinarians who examined and treated the patients and assisted in surgery during the study period.

**Competing interests**
The authors declare that they have no competing interests.

**Funding**
Not applicable since it was a retrospective analysis of medical records.

**References**

1. Dirksen G. Traumatische Hauben-Bauchfell-Entzündung (Reticuloperitonitis traumatica). In: Rosenberger G, editor. Krankheiten des Rindes. Berlin: Paul Parey; 1970. p. 217–32.
2. Dirksen G. Traumatische Hauben-Bauchfellentzündung. In: Dirksen G, Gründer HD, Stöber M, editors. Innere Medizin und Chirurgie des Rindes. Berlin: Parey Buchverlag; 2002. p. 400–14.
3. Del Seppia C. Ricerche ed estrzione dei corpi estranei degli stomaci die bovine. Allevatore. 1948;4:15.
4. Rost H. Untersuchungen über die Brauchbarkeit der Captometallsonde zur Entfernung von metallischen Fremdkörpern aus der Haube des Rindes. Dr. Med Vet Thesis: University of Veterinary Medicine Hannover; 1957.
5. Siegfried JP. Betrachtungen zur Fremdkörper-Behandlung mit dem Metallevaquator „System Eisenhut". Tierärztl Umschau. 1960;15:125–8.
6. Schmutzer A, Rosenmayr E. Magnetsonde, Fremdkörperoperation, konservative Therapie. Tierärztl Umschau. 1959;14:164–8.
7. Francoz D, Guard CL. Traumatic reticuloperitonitis (hardware disease, traumatic reticulitis). In: Smith BP, editor. Large animal internal medicine. St. Louis: Elsevier Mosby; 2015. p. 805–7.
8. Constable PD, Hinchliff KW, Done SH, Grünberg W. Diseases of alimentary tract—Ruminant. In: Constable PD, Hinchliff KW, Done SH, Grünberg W, editors. Veterinary medicine. A textbook of the diseases of cattle, horses, sheep, pigs and goats. St. Louis: Elsevier; 2017. p. 436–621.
9. Federer O. Beitrag zur Behandlung der traumatischen Indigestion des Rindes. Schweiz Arch Tierheilk. 1965;107:462–8.
10. Wittwer F. Erfahrungen mit dem Käfigmagneten in der Fremdkörpertherapie. Schweiz Arch Tierheilk. 1966;108:621–4.
11. Spadiut H. Zur Therapie der Reticulitis traumatica mit dem Käfigmagneten (Modell Rinderklinik Hannover). Wien Tierärztl Monatsschr. 1972;59:326–8.
12. Kalmar G. Untersuchungen zum therapeutischen Einsatz des Käfig-Magneten, mit und ohne Atropinprämedikation, bei fremdkörperkranken Rindern. Dr. Med Vet Thesis: University of Veterinary Medicine Hannover; 1984.
13. Dorresteijn J. Een nader onderzoek omtrent de acute indigestie en de reticuloperitonitis traumatica bij het rund. Tijdschr Diergeneeskd. 1973;98:831–9.
14. Der Schneider E. Verweilmagnet in der Therapie der Reticulitis traumatica des Rindes. Schweiz Arch Tierheilk. 1982;124:97–105.
15. Leuenberger W, Martig J, Schneider E. Untersuchungen zur Diagnose und Therapie der Reticulitis traumatica des Rindes. 2. Teil. Schweiz Arch Tierheilk. 1978;120:281–90.
16. Kleint M. Untersuchungen der Brauchbarkeit eines neuartigen Käfig-Magnetes zur Vorbeuge und Behandlung der Fremdkörpererkrankung des Rindes. Dr. Med Vet Thesis: University of Veterinary Medicine Hannover; 1987.
17. Taffe B. Untersuchungen der Brauchbarkeit des Käfig-Magneten CAP SUPER II zur Vorbeuge und Behandlung der Fremdkörpererkrankung des Rindes. Dr. Med Vet Thesis: University of Veterinary Medicine Hannover; 1993.
18. Gansohr B. Untersuchungen zur Eingabe von Fremdkörper-Nacktmagneten beim Rind. Dr. Med Vet Thesis: University of Zurich; 2001.
19. Braun U, Gansohr B, Flückiger M. Effects of atropine, scopolamine and xylazine on the placement of an orally administered magnet in cows. Vet Rec. 2003;152:258–60.
20. Braun U, Gansohr B, Hässig M. Ultrasonographic evaluation of reticular motility in cows after administration of atropine, scopolamine and xylazine. J Vet Med A. 2002;49:299–302.
21. Ducharme NG. Surgery of the bovine forestomach compartments. Vet Clin North Am Food Anim Pract. 1990;6:371–97.
22. Dehghani SN, Ghadrdani AM. Bovine rumenotomy: comparison of four surgical techniques. Can Vet J. 1995;36:693–7.
23. Niehaus AJ. Rumenotomy. Vet Clin North Am Food Anim Pract. 2008;24:341–7.
24. Hartnack AK, Niehaus AJ, Rousseau M, Pentecost RL, Miesner MD, Anderson DE. Indications for and factors relating to outcome after rumenotomy or rumenostomy in cattle: 95 cases (1999–2011). J Am Vet Med Assoc. 2015;247:659–64.
25. Warislohner S. Reticuloperitonitis traumatica beim Rind-eine Analyse von 503 Krankengeschichten. Dr. Med Vet Thesis: University of Zurich; 2017.
26. Braun U, Warislohner S, Torgerson P, Nuss K, Gerspach C. Clinical and laboratory findings in 503 cattle with traumatic reticuloperitonitis. BMC Vet Res. 2018;14:66.
27. Braun U, Gerspach C, Warislohner S, Nuss K, Ohlerth S. Ultrasonographic and radiographic findings in 503 cattle with traumatic reticuloperitonitis. Res Vet Sci. 2018;119:154–61.
28. Nägeli F. Die Röntgendiagnostik bei der Reticuloperitonitis des Rindes: Technik, Befunde, Interpretation und diagnostische Bedeutung. Dr. Med Vet Thesis: University of Zurich; 1991.
29. Braun U, Flückiger M, Nägeli F. Radiography as an aid in the diagnosis of traumatic reticuloperitonitis in cattle. Vet Rec. 1993;132:103–9.
30. Braun U, Gansohr B, Flückiger M. Radiographic findings before and after oral administration of a magnet in cows with traumatic reticuloperitonitis. Am J Vet Res. 2003;64:115–20.
31. Braun U, Tschoner T, Hässig M, Nuss K. Eating and rumination behaviour in cows with traumatic reticuloperitonitis. Schweiz Arch Tierheilk. 2017;159:101–8.
32. Herzog K, Kaske M, Bischoff C, Kehler W, Hoeltershinken M, Starke A, et al. Post surgical development of inflammatory adhesions and reticular function in cows suffering from traumatic reticuloperitonitis. Dtsch tierärztl Wschr. 2004;111:57–62.
33. Fraser CM. Conservative treatment of traumatic reticulitis. Can Vet J. 1961;2:65–8.
34. Hjerpe CA. Studies on acute bovine traumatic reticuloperitonitis. II. Signs of traumatic reticuloperitonitis. J Am Vet Med Assoc. 1961;139:230–2.
35. Maddy KT. Incidence of perforation of the bovine reticulum. J Am Vet Med Assoc. 1954;124:113–5.
36. Jagos P. The characteristics of foreign bodies in traumatic inflammations of cattle. Acta Vet (Brno). 1969;38:545–52.
37. Neumann N. Untersuchungen über das Vorkommen von Netzmagen Fremdkörpern bei Schlachtrindern in Bayern. Dr. Med Vet Thesis: University of Munich; 1979.
38. Cramers T, Mikkelsen KB, Andersen P, Enevoldsen C, Jensen HE. New types of foreign bodies and the effect of magnets in traumatic reticulitis in cows. Vet Rec. 2005;157:287–9.
39. Harwood D. Alimentary tract perforation in cattle caused by tyre wire. Vet Rec. 2004;154:574–5.
40. Monies B. Alimentary tract perforation in cattle caused by tyre wire. Vet Rec. 2004;154:735.

# Biosecurity and animal disease management in organic and conventional Swedish dairy herds

Ulf Emanuelson*, Karin Sjöström and Nils Fall

**Abstract**

**Background:** Good animal health is a notion that is germane to organic dairy production, and it is expected that such herds would pay significant attention on the health of their animals. However, it is not known if the applied animal disease management is actually more adequate in organic dairy cattle herds than in conventional dairy herds. A questionnaire study on biosecurity and animal disease management activities was therefore conducted among Swedish farmers with organic and conventional dairy cattle herds.

**Results:** A total of 192 useable questionnaires were returned; response rates of 30.3 and 20.2% for organic and conventional farmers, respectively. Herd characteristics of the two herd types were very similar, except that pipeline/tie-stall systems were less common in organic farms and that organic farmers had a higher education level than their conventional counterparts. Also, very few systematic differences in general or specific disease management activities were observed between the two types of farms. The main exceptions being how milk from cows during antibiotic treatment was used, views on policy actions in relation to antibiotic use, and attitudes towards calling for veterinary support. Using milk from cows during antibiotic treatment was more common in conventional herds, although it was mainly given to bull calves. Farmers of organic herds were more positive to policy actions to reduce the use and need for antibiotics, and they reported waiting longer before contacting a veterinarian for calves with diarrhoea and cows with subclinical mastitis.

**Conclusions:** The stated biosecurity and animal disease management was relatively equal in Swedish organic and conventional dairy herds. Our results thus indicate that animal health is as important in conventionally managed dairy herds in Sweden as in organically managed herds.

**Keywords:** Animal disease management, Animal health, Conventional, Dairy herds, Organic, Questionnaire study

## Background

The European Union Animal Health Strategy 2007–2013 clearly expressed that prevention is better than cure [1]. The necessary components of such a strategy are to monitor and to identify problems, but also to take relevant actions. Prevention would seem to be even more important in organic production because organic foods are commonly marketed as being healthier foods from healthier animals. Also, European regulations on organic production state that animal health should be promoted by the use of preventive measures [2], and the Swedish Control Association for Organic Agriculture (Kontrollföreningen för ekologisk odling, KRAV) follows the EU regulations for organic dairy production and puts particular emphasis on animal health [3].

Although the production conditions in organic farms aim to promote animal health, the health situation is not always better than in conventional farms [4]. Indeed, studies on animal disease in dairy cattle herds have shown somewhat divergent results, but there has generally not been any major or consistent advantage for organic over conventional production [5–12].

*Correspondence: ulf.emanuelson@slu.se
Department of Clinical Sciences, Swedish University of Agricultural Sciences, P.O. Box 7054, 750 07 Uppsala, Sweden

The reasons for this are probably many, but little is known about how animal diseases are managed in organic herds and if such management differs between organic and conventional herds. The few studies that compare management in organic and conventional dairy cattle herds found little evidence of fundamental differences [13–18]. However, most of these studies are relatively old, and organic dairy production has undergone significant changes over the last decade. Also, several studies were performed in the US, and organic production is very different in the US and Europe. Knowing how disease is actually managed is necessary to be able to identify appropriate actions to improve animal health. There is therefore a need to identify how dairy cow diseases are managed today under European conditions.

The aim of this study was therefore to investigate Swedish organic and conventional dairy cattle farmers' attitudes and knowledge towards biosecurity and animal disease management.

## Methods

A questionnaire was developed to acquire information on management routines that were hypothesised to be related to biosecurity and animal disease in dairy cattle herds. The questionnaire also addressed antibiotic use and resistance, but this will not be covered in the current paper. A draft questionnaire was developed based on discussions with researchers and veterinarians at the Swedish University of Agricultural Sciences (SLU), the National Veterinary Institute (SVA), Växa Sverige (the Swedish dairy association), and the staff at the food quality certification agency Kvalitetssystem Sigill AB. The draft was pre-tested on three animal science students at SLU and, after adjustments, pilot-tested on ten dairy farmers. The responses were studied to identify any confusing questions or questions that would not add any valuable information, and the questionnaire was further rephrased as needed. The final questionnaire was eight pages long, and most questions were closed, either multiple-choice or scored on a visual analogue scale (VAS).

Based on sample size calculations and practical considerations our goal was to receive 100 replies each from organic and conventional dairy farms and, considering our prior experience with distributing questionnaires to dairy farmers, a random sample of 300 organic and 500 conventional cattle farmers was drawn from the register kept by Växa Sverige.

The questionnaires were posted in the beginning of June 2014 by Växa Sverige, and the identities of the recipients were known only to them. A letter with information about the study was included with the survey, inviting the farmers to participate voluntarily. The respondents were informed that all information they provided would be treated confidentially. In September 2014, a postcard was sent to all farmers thanking them for participating in the survey and also reminding those who had not yet responded to fill in the survey and that it was possible to do so online. A note about the survey, with a link to the online version, was published at the same time in the Swedish agricultural magazine Land Lantbruk in order to increase the number of responses.

In October 2014, after the reply deadline, all data from the respondents were entered manually in Netigate (Netigate Ltd., Stockholm, Sweden). Ten surveys were randomly chosen after the data had been entered, to be used as a control of the recording process, and no errors were found. Comparisons of answers between organic and conventional farmers were performed with Kruskal–Wallis tests for replies on a continuous or and with $Chi^2$ tests for categorical answers. The statistical analyses were performed using SAS (version 9.4, SAS Institute Inc., Cary, NC, USA).

## Results

A total of 198 questionnaires were returned, but four were almost completely empty and another two did not indicate if they were from organic or conventional dairy cattle farmers. The number of usable questionnaires was thus 192, of which 91 were from organic farmers. The response rates were 30.3% among the organic farmers and 20.2% among the conventional farmers. Herd characteristics of the organic and conventional farms that replied are presented in Table 1. The two types were similar in all aspects, except that organic farms used pipeline/tie-stall systems to a much lower degree and that a higher proportion of the organic farmers had post-secondary school education than the conventional farmers.

Answers linked to general disease-related aspects are given in Table 2. Again, the two types were similar, except that a larger proportion of conventional farmers fed milk from cows during antibiotic treatment to calves and answered "other" for the use of such milk compared to organic farmers. The most common free-text answer explaining the "other" reply was that the milk was only fed to bull calves.

There were no differences between the two types of herds with respect to biosecurity (Table 3). Checking the climate and size of the stable was applied to a high degree in both types of herd. In contrast, there were significant differences in the respondents' intents related to prevention of disease between the two types (Table 4). The organic farmers were especially more favourable towards policy actions to reduce the use or need of antibiotics compared to conventional farmers.

Management of a calf with diarrhoea (Table 5) or a cow considered to be at risk of having subclinical mastitis

**Table 1 Characteristics [percentage of observations for categorical variables and median (range) for continuous variables] of Swedish dairy herds participating in a questionnaire study of biosecurity and disease management in organic and conventional dairy production**

| Variables | Organic n=91 | Conventional n=101 | P value[a] |
|---|---|---|---|
| Age (years) | 50 (20–69) | 53 (23–70) | 0.07 |
| Years in profession | 25 (4–45) | 28 (1.5–77) | 0.63 |
| Number of milking cows | 80 (40–460) | 75 (25–400) | 0.13 |
| Gender of the respondent | | | |
| Female | 43.3 | 43.6 | 0.97 |
| Geographical distribution[b] | | | |
| SE1 | 29.7 | 22.0 | 0.24 |
| SE21 | 19.8 | 22.0 | |
| SE22 | 5.5 | 15.0 | |
| SE23 | 27.5 | 22.0 | |
| SE3 | 17.6 | 15.0 | |
| Milking system | | | |
| Parlour/rotary | 41.1 | 30.7 | < 0.001 |
| Automatic milking system | 47.8 | 28.7 | |
| Pipeline/tie-stall | 11.1 | 40.6 | |
| Elementary agricultural school education | | | |
| Yes | 75.3 | 62.4 | 0.06 |
| Post-secondary school education | | | |
| Yes | 62.5 | 45.5 | 0.02 |

[a] Kruskal–Wallis/Chi$^2$

[b] NUTS (Nomenclature of Territorial Units for Statistics) regions SE1 East Sweden, SE21 Småland and the islands, SE22 South Sweden, SE23 West Sweden, and SE3 North Sweden http://ec.europa.eu/eurostat/documents/345175/7451602/nuts-map-SE.pdf

(Table 6) was also very similar between the two types of herds, with the only exception being that conventional cattle farmers tended to contact a veterinarian earlier than organic farmers; mean 2.8 and 2.3 ($P=0.05$), respectively, where six corresponds to always and one to never contact the veterinarian immediately upon signs.

## Discussion

There were no major differences in disease-related management activities between organic and conventional dairy cattle farms in Sweden. This is consistent with our previous results where we have shown that there is little difference in disease occurrence between organic and conventional dairy cattle herds in Sweden [7–10, 12]. Our results thus indicate that animal health and disease management may be just as important in conventionally managed as in organically managed dairy cattle herds in Sweden. These results also agree with other studies comparing management in the two production systems in Europe and the USA [13–18], indicating that this conclusion is not limited to Swedish conditions. The very small systematic differences between, but relatively large variation within, both groups indicate that management choices are more farm specific than dependent on the organic or conventional status of the herds.

Actions related to calves with diarrhoea or cows with subclinical mastitis were scored almost the same for the two types of herds, although organic herds tended to wait a bit longer before contacting a veterinarian. A dedicated herd veterinarian was also less common in organic herds. These results are consistent with previous studies showing that Norwegian organic dairy cattle farmers feel less in need of veterinary advisory services than conventional farmers [15]. Delayed antibiotic treatment of cows with mastitis might not be positive with respect to treatment effects and might be detrimental to animal welfare, and such delays have been reported to be a concern among practicing veterinarians [19, 20]. A contact with a veterinarian does not necessarily lead to a treatment decision, but in such cases a delayed contact will also lead to a delayed treatment because only veterinarians are allowed to initiate an antibiotic treatment in Sweden. We are not aware of any studies comparing treatment efficiencies between organic and conventional farms, but the on-farm mortality was found to be lower for organic than for conventional Swedish farms [21]. Because on-farm mortality might be a consequence of delayed veterinary treatment of diseases, the differences in actions we observed in this study might not have a negative consequence for animal health. Thus, the different use of veterinarians in organic herds might be balanced by more active handling of health disorders among their cattle by the farmers themselves, as was observed by Valle et al. [15].

The organic farmers indicated a stronger intention to prevent diseases and were more positive towards implementing policy measures to reduce the use of antibiotics than conventional farmers, although it should be noted that the readiness was relatively low on both farm types. The difference might be a result of the stronger requirements of Swedish Control Association for Organic Agriculture and the realisation among organic farmers of the value and feasibility of reducing antibiotic use. The response rate was, however, higher among the organic farmers, which might indicate higher levels of engagement in animal health issues. We also observed a significantly higher education level among the organic farmers, which might indicate a selection bias towards more well educated and interested farmers, leading to a higher awareness of preventive actions and acceptance of policy measures. However, the differences in attitudes might also be a true difference caused by the greater personal involvement that organic dairy cattle production requires.

**Table 2 Distribution (percentage) of variables linked to general disease-related aspects for Swedish dairy herds participating in a questionnaire study of biosecurity and disease management in organic and conventional dairy production**

| Variables | Category | Organic | Conventional | P value[a] |
|---|---|---|---|---|
| Herd veterinarian | Yes | 52.5 | 68.1 | 0.03 |
| Visits from livestock production advisor | At least once per month | 34.1 | 38.6 | 0.66 |
| | At least 3 times per year | 24.2 | 21.8 | |
| | At least once per year | 24.2 | 16.8 | |
| | Once every second year | 7.7 | 8.9 | |
| | Never | 9.9 | 15.6 | |
| Records kept of treated animals | Yes | 91.1 | 83.0 | 0.21 |
| | No | 8.9 | 16.0 | |
| | Do not know | 0.0 | 1.0 | |
| Hospital pen used only for sick animals | Yes | 39.6 | 34.7 | 0.48 |
| | No | 60.4 | 65.3 | |
| Milk from cows during antibiotic treatment[b] | Disposed of in manure | 68.1 | 59.4 | 0.21[c] |
| | Disposed of in sewer | 18.7 | 11.9 | 0.19 |
| | Fed to calves | 20.9 | 33.7 | 0.05 |
| | Other | 2.2 | 11.9 | 0.01 |
| Milk from cows after antibiotic treatment and during the withdrawal period[b] | Disposed of in manure | 39.6 | 36.6 | 0.67[c] |
| | Disposed of in sewer | 11.0 | 7.9 | 0.47 |
| | Fed to calves | 59.3 | 60.4 | 0.88 |
| | Other | 9.9 | 15.8 | 0.22 |

[a] $Chi^2$

[b] Multiple answers allowed

[c] Comparisons between "yes" and "no" for each row

**Table 3 Distribution (percentage) of variables linked to biosecurity for Swedish dairy herds participating in a questionnaire study of biosecurity and disease management in organic and conventional dairy production**

| Variables | Category | Organic | Conventional | P value[a] |
|---|---|---|---|---|
| Check the climate in the stable with respect to ventilation, humidity and temperature | Not done | 15.4 | 12.0 | 0.28 |
| | Might be done | 22.0 | 32.0 | |
| | It is done | 62.6 | 56.0 | |
| (Re-)Evaluate that the interior of the stable is adapted for animal size and need | Not done | 8.8 | 10.2 | 0.55 |
| | Might be done | 18.7 | 24.5 | |
| | It is done | 72.5 | 65.3 | |
| Let visitors only use clothes and shoes belonging to the farm | Not done | 3.3 | 8.1 | 0.37 |
| | Might be done | 30.0 | 27.3 | |
| | It is done | 66.7 | 64.6 | |
| Closing farm to others other than veterinarians, advisors, and family members | Not done | 60.4 | 44.5 | 0.12 |
| | Might be done | 27.5 | 36.6 | |
| | It is done | 12.1 | 17.8 | |
| Regular cleaning and disinfection of stables | Not done | 0.0 | 1.0 | 0.52 |
| | Might be done | 6.6 | 9.0 | |
| | It is done | 93.4 | 90.0 | |

[a] $Chi^2$

Our results show that feeding waste milk, i.e. milk from cows not permitted for human consumption due to antibiotic treatment, to calves was more common in conventional than in organic dairy cattle herds. This was especially pronounced considering the "other" use, which was mainly indicated as such milk being fed only

**Table 4 Respondents' ratings of statements linked to preventive intents on a scale from 1 to 6, where 1 is "never" and 6 is "always", from a questionnaire study of biosecurity and disease management in organic and conventional dairy production**

| Variables | Organic | | Conventional | | P value[a] |
|---|---|---|---|---|---|
| | Median (min–max) | Mean | Median (min–max) | Mean | |
| I want to try to prevent disease to a greater extent | 6 (1–6) | 5.5 | 6 (1–6) | 5.2 | 0.03 |
| If the use of antibiotics in a herd is higher than a predetermined level, a penalty and requirements for reduced usage should be required | 3 (1–6) | 2.9 | 1 (1–6) | 2.0 | < 0.001 |
| Animal owners should be responsible for forming a plan together with a veterinarian on how to reduce the use of antibiotics in their herd to a certain level | 4 (1–6) | 3.1 | 3 (1–6) | 2.9 | < 0.001 |

[a] Kruskal–Wallis

**Table 5 Respondents' ratings of statements linked to management of a calf showing signs of diarrhoea on a scale from 1 to 6, where 1 is "never" and 6 is "always", from a questionnaire study of biosecurity and disease management in organic and conventional dairy production**

| Variables | Organic | | Conventional | | P value[a] |
|---|---|---|---|---|---|
| | Median (min–max) | Mean | Median (min–max) | Mean | |
| Isolate the calf | 3 (1–6) | 3.6 | 3 (1–6) | 3.3 | 0.15 |
| Check the calf's temperature | 4 (1–6) | 4.3 | 4 (1–6) | 4.2 | 0.73 |
| Check the calf's general condition | 6 (2–6) | 5.6 | 6 (4–6) | 5.7 | 0.20 |
| Give the calf extra comfort—blanket, more litter, or a heat lamp | 4 (1–6) | 4.0 | 4 (1–6) | 4.0 | 0.92 |
| Give the calf water/fluid replacement | 6 (1–6) | 5.5 | 6 (1–6) | 5.5 | 0.98 |
| Contact the veterinarian immediately | 2 (1–5) | 2.3 | 2 (1–5) | 2.1 | 0.39 |
| Wait and contact the veterinarian at the earliest after 1–2 days | 3 (1–6) | 3.8 | 3 (1–6) | 3.3 | 0.02 |
| Contact the veterinarian only if the calf has fever/the general condition is affected | 5 (1–6) | 4.7 | 5 (1–6) | 4.6 | 0.68 |

[a] Kruskal–Wallis

to bull calves. This use agrees with general observations by Duse et al. [22], and it is therefore possible that antibiotic resistance is more common in conventional dairy cattle farms because feeding this kind of milk, even just to bull calves, is associated with increased occurrence of antimicrobial resistant bacteria in the herd [23]. Future research in this regard is warranted because lower antibiotic resistance in organic dairy cattle herds would indicate a competitive advantage for organic production. It is important to realize that also other ways to dispose of waste milk may impose increased risks for development of antimicrobial resistance, also in the environment, and any use of antibiotics should therefore be well justified.

The questionnaire study was anonymous and the distribution was not under our control, so we could not perform a formal non-response analysis. However, our sample agrees with official statistics with respect to age, gender, herd size, and geographical distribution [24], and we therefore consider it reasonably representative of the Swedish dairy cattle farmer community. It is possible, however, that the responders were more positive towards animal health and disease management than the general population of dairy farmers because answering the questionnaire required some interest in the question. A questionnaire study may also suffer from response bias, where replies are not completely truthful, and we cannot verify that the answers correspond to actual actions. The limitations of studies such as this should be kept in mind when interpreting the results, but there is no reason to believe that possible biases would be differential, i.e. invalidate the comparisons between organic and conventional farmers.

There were no major differences in the general characteristics of the herds in the sample, except that tie-stalls were more common in conventional herds and that automatic milking systems (AMS) were more common in organic herds. This is probably rather unique to the Swedish situation because a comparison between organic dairy farms in France, Germany, Spain, and Sweden showed that AMS was rarely used in these other countries [25]. However, tie-stalls were also found to be more common among equally sized conventional herds than organic herds in the US [18], but the extent of AMS systems in that sample is not known. We have

**Table 6 Respondents' ratings of statements linked to management of a dairy cow considered to be at risk of having subclinical mastitis on a scale from 1 to 6, where 1 is "never" and 6 is "always", from a questionnaire study of biosecurity and disease management in organic and conventional dairy production**

| Variable | Organic | | Conventional | | P value[a] |
|---|---|---|---|---|---|
| | Median (min–max) | Mean | Median (min–max) | Mean | |
| Put the cow in a hospital pen | 2 (1–6) | 2.1 | 2 (1–6) | 2.2 | 0.26 |
| Increase cow-comfort by adding more litter/straw | 3 (1–6) | 2.9 | 3 (1–6) | 3.2 | 0.18 |
| Check the cell count of the milk | 5 (1–6) | 5.0 | 5 (1–6) | 4.8 | 0.53 |
| Send milk for bacteriological analysis | 4 (1–6) | 3.4 | 3 (1–6) | 2.9 | 0.06 |
| Contact the veterinarian immediately | 2 (1–6) | 2.3 | 2 (1–6) | 2.8 | 0.05 |
| Contact the veterinarian earliest after 1–2 days | 4 (1–6) | 3.5 | 3 (1–6) | 3.4 | 0.64 |
| Dry up the inflamed quarter and milk the other quarters as usual | 4 (1–6) | 3.5 | 3 (1–6) | 3.2 | 0.12 |
| Milk that cow separately and/or last | 5 (1–6) | 4.5 | 5 (1–6) | 4.9 | 0.06 |
| Milk the cow with shorter intervals | 4 (1–6) | 4 | 4 (1–6) | 4.1 | 0.72 |
| Milk the inflamed quarter completely | 6 (2–6) | 5.3 | 6 (1–6) | 5.3 | 0.66 |
| Dry off the cow earlier than planned (the whole udder) and apply dry-cow therapy | 4 (1–6) | 3.3 | 3 (1–6) | 3.2 | 0.57 |
| Treat the cow during the planned dry period | 5 (1–6) | 4.5 | 5 (1–6) | 4.7 | 0.35 |
| Dry the affected quarter if the cell count remains high after (antibiotic) treatment | 5 (1–6) | 4.3 | 5 (1–6) | 4.4 | 0.76 |
| Do not inseminate the cow and cull it at the next planned dry off | 4 (1–6) | 3.9 | 4 (1–6) | 3.9 | 0.66 |
| Cull the cow immediately | 2 (1–5) | 2.1 | 2 (1–5) | 2.2 | 0.47 |
| Cull the cow if an (antibiotic) treatment does not work | 4 (1–6) | 4.0 | 5 (1–6) | 4.3 | 0.11 |
| Cull the cow if the cell count remains high after (antibiotic) treatment | 5 (1–6) | 4.5 | 5 (1–6) | 4.6 | 0.59 |
| Check cell count of the whole herd | 5 (1–6) | 4.9 | 6 (1–6) | 5.1 | 0.19 |

[a] Kruskal–Wallis

previously shown that there are differences in implemented mastitis management options between Swedish dairy farms with and without AMS [26], so the differences in milking systems might impose differences in management between the two types of herds. However, few of the questions in this study were directed to mastitis management, and any such differences are thus not likely to have influenced the comparisons to any significant degree.

## Conclusions

The stated biosecurity and animal disease management was relatively similar in Swedish organic and conventional dairy cattle herds, although farmer attitude towards health improvement might be somewhat different. Future research should study if the different use of veterinarians might have an impact on treatment success and if the different use of waste milk might have an impact on antibiotic resistance in these types of herds.

#### Authors' contributions

All authors participated in the design of the study and collection of data. UE performed the analysis and drafted the manuscript. All authors read and approved the final manuscript.


#### Acknowledgements

We acknowledge Sofie Winding for drafting the questionnaire and performing the data collection. We also thank the researchers and veterinarians at SLU, SVA, and Kvalitetssystem Sigill AB; the three anonymous animal science students; and the 10 pre-pilot farmers for their help in developing the questionnaire. All responding farmers are thanked for their contributions.

#### Competing interests

The authors declare that they have no competing interests.

#### Funding

Funds for the study were provided by the Swedish Board of Agriculture, but they did not have any influence on the design of the study; the collection, analysis, and interpretation of the data; or in writing the manuscript.


#### References


1. European Commission. A new Animal Health Strategy for the European Union (2007–2013) where "Prevention is better than cure". Luxembourg: Office for Official Publications of the European Communities; 2007.
2. European Commission. Commission regulation (EC) No 889/2008. Off J Eur Union. vol. 51; 2008.
3. The KRAV Association. Standards for KRAV-certified production, 2015 Version. Uppsala: KRAV; 2015.
4. Sundrum A. Organic livestock farming. Livest Prod Sci. 2001;67:207–15.
5. Hardeng F, Edge VL. Mastitis, ketosis, and milk fever in 31 organic and 93 conventional Norwegian dairy herds. J Dairy Sci. 2001;84:2673–9.

6. Roesch M, Doherr MG, Blum JW. Management, feeding, production, reproduction and udder health on organic and conventional Swiss dairy farms. Schweiz Arch Tierheilkd. 2006;148:387–95.
7. Fall N, Emanuelson U, Martinsson K, Jonsson S. Udder health at a Swedish research farm with both organic and conventional dairy cow management. Prev Vet Med. 2008;83:186–95.
8. Fall N, Forslund K, Emanuelson U. Reproductive performance, general health, and longevity of dairy cows at a Swedish research farm with both organic and conventional production. Livest Sci. 2008;118:11–9.
9. Fall N, Grohn YT, Forslund K, Essen-Gustafsson B, Niskanen R, Emanuelson U. An observational study on early-lactation metabolic profiles in Swedish organically and conventionally managed dairy cows. J Dairy Sci. 2008;91:3983–92.
10. Fall N, Emanuelson U. Milk yield, udder health and reproductive performance in Swedish organic and conventional dairy herds. J Dairy Res. 2009;76:402–10.
11. Garmo RT, Waage S, Sviland S, Henriksen BIF, Osteras O, Reksen O. Reproductive performance, udder health, and antibiotic resistance in mastitis bacteria isolated from Norwegian Red cows in conventional and organic farming. Acta Vet Scand. 2010;52:11.
12. Blanco-Penedo I, Lundh T, Holtenius K, Fall N, Emanuelson U. The status of essential elements and associations with milk yield and the occurrence of mastitis in organic and conventional dairy herds. Livest Sci. 2014;168:120–7.
13. Zwald AG, Ruegg PL, Kaneene JB, Warnick LD, Wells SJ, Fossler C, et al. Management practices and reported antimicrobial usage on conventional and organic dairy farms. J Dairy Sci. 2004;87:191–201.
14. Sato K, Bartlett PC, Erskine RJ, Kaneene JB. A comparison of production and management between Wisconsin organic and conventional dairy herds. Livest Prod Sci. 2005;93:105–15.
15. Valle PS, Lien G, Flaten O, Koesling M, Ebbesvik M. Herd health and health management in organic versus conventional dairy herds in Norway. Livest Sci. 2007;112:123–32.
16. Langford FM, Rutherford KMD, Jack MC, Sherwood L, Lawrence AB, Haskell MJ. A comparison of management practices, farmer-perceived disease incidence and winter housing on organic and non-organic dairy farms in the UK. J Dairy Res. 2009;76:6–14.
17. Stiglbauer KE, Cicconi-Hogan KM, Richert R, Schukken YH, Ruegg PL, Gamroth M. Assessment of herd management on organic and conventional dairy farms in the United States. J Dairy Sci. 2013;96:1290–300.
18. Sorge US, Moon R, Wolff LJ, Michels L, Schroth S, Kelton DF, et al. Management practices on organic and conventional dairy herds in Minnesota. J Dairy Sci. 2016;99:3183–92.
19. Hansson I, Hamilton C, Ekman T, Forslund K. Carcass quality in certified organic production compared with conventional livestock production. J Vet Med Series B Infect Dis Vet Public Health. 2000;47:111–20.
20. von Borell E, Sorensen JT. Organic livestock production in Europe: aims, rules and trends with special emphasis on animal health and welfare. Livest Prod Sci. 2004;90:3–9.
21. Alvåsen K, Mörk MJ, Hallén Sandgren C, Thomsen PT, Emanuelson U. Herd-level risk factors associated with cow mortality in Swedish dairy herds. J Dairy Sci. 2012;95:4352–62.
22. Duse A, Persson Waller K, Emanuelson U, Unnerstad HE, Persson Y, Bengtsson B. Farming practices in Sweden related to feeding milk and colostrum from cows treated with antimicrobials to dairy calves. Acta Vet Scand. 2013;55:49.
23. Duse A, Waller KP, Emanuelson U, Unnerstad HE, Persson Y, Bengtsson B. Risk factors for antimicrobial resistance in fecal *Escherichia coli* from preweaned dairy calves. J Dairy Sci. 2015;98:500–16.
24. SCB. Farm labour force in 2013 [Sysselsättning i jordbruket 2013]. Statistiska Centralbyrån. 2014. http://www.scb.se/Statistik/JO/JO0401/2013A01/JO0401_2013A01_SM_JO30SM1401.pdf. Accessed 30 July 2017.
25. Krieger M, Sjöström K, Blanco Penedo I, Madouasse A, Duval JE, Bareille N, Fourichon C, et al. Prevalence of production disease related indicators in organic dairy herds in four European countries. Livest Sci. 2017;198:104–8.
26. Nielsen C, Emanuelson U. Mastitis control in Swedish dairy herds. J Dairy Sci. 2013;96:6883–93.

23

# Scorer and modality agreement for the detection of intervertebral disc calcification in Dachshunds

Alana Jayne Rosenblatt[1,4*], Anu Katriina Lappalainen[2], Nina Alice James[1], Natalie Siu Ling Webster[3] and Charles Grégoire Bénédict Caraguel[1]

**Abstract**

**Background:** The Dachshund is a chondrodystrophic breed of dog predisposed to premature degeneration and calcification, and subsequent herniation, of intervertebral discs (IVDs). This condition is heritable in Dachshunds and breeding candidates are screened for radiographically detectable intervertebral disc calcification (RDIDC), a feature of advanced disc degeneration and a prognostic factor for clinical disease. RDIDC scoring has been previously shown to be consistent within scorers; however, strong scorer effect (subjectivity) was also reported. The aim of this study was to estimate the within- and between-scorer agreement (repeatability and reproducibility, respectively) of computed tomography (CT) scanning and magnetic resonance imaging (MRI) for scoring IVD calcification, and to compare these modalities with radiographic scoring.

**Results:** Twenty-one Dachshund dogs were screened for IVD calcification using the three imaging modalities. Three scorers scored each case twice, independently. Repeatability was highest for radiography (95.4%), and significantly higher than for CT (90.4%) but not MRI (93.8%). Reproducibility was also highest for radiography (92.9%), but not significantly higher than for CT or MRI (89.4% and 86.4%, respectively). Overall, CT scored IVDs differently than radiography and MRI (64.8% and 62.7% agreement, respectively), while radiography and MRI scored more similarly (85.7% agreement).

**Conclusions:** Despite high precision for radiography, previous evidence of scorer subjectivity was confirmed, which was not generally observed with CT and MRI. The increased consistency of radiography may be related to prior scorer experience with the modality and RDIDC scoring. This study does not support replacing radiography with CT or MRI to screen for heritable IVD calcification in breeding Dachshunds; however, evaluation of dog-level precision and the accuracy of each modality is recommended.

**Keywords:** CT, Dachshund, Intervertebral disc calcification, MRI, Radiography, Repeatability, Reproducibility, Scoring

## Background

Of all the dog breeds, the Dachshund has the highest lifetime incidence of intervertebral disc disease (IVDD) [1, 2]. The results of a recent study in the UK, based on a survey of Dachshund owners ("Dachs-Life 2015"), found an overall IVDD prevalence of 15.7% in the surveyed Dachshund population of 1975 dogs, with a significant prevalence range between different breed variants (7.1–24.4%) [3]. This high prevalence may be due to a variety of genetic, physical and lifestyle-related factors [3], but is likely primarily attributable to their chondrodystrophic morphology. Dogs with chondrodystrophy undergo chrondroid metaplasia, the premature maturation and degeneration of intervertebral discs (IVDs) that often results in calcification, an indicator of severe degeneration [2, 4, 5]. These degenerated IVDs are predisposed to herniate into the spinal canal under minimal stress, resulting in spinal cord compression and injury

*Correspondence: a.rosenblatt@uq.edu.au
[4] Present Address: School of Veterinary Science, The University of Queensland, Gatton, QLD 4343, Australia

[4]. Dachshunds with IVD herniation have a high level of morbidity and mortality, and despite treatment that often includes complex and costly surgical intervention, a substantial proportion of dogs retain neurologic deficits [6–8]. IVDD is widely accepted as the Dachshund breed's greatest health problem.

A scheme for radiographic scoring of intervertebral disc calcification in Dachshunds has been developed, and recently reviewed [9]. Radiographically detectable intervertebral disc calcification (RDIDC) is highly heritable in Dachshunds [10–14], and the development of RDIDC at a young adult age corresponds with an increased risk of developing clinical IVDD during the lifetime of the dog [8, 10, 15–18]. Therefore, screening young adult breeding candidates for RDIDC, ideally at 24–30 months of age, can reduce the prevalence of the disease in the breed [11, 18, 19]. RDIDC is scored from 0 to a maximum of 26 (i.e. 26 total IVDs in the canine cervical, thoracic and lumbar spine). Current screening programs recommend that Dachshunds with RDIDC scores of $\leq 2$ are suitable for breeding, dogs with scores of 3–4 should be bred judiciously, and animals with scores $\geq 5$ should be excluded for breeding purposes [8, 11, 12, 17, 18].

For a screening test to be useful in a selective breeding program, it must be precise (i.e. very reproducible). Recent evaluation of within- and between-scorer agreement for RDIDC scoring identified an overall high level of repeatability and reproducibility, but also identified some limitations of radiography as a screening tool [20]. Test precision was influenced by scorer experience level (expert scorer > specialist radiologist > general practitioner), which in turn affected the consistency (agreement) of the results. Individual scorer-dependent subjectivity was also identified.

The absence of RDIDC does not exclude a disc from being degenerative nor calcified, and only a portion of IVD calcifications present in a spine would be expected to be detected radiographically [17, 21]. It is postulated that a cross-sectional imaging modality such as computed tomography (CT) scanning would be a superior alternative for screening dogs for IVD calcification compared to radiography, as CT reduces challenges associated with anatomic superimposition and has improved contrast resolution [22, 23]. Alternatively, magnetic resonance imaging (MRI) is a cross-sectional modality with superior contrast resolution to both CT and radiography, and high-field MRI is considered the optimal modality for imaging the spine [24, 25]. MRI of intervertebral discs allows identification of earlier stages of disc degeneration than calcification, due to its ability to detect biochemical changes in tissues including loss of water and proteoglycan content and decreased chondroitin-keratan sulfate ratio in the nucleus pulposus, such that both degenerative and calcified IVDs have decreased MR signal intensity [22, 26–29]. That is, MRI detects a spectrum of IVD degeneration but cannot differentiate between calcified and non-calcified degenerative discs, compared to radiography and CT which can only detect disc calcification as an indicator of (advanced) degeneration. IVD degeneration in the canine spine can be reliably graded using low-field MRI and the Pfirrmann classification system, which is based on lumbar IVD degeneration in people and has been verified with the gross pathology-based Thompson system [30–33].

The precision of CT and MRI scoring of IVD calcification in Dachshunds has not been assessed. Thus, the objectives of this study were to: (i) compare the precision of three diagnostic imaging modalities (radiography, CT and MRI) by estimating their repeatability and reproducibility, (ii) estimate and compare the robustness (i.e. scorer independence) of each modality, and (iii) estimate the agreement across the three modalities for the detection of IVD calcification. It was anticipated that both CT and MRI would be more precise than radiography due to the cross-sectional nature of these modalities. However, it was expected that MRI would not completely agree with the two other modalities because this modality assesses various stages of IVD degeneration, not only calcification.

## Methods

### Study subjects

Dogs were prospectively recruited from Finnish Dachshund breeders through The Dachshund Club of Finland, between 22 November 2011 and 7 March 2012. Eligibility criteria included: purebred registered Standard Dachshund dog, young adult age (24–48 months old), and clinically healthy. Dogs were excluded if they had prior or current signs of intervertebral disc disease (IVDD) or other illness. Dogs were enrolled in the study with informed owner consent and the study was approved and conducted with animal ethics approval.

#### *Diagnostic imaging*

The imaging was performed at the University of Helsinki Veterinary Teaching Hospital. Three diagnostic imaging modalities were employed to image the dogs' spines—radiography, CT scanning and low-field MRI (Fig. 1). All imaging was performed within a single hospital visit, with the dogs under heavy sedation or general anaesthesia. Radiography and CT were conducted on all dogs, while MRI was optional and based on owner preference given it would substantially prolong anaesthetic time for an elective procedure.

**Radiography**

Lateral radiographs of the cervical, thoracic and lumbar spine regions were obtained for each dog using a previously described protocol [20] and a digital radiographic system (CPI Indico 100, Ontario, Canada). A minimum of five diagnostic quality radiographs were acquired for each dog.

**Computed tomography**

CT was performed using a 2-slice helical scanner (Siemens Somatom Emotion Duo, Forchheim, Germany) with the following scan parameters: 100 mA, 110 kV, 1.0 mm acquisition slice thickness, feed/rotation 2 mm, rotation time 0.8 s, reconstruction interval 0.5 mm, bone algorithm (WL, 500; WW, 3500). CT scanner limitations (i.e. excess tube heat) did not allow for scanning of the entire spine. The thoracolumbar spine was of greatest interest due to the propensity for clinical IVDD in this region. Therefore, T5-L7 (or a portion thereof) was scanned in all dogs. Where possible, the cervicothoracic (C6-T2) and/or the lumbosacral (L7-S1) spine junctions were also scanned; these regions were selected as they are anecdotally challenging to score radiographically for IVD calcification due to issues with superimposition of anatomy.

**Magnetic resonance imaging**

MRI studies of the thoracolumbar spine were obtained using a low-field scanner (Vet-MR 0.23T, Esaote S.p.A,

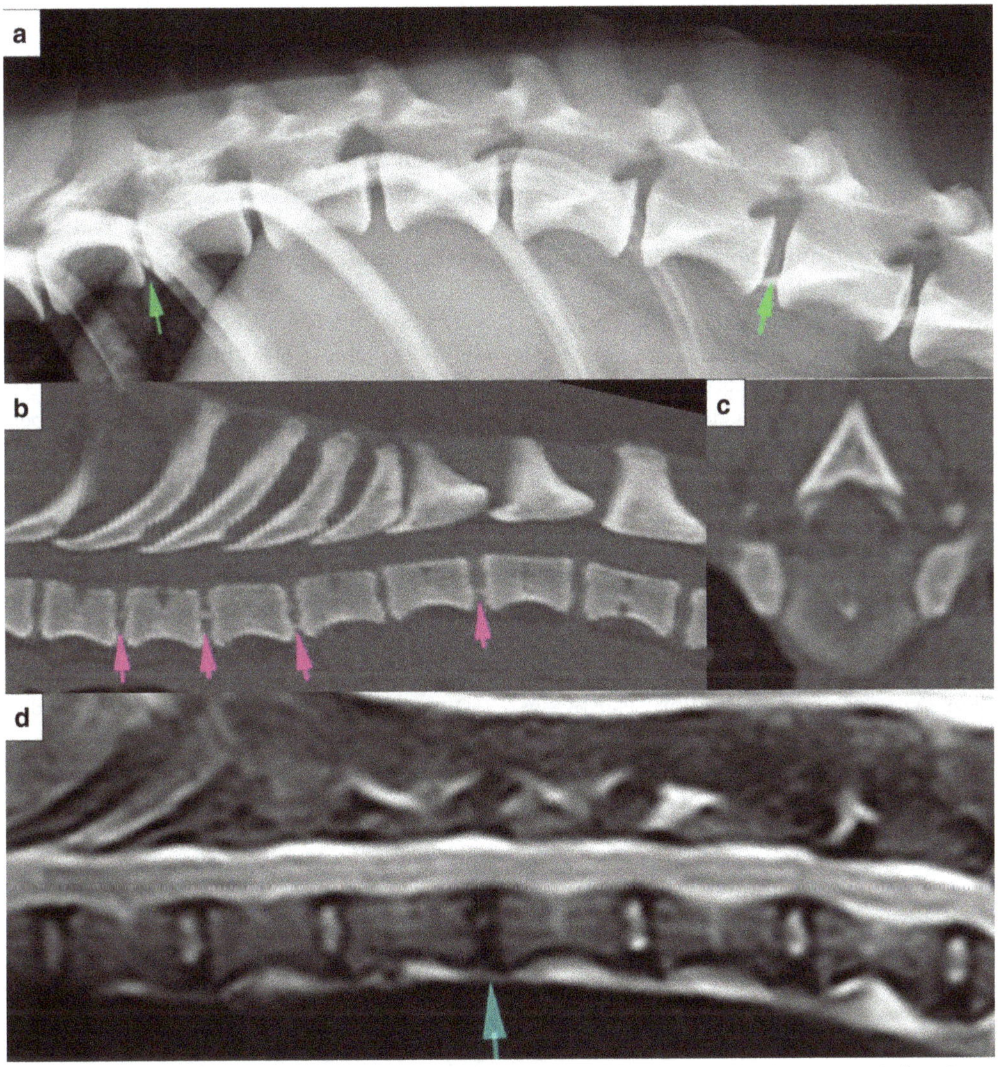


**Fig. 1** Example radiographic (**a**), CT (**b, c**) and MR (**d**) images obtained for intervertebral disc (IVD) scoring (not necessarily from the same Dachshund). The images are centered on the caudal thoracic spine. Example intervertebral disc calcifications are indicated on the lateral spinal radiograph (**a**; green arrows), and on the sagittal (**b**; pink arrows) and transverse (**c**) CT images which are displayed in a bone window. On the T2W sagittal MR image (**d**), the blue arrow indicates an MRI Pfirrmann grade 3 degenerative IVD. *CT* computed tomography, *MRI* magnetic resonance imaging

Genoa, Italy) and the following pulse sequences: sagittal plane T1W (TR, 510; TE, 18), sagittal plane T2W (TR, 2800; TE, 80), and transverse plane T1W (TR, 830; TE, 18). As with the CT imaging, the limitations of using a low-field magnet (specifically, acquisition time) did not allow for imaging of the entire spine, so the thoracolumbar spine (T5-S1, or part thereof) was scanned, being the region of greatest clinical interest.

### Scoring

Three veterinarians who all had diagnostic imaging backgrounds and training, but varying levels of RDIDC scoring experience, performed the scoring of the intervertebral discs. All cases were duplicated, coded (with individual identifying information removed from the images), and randomly ordered prior to distribution to ensure blinding of the scorers. The imaging studies were viewed in Digital Imaging and Communications in Medicine (DICOM) format using OsiriX image viewing software (Pixmeo, Geneva, Switzerland) and high resolution/brightness, commercial-grade monitors, with freedom to post-process images as preferred by the individual.

Each radiographic study was scored for the presence or absence of IVD calcification. The CT cases were distributed 1 month after the radiographic scoring had been completed to facilitate scorer blinding. The subjective presence or absence of IVD calcification was recorded, as was scorer confidence in their decision and approximate percentage of calcification of the total disc cross-sectional area (in 10% increments, 0–100%). Again, MRI cases were distributed 1 month after all scorers had completed the CT scoring. Based primarily on the sagittal T2W images [32], IVDs were graded for any sign of degeneration (i.e. not specifically calcification) following the Pfirrmann classification scheme [30, 33], which uses visual analysis of the IVD structure, distinction between nucleus pulposus and annulus fibrosis, MR signal intensity, and height of the IVD, to grade a disc on a scale of 1 (normal) to 5 (severe degeneration). Scorers were provided with example images and written description of the characteristics of each grade, as a reference. The scorers recorded results for each imaging study using custom scoring templates, as per a previous study [20]. Scoring decisions were made by independent opinion. Observers were aware that the dogs were clinically healthy but were otherwise blinded to patient details and other identifiers.

### Statistical analysis

Scores were collected, collated and formatted using Microsoft Excel (Microsoft Corporation, Redmond, WA, USA). An IVD score was classified as positive for calcification when calcification ($\geq$ 10% of IVD area) was observed (radiographs and CT) or when the Pfirrmann grade was $\geq$ 3 (MRI), and classified as negative otherwise. Analyses for study objectives (i) and (iii) were conducted using the statistical package Stata version 14.2 (Stata Corp, College Station, TX, USA), and analysis for objective (ii) was conducted using the phylogenetic package MEGA version 7 [34].

### Modalities' precision (repeatability and reproducibility)

Precision was evaluated by estimating the repeatability and reproducibility of the three modalities. For a given modality, repeatability was estimated as the proportion of pairs of scores that agreed within a given scorer. The reproducibility was measured as the proportion of pairs of scores that agreed between two scorers. To compare precision across modalities, separate datasets and logistic models were developed for repeatability and reproducibility. The datasets were reformatted in a long format with each observation reporting an agreement (coded as "1") or a disagreement (coded as "0") between two scorer iterations for a given dog's IVD from a same scorer (repeatability dataset) or from two separate scorers (reproducibility dataset) of a given modality. Covariate factors included dog, IVD, modality, and scorer for each observation. Given that agreement observations were clustered within IVDs and IVDs were clustered within dogs, random effects for dog and IVD were added to the models to account for the lack of independence across observations. Also, given that the study dogs and their IVDs were scored up to 6 times by a same scorer (clustered within scorers), scorer was included as a random effect cross-classified with dog and IVD. When modeling reproducibility, models with cross-classified structure could not converge and the reproducibility was modeled using scorers' pair, dog, and IVD random effect without cross-classification. Repeatability and reproducibility across modalities were estimated and compared by including modality as a fixed effect in the respective models.

The direct interpretation of the models' coefficients (intercepts and/or effect coefficient), ignoring random effects, provides cluster-specific estimates of agreement. To obtain average estimates across dogs, scorers and IVDs (i.e. population-averaged interpretation), cluster-specific predicted agreements and the limits of the 95% confidence interval were converted to population-averaged values using the following approximation formula [35]:

$$Prob(agreement) \approx logit^{-1}\Big(\big(\beta_0 + \beta_1 Modality\big) / \sqrt{\Big(1 + 0.346 * \big(\sigma^2_{scorer} + \sigma^2_{dog} + \sigma^2_{IVD}\big)\Big)}\Big) \quad (1)$$

where $\beta_0$ is the model intercept coefficient; $\beta_1$ *Modality* is the modality fixed effect (radiography set as default category); $\sigma^2_{scorer}$, $\sigma^2_{dog}$ and $\sigma^2_{IVD}$ are the scorer, dog and IVD within dog random effect variance, respectively; and $\text{logit}^{-1}$ is the inverse of the logit function ($logit^{-1}(x) = 1/(1+e^{-x})$). Post-regression inferences were two-sided and adjusted using the Bonferroni method (alpha, set at 5%, divided by the number of pairwise comparisons between modalities, $\text{alpha}_{\text{Bonferroni}} = 1.7\%$).

#### Modalities' robustness (scorer independence)

The ruggedness of a test is defined as the capacity of the test to resist expected variation across users [36]. In other words, ruggedness measures how dependent the outcome of the test is on the person running or interpreting the test. Here, the ruggedness of each modality was investigated by determining the existence of scorer subjectivity when interpreting IVDs using a diagnostic imaging test. Similar to a previous report [20] and following the principle of a cluster analysis, distance-based Neighbor-Joining phylograms were built from an alignment of IVD scores (IVDs in columns and scoring iterations in rows) to identify the presence of iteration cluster(s) corresponding to distinct scoring patterns. If the two scoring iterations from a same scorer cluster together, there is evidence that the scoring from this scorer is distinct from the other scorers. To assess the robustness of the node linking two iterations together, bootstrap support values (proportion of resampled trees that include the node of interest) were generated using bootstrap-resampling 1000 times and reported as a percentage on the nodes of the original tree [37]. A node with a bootstrap support value of $\geq 70\%$ was considered robust. The advantage of this approach is that it accounts for both the quantitative distance and the qualitative pattern across scoring iterations.

#### Agreement across modalities

Agreement across modalities was estimated as the proportion of pairs of scores between modalities' iterations that agreed within a given scorer. Comparisons between scorer iterations were ignored to exclude between-scorer effect. The same data structure, model building, and population-averaged interpretation as for repeatability and reproducibility were used. Agreement across modalities was explored across all MRI Pfirrmann grade cut-offs (i.e. $\geq 1$ to $= 5$).

## Results

### Study subjects

Twenty-one young adult (age range, 26–45 months; median, 30 months; SD, 4.8 months) Dachshund dogs were recruited. The study population was relatively homogeneous, with dogs being intact females (n = 10), intact males (9), neutered female (1) and neutered male (1); breed variants being standard long-haired (11) or standard wire-haired (10); and dogs weighing 7.6–12.6 kg (mean, 9.8 kg; SD, 1.3 kg).

#### Precision and robustness of each modality

A summary of the score for each available IVD in each dog, for each scorer, each iteration and each modality, is presented in Fig. 2. Estimates and 95% confidence intervals (95% CI) of repeatability (within-scorer agreement) and reproducibility (between-scorer agreement) are reported (Table 1).

#### Radiography

Except for the C2-3 IVD of dogs #4 and #21 (Fig. 2), all 26 potential IVDs from the 21 participating dogs (544 IVDs in total) were examined radiographically by each of the three scorers, two times independently (total, 3264 scores). The repeatability of radiography was slightly higher than its reproducibility suggesting at first little scorer effect (Table 1). However, the phylogram (distance tree) of IVD scoring using radiography identified three clear clusters, corresponding to each individual scorer, supported by high bootstrap values (>70%) (Fig. 3). This revealed that each scorer had a scoring pattern that was unique enough to be discriminated from the other scorers. The length of the branches between two iterations reflects the amount of disagreement between these iterations (i.e. the shorter the branch length, the stronger the agreement between two iterations). Within each scorer, the distance between the iterations of scorer B were clearly longer than for scorers A and C, showing a lower repeatability for scorer B. Across scorers, scorer B was further away from the other two scorers corresponding to poorer reproducibility for this scorer.

(See figure on next page.)

**Fig. 2** Scoring alignment of individual intervertebral discs (IVDs) scored (column) by each scorer (A, B and C) for each iteration (1 and 2) and each modality (X-ray, CT and MRI) (row). The intervertebral discs (IVDs) of each of the 21 participating Dachshund dogs are ordered per their location in the vertebral column i.e. position 1 (C2-3) to 26 (L7-S1). An "a" codes for a negative score, a "g" codes for a positive score, a "dot" codes for a score that agrees with the first row (X-ray iteration 1 of scorer A), and a "blank" codes for an absent IVD score due to missing data. "X-ray" denotes radiography; "CT" denotes computed tomography; "MRI" denotes magnetic resonance imaging

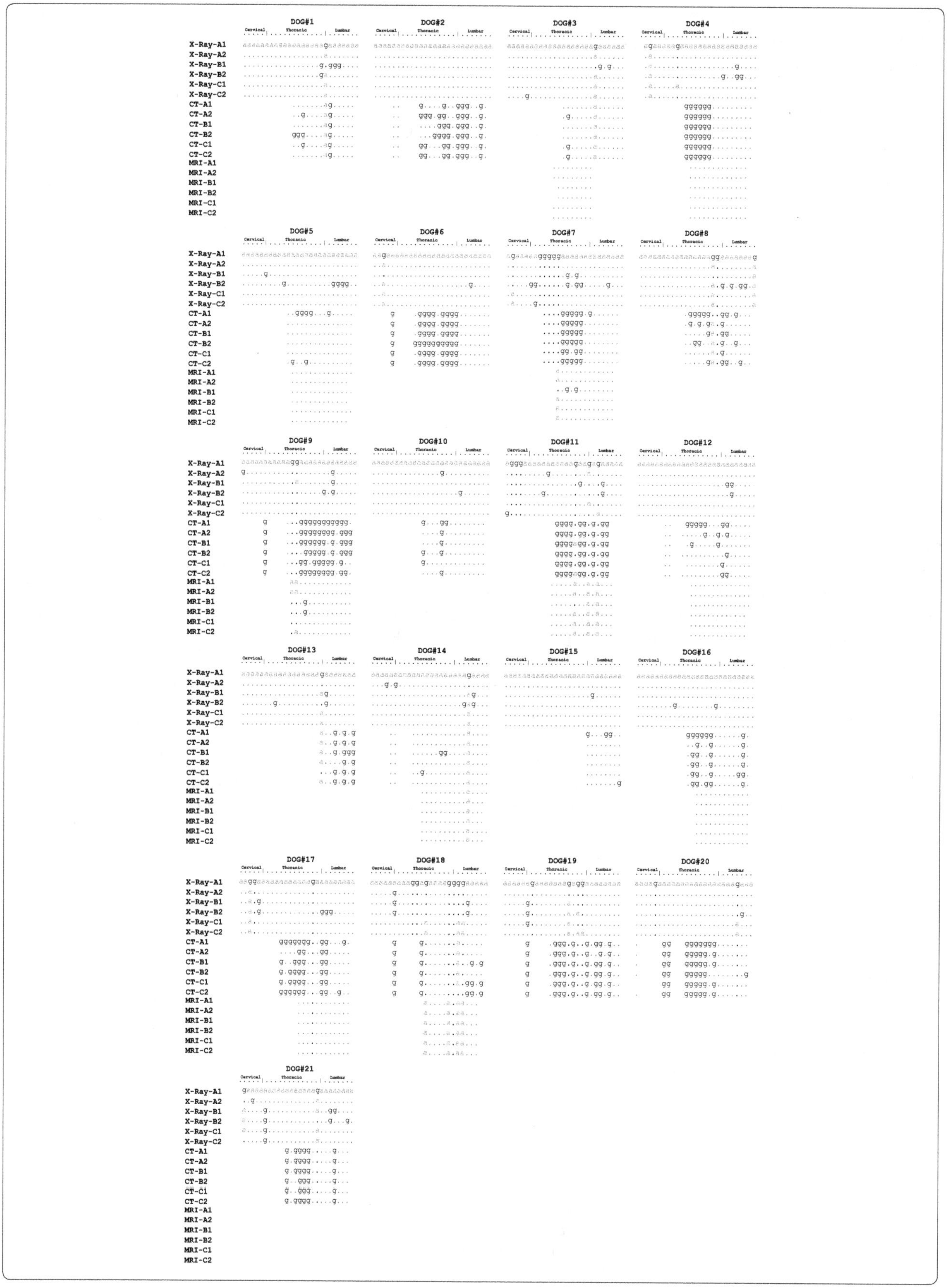
DOG#1
DOG#2
DOG#3
DOG#4
DOG#5
DOG#6
DOG#7
DOG#8
DOG#9
DOG#10
DOG#11
DOG#12
DOG#13
DOG#14
DOG#15
DOG#16
DOG#17
DOG#18
DOG#19
DOG#20
DOG#21
Cervical
Thoracic
Lumbar
X-Ray-A1
X-Ray-A2
X-Ray-B1
X-Ray-B2
X-Ray-C1
X-Ray-C2
CT-A1
CT-A2
CT-B1
CT-B2
CT-C1
CT-C2
MRI-A1
MRI-A2
MRI-B1
MRI-B2
MRI-C1
MRI-C2

**Table 1 Imaging modalities' repeatability and reproducibility**

| Modality | Repeatability (95% CI) | Reproducibility (95% CI) |
|---|---|---|
| Radiography | 95.4%$^{b}$ (92.4–97.3) | 92.9%$^{c}$ (67.8–98.8) |
| CT | 90.4%$^{a}$ (84.8–94.1) | 89.4%$^{c}$ (62.8–97.7) |
| MRI | 93.8%$^{a,b}$ (88.9–96.6) | 86.4%$^{c}$ (60.4–96.4) |

Model estimates of the repeatability and reproducibility for intervertebral disc (IVD) calcification scoring by radiography, computed tomography (CT) and magnetic resonance imaging (MRI) (interpreted as positive if MRI Pfirrmann grade ≥3), with 95% confidence intervals reported in brackets. Within a column, different superscript letters indicate significant differences between modalities

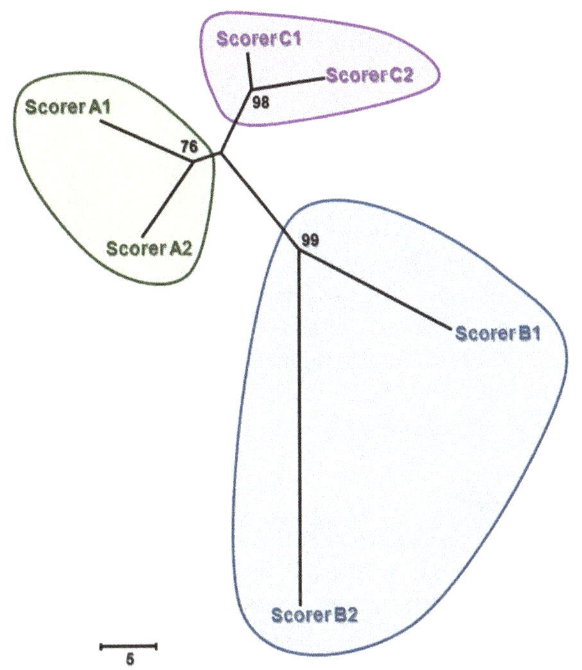


**Fig. 3** Phylogram demonstrating the agreement within and between scorers for radiographic scoring of intervertebral disc (IVD) calcification in 21 Dachshunds. The length of the branches between different scorers (A, B, C) represent the disagreement between scorers. The length of the branches between two scorer iterations (1, 2) represents the within-scorer disagreement. The scale is based on the number of differing scores out of the 544 IVDs assessed by an individual scorer. Numerical bootstrap values indicate strength. Scale bar = 5 IVD scoring differences

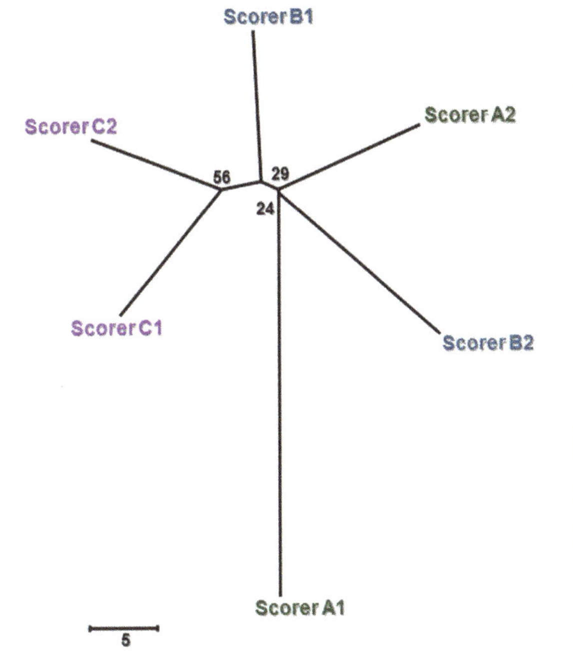


**Fig. 4** Phylogram demonstrating the agreement within and between scorers for computed tomographic (CT) scoring of intervertebral disc (IVD) calcification. The length of the branches between two scorer iterations (1, 2), and between each of the three scorers (A, B, C), represents the within-scorer disagreement and between-scorer disagreement, respectively. The scale is based on the number of differing scores out of the 314 IVDs assessed by an individual scorer. Numerical bootstrap values indicate strength. Scale bar = 5 IVD scoring differences

### Computed tomography

Only a fraction of the IVDs (range, 8 to 19 per dog) were scanned using CT, providing a total of 314 IVDs scored. Overall, a total of 1880 CT scores were obtained from the six scoring iterations, with four scores missing (Fig. 2). The reproducibility of CT for scoring IVD calcification approximated its repeatability, which suggested no scorer effect (Table 1). Indeed, the CT phylogram (Fig. 4) indicated no evidence of clear clusters (all bootstrap values <70%), confirming a lack of evidence of scorer effect (subjectivity) with CT. The distances between iterations within a scorer and between scorers were similar but long, producing a starfish-shaped tree. This reflects lower within-scorer agreement (repeatability) across all scorers compared to radiography, which subsequently resulted in lower between-scorer agreement (reproducibility).

### Magnetic resonance imaging

MRI scans were only available for 11 of the participating dogs and, at most, 14 IVDs per dog were examined. Overall, 142 IVDs were scored with a total of 840 MRI scores obtained from the six scoring iterations. The repeatability of MRI was moderately higher than its reproducibility (Table 1). The MRI phylogram (Fig. 5) identified one strong cluster (bootstrap value 100%) corresponding to scorer B. This suggested that scorer B's interpretation of MR images was significantly different from the other two scorers (i.e. lower reproducibility for this scorer). The distance between the iterations within scorer B were also

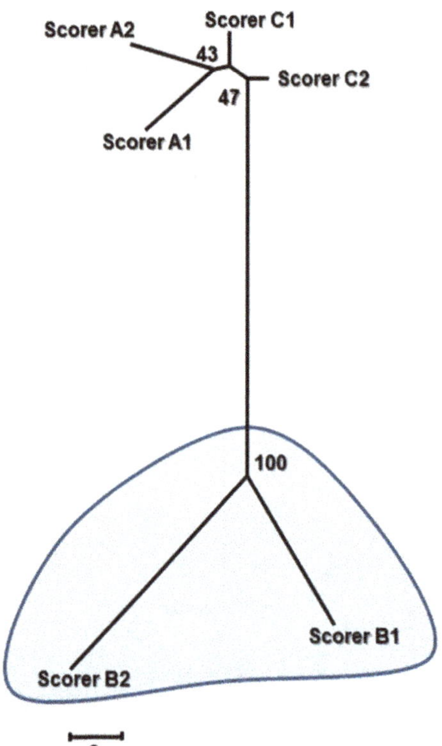


**Fig. 5** Phylogram demonstrating the agreement within and between scorers for magnetic resonance imaging (MRI) scoring of intervertebral disc (IVD) calcification. The length of the branches between two scorer iterations (1, 2), and between each of the three scorers (A, B, C), represents the within-scorer disagreement and between-scorer disagreement, respectively. The scale is based on the number of differing scores out of the 142 IVDs assessed by an individual scorer. Numerical bootstrap values indicate strength. Scale bar = 2 IVD scoring differences

clearly longer compared to the iterations within each of the other two scorers, reflecting a lower repeatability for scorer B.

### Comparison of modalities' precision

Across the three diagnostic imaging modalities, radiography showed the highest repeatability (95.4%) for scoring IVD calcification, and was significantly higher than CT (90.4%) but not significantly higher than MRI (93.8%) (Table 1). There was no significant difference in reproducibility across the three modalities; however, a trend was present with decreasing between-scorer agreement for radiography, followed by CT and then MRI (92.9, 89.4 and 86.4%, respectively).

### Agreement between modalities

Of all three modalities, considerably more IVD calcification was identified by CT (38.8% of all CT scores were positive for calcification) than radiography (8.2% of all radiography scores) and MRI (11.6% of all MRI scores interpreted at Pfirrmann Grade ≥ 3). Regardless of the Pfirrmann grade cut-off used to binarize data into a 'positive' or 'negative' score for IVD calcification, CT moderately agreed with radiography (approximately 65% agreement) (Table 2). Agreement between MRI and the other two modalities substantially increased at the Pfirrmann grade cut-off ≥ 3 and was highest at the cut-off ≥ 4. However, agreements between modalities at the cut-offs between ≥ 3 and = 5 approximated. At cut-off ≥ 4, MRI and radiography agreed 85.4% of the time (95% CI 80.3–89.3%), while MRI and CT agreed 64.9% of the time (95% CI 56.5–72.4%).

## Discussion

Due to the heritability of IVDD and IVD calcification in Dachshunds, selective breeding is important to reduce transmission to offspring [11, 14, 38]. Scoring IVDs for calcification is a reliable predictor of future IVDD development [18], and IVD calcification is currently screened for using conventional radiography. It was predicted that CT and MRI would provide better precision (repeatability and reproducibility) and less subjectivity than radiography when scoring for IVD calcification, as these cross-sectional imaging modalities reduce the confounding effects of anatomic superimposition and provide superior contrast resolution [25]. Despite expectations, neither the repeatability nor reproducibility of CT or MRI was better than the repeatability and reproducibility

**Table 2 Agreement between scoring modalities relative to MRI Pfirrmann grade cut-off**

| Compared modalities | Pfirrmann grade ≥ 1 | Pfirrmann grade ≥ 2 | Pfirrmann grade ≥ 3 | Pfirrmann grade ≥ 4 | Pfirrmann grade = 5 |
|---|---|---|---|---|---|
| Radiography vs. CT | 64.2% (58.5–69.4) | 64.4% (58.5–69.9) | 65.6% (58.0–72.5) | 67.0% (59.0–74.2) | 67.1% (58.9–74.3) |
| Radiography vs. MRI | 20.1% (16.2–24.6) | 46.4% (40.1–52.8) | 80.8% (75.1–85.4) | 85.4% (80.3–89.3) | 83.9% (78.1–88.2) |
| CT vs. MRI | 45.9% (39.9–52.0) | 51.1% (44.6–57.5) | 62.8% (54.8–70.0) | 64.9% (56.5–72.4) | 62.8% (54.2–70.7) |

Model estimates (95% CI) of pairwise agreement between scoring modalities for each MRI Pfirrmann grade cut-off used to binarize data into a 'positive' or 'negative' score for intervertebral disc (IVD) calcification

*CT* computed tomography, *MRI* magnetic resonance imaging

of radiography. While the repeatability of MRI was similar to that of radiography, the repeatability of CT was significantly less. The reproducibility of both CT and MRI were less than that of radiography, however these were not significantly different. As anticipated for all modalities, estimates of repeatability were higher than estimates of reproducibility, although the two values were very similar for CT. The similar repeatability and reproducibility for CT indicates a lack of individual scorer subjectivity for this modality. Challenges with scoring IVD calcification using CT could have been due to less experience and/or training using this method of screening compared to radiography. Further, CT detected substantially greater overall numbers of calcified IVDs than the other modalities, including discs with smaller total proportion of calcification. This may have led to decreased scorer confidence in assigning a positive or negative score to a given IVD and thus greater variability between scoring iterations.

While the repeatability and reproducibility estimates were similar for both radiography and CT, MRI showed a larger discrepancy between repeatability and reproducibility. The lower level of reproducibility for MRI could be explained by the clear difference in scoring pattern of scorer B compared to scorers A and C (Fig. 5). It is unclear which of the scorers were scoring most correctly (i.e. accurately); regardless, it could be concluded that a degree of difficulty arose when using MRI to screen for IVD calcification, possibly attributable to a lack of experience or training using MRI and the Pfirrmann grading system. On the other hand, our findings are similar to those of others who have evaluated the reliability of the Pfirrmann MRI classification system [30, 33, 39]. When the system was initially evaluated in people, the intra- and inter-observer agreement yielded average kappa scores of 0.88 and 0.77, respectively, with percentage agreements that approximated our results (90.8% and 83.0%, respectively) [33]. A subsequent reliability study was conducted using a modified Pfirrmann grading system, and the intra- and inter-reader agreement remained good but comparatively less (Avg. K scores, 0.86 and 0.66, respectively; Avg. % agreement, 84.9% and 66.8%, respectively) [39]. Variable intra- and inter-observer agreement for scoring canine IVDs for degeneration using the Pfirrmann grading system has been identified (K score range, 0.58 to 0.93) [30, 40]. We chose not to use conventional kappa values because of the recognised limitations of this method including its sensitivity to prevalence [41], which limits direct comparison between our agreement estimates and the kappa results obtained in earlier studies.

The Pfirrmann grading system is based on identifying progressive phases of IVD degeneration [30, 33], not specifically IVD calcification. Although this means that our estimates of agreement for scoring IVD calcification between the different modalities cannot be considered equal, a cut-off Pfirrmann grade $\geq 3$ was selected to assign a 'positive' score for IVD calcification on MRI. We chose this cut-off as grades of 3, 4 and 5 are assigned to IVDs with changes (reduced MR signal intensity and distinction between nucleus pulposus and annulus fibrosus) that would be expected with more severe IVD degeneration, potentially including some degree of calcification [32, 42]. Further, it is recognised that discriminating between Pfirrmann grades 1 and 2, and between grades 3 and 4, can be challenging and subjective [30, 33, 39], supporting the choice to categorise scores of $\leq 2$ as negative and $\geq 3$ as positive for calcification. The agreement estimates between modalities at cut-off $\geq 3$ approximated those at cut-offs $\geq 4$ and $= 5$ (Table 2).

The recommendation that RDIDC scoring be performed by experts is further supported by the higher precision found in this study for scorers that had specific experience in diagnostic imaging, compared to our prior study using a heterogeneous group of scorers with variable backgrounds [20]. Based on the agreement estimates identified herein, the chance of every IVD within a given dog being scored identically when evaluated twice by the same person (repeatability) is 29.4% ($0.954^{26}$), compared to 12.5% seen previously [20]. Similarly for reproducibility, when a given dog is scored twice by two different scorers the chance of every IVD within that dog being identically scored is 14.7% ($0.929^{26}$), compared to 5.1%. These calculations assume complete independence of individual IVD scoring, which is the worst-case scenario.

Radiography was the only modality of the three to show a clear scorer pattern (i.e. subjectivity), demonstrated as three distinct scoring clusters (Fig. 3). These findings agree with those from our earlier work [20]. The scorer-dependent patterns demonstrated in that study were attributed to scorer differences that might be explained by variation in scoring ability and experience (general practitioner, specialist radiologist, and expert scorer). Comparatively, in the present experiment the scorers had a more similar background and training in diagnostic imaging; therefore, the observed subjectivity is less likely to be attributed to scorer ability but instead may be due to distinct individual scoring styles that could feasibly develop with greater experience. Nevertheless, of the three modalities evaluated, radiography provides consistently higher within- and between-scorer agreement across all 26 potential IVDs, and when the highest level of precision in IVD calcification scoring is desired, radiography should be considered above CT and MRI.

The agreement estimates across the three modalities showed that MRI and radiography agreed more with each other than CT did with either modality. More agreement between radiography and CT might be initially expected as both modalities assess IVD calcification specifically, whereas MRI scoring is based on a wider spectrum of IVD degeneration. However, the lack of modality agreement between radiography and CT, and MRI and CT, is likely due to the substantially larger number of IVD calcifications detected using CT versus the other two modalities. The potential benefits of this higher detection rate using CT need further investigation. Although the relatively good agreement between radiography and low-field MRI (85.7%) could make MRI an acceptable alternative to RDIDC scoring when performed by an individual who is experienced using the Pfirrmann grading system, MRI is substantially more expensive and time consuming to perform than radiography, making it an impractical screening tool for dog breeders.

The results of this study suggest that further insight into the accuracy of each modality is required before considering replacement of radiography with CT or MRI for IVD calcification screening in Dachshunds. As might be expected, the three modalities appeared to detect distinct features of IVD degeneration. While it seems that radiography is the best method of IVD screening in terms of precision, it is suspected that CT is in fact scoring more correctly—that is, CT is more accurate—than radiography and MRI, resulting in the disagreement of CT scores with radiography and MRI. Use of a modified Pfirrmann grading system that is more discriminatory in determining severity of disc degeneration, such as the one developed for elderly people [39], may be warranted in Dachshunds. If CT or MRI were shown to be more accurate than radiography, any gains achieved would need to be balanced with the increased cost, reduced access to the modality in veterinary practice, and overall feasibility for breeders.

Potential limitations of this study might be related to the CT and MRI equipment used, as whole dog spines could not be imaged because of technical limitations, thereby reducing the number of IVDs that were sampled and scored. However, the total number of scores obtained for each modality by the duplicate iterations for each of three scorers was sufficiently high for analysis at the individual IVD level. Analysis of scorer precision at the whole dog level was not performed due to the aforementioned limitations. Further, low-field MRI has known limitations in terms of image quality compared to high-field MRI; nevertheless, the literature indicates that low-field MRI is suitable for grading IVD degeneration in dogs [28, 30–32]. The moderately inconsistent number and position of IVDs imaged by the various modalities in different dogs could have caused human counting error when identifying which IVD was being scored at a given time. However, visual examination of the score summary diagram (Fig. 2) did not identify patterns suggestive of frequent counting or localisation errors.

## Conclusions

While it might be anticipated that more advanced screening modalities, namely CT and MRI, would improve diagnosis of IVD calcification compared to radiographic scoring, this study did not find any improvement in repeatability or reproducibility of those modalities. If an alternative modality were to replace radiography, training in modality-specific scoring should be implemented to increase within- and between-scorer agreement and test robustness. With correct scorer instruction, CT and MRI have the potential to increase the precision of IVD calcification screening. However, it is important to first evaluate the accuracy of CT and MRI to provide appropriate recommendations regarding which, if any, of the alternative modalities should replace radiography for the screening of IVD calcification in Dachshunds.

### Abbreviations

CT: computed tomography; IVD: intervertebral disc; IVDD: intervertebral disc disease; MRI: magnetic resonance imaging; RDIDC: radiographically detectable intervertebral disc calcification.

### Authors' contributions

AR is the primary investigator, collected data, was a scorer in the study, contributed to data interpretation, and was a major contributor to manuscript writing. AL developed the study topic, was the key facilitator in data collection, and was a scorer in the study. NJ assisted data collation and statistical analysis, and contributed to manuscript writing. NW was a scorer in the study, contributed to experimental methodology, and reviewed the manuscript. CC contributed to study design, performed data analysis and interpretation, and contributed to manuscript writing. All authors read and approved the final manuscript.

### Author details

[1] School of Animal and Veterinary Sciences, The University of Adelaide, Roseworthy Campus, Adelaide, SA 5005, Australia. [2] Faculty of Veterinary Medicine, University of Helsinki, Viikki Campus, Agnes Sjöberginkatu 2, 00014 Helsinki, Finland. [3] Darkroom Veterinary Imaging, 7/489A Warrigal Rd, Moorabbin, VIC 3189, Australia. [4] Present Address: School of Veterinary Science, The University of Queensland, Gatton, QLD 4343, Australia.

### Acknowledgements

Not applicable.

### Competing interests

The authors declare that they have no competing interests.

### Funding

The authors would like to thank The Faculty of Veterinary Medicine at the University of Helsinki, The School of Animal and Veterinary Sciences at the University of Adelaide, and The Dachshund Club of Finland, for their financial support of the project.

## References


1. Bergknut N, Egenvall A, Hagman R, Gustas P, Hazewinkel HA, Meij BP, et al. Incidence of intervertebral disk degeneration-related diseases and associated mortality rates in dogs. J Am Vet Med Assoc. 2012;240:1300–9.
2. Simpson ST. Intervertebral disc disease. Vet Clin North Am Small Anim Pract. 1992;22:889–97.
3. Packer RM, Seath IJ, O'Neill DG, De Decker S, Volk HA. DachsLife 2015: an investigation of lifestyle associations with the risk of intervertebral disc disease in Dachshunds. Canine Genet Epidemiol. 2016;3:8.
4. Hansen HJ. A pathologic-anatomical study on disc degeneration in dog, with special reference to the so-called enchondrosis intervertebralis. Acta Orthop Scand. 1952;11(Suppl):1–17.
5. Verheijen J, Bouw J. Canine intervertebral disc disease: a review of etiologic and predisposing factors. Vet Q. 1982;4:125–34.
6. Scott HW. Hemilaminectomy for the treatment of thoracolumbar disc disease in the dog: a follow-up study of 40 cases. J Small Anim Pract. 1997;38:488–94.
7. Aikawa T, Fujita H, Kanazono S, Shibata M, Yoshigae Y. Long-term neurologic outcome of hemilaminectomy and disk fenestration for treatment of dogs with thoracolumbar intervertebral disk herniation: 831 cases (2000–2007). J Am Vet Med Assoc. 2012;241:1617–26.
8. Lappalainen AK, Vaittinen E, Junnila J, Laitinen-Vapaavuori O. Intervertebral disc disease in Dachshunds radiographically screened for intervertebral disc calcifications. Acta Vet Scand. 2014;56:89.
9. Rosenblatt AJ, Bottema CD, Hill PB. Radiographic scoring for intervertebral disc calcification in the Dachshund. Vet J. 2014;200:355–61.
10. Havranek-Balzaretti B: Beitrag zur Aetiologie der Dackellahme und Vorschlag zur zuchterischen Selektion. (The etiology of intervertebral disc disease in the Dachshund and the proposal of an eradication programme). Inaugural Dissertation. Universitat Zurich, Switzerland, Veterinar-Chirurgischen Klinik und Institut fur Veterinar-patologie; 1980.
11. Jensen VF, Christensen KA. Inheritance of disc calcification in the dachshund. J Vet Med A. 2000;47:331–40.
12. Mogensen MS, Karlskov-Mortensen P, Proschowsky HF, Lingaas F, Lappalainen A, Lohi H, et al. Genome-wide association study in dachshund: identification of a major locus affecting intervertebral disc calcification. J Hered. 2011;102(Suppl 1):81–6.
13. Mogensen MS, Scheibye-Alsing K, Karlskov-Mortensen P, Proschowsky HF, Jensen VF, Bak M, et al. Validation of genome-wide intervertebral disk calcification associations in dachshund and further investigation of the chromosome 12 susceptibility locus. Front Genet. 2012;3:225.
14. Lappalainen AK, Maki K, Laitinen-Vapaavuori O. Estimate of heritability and genetic trend of intervertebral disc calcification in Dachshunds in Finland. Acta Vet Scand. 2015;57:78.
15. Stigen O. Calcification of intervertebral discs in the dachshund: a radiographic study of 115 dogs at 1 and 5 years of age. Acta Vet Scand. 1996;37:229–37.
16. Lappalainen A, Norrgard M, Alm K, Snellman M, Laitinen O. Calcification of the intervertebral discs and curvature of the radius and ulna: a radiographic survey of Finnish miniature dachshunds. Acta Vet Scand. 2001;42:229–36.
17. Rohdin C, Jeserevic J, Viitmaa R, Cizinauskas S. Prevalence of radiographic detectable intervertebral disc calcifications in Dachshunds surgically treated for disc extrusion. Acta Vet Scand. 2010;52:24.
18. Jensen VF, Beck S, Christensen KA, Arnbjerg J. Quantification of the association between intervertebral disk calcification and disk herniation in Dachshunds. J Am Vet Med Assoc. 2008;233:1090–5.
19. Jensen VF, Arnbjerg J. Development of intervertebral disk calcification in the dachshund: a prospective longitudinal radiographic study. J Am Anim Hosp Assoc. 2001;37:274–82.
20. Rosenblatt AJ, Hill PB, Davies SE, Webster NS, Lappalainen AK, Bottema CD, et al. Precision of spinal radiographs as a screening test for intervertebral disc calcification in Dachshunds. Prev Vet Med. 2015;122:164–73.
21. Stigen O, Kolbjornsen O. Calcification of intervertebral discs in the dachshund: a radiographic and histopathologic study of 20 dogs. Acta Vet Scand. 2007;49:39.
22. Modic MT, Masaryk TJ, Ross JS, Carter JR. Imaging of degenerative disk disease. Radiology. 1988;168:177–86.
23. Hecht S, Thomas WB, Marioni-Henry K, Echandi RL, Matthews AR, Adams WH. Myelography vs. computed tomography in the evaluation of acute thoracolumbar intervertebral disk extrusion in chondrodystrophic dogs. Vet Radiol Ultrasound. 2009;50:353–9.
24. Dennis R. Optimal magnetic resonance imaging of the spine. Vet Radiol Ultrasound. 2011;52:S72–80.
25. Robertson I, Thrall DE. Imaging dogs with suspected disc herniation: pros and cons of myelography, computed tomography, and magnetic resonance. Vet Radiol Ultrasound. 2011;52:S81–4.
26. Levitski RE, Lipsitz D, Chauvet AE. Magnetic resonance imaging of the cervical spine in 27 dogs. Vet Radiol Ultrasound. 1999;40:332–41.
27. Sharp NJH, Wheeler SJ, editors. Diagnostic aids. In: Small animal spinal disorders—diagnosis and surgery. 2nd ed. Edinburgh: Elsevier Mosby; 2005. p. 41–64.
28. Karkkainen M, Punto LU, Tulamo RM. Magnetic resonance imaging of canine degenerative lumbar spine diseases. Vet Radiol Ultrasound. 1993;34:399–404.
29. Tertti M, Paajanen H, Laato M, Aho H, Komu M, Kormano M. Disc degeneration in magnetic resonance imaging. A comparative biochemical, histologic, and radiologic study in cadaver spines. Spine. 1991;16:629–34.
30. Bergknut N, Auriemma E, Wijsman S, Voorhout G, Hagman R, Lagerstedt AS, et al. Evaluation of intervertebral disk degeneration in chondrodystrophic and nonchondrodystrophic dogs by use of Pfirrmann grading of images obtained with low-field magnetic resonance imaging. Am J Vet Res. 2011;72:893–8.
31. Bergknut N, Grinwis G, Pickee E, Auriemma E, Lagerstedt AS, Hagman R, et al. Reliability of macroscopic grading of intervertebral disk degeneration in dogs by use of the Thompson system and comparison with low-field magnetic resonance imaging findings. Am J Vet Res. 2011;72:899–904.
32. Seiler G, Hani H, Scheidegger J, Busato A, Lang J. Staging of lumbar intervertebral disc degeneration in nonchondrodystrophic dogs using low-field magnetic resonance imaging. Vet Radiol Ultrasound. 2003;44:179–84.
33. Pfirrmann CW, Metzdorf A, Zanetti M, Hodler J, Boos N. Magnetic resonance classification of lumbar intervertebral disc degeneration. Spine. 2001;26:1873–8.
34. Tamura K, Stecher G, Peterson D, Filipski A, Kumar S. MEGA6: molecular evolutionary genetics analysis version 6.0. Mol Biol Evol. 2013;30:2725–9.
35. Dohoo I, Martin W, Stryhn H. Screening and diagnostic tests. In: Margaret McPike S, editor. Veterinary epidemiologic research. 2nd ed. Charlottetown: VER Inc.; 2009. p. 99–127.
36. Manual of Diagnostic Tests for Terrestrial Animals. 12 rue de Prony, 75017 Paris, France. World Organisation for Animal Health: OIE (Office International des Epizooties); 2009.
37. Felsenstein J. Confidence limits on phylogenies: an approach using the bootstrap. Evolution. 1985;39:783–91.
38. Stigen O, Christensen K. Calcification of intervertebral discs in the dachshund: an estimation of heritability. Acta Vet Scand. 1993;34:357–61.
39. Griffith JF, Wang YX, Antonio GE, Choi KC, Yu A, Ahuja AT, et al. Modified Pfirrmann grading system for lumbar intervertebral disc degeneration. Spine. 2007;32:708–12.
40. Harder L, Ludwig D, Galindo-Zamora V, Wefstaedt P, Nolte I. Classification of canine intervertebral disc degeneration using high-field magnetic resonance imaging and computed tomography. Tierarztl Prax K H. 2014;42:374–82.
41. Byrt T, Bishop J, Carlin JB. Bias, prevalence and kappa. J Clin Epidemiol. 1993;46:423–9.
42. Sether LA, Nguyen C, Yu SW, Haughton VM, Ho KC, Biller DS, et al. Canine intervertebral disks—correlation of anatomy and MR Imaging. Radiology. 1990;175:207–11.

# Bronchopneumonia in Swedish lambs: a study of pathological changes and bacteriological agents

Lisa Lindström*, Felicia Asp Tauni and Karin Vargmar

**Abstract**

**Background:** One of the most common post-mortem inspection finding of sheep and lambs in Sweden, following routine slaughter is pneumonia and its prevalence is increasing. To our knowledge, the aetiology of pneumonia in lambs is not well-known for Swedish conditions. Chronic bronchopneumonia, also known as "atypical" or chronic non-progressive pneumonia, is a common disease worldwide, affecting lambs up to 12 months old. It is therefore of interest to elucidate if this disease complex is also a common cause of pneumonia among Swedish lambs. Chronic bronchopneumonia has a characteristic macroscopic and histopathologic appearance, and *Mycoplasma ovipneumoniae* is the microbial agent most frequently found. Although this bacterium is important for the pathogenesis, multiple agents are presumed to be involved. The aim of this study was to describe the macroscopic and histopathologic lung lesions in routinely slaughtered lambs with pneumonia, and to determine the bacterial agents involved.

**Results:** A total of 41 lungs with gross lesions consistent with pneumonia were examined. Of these, 35 lungs displayed the typical gross appearance of chronic bronchopneumonia, with several or all of the characteristic histological features. *M. ovipneumoniae* was detected in 83% of the 35 lungs and *Mannheimia haemolytica* was isolated in 71%. Pneumonia associated with *M. ovipneumoniae* could be correlated to specific gross lesions consistent with the gross description of chronic bronchopneumonia in lambs.

**Conclusion:** In this study, chronic bronchopneumonia was the most common lung disease in routinely slaughtered Swedish lambs. This diagnosis was based on the characteristic macroscopic and histopathologic pulmonary findings and the frequent presence of the bacterium *M. ovipneumoniae*. The macroscopic appearance of chronic bronchopneumonia could therefore be used during routine investigation of the lamb carcasses at slaughter, to determine the most likely cause of pneumonia.

**Keywords:** Chronic bronchopneumonia, Atypical pneumonia, Lamb, *Mycoplasma ovipneumoniae*, Respiratory disease

## Background

Swedish lamb production is growing, with both the number of animals and farmers steadily increasing. Although Swedish sheep and lambs are generally healthy, pneumonia and pleuritis are two of the most common findings during routine slaughter of lambs. The prevalence of these illnesses increased from 1.2% in 2005 to 2.8% in 2015 [1]. Between 2011 and 2013 Gård and Djurhälsan (Farm and Animal Health) financed 2200 necropsies of sheep and lambs. They showed that 20% of the sheep and 15% of the lambs (2–12 months old) suffered from pneumonia [2]. However, since the data were collected from animals sent for necropsy, it could be assumed that they had presented with severe signs of disease, had a therapeutic failure, or had been found dead. To our knowledge, the aetiology causing pneumonia in lambs is not well-known for Swedish conditions.

*Correspondence: lisa.lindstrom@slu.se
Department of Biomedical Sciences and Veterinary Public Health, Faculty of Veterinary Medicine and Animal Science, Swedish University of Agricultural Sciences (Ulls väg 26), 757 56 Uppsala, Sweden

In lambs that are up to 12 months old, chronic bronchopneumonia (also called atypical pneumonia, chronic non-progressive bronchopneumonia, and mycoplasmosis), is a common, often subclinical disease, worldwide. Multiple infectious agents are implicated, including *Mycoplasma ovipneumoniae, Mannheimia haemolytica*, and possible viral agents, like parainfluenza type 3 virus, and respiratory syncytial virus [3–5]. *M. ovipneumoniae* is the agent most frequently found [6–8]. Thus, it can be assumed to play an important role in the pathogenesis of atypical pneumonia. *M. ovipneumoniae* is mainly transmitted via the respiratory tract through close contact between the animals [6], and lambs are infected within a few days of birth [4]. The bacteria can be isolated in the respiratory tract of healthy animals, suggesting it is part of the normal bacterial flora [9, 10]. However, primary infection with the bacteria might predispose invasion by other organisms, such as *M. haemolytica* [6, 10]. *M. ovipneumoniae* can predispose to secondary infection by producing hydrogen peroxide, causing ciliostasis [11] and facilitating the mycoplasma infection. The pathogenesis of *M. ovipneumoniae* involves a polysaccharide capsule, which could promote adherence of the organisms to the ciliated epithelium, thus promoting bacterial colonization [12, 13]. Furthermore, the polysaccharide capsule may have cytotoxic effects on the epithelial cells, inducing apoptosis [14, 15], which would also contribute to the pathogenesis of the disease. *Mycoplasma* spp. lack cell walls, making the bacteria resistant to penicillin, so treatment would require broad-spectrum antibiotics [16, 17]. Because of the risk of antibiotic resistance, unnecessary use of antibiotics should be avoided. Stress, poor air quality and adverse weather conditions may also contribute to the development of the disease [3, 6]. Apart from the effect on the individual animal's health, chronic bronchopneumonia has economic impacts due to reduced growth rates in the lambs [18–20].

Chronic bronchopneumonia causes lesions in the cranial lung lobes. These can be observed as red-brown discolorations with clearly demarcated regions of consolidation and occasional pleuritis [6, 21, 22]. The typical finding in histopathological examinations is a chronic active inflammation. It is characterized by lymphoid proliferation around airways, bronchiolar epithelial hyperplasia, neutrophil accumulation in airspaces, and the unique lesion of hyaline scars. The hyaline scars consist of nodular masses of collagen and fibroblasts in the wall of bronchioles that protrude into the lumen [3, 22, 23].

In Sweden, all lungs from sheep and lambs rejected at slaughter are coded with one of three specific codes representing the cause of pneumonia. These are: lesion from lungworm (code 73/74), pleuritis and pericarditis (code 75/76) and "other pneumonia" (code 63/64). Previously there was also a code for chronic bronchopneumonia or "mycoplasma-like pneumonia" (code 61/62). It was assigned to lungs with a gross appearance of moderate pneumonia in at least three lung lobes, or severe pneumonia in one lung lobe. However, this code is no longer in use.

Studies from other countries have shown that chronic bronchopneumonia is common in slaughtered lambs [6, 7, 24]. Therefore, it is of interest to investigate if the disease complex is also common in the Swedish lamb population. The aim of this study was to investigate the bacterial agents found in lungs with pneumonia detected at routine slaughter of lambs, and to describe the macroscopic and histopathological appearance of the lesions. The study also aimed to elucidate if the macroscopic appearance of chronic bronchopneumonia could establish the cause of disease when applied to Swedish flocks. If it can be determined during routine investigations of carcasses at slaughter the farmer would gain valuable information about flock health and it would contribute to national disease surveillance.

## Methods

### Sample collection

During the period of September–October 2016, all lamb lungs with pneumonic lesions at post-mortem inspection were collected from two slaughterhouses located in the province of Uppland, Sweden. In total, 44 sets of lungs with lesions were collected. Of these, 41 had gross lesions suggestive of pneumonia and were included in the study. The lungs were stored at maximum +4 °C until starting the examination and sampling, which were performed within 2 days of slaughtering. The lambs in the study passed the ante-mortem inspection performed by a veterinarian. Therefore, it was assumed that the animals had shown few or no clinical signs of disease prior to slaughter. No details of the sex, breed or husbandry conditions were available.

### Pathological investigation

The pulmonary lesions were photographed and described using the following attributes: distribution, demarcation, contour, shape, colour, size, texture, consistency, and extent. A schematic illustration was used to get an objective estimate of the extent of consolidation (Fig. 1). The affected areas were marked with red, and the graphics editor GNU Image Manipulation Program (GIMP 2.10.2) was used to calculate the areas of the red markings. The pneumonia was then scored as mild, moderate, or severe, depending on the extent of the consolidation. If $< 10\%$ was affected the pneumonia was scored as mild, 10–20% as moderate and $> 20\%$ as severe. The same categories were used by Sheehan et al. [24]. Type 1 lungs were classified as having at least the right cranial lung lobe exhibiting the following attributes: well-demarcated homogeneous consolidation, red-brown discolorations, and meaty consistency. These lesions are characteristic of chronic bronchopneumonia [6, 22]. The lungs with lesions that did not fit the description were grouped as Type 2. Representative samples of grossly affected lung tissue were fixed in 10% buffered formalin.

The formalin fixed tissue was embedded in paraffin and cut in 4-μm sections. These were stained with haematoxylin and eosin and examined with light microscopy. If fibrosis was suspected, the slides were stained with Masson's trichrome [25]. The histopathological investigations were blinded. Thus, no information about the gross appearance of the lungs or microbiological results were available at the time of histopathological examination. General characteristics of the inflammatory process that were recorded included pattern, chronicity, and extent of the lesion. It was also recorded if there was pleuritis, hyperplasia of the bronchiolar epithelium, hyperplasia of lymphoid tissue, exudate in the lumen of the airways, or hyaline scars.

### Microbiological investigation

Affected lung tissue, (usually the right cranial lobe) was cut, using a sterile scalpel. Thereafter a Liquid-based Collection and Transport System (E-Swab, COPAN Diagnostics) was used to collect samples from the lung parenchyma at the cut surface. One E-swab was used for bacterial isolation and one for detection of mycoplasma by polymerase chain reaction (PCR).

The bacterial isolations were performed at the diagnostic laboratory at SVA (the Swedish National Veterinary Institute) using accredited methods including bacterial culture for MALDI-TOF MS (Matrix Assisted Laser Desorption Ionization Time-of-Flight Mass Spectrometry) (Bruker Daltonic GmbH, Bremen, Germany). The analyses started within 24 h of sample collection. The laboratory was requested to pay particular attention to any growth of *Pasteurella multocida, M. haemolytica, and Bibersteinia trehalosi* and an antimicrobial susceptibility test was performed on collected bacterial agents. The same breakpoints for resistance were used as in the report from the Swedish Veterinary Antimicrobial Resistance Monitoring [26]. One of the samples taken from the cut surface using the Liquid-based Collection and Transport System (E-Swab) was sent to the Animal and Plant Health Agency (Department of Bacteriology, Mycoplasma Group, Weybridge, UK) where the PCR detection of *Mycoplasma* spp. was performed [27].

### Statistics

The statistical analyses were done at SLU (Swedish University of Agricultural Sciences) Centre for Statistics using Fischer's exact test (SAS® System for Windows, version 9.3; SAS Institute Inc., Cary, NC, USA) and the result was interpreted as significant at a P-value of $<0.05$.

## Results

### Pathological investigation

#### *Gross pathological investigation*

During the sampling period, a total of 44 lamb lungs displayed signs of lung pathology and were collected from the slaughterhouses. Three lungs did not show the characteristics of pneumonia and were excluded from the study. The gross appearances for the remaining 41 lungs were described and the extent of the consolidated area

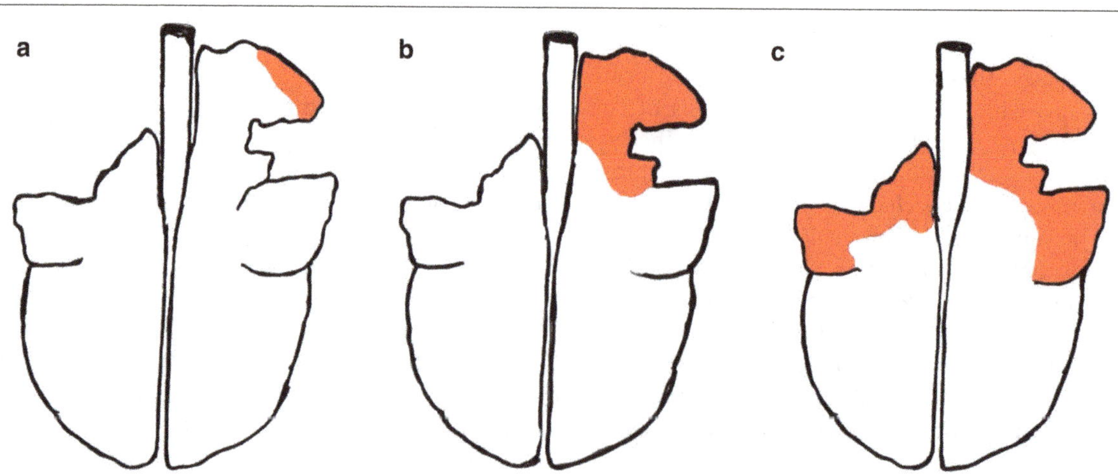


**Fig. 1** Examples of the grading system of the pneumonia. **a** Less the 10% of the tissue affected, pneumonia scored as mild. **b** 10–20% of the tissue affected, pneumonia scored as moderate. **c** More than 20% of the tissue affected, pneumonia scored as severe

was calculated to evaluate the severity. The severity of the pneumonia was scored as mild in 12%, moderate in 73%, and severe in 17% of the lungs. Examples of the grading system are demonstrated in Fig. 1.

Out of the 41 lungs, 35 showed well demarcated consolidated areas with cranial distribution affecting one or several lobules. The lesions were red-brown to purple-grey and had a firm, meaty consistency. The texture was solid, and the cut surfaces varied from dark red and oedematous to greyish and firm, occasionally with pale grey areas (Fig. 2a, b). In five cases multifocal abscesses were observed (Fig. 2b). All 35 lungs fitted the classification criteria of Type 1. The gross appearances of Type 1 lesions were consistent with the characteristics of chronic bronchopneumonia [3, 6, 23]. Out of the 41 lungs, six did not fulfil the Type 1 criteria and were therefore classified as Type 2. For example, the Type 2 lungs had lesions with multifocal distribution affecting both cranial and caudal lung lobes (Fig. 2c), and lesions mainly affecting subpleural areas of the lungs (Fig. 2d). Out of the 41 lungs, 19 (46%) had grossly visible pleuritis (Fig. 2e), and in 25 (61%) clearly visible mucous to mucopurulent exudate was present in the airways (Fig. 2f). The macroscopic appearances are summarised in Table 1.

### Histopathological investigation

All 41 lung slides were dominated by severe consolidation (Fig. 3a). The inflammation was interpreted as either chronic or chronic active. Apart from consolidation, the most common findings were bronchiolar epithelial hyperplasia (98%), peribronchial/peribronchiolar lymphoid hyperplasia (98%), and exudate dominated by neutrophils within the airspaces (95%) (Fig. 3a, b). Hyaline scars were observed in 14 lungs (34%) (Fig. 3c). The scars were most easily detected with the Masson's trichrome stain (Fig. 3d). Pleuritis was evident in 28 of the lungs (68%), and in most, it was mild and chronic.

Other, less frequently observed lesions, included proliferation of type II pneumocytes and bronchiectasis. An incidental finding was present in one lung; it had remnants of lungworms but with no inflammatory lesions

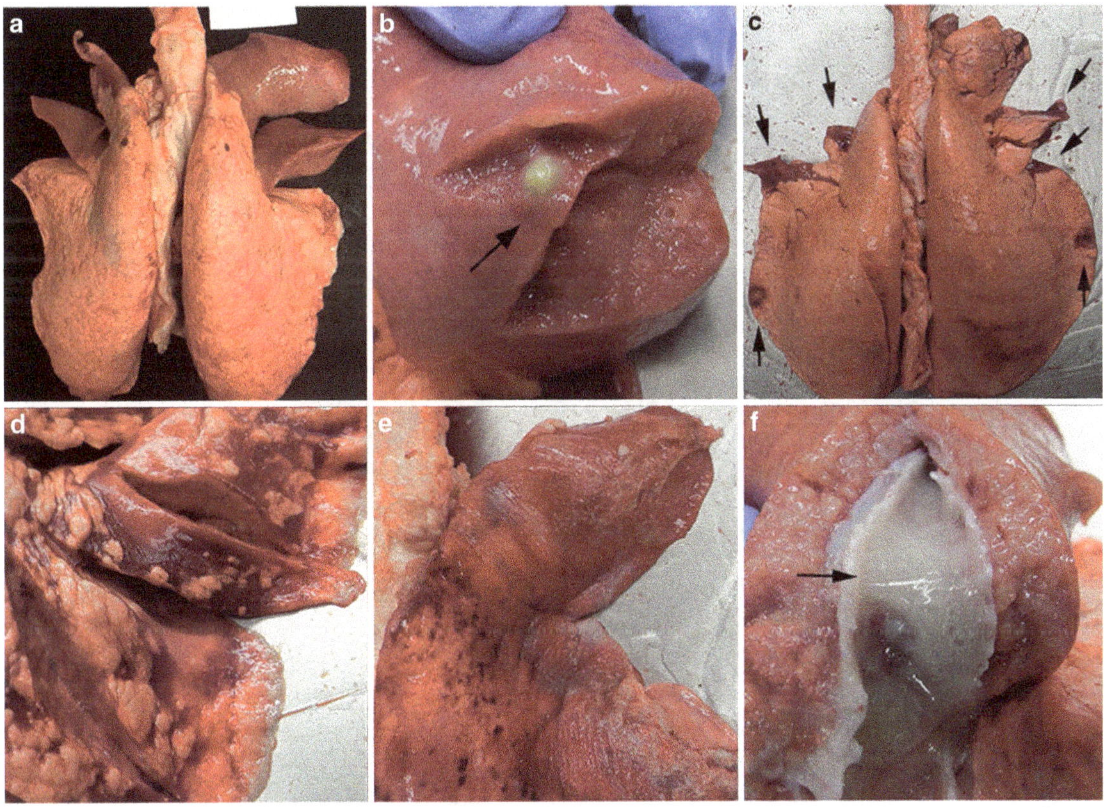


**Fig. 2** Examples of macroscopic lesions in the lungs. **a** Type 1 lung. Well-demarcated consolidated areas and red-grey discoloration affecting the cranial lung lobes, lung number 1. **b** Type 1 lung. Well-demarcated consolidated areas and red-grey discoloration and abscess (black arrow), lung number 19. **c** Type 2 lung. Multifocal consolidated areas affecting both cranial and caudal lung lobes (black arrows), lung number 6. **d** Type 2 lung. Mainly subpleural consolidation of the tissue, lung number 9. **e** Pleuritis, lung number 8. **f** Mucopurulent exudate within airways (black arrow), lung number 18

**Table 1 Summary of pathological and microbiological findings**

| No. | Gross pathology | | | | | Histopathology | | | | | Microorganisms | | |
|---|---|---|---|---|---|---|---|---|---|---|---|---|---|
| | S | T | GPI | GEx | Ab | HPI | EH | LH | HEx | HS | Isolation | PcS | Myc PCR |
| 1 | sev | 1 | − | + | − | − | + | + | + | + | *M.h* | S | *M.o* |
| 2 | sev | 1 | + | + | + | + | + | + | + | + | − | | − |
| 3 | mod | 2 | − | + | − | − | + | + | + | + | *S.e* | S | *M.o, M.a* |
| 4 | mod | 1 | − | + | − | − | + | + | + | − | *M.h* | S | *M.o* |
| 5 | mod | 1 | − | − | − | − | + | + | + | − | − | | − |
| 6 | mod | 2 | − | − | + | − | − | + | − | − | − | | − |
| 7 | mod | 1 | − | − | − | + | + | + | + | − | *M.h* | S | *M.o* |
| 8 | sev | 1 | + | + | − | + | + | + | + | + | *M.h* | S | *M.o* |
| 9 | mld | 2 | + | − | − | + | + | + | + | − | − | | − |
| 10 | mod | 1 | + | + | − | + | + | + | + | + | *M.h* | S | *M.o* |
| 11 | sev | 1 | − | + | − | + | + | + | + | − | − | | *M.o* |
| 12 | mod | 1 | − | − | − | + | + | + | + | − | *M.h* | S | *M.o* |
| 13 | mld | 1 | + | + | − | + | + | − | + | − | − | | *M.o* |
| 14 | mld | 1 | + | − | − | + | + | + | + | − | − | | *M.o* |
| 15 | mod | 1 | + | + | − | + | + | + | + | − | *M.h* | S | *M.o* |
| 16 | mld | 2 | + | − | − | + | + | + | − | − | − | | − |
| 17 | mod | 1 | + | − | − | + | + | + | + | − | *M.h* | S | *M.o* |
| 18 | mod | 1 | − | + | − | + | + | + | + | − | *M.h* | S | *M.o* |
| 19 | mod | 1 | + | + | + | + | + | + | + | − | − | | *M.o* |
| 20 | mod | 2 | − | − | − | + | + | + | + | − | − | | − |
| 21 | sev | 1 | + | + | − | + | + | + | + | − | − | | − |
| 22 | mod | 1 | − | + | − | − | + | + | + | + | *M.h* | S | *M.o, M.a* |
| 23 | mod | 1 | − | + | − | + | + | + | + | − | *M.h* | S | *M.o, M.a* |
| 24 | mod | 1 | − | − | − | − | + | + | + | + | − | | *M.o* |
| 25 | sev | 1 | − | − | − | − | + | + | + | − | *M.h* | S | *M.o* |
| 26 | mld | 2 | − | + | − | + | + | + | + | − | *M.h* | S | *M.o* |
| 27 | mod | 1 | + | + | − | − | + | + | + | − | *M.h* | S | *M.o, M.a* |
| 28 | mod | 1 | − | + | − | − | + | + | + | − | − | | *M.o* |
| 29 | sev | 1 | + | − | − | − | + | + | + | + | *M.h* | S | *M.o* |
| 30 | mod | 1 | + | + | + | + | + | + | + | + | *B.t* | S | *M.a* |
| 31 | mod | 1 | + | + | + | + | + | + | + | + | *M.h* | S | *M.a* |
| 32 | mod | 1 | − | + | − | + | + | + | + | + | *M.h* | S | *M.o* |
| 33 | mod | 1 | − | − | − | + | + | + | + | − | *M.h* | S | *M.o* |
| 34 | mod | 1 | + | − | − | + | + | + | + | − | *M.h* | S | *M.a* |
| 35 | mod | 1 | − | + | − | − | + | + | + | + | *M.h* | S | *M.o* |
| 36 | mod | 1 | − | + | − | − | + | + | + | − | *M.h* | S | *M.o* |
| 37 | mod | 1 | − | + | − | + | + | + | + | + | *M.h* | S | *M.o, M.a* |
| 38 | mod | 1 | − | − | − | + | + | + | + | − | *M.h* | S | *M.o* |
| 39 | mod | 1 | + | + | − | + | + | + | + | + | *M.h* | S | *M.o* |
| 40 | mod | 1 | + | − | − | + | + | + | + | − | *M.h* | S | *M.o* |
| 41 | mod | 1 | + | + | − | + | + | + | + | − | *M.h* | S | *M.o* |

S, severity of lesions; mld, mild; mod, moderate; sev, severe; T, type of appearance; 1, Type 1; 2, Type 2; +, present; −, absent; GPI, evidence of pleuritis at gross examination; GEx, signs of exudate in airways at gross examination; Ab, abscess; HPI, visible pleuritis in histopathological examination; EH, bronchiolar epithelial hyperplasia; LH, peribronchial/peribronchiolar lymphoid hyperplasia; HEx, Exudate whitin airways; HS, hyalin scar; Isolation, isolation of bacteria; PcS, penicillin sensitivity of isolated bacteria (S, sensitive); Myc PCR, Mycoplasma PCR; *M.h, M. haemolytica* isolated; *S.e, S. equisimilis* isolated; *B.t, B. trehalosi* isolated; *M.o, M. ovipneumoniae* detected; *M.a, M. arginini* detected

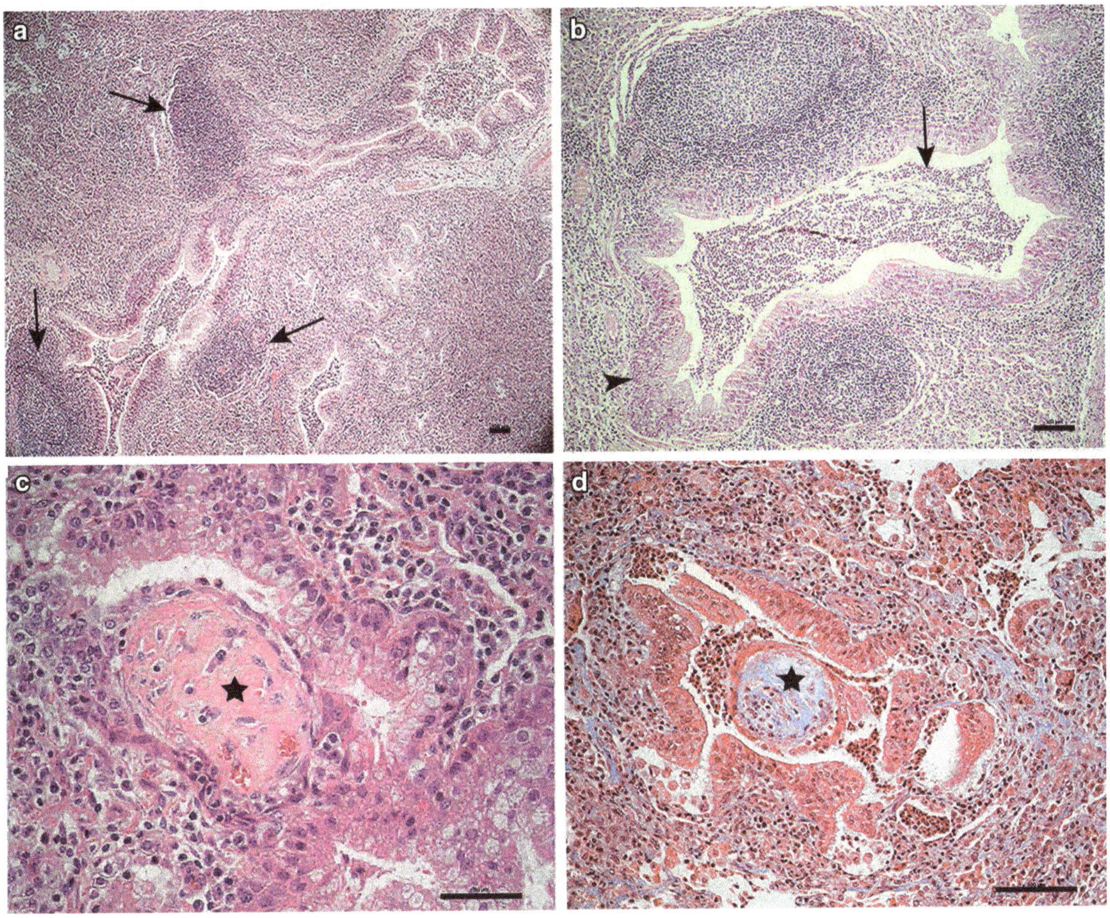


**Fig. 3** Examples of the histopathological changes in the lungs. **a** Severe consolidation of the tissue and lymphoid proliferation (black arrows) around airways, HE, bar 100 μm. **b** Hyperplasia of the bronchiolar epithelium (black arrowhead) and neutrophilic exudate within airspaces (black arrow) HE, bar 100 μm. **c** Hyaline scar (black star) HE, bar 50 μm. **d** Hyaline scar (black star). Masson Trichrome (connective tissue stains with blue colour), bar 100 μm

adjacent to the parasite. A summary of the results from the histopathological examination is presented in Table 1.

### *Microbiological investigation*

*Mycoplasma ovipneumoniae* was detected in 76% (31/41) and *Mycoplasma arginini* in 20% (8/41) of the lungs. *M. ovipneumoniae* was present in 83% (29/35) of the lungs classified as Type 1. *M. haemolytica* was isolated in 63% (26/41), always together with a *Mycoplasma* spp. (*M. ovipneumoniae* and/or *M. arginini*), most often with *M. ovipneumoniae*. *Streptococcus dysgalactiae* subsp. *equisimilis* was isolated from one lung.

Lungs number 30 and 31 had multiple abscesses. In these two cases, two samples were taken, one from the cut surface of the consolidated parenchyma and one from the abscess. In lung number 30, *M. arginini* was detected from the parenchyma and *B. trehalosi* was isolated from the abscess. In lung number 31, *M. haemolytica* was isolated and *M. arginini* was detected from the parenchyma. No specific bacterial agent could be isolated from the abscess.

In seven lungs (three Type 1 lungs, and four Type 2 lungs), no bacterial agent was found. The isolates of *M. haemolytica*, *B. trehalosi* and *S. dysgalactiae* found in the affected tissue were all sensitive to penicillin. A summary of the results from the microbiological investigation is presented in Table 1.

There was a statistically significant association between PCR positive samples for *M. ovipneumoniae* and the gross appearance classified as Type 1 (Fischer's exact test $P = 0.0217$). There was no significant association between *M. ovipneumoniae* and any of the specific histological attributes. No significant correlations were found between the presence of *M. haemolytica* and any of the gross or histopathological findings.

## Discussion

Out of the collected lungs, 85% were classified as Type 1, macroscopically suggestive of chronic bronchopneumonia. *M. ovipneumoniae* was the most frequent bacterium found (83%), followed by *M. haemolytica* (71%). These bacteria, particularly *M. ovipneumoniae*, are part of the aetiology of chronic bronchopneumonia in lambs [3, 6, 23], further supporting the diagnosis. Previous studies have pointed out that *M. ovipneumoniae* can be found in lungs without gross evidence of pneumonia. However, the prevalence of this bacterium is higher in diseased lungs [6, 7], and with larger amounts of bacteria [6, 22]. In our study, *M. ovipneumoniae* was detected using PCR, which does not provide information about the amount of bacteria in the affected tissue. Due to limited possibility for sampling of healthy lungs as paired controls, our study lacks information concerning prevalence. Nevertheless, *M. ovipneumoniae* was found in a high proportion of affected lungs, suggesting a non-negligible role in the disease complex. Type 1 lungs exhibited all, or several, of the histopathological lesions strongly associated with chronic bronchopneumonia including: lymphoid proliferation, bronchiolar epithelial hyperplasia, hyaline scars, and exudate in airways [22, 23].

Out of the six lungs classified as Type 2, *M. ovipneumoniae* was identified in two lungs, and in one of these in combination with *M. haemolytica*. During microscopic evaluation, all six cases exhibited several of the different histological lesions described in chronic bronchopneumonia. One cannot therefore exclude that those lungs, although lacking the typical gross appearance, represent this disease complex. The deviant gross appearance might represent older stages of a healing process. Furthermore, Type 2 lungs were an exclusion category, and other aetiologies are conceivable.

*Mycoplasma arginini* was present in 20% (8/41) of the lungs examined. In five cases it was found together with *M. ovipneumoniae* and *M. haemolytica*. In two cases it was found solely with *M. haemolytica*. Finally, it was found in the parenchyma of the single lung where *B. trehalosi* was isolated from an abscess. The pathogenicity of *M. arginini* is not completely known, and most often the organism is considered non-pathogenic [10, 28, 29]. The bacterium has been shown to cause elevation in rectal temperature, circulating monocytes, neutrophils and blood fibrinogen [28]. However, the bacterium did not induce any tissue lesion in the same study. In our study, *M. arginini* was observed in all of our cases in the presence of additional bacteria, supporting its role as a non- or minimally pathogenic bacterium.

Seven of the lungs in this study were found to have no bacterial agent. The gross classifications of these lungs were both of Type 1 (three lungs) and Type 2 (four lungs). Possible reasons could be that there were no viable bacteria in the sampled area, the sample handling had been inadequate, or the pneumonia was of viral aetiology. Chronic bronchopneumonia in lambs is described as a multifactorial disease and both parainfluenza virus type 3 and respiratory syncytial virus are suggested to be part of the aetiology. These viruses cause mild respiratory disease with fever, anorexia, and sporadic coughing [30]. Parainfluenza virus type 3 [30, 31] and respiratory syncytial virus are only reported to cause serious diseases in co-infections with additional pathogens [30]. Because of the suggested minor role of viruses, we decided to focus on bacterial agents, as these are believed to be the most important cause of disease. However, the lungs were not tested for viruses, so we cannot exclude that a concurrent viral infection may have contributed to some of the lung lesions.

The pneumonia was evaluated as moderate (73%) or severe (17%) in a high proportion of the lungs, and 95% had neutrophilic exudate within airspaces. This might have been a consequence of the common co-infection with *M. haemolytica*. *M. ovipneumoniae* causes mild suppuration [32] and in co-infection with *M. haemolytica*, the neutrophilic exudation is enhanced [21, 24]. The high incidence of pneumonic lesions classified as moderate or severe is noteworthy since the lambs passed the ante-mortem inspection and might reflect the difficulty in recognizing sick animals. This further highlights the importance of adequate post-mortem registration of lesions in disease surveillance.

## Conclusions

In this study, chronic bronchopneumonia was the most common lung disease in routinely slaughtered lambs in the province of Uppland, Sweden. In affected lungs, *M. ovipneumoniae* was a common pathogen and often occurred in combination with *M. haemolytica*. In the literature, these bacteria, in particular *M. ovipneumoniae*, are frequently associated with the disease complex [4, 6, 8]. A high proportion of the lungs showed the characteristic macroscopic appearance of chronic bronchopneumonia and the lungs exhibited all or several of the typical histological features described for the disease, further supporting the diagnosis. The macroscopic appearance of chronic bronchopneumonia could therefore be used as an indicator of the most likely cause of pneumonia during post-mortem investigation of the carcasses of Swedish lambs.

#### Authors' contributions

KV, LL and FAT planned the study design. FAT collected all lamb lungs from slaughterhouses. FAT examined, photographed, described and summarized the macroscopic and microscopic lung lesion in collaboration with LL and in part with KV. LL, KV and FAT analysed and interpreted the data. LL, KV and FAT wrote the manuscript. All authors read and approved the final manuscript.

**Acknowledgements**
The study was designed in collaboration with, and on request by Ulrika König at Gård & Djurhälsan (Farm and Animal Health), who came up with the initial idea for the project.

**Competing interests**
The authors declare that they have no competing interests.

**Funding**
The study was part of a Master thesis in veterinary medicine founded by the Swedish University of Agriculture Sciences. Bacteriological tests and histopathological laboratory work was financed by SvarmPat. SvarmPat is a programme run in collaboration between the Swedish National Veterinary Institute and Farm & Animal Health, and is financed by the Swedish Board of Agriculture.

**References**

1. Jordbruksverket statistikdatabas (statistical database) Jordbruksverket; 2018. http://statistik.sjv.se. Accessed 5 Sept 2018.
2. Lundström J. Vad hittar vi vid obduktioner hos får? In: Gård och Djurhälsan. 2015; http://www.gardochdjurhalsan.se/sv/far/kunskapsbank/artiklar/2015/e/642/vad-hittar-vi-vid-obduktioner-av-far. Accessed 5 Sept 2018.
3. Caswell JL, Williams KJ. Respiratory system: infectious respiratory diseases of sheep and goats. In: Grant Maxie M, editor. Jubb, Kennedy and Palmer's pathology of domestic animals, vol. 2. 6th ed. Missouri: Elsevier; 2016. p. 557–66.
4. Nicholas R, Ayling R, McAuliffe L. Respiratory disease of small ruminants. In: Nicholas R, Ayling R, McAuliffe L (eds) Mycoplasma diseases of ruminants. Wallingford: CABI; 2008. p. 169–98.
5. Sharp JM, Nettleton PF. Acute respiratory infections. In: Aitken ID, editor. Diseases of sheep. 4th ed. Oxford: Blackwell Publishing; 2007. p. 207–21.
6. Alley MR, Jones G, Clarke JK. Chronic non-progressive pneumonia of sheep in New Zealand—a review of the role of *Mycoplasma ovipneumoniae*. N Z Vet J. 1999;47:155–60.
7. Bakke T, Nøstvold S. An investigation of ovine pneumonia in four herds from Central Norway. I. Prevalence of pneumonia and microbiological findings. Acta Vet Scand. 1982;23:248–58.
8. Bakke T. The occurrence of mycoplasmas and bacteria in lungs from sheep in Southern Norway. Acta Vet Scand. 1982;23:235–47.
9. Brogden KA, Rose D, Cutlip RC, Lehmkuhl HD, Tully JG. Isolation and identification of mycoplasmas from the nasal cavity of sheep. Am J Vet Res. 1988;49:1669–72.
10. DaMassa J, Patricia S, Wakenell S, Brooks DL. Review article. Mycoplasma of goats and sheep. J Vet Diagn Invest. 1992;4:101–13.
11. Al-Kaissi A, Alley MR. Electron microscopic studies of the interaction between ovine alveolar macrophages and *Mycoplasma ovipneumoniae* in vitro. Vet Microbiol. 1983;8:571–84.
12. Niang M, Rosenbusch RF, Andrews JJ, Kaeberle ML. Demonstration of a capsule on *Mycoplasma ovipneumoniae*. Am J Vet Res. 1998;59:557–62.
13. Niang M, Rosenbusch RF, Debey MC, Niyo Y, Andrews JJ, Kaeberle ML. Field isolates of *Mycoplasma ovipneumoniae* exhibit distinct cytopathic effects in ovine tracheal organ cultures. Zentralbl Veterinarmed A. 1998;45:29–40.
14. Jiang Z, Song F, Li Y, Xue D, Zhao N, Zhang J, et al. Capsular polysaccaride of *Mycoplasma ovipneumoniae* induces sheep airway epithelial cell apoptosis via ROS-dependent JNK/P38 MAPK pathways. Oxid Med Cell Longev. 2017;5:1–15.
15. Xue D, Li Y, Jiang Z, Deng G, Li M, Liu X, et al. A ROS-dependent and Caspase-3-mediated apoptosis in sheep bronchial epithelial cells in response to *Mycoplasma ovipneumoniae* infections. Vet Immunol Immunopathol. 2017;187:55–63.
16. Radostits OM, Gay CC, Hinchcliff KW, Constable PD. Diseases associated with bacteria. In: Radostits OM, Gay CC, Hinchcliff KW, Constable PD, editors. Veterinary medicine, 10th edn. Philadelphia: Elsevier; 2007. p. 1124–5.
17. Scott PR. Treatment and control of respiratory disease in sheep. Vet Clin North Am Food Anim Pract. 2011;27:175–86.
18. Baird HJ, Clarke SM, Johnson PL. Brief communication: development of visual scoring system of ovine pneumonia at the processing plant. Proc N Z Soc Anim. 2012;72:169–71.
19. Goodwin KA, Jackson R, Brown C, Davies PR, Morris R, Perkins NR. Pneumonic lesions in lambs in New Zealand: patterns of prevalence and effect on production. N Z Vet J. 2004;52:175–9.
20. Jones GE, Field AC, Gilmour JS, Rae AG, Nettleton PF, McLauchland M. Effects of experimental chronic pneumonia on body weight, feed intake and carcass composition of lambs. Vet Rec. 1982;110:168–73.
21. Gilmour JS, Jones GE, Keir WA, Rae AG. Long-term pathological and microbiological progress in sheep of experimental disease resembling atypical pneumonia. J Comp Pathol. 1982;92:229–38.
22. Nøstvold S, Bakke T. An investigation of ovine pneumonia in four herds from Central Norway. II. Relation between pathomorphology and presence of micro-organisms. Acta Vet Scand. 1982;23:259–74.
23. Ruffin DC. Mycoplasma infections in small ruminants. Vet Clin North Am Food Anim Pract. 2001;17:315–32.
24. Sheehan M, Cassidy JP, Brady J, Ball H, Doherty ML, Quinn PP, et al. An aetiopathological study of chronic bronchopneumonia in lambs in Ireland. Vet J. 2007;173:630–7.
25. Lee GL. The manual of histological staining methods of the armed forces institute of pathology. 3rd ed. New York: McGraw-Hill Book company; 1968.
26. Swedish veterinary antimicrobial resistance monitoring. Swarm/swedres 2014. National Veterinary Institute. http://www.sva.se/en/antibiotics/svarm-reports. Accessed 5 Sept 2018.
27. McMauliffe L, Ellis RJ, Lawes, Ayling RD, Nicholas RA. 16S rDNA PCR and denaturing gradient gel electrophoresis; a single generic test for detecting and differentiating Mycoplasma species. J Med Microbiol. 2005;54:731–9.
28. Goltz JP, Rosendal S, McCraw BM, Ruhnke HL. Experimental studies on the Pathogenicity of *Mycoplasma ovipneumoniae* and *Mycoplasma arginine* for the respiratory tracts of goats. Can J Vet Res. 1986;50:59–67.
29. Lin YC, Miles RJ, Nicholas RAJ, Kelly DP, Wood AP. Isolation and immunological detection of *Mycoplasma ovipneumoniae* in sheep with atypical pneumonia, and lack of a role for *Mycoplasma arginini*. Res Vet Sci. 2008;84:367–73.
30. Robinson RA. Respiratory diseases of sheep and goats. Vet Clin North Am Large Anim Pract. 1983;5:539–55.
31. Davies DH, Jones BAH, Thurley DC. Infection of specific-pathogen-free lambs with para-influenza virus type 3, *Pasteurella haemolytica* and *Mycoplasma ovipneumoniae*. Vet Microbiol. 1981;6:295–308.
32. Foggie A, Jones GE, Buxton D. The experimental infection of specific pathogen-free lambs with Mycoplasma ovipneumoniae. Res Vet Sci. 1976;21:28–35.

# Permissions

All chapters in this book were first published in AVS, by BioMed Central; hereby published with permission under the Creative Commons Attribution License or equivalent. Every chapter published in this book has been scrutinized by our experts. Their significance has been extensively debated. The topics covered herein carry significant findings which will fuel the growth of the discipline. They may even be implemented as practical applications or may be referred to as a beginning point for another development.

The contributors of this book come from diverse backgrounds, making this book a truly international effort. This book will bring forth new frontiers with its revolutionizing research information and detailed analysis of the nascent developments around the world.

We would like to thank all the contributing authors for lending their expertise to make the book truly unique. They have played a crucial role in the development of this book. Without their invaluable contributions this book wouldn't have been possible. They have made vital efforts to compile up to date information on the varied aspects of this subject to make this book a valuable addition to the collection of many professionals and students.

This book was conceptualized with the vision of imparting up-to-date information and advanced data in this field. To ensure the same, a matchless editorial board was set up. Every individual on the board went through rigorous rounds of assessment to prove their worth. After which they invested a large part of their time researching and compiling the most relevant data for our readers.

The editorial board has been involved in producing this book since its inception. They have spent rigorous hours researching and exploring the diverse topics which have resulted in the successful publishing of this book. They have passed on their knowledge of decades through this book. To expedite this challenging task, the publisher supported the team at every step. A small team of assistant editors was also appointed to further simplify the editing procedure and attain best results for the readers.

Apart from the editorial board, the designing team has also invested a significant amount of their time in understanding the subject and creating the most relevant covers. They scrutinized every image to scout for the most suitable representation of the subject and create an appropriate cover for the book.

The publishing team has been an ardent support to the editorial, designing and production team. Their endless efforts to recruit the best for this project, has resulted in the accomplishment of this book. They are a veteran in the field of academics and their pool of knowledge is as vast as their experience in printing. Their expertise and guidance has proved useful at every step. Their uncompromising quality standards have made this book an exceptional effort. Their encouragement from time to time has been an inspiration for everyone.

The publisher and the editorial board hope that this book will prove to be a valuable piece of knowledge for researchers, students, practitioners and scholars across the globe.

# List of Contributors

**Trine Hammer Jensen, Mariann Chriél and Mette Sif Hansen**
National Veterinary Institute, Technical University of Denmark, Bülowsvej 27, 1870 Frederiksberg C, Denmark

**Trine Hammer Jensen**
Department of Chemistry and Bioscience, Aalborg University/Aalborg Zoo, Frederik Bajers Vej 7H, 9100 Aalborg, Denmark
Aalborg Zoo, Mølleparkvej 63, 9000 Aalborg, Denmark

**Efrem Degneh, Getachew Terefe and Hagos Ashenafi**
Department of Pathology and Parasitology, College of Veterinary Medicine and Agriculture, Addis Ababa University, Debre Zeit, Ethiopia

**Workineh Shibeshi**
Department of Pharmacology and Clinical Pharmacy, School of Pharmacy, College of Health Sciences, Addis Ababa University, Addis Ababa, Ethiopia

**Kaleab Asres**
Department of Pharmaceutical Chemistry and Pharmacognosy, School of Pharmacy, College of Health Sciences, Addis Ababa University, P.O.Box 9086, Addis Ababa, Ethiopia

**Adnan Hassan Tahir, Juan Wan, Manoj Kumar Shah, Habibullah Janyaro, Xiao-Jing Li and Ming-Xing Ding**
College of Veterinary Medicine, Huazhong Agricultural University, No. 1, Shizishan Street, Hongshan District, Wuhan, Hubei 430070, People's Republic of China

**Bernadette Earley**
Animal and Bioscience Research Department, Animal & Grassland Research and Innovation Centre, Teagasc, Grange, Dunsany, Co. Meath C15 PW93, Ireland

**John D. McNamara and Stephen J. Jerrams**
Centre for Elastomer Research (CER), School of Manufacturing and Design Engineering, Dublin Institute of Technology (DIT), Dublin, Ireland

**Edward G. O'Riordan**
Livestock Systems Research, Department Animal & Grassland Research and Innovation Centre, Teagasc, Grange, Dunsany, Co. Meath C15 PW93, Ireland

**Katarzyna Zabielska-Koczywąs, Anna Wojtalewicz and Roman Lechowski**
Department of Small Animal Diseases with Clinic, Faculty of Veterinary Medicine, Warsaw University of Life Sciences, Nowoursynowska 159c, 02-776 Warsaw, Poland

**Monika Sikora and Roland Kozdrowski**
Department of Reproduction and Clinic of Farm Animals, Faculty of Veterinary Medicine, Wroclaw University of Environmental and Life Sciences, Plac Grunwaldzkistreet 49, 50366 Wroclaw, Poland

**Jarosław Król and Marcin Nowak**
Department of Pathology, Faculty of Veterinary Medicine, Wroclaw University of Environmental and Life Sciences, C. K. Norwidastreet 31, 50375 Wroclaw, Poland

**Tadeusz Stefaniak**
Department of Immunology, Pathophysiology and Veterinary Preventive Medicine, Faculty of Veterinary Medicine, Wroclaw University of Environmental and Life Sciences, C. K. Norwidastreet 31, 50375 Wroclaw, Poland

**Gudmar Aubertsson**
Dýralæknir Sandhólaferja, 851 Hella, Iceland

**Tiina Nokireki and Miia Jakava-Viljanen**
Finnish Food Safety Authority Evira, Mustialankatu 3, 00790 Helsinki, Finland

**Anna-Maija Virtala and Liisa Sihvonen**
Department of Veterinary Biosciences, Faculty of Veterinary Medicine, University of Helsinki, 00014 Helsinki, Finland

**Miia Kontturi, Minna Kujala, Reijo Junni, Timo Soveri and Heli Simojoki**
Department of Production Animal Medicine, Faculty of Veterinary Medicine, University of Helsinki, Paroninkuja 20, 04920 Saarentaus, Finland

**Erja Malinen and Eija Seuna**
Veterinary Bacteriology Research Unit, Finnish Food Safety Authority Evira, Mustialankatu 3, 00790 Helsinki, Finland

**Sinikka Pelkonen**
Veterinary Bacteriology Research Unit, Finnish Food Safety Authority Evira, Neulaniementie 4, 70210 Kuopio, Finland

**Hussein Awad Hussein**
Internal Veterinary Medicine, Department of Animal Medicine, Faculty of Veterinary Medicine, Assiut University, Assiut 71526, Egypt

**Rudolf Staufenbiel**
Klinik für Klauentiere, Freie Universität Berlin, 14163 Berlin, Germany

**Hai-Feng Liu, Li Gao, Tao Liu and Hong-Bin Wang**
Department of Veterinary Surgery, College of Veterinary Medicine, Northeast Agricultural University, No. 59 Mucai Street, Gongbin Road, Xiangfang District, Harbin 150030, People's Republic of China

**Yan-Jiang**
College of Veterinary Medicine, Northeast Agricultural University, Harbin 150030, People's Republic of China

**Mai Louise Grandsgaard Mikkelsen, James Edward Miles, Helle Harding Poulsen, Finn Borgbjerg Moltke and Thomas Eriksen**
Department of Veterinary Clinical and Animal Sciences, University of Copenhagen, 16 Dyrlægevej, 1870 Frederiksberg C, Denmark

**Rikard Ambrus**
Department of Surgical Gastroenterology C, Rigshospitalet, University of Copenhagen, 9 Blegdamsvej, 2100 Copenhagen Ø, Denmark

**Finn Borgbjerg Moltke**
Department of Neuroanaesthesia, Rigshospitalet, University of Copenhagen, 9 Blegdamsvej, 2100 Copenhagen Ø, Denmark

Department of Anaesthesia, Sealand Hospital, University of Copenhagen, 1 Lykkebækvej, 4600 Køge, Denmark

**Reija Junkkari, Satu Sankari, Riitta-Mari Tulamo and Anna Mykkänen**
Department of Equine and Small Animal Medicine, University of Helsinki, Helsinki 00014, Finland

**Heli Simojoki**
Department of Production Animal Medicine, University of Helsinki, Helsinki 00014, Finland

**Minna-Liisa Heiskanen**
Equine Information Centre, Neulaniementie 5, Kuopio 70210, Finland

**Sinikka Pelkonen**
Research and Laboratory Department, Veterinary Bacteriology Research Unit, Finnish Food Safety Authority Evira, Neulaniementie 4, Kuopio 70701, Finland

**Anna Ordell, Hans Gustafsson and Renée Båge**
Department of Clinical Sciences, Swedish University of Agricultural Sciences, SE-750 07 Uppsala, Sweden

**Helle Ericsson Unnerstad and Ann Nyman**
Department of Animal Health and Antimicrobial Strategies, National Veterinary Institute, SE-751 89 Uppsala, Sweden

**Hans Gustafsson and Renée Båge**
Development and Services for Farmers, Växa Sverige, SE-104 25 Stockholm, Sweden

**Alexander J. German**
Institute of Ageing and Chronic Disease, University of Liverpool, Leahurst Campus, Chester High Road, Neston, Wirral CH64 7TE, UK

**Lovisa Orleifson, Ingrid Ljungvall and Jens Häggström**
Department of Clinical Sciences, Faculty of Veterinary Medicine, Swedish University of Agricultural Sciences, Uppsala, Sweden

**Katja Höglund**
Department of Anatomy, Physiology and Biochemistry, Faculty of Veterinary Medicine, Swedish University of Agricultural Sciences, Uppsala, Sweden

**Sanna Lindåse, Katarina Nostell and Johan Bröjer**
Department of Clinical Sciences, Swedish University of Agricultural Sciences, Box 7054, 750 07 Uppsala, Sweden

**Siobhan Simpson, Mark David Dunning, Simone de Brot, Llorenç Grau-Roma, Nigel Patrick Mongan and Catrin Sian Rutland**
Faculty of Medicine and Health Sciences, School of Veterinary Medicine and Science, The University of Nottingham, Sutton Bonington Campus, Loughborough LE12 5RD, UK

**Nigel Patrick Mongan**
Department of Pharmacology, Weill Cornell Medicine, 1300 York Avenue, New York, NY 10065, USA

**Joanna Katarzyna Bujak, Rafał Pingwara and Kinga Majchrzak**
Department of Physiological Sciences, Faculty of Veterinary Medicine, Warsaw University of Life Sciences, ul. Nowoursynowska 159, 02-776 Warsaw, Poland

**Michelle Hase Nelson**
Department of Microbiology and Immunology, Medical University of South Carolina, 86 Jonathan Lucas Street HCC-612, Charleston, SC 29425, USA

**Karin Alvåsen and Ulf Emanuelson**
Department of Clinical Sciences, Swedish University of Agricultural Sciences, 75007 Uppsala, Sweden

**Ian Dohoo**
Department of Health Management, Atlantic Veterinary College, University of Prince Edward Island, Charlottetown, PEI C1A 4P3, Canada

**Anki Roth**
Växa Sverige, 63220 Eskilstuna, Sweden

**Jane Margaret Morrell, Andra Sabina Valeanu and Anders Johannisson**
Division of Reproduction, Department of Clinical Sciences, Faculty of Veterinary Medicine and Animal Science, Swedish University of Agricultural Sciences (SLU), 75007 Uppsala, Sweden

**Andra Sabina Valeanu**
University of Agricultural Sciences and Veterinary Medicine Iaşi, 3, Mihail Sadoveanu Alley, 700490 Iaşi, Romania

**Nils Lundeheim**
Department of Animal Breeding and Genetics, Faculty of Veterinary Medicine and Animal Science, Swedish University of Agricultural Sciences, 75007 Uppsala, Sweden

**Ueli Braun, Sonja Warislohner, Christian Gerspach and Karl Nuss**
Department of Farm Animals, Vetsuisse Faculty, University of Zurich, Zurich, Switzerland

**Stefanie Ohlerth**
Clinic of Diagnostic Imaging, Vetsuisse Faculty, University of Zurich, Zurich, Switzerland

**Ulf Emanuelson, Karin Sjöström and Nils Fall**
Department of Clinical Sciences, Swedish University of Agricultural Sciences, Uppsala, Sweden

**Alana Jayne Rosenblatt, Nina Alice James and Charles Grégoire Bénédict Caraguel**
School of Animal and Veterinary Sciences, The University of Adelaide, Roseworthy Campus, Adelaide, SA 5005, Australia

**Anu Katriina Lappalainen**
Faculty of Veterinary Medicine, University of Helsinki, Viikki Campus, Agnes Sjöberginkatu 2, 00014 Helsinki, Finland

**Natalie Siu Ling Webster**
Darkroom Veterinary Imaging, 7/489A Warrigal Rd, Moorabbin, VIC 3189, Australia

**Alana Jayne Rosenblatt**
School of Veterinary Science, The University of Queensland, Gatton, QLD 4343, Australia

**Lisa Lindström, Felicia Asp Tauni and Karin Vargmar**
Department of Biomedical Sciences and Veterinary Public Health, Faculty of Veterinary Medicine and Animal Science, Swedish University of Agricultural Sciences (Ulls väg 26), 757 56 Uppsala, Sweden

# Index

## R



## S



## T



## U



## V

CPSIA information can be obtained
at www.ICGtesting.com
Printed in the USA
LVHW011958260423
745396LV00005B/483

9 781639 275250